Peroral Endoscopy and Laryngeal Surgery - Primary Source Edition

Chevalier Jackson, Gustav Killian

Peroral Endoscopy and Laryngeal Surgery

BY

CHEVALIER JACKSON, M. D.

Professor of Laryngology, University of Pittsburgh; Consulting Laryngologist Bronchoscopist, Esophagoscopist, and Gastroscopist, Western Pennsylvania Hospital; Laryngologist, Presbyterian Hospital; Laryngologist, Eye and Ear Hospital; Consulting Laryngologist, Western Pennsylvania Hospital for the Insane; Consulting Laryngologist, Bronchoscopist, Esophagoscopist and Gastroscopist, Montefiore Hospital; Consulting Laryngologist, Bronchoscopist, Esophagoscopist and Gastroscopist, St. Francis Hospital; Consulting Laryngologist, Bronchoscopist, Esophagoscopist and Gastroscopist, Passavant Hospital; Bronchoscopist and Esophagoscopist, Allegheny General Hospital; Bronchoscopist and Esophagoscopist, Pittsburgh Hospital for Children.

WITH SIX COLORED PLATES AND
490 ILLUSTRATIONS.

SAINT LOUIS, MO., U. S. A.
THE LARYNGOSCOPE COMPANY, PUBLISHERS.
1915

To

My Mother

To Whose Interest in Medical Science

The Author Owes His Incentive,

And to

My Father

Whose Constant Advice to

"Educate the Eye and the Fingers"

Spurred the Author to Continual Effort,

This Book is Affectionately Dedicated.

Preface.

A number of repetitions of fundamental facts have been necessary in order to facilitate ready reference in the limited time available for the busy surgeon without perusing the entire book. But, as full repetitions were impossible, it is hoped that, for full comprehension, the entire book shall have been previously read. Symptoms are referred to only in so far as they concern indications or contraindications for endoscopy. Diagnosis is referred to only in so far as it is to be made endoscopically. An earnest effort has been made to give due credit to everyone so far as possible within the limits of a practical manual. This effort resulted in such an enormous number of references that, to save repetition, the references are all compressed into a numerical "Bibliography" at the end of the book, referred to in the text as "Bib." followed by the number. The author cites his personal experiences for what they may be worth; and he apologizes for the frequency of these citations, which is necessitated by the newness of the field, and the nature of the book. The French saying: "Neither never nor always" is particularly applicable to surgery. The author has tried to make the use of these words as rare as possible because "circumstances alter cases," and great injustice might follow dogmatic assertions. For literary shortcomings, the author asks indulgence because, even if he were more capable, literary work, as with all clinicians, is done under stress of limited time and opportunity. Unless otherwise credited, the illustrations are photographic reproductions of drawings and paintings by the author who solely is responsible for illustrative errors and shortcomings.

Thanks are due, first of all, to the great master, Prof. Killian, for kindly consideration and for doing me the honor of writing the Chapter on Suspension Laryngoscopy. For the translation of that Chapter the author is indebted to Dr. J. A. Hageman, and for editing the translation, as well as for valuable advise and assistance, to Dr. M. A. Goldstein. For aid in the literary work the author acknowledges his great obligations to Miss Josephine W. White. Thanks are due to Miss Babette Kahn for the careful preparation of the very complete index. For the accuracy of case records and for assistance in all phases of the work, clinical and literary, thanks are due to that able endoscopist, Dr. Ellen J. Patterson. The author wishes here to express his appreciation of the part taken by the following associates with whom he has for years worked shoulder to shoulder and without whose aid whatever measures of success that may have been attained would have been impossible:

Drs. Patterson, Boyce, Price, Clark, McCready, Lichtenfels, McKee, Fisher, Simpson, Upham, Spiro; Mrs. Braddow; Misses Ketcham, Saunders. Eissler, Bear, Dice, Talbot, Lewellyn, Symes and Bird.

Last, and not the least important, the author's thanks are due to the profession, general and special, at home and abroad, for the clinical material and the hearty support which have rendered this book possible. Especial assurances of appreciation are due the staffs of various hospitals with which the author was not connected, for their broadmindedness in sanctioning the author's aid in the relief of ward sufferers.

CHEVALIER JACKSON.

Pittsburgh, Pa., July, 1914.

Contents.

CHAPTER I.

Instruments.

Since the author's earlier work was published a large number of new instruments and modifications of old forms have been devised. Each of them is probably useful to others besides the originators; but it is clear that there will never be a universal instrument. Each endoscopist will work successfully with those instruments to which he is accustomed. By this it is not meant that a wise selection is of no importance; quite the contrary. In general surgery, if knives are sharp, instrumental equipment is of minor importance. In endoscopy, however, the instrumentarium is an absolutely fundamental element for success. It is no wonder that some of the laryngologists who have taken up endoscopy have been discouraged, when one looks at the miserably inefficient, clumsy instruments with which their first attempts were made. Unfortunately there are many bad mechanics in the world, and surgeons who have originated excellent, practical ideas are chagrined to find that failures due to faulty workmanship are blamed, not on the incompetent mechanic who made the particular instrument that failed, but upon the originator who is getting excellent results from a well-made instrument of correct model. All long instruments, such as forceps, cannulae, stylets, probes, sponge holders, and the like, should be of spring tempered steel or spring brass in order not to get bent, as a bent instrument is much more difficult to manage accurately. On the other hand the temper of steel must not be so hard as to risk breaking, which might be a disaster. There is a "happy medium" in the temper of steel that a reliable workman can be depended upon to produce, that will bend slightly to extreme pressure without breaking.

Tubes and illuminating devices. The personal equation enters so largely into the choice of instruments that the author urges the reader to get for selection differently illuminated instruments and try them on the dog, using first the largest tubes and then the smallest, keeping in mind that it is in the use of small tubes that the greatest difficulties lie; and. unfortunately, most of the cases encountered are in children where small tubes are obligatory. All forms of illumination have been greatly improved by the development of the tungsten lamp. Quite a number of new forms of illumination and new tubes have been devised, and they practically all have done good service in the hands of skillful men. In the statistics which the author gathered, there is practically no difference either in the mortality or the percentage of successful removals of foreign bodies between the different kinds of tubes and illum-

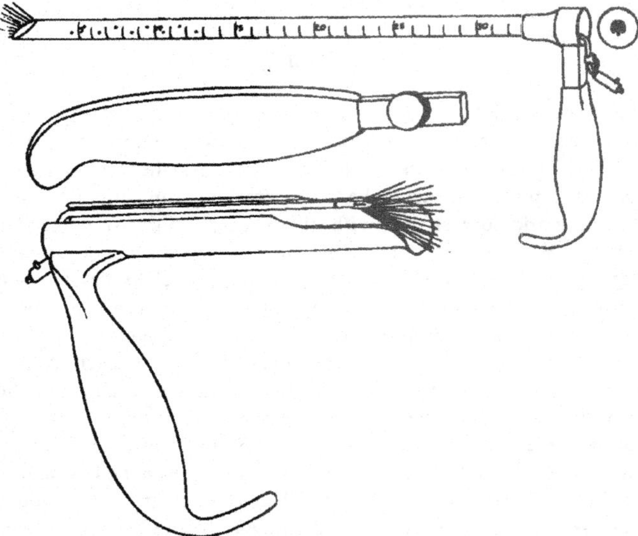

FIG. 1. Ingals' bronchoscope and open laryngeal speculum.

ination. Far more depended on the individual skill of the operator. Doubtless, the best instrument for each operator is the one with which he has practiced most.

Killian still uses the Kirstein headlamp except for demonstration purposes. The lamp is very much improved in construction and has enormously greater illuminating power.

Guisez has abandoned his triple endoscopic headlamp, and now uses the Claar reflector (Fig. 6).

The Brünings sliding tubes described in the appendix of the earlier book have been much improved and are extensively used. (Figs. 2. 3. and 4.)

D. R. Patterson has modified the Brünings tubes by placing the beak on the inner tube and the cylindrical end on the outer tube, always introducing the instrument with the distal end of the inner tube extended beyond the distal end of the outer tube.

Excellent work is being done in Chiari's clinic and elsewhere with Kahler's bronchoscopes and esophagoscopes. They are double tubes, one sliding within the other like the Brünings instruments, but the illuminating mechanism is different. (Fig. 8.)

Schoonmaker has devised an excellent sliding double-tube bronchoscope.

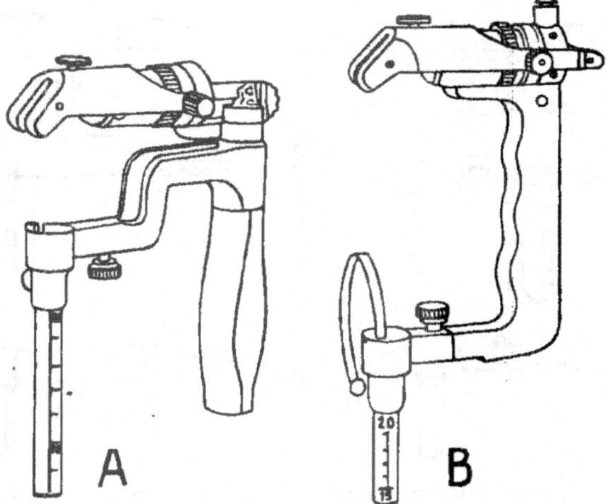

FIGS. 2 and 3. Brünings' two illuminating handles for laryngoscopes, bronchoscopes, and esophagoscopes.

Ingals uses an improved form of his original distally illuminated bronchoscope (Fig. 1), with which he has done some remarkably successful work.

Mosher uses esophagoscopes of very large transverse diameter with distal illumination. (Fig. 5.)

Efforts to produce jointed and angular esophagoscopes and gastroscopes continue, and all such should be encouraged (provided great care is exercised) because all effort results in increased attention to the esophagus and its diseases. There is absolutely no hope that any esophageal instrument will ever be devised that will be safe unless carefully used, because even the soft rubber stomach tube has been known to cause fatal perforation. One of the most successful of the angular esophago-

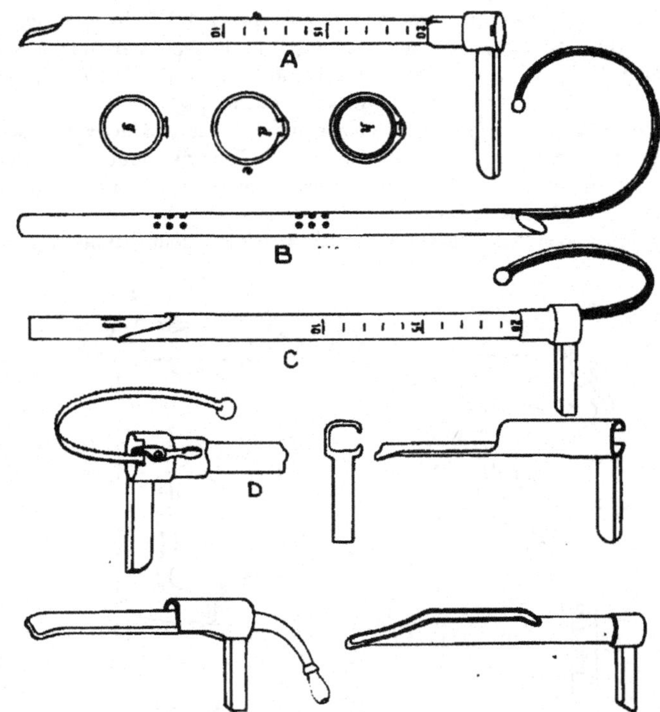

Fig. 4. Brünings' spatulae and tubes for use with the illuminating handles shown in the preceding illustration. A, tube to be attached to handle. B, inner tube sliding into A, as shown at C, the inner tube being locked at the required depth by the ratchet shown at D. The other illustrations are laryngeal spatulae.

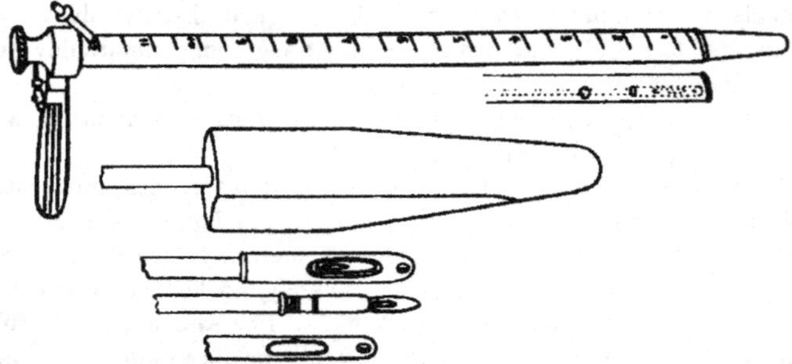

Fig. 5. Mosher's esophagoscope showing distal light and mandrin for introduction.

scopes is the indirect one of Lewisohn. The author saw it passed upon a patient with practically no discomfort and the view was good. In its present form it is, of course, adapted to simple inspection, not for the

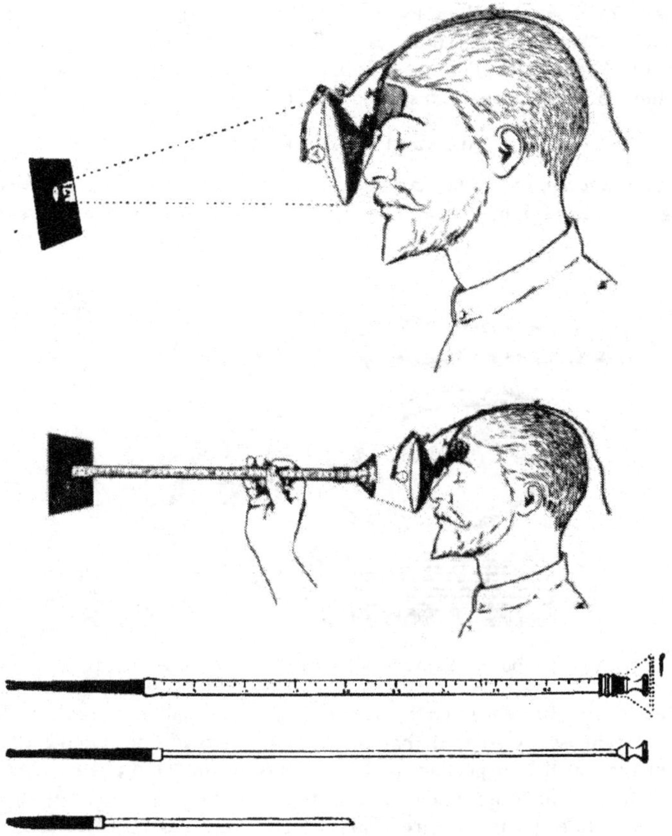

FIG. 6. Guisez's esophagoscope. Guisez, as shown in the upper illustration, uses a Claar headlight for illumination and a soft-ended mandrin for introduction as shown in the lower illustration.

removal of foreign bodies or specimens, nor for probing or palpation, wiping or medication.

A number of laryngeal speculae have been devised. Ingals' (Fig. 1), Hill's (Fig. 9), Dickinson's (Fig. 13), and Pratt's use a distal light. Pratt's has a battery contained in the handle. Richard H. Johnston prefers a narrow tube and has done wonderful work with the author's original tubular speculum (Fig. 6, p. 19, of the earlier book, Bib. 269). Johnston attached a handle as shown in Fig. 11. Mosher devised an open speculum for use with the headlight or head mirror, Fig. 12. The Boyce speculum is quite simple and effective when used with the Wendell C. Phillips headlight, worn between the eyes, where the luminous and visual axes almost correspond.

THE AUTHOR'S INSTRUMENTS.

Laryngoscopes. The laryngeal speculum or direct laryngoscope (Fig. 14) devised by the author in 1903 and shown in Fig. 7 of the

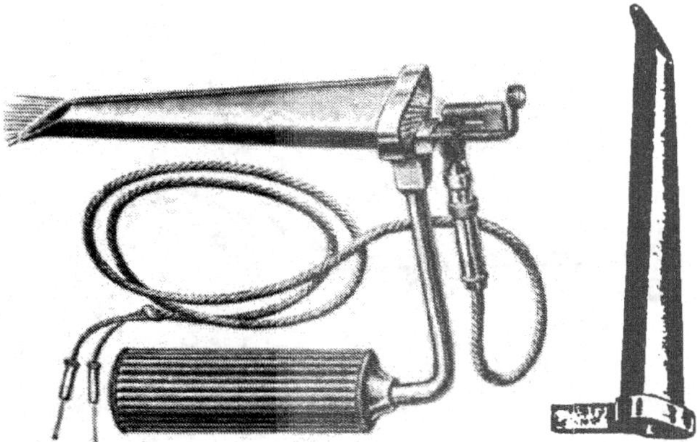

FIG. 7. Yankauer's laryngeal tube-spatula.

earlier book (Bib. 269) has been found to answer all requirements for direct laryngoscopy so well that the author has made no modifications, except that, at the suggestion of R. H. Johnston the handle is now made detachable. This instrument has received various names: laryngeal speculum, slide speculum, direct laryngoscope, etc. Being used for examination of the larynx, it would seem that the now generally used term "laryngoscope" is preferable. The method of introducing bronchoscopes through this laryngoscope has the great advantage that no septic instrument need be introduced into the trachea, because, as abundantly proven by laboratory examinations of secretions withdrawn from the bronchi through the bronchoscope, the bronchoscope need not be contaminated in introduction. Laboratory work has shown that there is, under normal conditions, a sharp line of limitation of oral sepsis at the orifice of the larynx. The first form of laryngoscope used by the author was modeled after the original Kirstein "autoscope" which had its transverse greater than its vertical diameter. A double handle was attached to a simple oval tube with half its periphery cut away for the distal two-thirds of its length (Fig. 15). Then, after Killian created bronchoscopy, the author added a slide at the side for bronchoscopy. Both of these

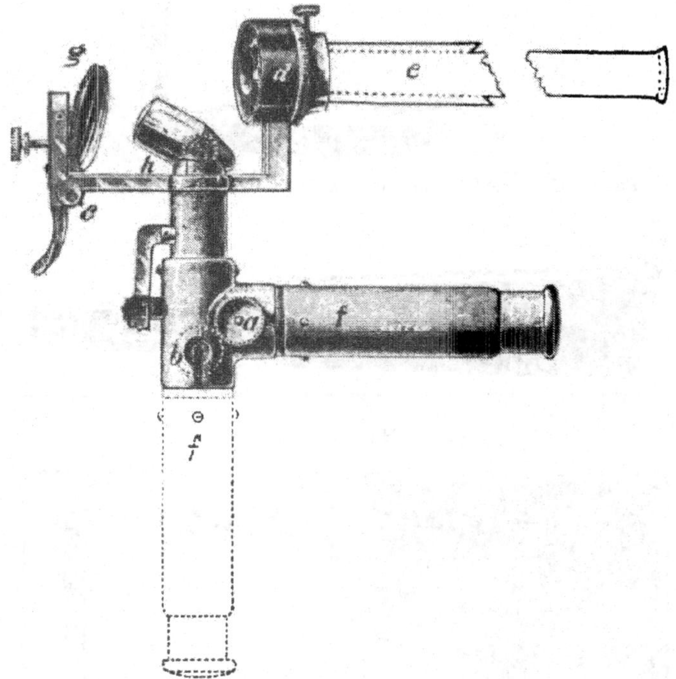

Fig. 8. Kahler panelectroscope. The tubes used with this are similar to the sliding tubes of Brünings. The rays of light from the lamp, h, are reflected by the mirror, g, into the tube, e. The endoscopist's eye is placed at the notch in the mirror, g. The mirror can be thrown out of the way for the introduction of instruments by pressure of the thumb on the arm, c.

laryngoscopes were used with the ordinary head-mirror, and with the Wendell C. Phillips head-lamp worn between the eyes. As the author found the oval lumen less convenient than the round for working at the side instead of over the dorsum of the tongue, as he frequently wished to do, he abandoned the oval lumen for the round lumen with the slide

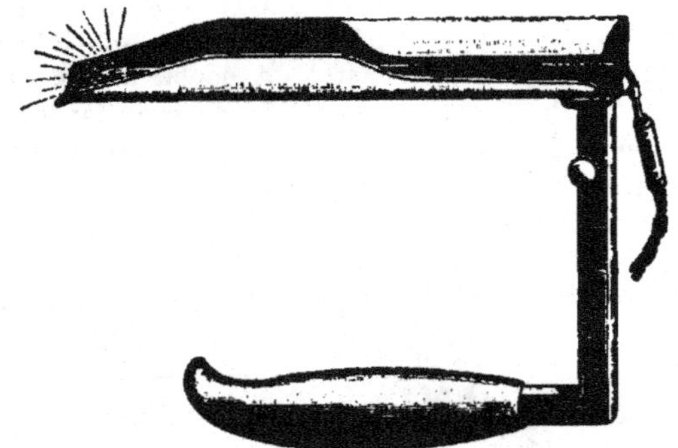

FIG. 9. Hill's modification of the Chevalier Jackson laryngoscope.

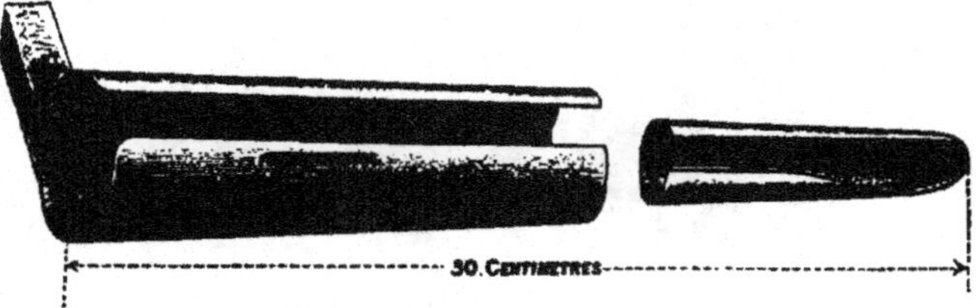

FIG. 10. Hill's esophagoscope.

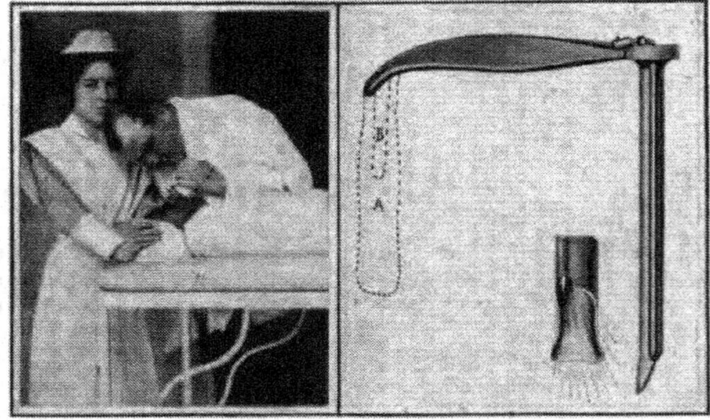

FIG. 11. The author's tubular speculum to which Dr. Richard H. Johnston added the laryngoscope detachable handle (A), preferring this narrow tube to the wider laryngoscope tube. At the left Dr. Johnston is using the tubular speculum with handle detached, the patient being in the straight position, without extenson of the head.

at the side. As the edges of the slide were then made they became rough in use, and to prevent this the slide was moved to the top and in this form, with the addition of the light carrier of the Einhorn esophagoscope, it has been in general use ever since. Recently some men who have done the author the honor to work with him have found the oval model so

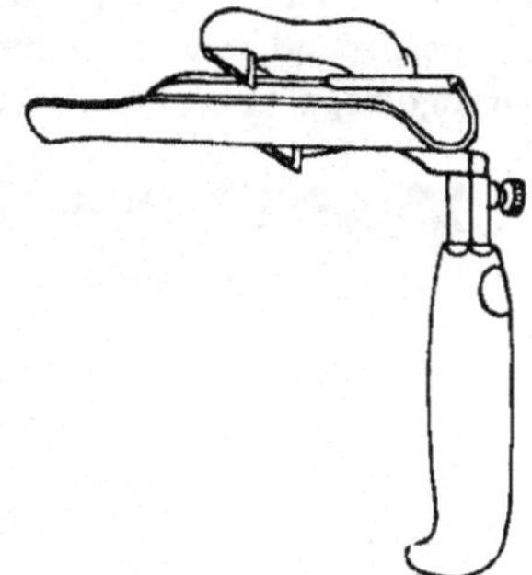

FIG. 12. Mosher's laryngeal spatula with dental protector.

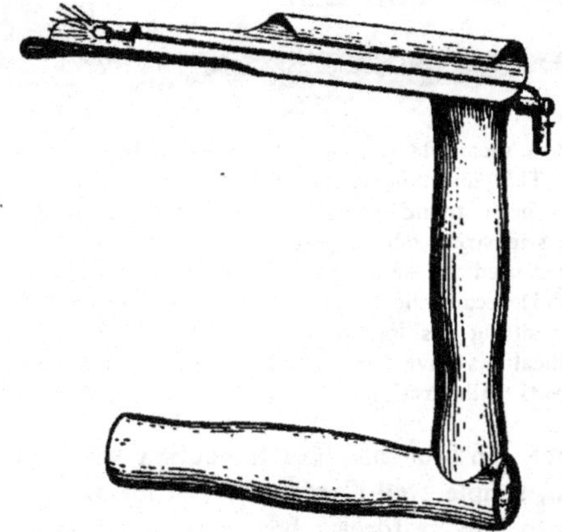

FIG. 13. B. M. Dickinson's laryngoscope.

convenient for the introduction of esophagoscopes, bronchoscopes, and especially intratracheal insufflation tubes, that it has been deemed worth while to resurrect the oval model. The slide can be left off altogether and thus removal of the laryngoscope after introduction of tubes of all kinds is facilitated, as in the Dickinson speculum. The oval lumen, giving a larger field, has the additional advantage of facilitating the identifications of land-marks and of affording more room for endolaryngeal operations. Probably many operators will prefer working through the oval laryngoscope to the method that has seemed easiest to me: namely, using the round lumen laryngoscope for vision only, the forceps and other instruments being passed alongside the laryngoscope.

The width of the oval lumen laryngoscope will be found greatly to increase the difficulty of exposing the anterior commissure. Everything considered, the regular laryngoscope (Fig. 14) will be found preferable.

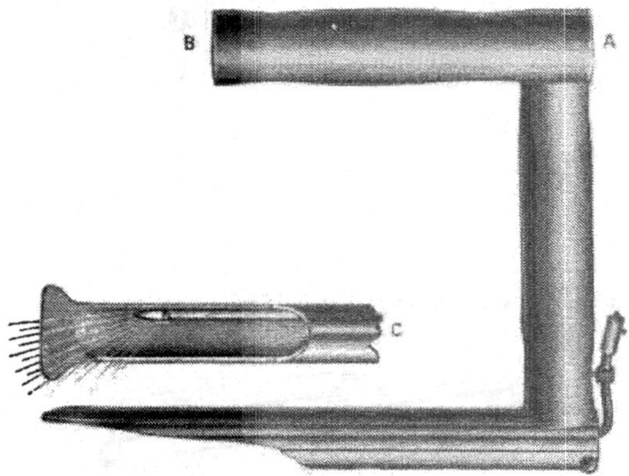

FIG. 14. Author's separable speculum for passing bronchoscopes and for direct laryngoscopy. This instrument, also called "direct laryngoscope," laryngeal speculum, etc., has been found perfectly satisfactory without modification in size or shape. Two sizes are needed, one for adults and one for children. The author personally never used the handle, A. B., in the child's size instrument, (substituting a hooked end) because he always examines children recumbent. For endoscopists who use the sitting position for children the handle is a great advantage. A number of modifications have been made by various endoscopists to suit their individual requirements. (Illustration reproduced from the author's earlier volume.*)

Bronchoscopes. In bronchoscopes the author has been unable to improve on the light, simple, well-illuminated instrument shown in Fig. 16. His only failures to remove foreign bodies from the bronchi since commencing to use this instrument a number of years ago, were due to failures to find four pins which were in minute bronchi beyond the limits reachable by a 4 mm. tube, in other words, beyond the limits of bronchoscopy. In no instance has this bronchoscope been found wanting.

Four sizes are sufficient for every possible case from a new-born infant to the largest adult.

*Tracheo-bronchoscopy, Esophagoscopy and Gastroscopy. Published at St. Louis, 1907.

The selection of a tube for the particular case no longer presents the difficulties that it did when a large number of tubes of various lengths were thought to be necessary. The bronchoscopes and esophagoscopes can, as a rule, be selected absolutely by the ages mentioned in the given list. Naturally there is a border-line between the older child and the young adult, where a slightly larger size than the child's size could be used where the adult instruments are slightly too large. In the case of the bronchoscope, this field is fully covered by the 7 mm. instrument, which can be used in such cases, and is plenty large enough for work in an adult also, though for adults of average-sized larynx and trachea it is much better to have the 9 mm. bronchoscope, as it gives a much larger

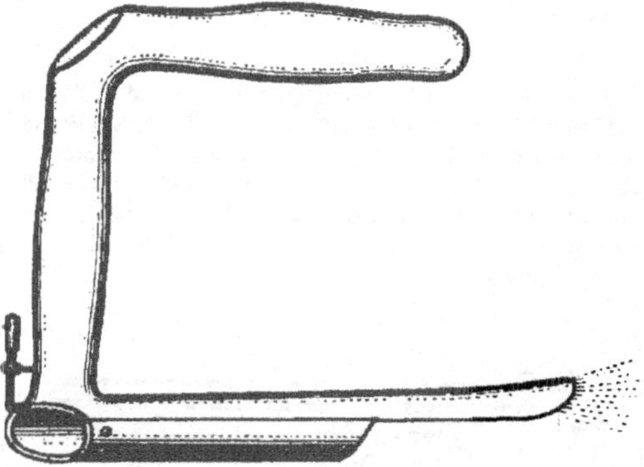

Fig. 15. Form of the first of the author's laryngoscopes originally used with the Wendell C. Phillips headlight. Here shown with Einhorn light carrier added. The slide at the side can be left off altogether, if desired, to facilitate the removal of the laryngoscope after the insertion of bronchoscopes, intratracheal insufflation anesthesia catheters, etc. The instrument shown in Fig. 14 is preferable.

field of view. In cases where it is desired to enter a very small branch bronchus, low down, it would be necessary to use the 7x40 bronchoscope in an adult. In children under one year of age the 5 mm. bronchoscope, is used by many American bronchoscopists, but as it does not ordinarily go through easily, some traumatism may be done to the larynx which will result afterward in subglottic edema. The author and Dr. Ellen J. Patterson always use, in such cases, 4 mm. bronchoscopes, through the mouth; but to those who have not practiced work with small tubes, this may prove rather difficult. From one to five years of age, a 5 mm. bronchoscope will be found perfectly satisfactory for use through the larynx. At six years of age and over, the 7 mm.

bronchoscope can be used through the larynx without risk of subglottic edema, if none has existed prior to the bronchoscopy, and if manipulations be gentle.

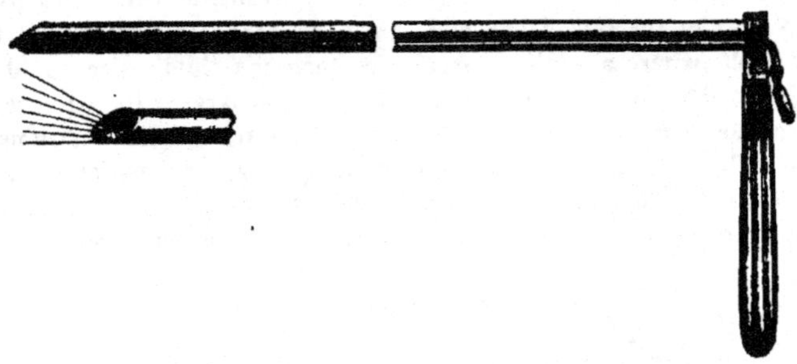

Fig. 16. Author's bronchoscope as originally devised. The author has had added to this the small branch tube suggested by T. Drysdale Buchanan. (Fig. 17). The slanted tube mouth gives a lip that not only facilitates introduction, but has manifold uses. All of the author's tubes are fitted with "cold" lamps, which lie in a recess out of harm's way and out of the line of vision. Aspirating canals were found occasionally useful before the author developed his "sponge-pumping" method of removing secretions.

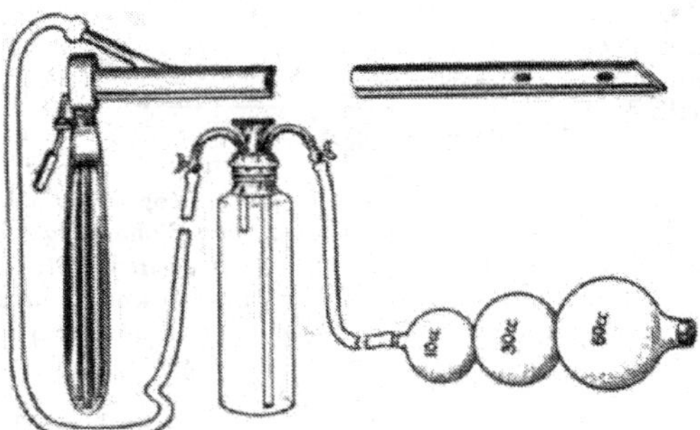

Fig. 17. Dosimetric anesthetizing attachment for the bronchoscope. Devised by Dr. T. Drysdale Buchanan. The small branch tube ends in the lumen of the bronchoscope, and not in an auxiliary canal. All of the author's bronchoscopes are now made with this small branch tube, as it has been found very useful for bronchoscopic oxygen insufflation.

If instruments are selected by the given suggestions, as to sizes, there will never be any need for withdrawing one bronchoscope and replacing it with a different size. Should there be any trouble with the lamp, which should not occur more than once or twice in a hundred bronchoscopies, the lamp can be withdrawn with the light carrier and replaced by a new one, without removing the bronchoscope. With the proper use of the sponges shown in Fig. 27, the light carrier never need be withdrawn for the purpose of cleaning the lamp, as the sponges wipe the lamp clean at the same time that they are used for removing secretions from the field of vision, as shown in Fig. 25. One of the author's assistants has called attention to the fact that it was unnecessary to remove a light carrier once in 72 consecutive cases. Secretions never bake on the lamp because the lamp does not get hot. The lamp is in a recess out of the way of instruments, so that it cannot be broken and cannot get caught on sponges.

The objections raised by operators who have never used distal illumination are unjust. One statement made that the distal light is quickly

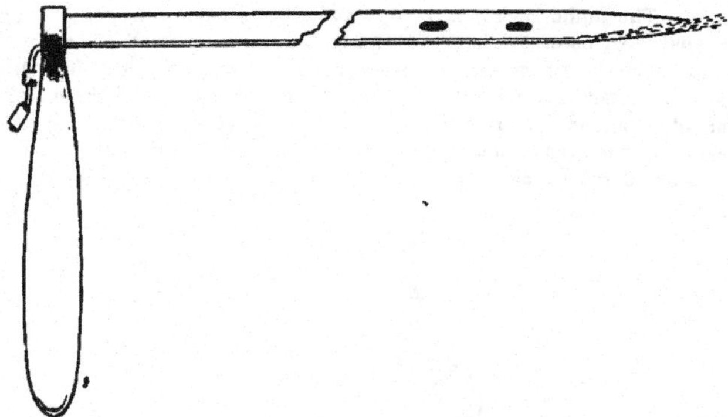

Fig. 18. Author's special small-ended bronchoscope for examining the orifices of very small bronchi. Not intended for regular work upon ordinary cases.

obscured by blood and secretions is based purely on theory. The author, as is well known by all who have honored his clinic with a visit, works for hours at a time without one moment's interruption for removal or cleansing of lamps other than the regular swabbing that is necessary for the removal of secretion from the field with any form of illumination. It is impossible to see, with any form of instrument, through a pool of secretions.

Esophagoscopes. The author has made no changes whatever in the esophagoscope devised by him in 1904. He has, however, abandoned the use of the mandrin altogether, the instrument being always passed by sight and the mandrin is never used unless it is desired to hold it on the outside of a patient to determine the point on the surface corresponding to the depth of insertion of the tube. For this purpose, the mandrin gives the exact length of the esophagoscope, and by holding it parallel to the esophagoscope, as indicated by the portion of the esophagoscope not yet inserted, a point can be found on the skin-surface of the chest or epigastrium that will correspond precisely to the distal end of the esophagoscope. The esophagoscope is always passed by sight, absolutely never any other way, for the following reasons: 1. Once the knack is acquired, it is just as easy to pass by sight. 2. In foreign-body cases, if a mandrin be used the foreign body, if small, is very apt to be overridden before the operator realizes that the distal end has reached the position

Fig. 19. The author's esophagoscope and gastroscope with distal light and drainage canal. An obturator is provided but is never used by the author. Only two sizes are needed. 10 mm. x 53 cm. for adults. 7 mm. x 45 cm. for children. Shorter sizes are made but are not used by the author because with the distal light there is no advantage in a short tube. This esophagoscope has been in constant use for 10 years and has been found to be in every way satisfactory without modification. The slanted end added (Fig. 426), for special purposes, facilitates introduction.

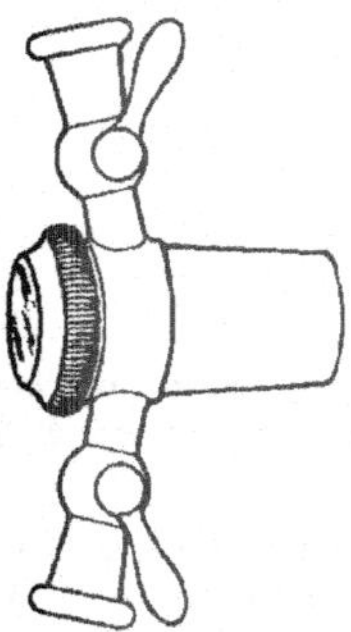

Fig. 20. Window-plug for occluding the proximal tube-mouth when it is desired to balloon the esophagus or stomach, as suggested by Mosher.

of the foreign body. 3. There may be in any case, lesions of the esophagus that can be seen and avoided, provided the instrument is being passed by sight. 4. The importance of the use of the open tube passed by sight in foreign-body extractions is so great that it is important that all esophagoscopies should be done in that manner, in order that skill may be acquired, so that when foreign-body cases are met with, the passage by sight will be easy. If this knack is not acquired, it is very much more difficult to pass by sight than with a mandrin.

An esophagoscope with a slanted end similar to the bronchoscope (Fig. 16), is useful for finding the subdiverticular opening, and for solving some of the mechanical problems of foreign-body extraction. It has no holes in the side and is longer and larger in diameter than the bronchoscope. (Fig. 126).

Complicated forms of tubes with extracting, excising, and dilating attachments have not seemed to the author as generally applicable as plain tubes through which, by manual manipulations, any procedure can be carried out with appropriate, independent instruments.

Measuring rule. It is customary with esophagoscopists to measure distance from the upper teeth. Some esophagoscopes have graduations marked on the outside. The author's tubes are too thin and light for this, and moreover, a smooth exterior is a great advantage. Therefore, he uses a 25 cm. steel rule, (obtainable at any machinist's supply house),

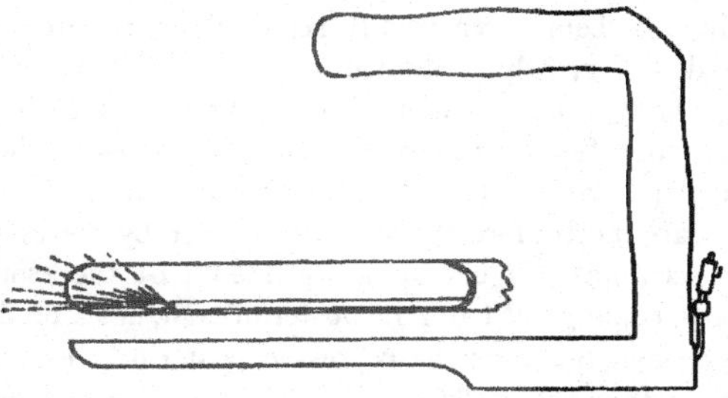

Fig. 21. Esophageal speculum for foreign body work and for operations upon the upper end of the esophagus. This instrument, by detaching the handle, becomes a very efficient pleuroscope because of the facility with which the flopping lung can be controlled. It can be thoroughly sterilized. The child's size is an excellent laryngoscope and subglottic laryngoscope for adults.

which is sterilized with the instruments and kept on the sterile instrument table. When the tube-mouth is at the lesion, an assistant places one end of the rule at the upper teeth (or alveolus if teeth are absent) and the distance to the proximal end of the esophagoscope is marked by holding the thumb at the point. The measurement is subtracted from the known tube length. Thus, when 20 cm. of the 53 cm. esophagoscope projects proximally from the teeth the lesion is known to be 33 cm. from the upper teeth. If it is desired to locate this point externally on the patient's chest after the esophagoscope is withdrawn, the patient sitting erect is told to look at the ceiling and the 23 cm. is measured downward from the upper teeth, and a mark is made on the skin of the chest. The same method is used in bronchoscopy.

Esophageal speculum. For dealing with foreign bodies and disease high up in the esophagus, the author has found an elongation of his laryngeal speculum exceedingly useful. This instrument is 25 cm. long for use in adults, 16 cm. for children, and with these instruments there is very much less risk of overriding foreign bodies in the high situation than with the esophagoscope. This esophageal speculum has also been found particularly useful for the breaking up of those rare congenital webs first described by Mosher and Clark, and of the high strictures of the esophagus following decubitus ulcers resulting from the mixed infections complicating enteric fever, scarlatina, diphtheria and like conditions, and those following gummata. These webs and strictures yield quite readily to the breaking up and stretching with this speculum. Cicatricial stenoses, especially those following the breaking down of gummata, have a tendency to recur, and it is necessary to repeat the treatment frequently, but in some of the conditions a very few treatments are sufficient. a divulser being occasionally required. Intricate instrumentation, when needed, is greatly facilitated by the wide exposure afforded.

In foreign body work it has seemed to the author to be preferable to an esophagoscope for the removal of foreign bodies at their favorite site of lodgment just above the upper thoracic aperture. Foreign bodies in this location are much more apt to be overridden by the esophagoscope than by this speculum. Of course at the mouth of the esophagus, the cricopharyngeus, coming out from the posterior wall, has a tendency to obstruct the view; and this must be repressed posteriorly by an elongated Mosher alligator forceps. (Plate III, Fig. 10.) The speculum can be used in either the recumbent or the sitting position of the patient. It is made in two sizes, one for adults and one for children. The child's size makes an excellent adult laryngoscope, especially for those who prefer a narrow spatular end. It also makes an excellent subglottic laryngoscope for adults, as the relatively narrow spatular end can be readily inserted through the glottic chink.

Batteries. No practical effort has yet been made to adapt the tallow candle or a kerosene lamp to endoscopy. We are compelled to use electric light of some kind. If the endoscopist is not of a sufficiently mechanical turn of mind to keep his electric lights burning properly, no matter what form of instrument he uses, he will not have the greatest success in foreign-body work, for endoscopic extraction is a question of mechanics from beginning to end. It does not require great brain power or high intellect, but in some cases mechanical ingenuity is taxed to the utmost to get out the foreign body without interfering with breathing and without traumatism to the tissues. If the surgeon is not a mechanical genius, he should have a trained surgical assistant who has the necessary mechanical ability. The simplest, best and safest source of current is a double dry battery arranged in two groups of four cells each. Each set should have two binding posts and a rheostat. Failure will result from an attempt to work with makeshift batteries, the current from which, with only a cell selector for control, jumps up from underillumination to overillumination and burns out the lamps. Ingals, who is a leading authority on bronchoscopy, and the author concur in the belief that all forms of rheostats devised for adapting commercial circuits to tube work involve a certain degree of risk because of the tube which makes a moist contact with tissues so close to more or less of the course of the vagi. No matter how

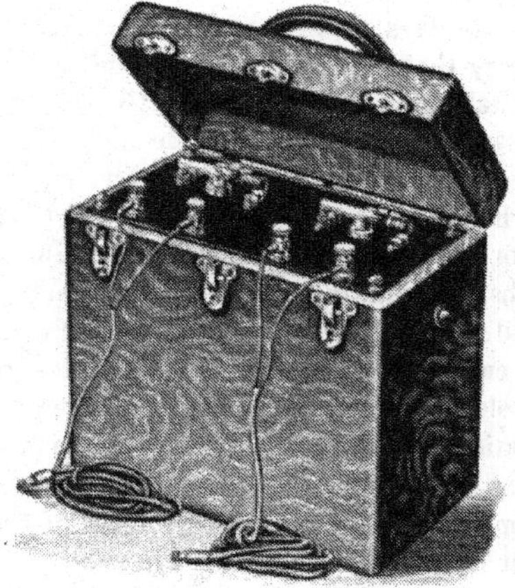

Fig. 22. Author's endoscopic battery heavily built for reliability. It contains 8 dry cells, series-connected in 2 groups of 4 cells each. Each group has its own rheostat and pair of binding posts.

thorough the construction, there is always a possibility of "grounding" of the circuit through the handle, tube, and patient. This danger is present, whether the lighting is proximally or distally applied. These remarks do not apply, of course, to the Kirstein lamp such as was originally used by Killian, and such as he still uses for all work other than demonstration. This lamp, being on the forehead of the operator, there is no chance of the current being communicated to the bronchoscope or esophagoscope. The operator may, at times, get a portion of the current on his head, but this being on the skin surface is of no consequence, and is a very different matter from the long moist contact of large area throughout nearly the full length of both vagi. The author is delighted to have the support of so eminent an authority as Ingals. (Bib. 226). The author's objection has been altogether theoretical, but Ingals has actually seen the sparking due to "short circuiting." The author has always used batteries and has found them quite satisfactory. All operators who have had any trouble with batteries have been working with an equipment that is not of substantial character. In his early days, the author had much trouble with batteries which were made in the same flimsy manner as the ignition system of the early automobiles. In the latter, freedom from trouble only came with heavy solid construction. With this in view, the author had built by Mr. Mueller, a substantial battery, the construction of which should be beyond failure. (Fig. 22). It contains two sets of four cells each of the ordinary dry battery, which can be obtained anywhere, day or night, Sundays and holidays, at any garage. It is free from the objection to the storage battery that, once exhausted, requires a number of hours for recharging. It takes but a moment to put in new cells. Dr. Ellen J. Patterson and the author have two of these batteries and in an experience of thousands of cases, they have never yet failed to obtain a light, nor has any bronchoscopy, esophagoscopy, or direct laryngoscopy failed or been delayed for want of illumination. The cells are changed once every three months without waiting for them to deteriorate. Small, flimsy batteries, and especially pocket batteries are a delusion and a snare, and their use for endoscopy is an injustice to the patient. Where the speculum is used solely for direct laryngoscopy, or in the introduction of silk-woven insufflation catheters which are non-conductors, the author believes that the use of commercial circuits with good rheostats is harmless, because the small area of contact at the base of the tongue involves no serious risk, but personally he prefers batteries.

Aspirators. Many new forms of aspirators have been devised. For the removal of secretions Yankauer has perfected an aspirator operated by a small exhaust-fan in connection with an electric motor. He has also used a jet of compressed air blowing sidewise across the proximal tube-mouth to blow away the secretions coughed out by the patient to prevent them soiling the mirror of the Brünings lamp or Kirstein headlight, and to prevent them reaching the endoscopist's face. Ingals uses an electric aspirating pump originally devised for massage of the ear. A number of endoscopists are using various forms of aspirators attached to a water-faucet. In using these, it is necessary to exercise precaution if commercial circuits are used for illumination, lest the current be "grounded" through the water pipes, especially when withdrawing long aspirating tubes. The author prefers, for esophagoscopy, an aspirating canal in the wall of the esophagoscope or gastroscope, the exhaust being by an aspirating syringe. (Fig. 23.) The positive pressure-side of the syringe also has a soft rubber tube, and in case the aspirating canal in the wall of the esophagoscope becomes obstructed, a change of the soft rubber tube from the negative pressure to the positive pressure will force out any clots or other obstructions which may have entered the canal. Contrary to many of the statements that have appeared, the form of aspiration used by the author has absolutely nothing to do with distal illumination. There is no form of illumination that will enable the operator to see through a pool of blood and secretion. How to remove the fluid in the least possible time is the study of all endoscopists, and the aspirator

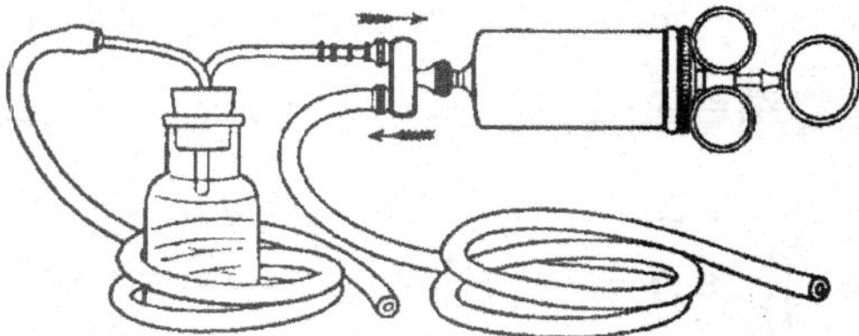

Fig. 23. Aspirator for esophagoscopy with additional tube connected with the plus pressure side for use in case of occlusion of the esophageal drainage tube. This aspirator is much more efficient than any soft rubber-ball aspirator can possibly be.

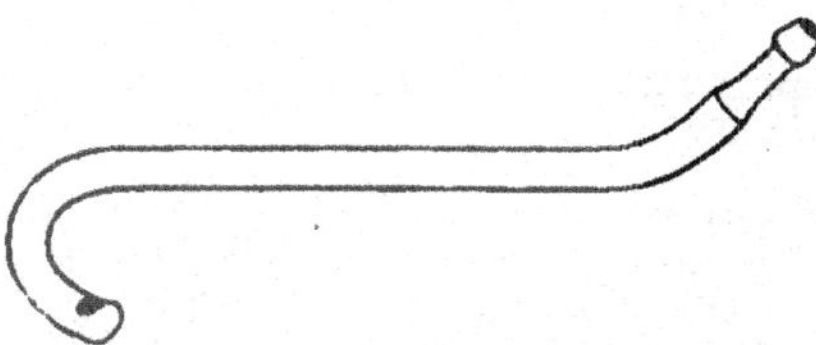

Fig. 24. Nozzle for attaching to the aspirator, for freeing the fauces and pharynx from secretion which otherwise would overflow into the larynx in peroral endoscopy, because the patient cannot swallow while endoscopic tubes are in place.

in the wall of the esophagoscope is used because there is no interruption of the work. It is a common thing at a gastroscopy to remove a pint of fluid without any interruption. An aspirating canal in the tube-wall can never become occluded by the indrawing of the mucosa as happens with an inserted independent tube, sometimes thus injuring the indrawn mucosa as well as occluding the aspirating tube. One great advantage of the syringe form of aspirator is its simplicity and portability. Most of the author's work has been done at the fourteen hospitals of Pittsburgh, and portability of the entire instrumentarium and organization made work in each as convenient as if all work had been done in one institution.

If the patient is being annoyed with secretions overflowing from the pharynx into the larynx in the recumbent position, the soft rubber aspirator tubing is detached from the esophagoscope and attached to the curved metal tube (Fig. 24), which is hooked over the upper alveolus (recumbent patient) and the pharyngeal secretions thus aspirated.

The author does not use any form of aspirator, either in the wall of the tube or otherwise in the bronchoscope. He has found that the best of all ways to remove abundant secretions and blood during bronchoscopy is to insert a large swab on the usual long Coolidge sponge-carrier, pushing it down until the large gauze sponge goes beyond the distal end of

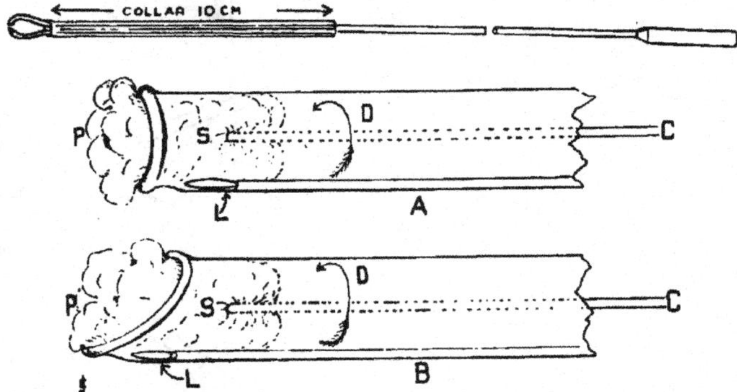

Fig. 25. Sponge carrier with long collar for carrying the small sponges shown in Fig. 27. The collar screws down as in the Coolidge cotton carrier. About a dozen of these are needed and they should all be small enough to go through the 4 mm. (diameter) bronchoscope and long enough to reach through the 53 cm. (length) esophagoscope, so that one set will do for all tubes. The schema shows method of sponging. The carrier C, armed with the sponge, S, when rotated as shown by the dart, D, wipes the field, P, at the same time wiping the lamp, L. The lamp does not need ever to be withdrawn for cleaning during bronchoscopy. It is protected in a recess so that it does not catch in the sponges.

the bronchoscope. Then the patient will cough the bronchoscope full of the fluid, and the withdrawal of the carrier and swab will pull up often as much as an entire tube full of secretions at a time, just as the plunger of an ordinary pump will lift the water which is above the plunger. This is one of the advantages in working under slight anesthesia or none at all. This method of aspiration in a case of bronchoscopy with profuse secretion may seem to the bystander to be less efficient than would be some form of pump, but it must be remembered that there is no great pool of secretion which can be completely and permanently emptied. The secretion is constantly being brought up from the bronchioles by the continued coughing efforts and must be removed intermittently from time to time as it is brought up to the neighborhood of the distal end of the tube. The effect of the sponge is to cause a fresh cough and to bring up more secretion to the point where it can be reached. Thus the continued swabbing with the gauze sponges removes not only the secretion which is already in the bronchus which is being explored, but it results in the removal of all the secretions from the minute bronchi, thus soon resulting in a relatively dry field.

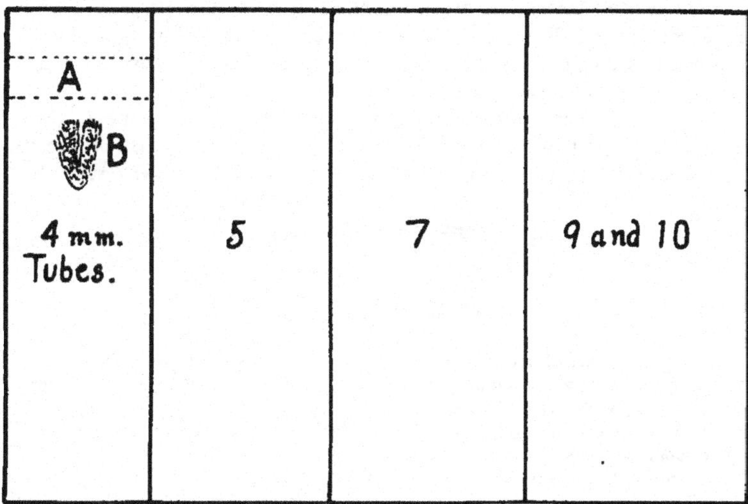

Fig. 26. Exact size to which the bandage-gauze is cut to make endoscopic sponges. Each rectangle is the size for the tubal diameter given. The dimensions of the respective rectangles are not given because it is easier for the nurse or anyone to cut a cardboard pattern of each size directly from this drawing. The gauze rectangles are folded up endwise as shown at A, then once in the middle as at B, then strung one dozen on a safety pin. In America gauze bandages run about 16 threads to the centimeter. Different material might require a slightly different size and the pattern could be made to suit.

Sponge carrier. The author has lengthened the collar of the Coolidge cotton carrier so that the collar never catches on the distal end of the bronchoscope or esophagoscope on withdrawal of the sponge holder, because the collar is too long for its proximal end to get beyond the tubemouth. The author uses in this holder the small folded sponges shown in Fig. 27.

Sponges. Small squares cut from a gauze roller bandage (ordinary surgical gauze is too large in the mesh) and folded into little pads and strung onto a safety-pin, as shown in Fig. 27, before sterilizing. These are prepared beforehand like any other operating room supplies, packed sterile, and kept in readiness. Four sizes are needed for the different tubes and they are numbered on the outside of the packages 4, 5, 7, 10. They are held securely in the sponge carrier shown in Fig. 25.

Foreign-body forceps. Years of experience have demonstrated that for foreign-body work in the larynx an alligator forceps with roughened jaws, known in America as Mosher's, in Great Britain as Paterson's, and in Germany and France as Mathieu's forceps, serve every purpose. Mathieu's is longer than the others and hence is better adapted to use through the esophageal speculum.

Experience has continued to demonstrate the fact that there is no form of forceps that has the power and the strength against breakage that pertains to the tube forceps. Hinged-jaw forceps are weakest at the

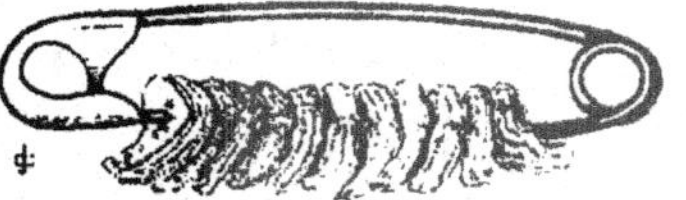

Fig. 27. Manner of keeping endoscopic sponges. About a dozen of one size are transfixed on a safety pin, wrapped, the size marked on the wrapper, and then sterilized, to be opened only as needed. About 5 dozen sponges of each of the 4 sizes should be kept on hand. Only one sponge is placed in the sponge-carrier at a time. These sponges are made for the author by Messrs. Johnston and Johnston, of New Brunswick, N. J., and are known as "bronchoscopic sponges."

rivet and do not begin to have the strength of grip, nor the strength against breakage when the forceps of necessity is long and slender, as in bronchoscopy and esophagoscopy, though for the larynx where a short and relatively heavy and rigid instrument is required, the alligator-jaw fulfills all purposes.

Instrument-makers, either through carelessness, or more likely from the taking of a later and still later instrument as a model, drift farther and farther away from the original design, so that very often the devisor of an instrument can scarcely recognize it when it comes to hand. In some instances forceps are made so far wrong that they will not go in the bronchoscope. More often the errors are in the little details, such as the serrations of forceps. Killian in his early forceps, such as the "bean" forceps (Fig. 32), especially designed the serrations to have a cant backward so as to make the forceps easy to push down over a foreign body but to grip firmly on withdrawal. Copying after Killian, the author's early forceps were all thus made; but instrument makers have drifted away from the original model until now they are turned out with evenly notched serrations that are very smooth on the top edges instead of being sharp and canted as shown in Fig. 30. The shape of serrations and their action can be readily understood by looking at the lower feed mechanism of any sewing machine or the gripping-jaw of any pipe-wrench. Such forceps, however, are capable of much traumatism if carelessly used, and under no circumstances whatever should such a forceps be placed blindly into a bronchus which is so small that the closure

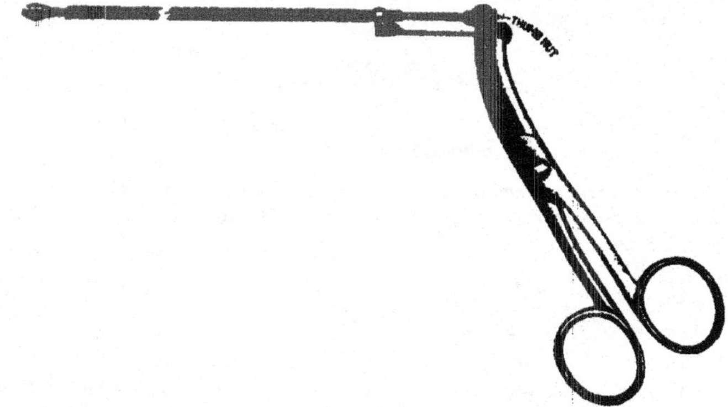

Fig. 28. Author's universal handle with one form of foreign-body jaws attached. This handle mechanism is so simple and delicate that the most exquisite delicacy of touch is possible. Unfortunately, instrument makers have often omitted the little thumb nut indicated above, with the result that the stylet was pulled through when strong traction was made. The cannulae are 45 cm. and 60 cm. long. There is a smaller size made for infant use, just half of the dimensions except those of the handle.

of the forceps cannot be watched. If blind groping in a small bronchus is ever justifiable, it is only so with forceps whose serrations are rounded and not canted. The author prefers all instruments, and especially forceps, in the lightest possible form consistent with the amount of strength necessary plus a sufficient factor of safety. Furthermore, for lightness of touch it is absolutely necessary to dispense with springs to throw the forceps open. A spring-opposed forceps cannot possibly communicate to the fingers the lightness of touch which is essential. For general work, the author has never found anything better than the forceps illustrated in his first work on bronchoscopy (Bib. 269). The ring handles do away with the necessity for opening springs. These forceps enable exceeding lightness of touch by which one can easily tell if the foreign body is properly grasped, and also enable the endoscopist to gauge precisely the degree of pressure that can be applied without crushing the foreign body in the case of friable bodies.

The selection of the forceps for use in a particular case is a very important matter and concerns the mechanical problems very closely. In

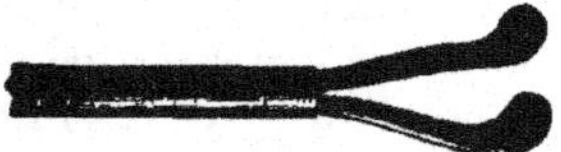

Fig. 29. Side-curved jaws for the author's forceps. Reproduced here to emphasize their usefulness. (Bib. 269.)

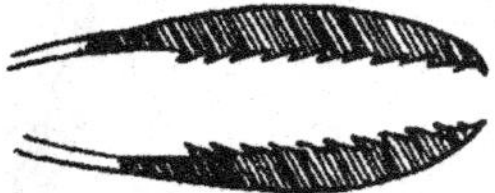

Fig. 30. Enlarged view of the author's foreign-body jaws, showing proper slant of serrations to prevent slipping. This slant is often lacking in the instruments in the shops.

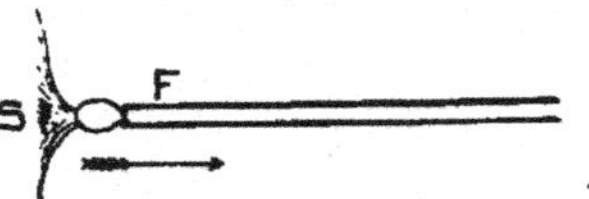

Fig. 31. Schema showing test of author's forceps. If properly adjusted, the point of the jaws of the forceps, F, will pick up the epithelium and elevate the skin from the palm of the hand (S) held vertically in contact with the point of the forceps jaws, when traction is made. This shows that the jaws come together first at the point in closing.

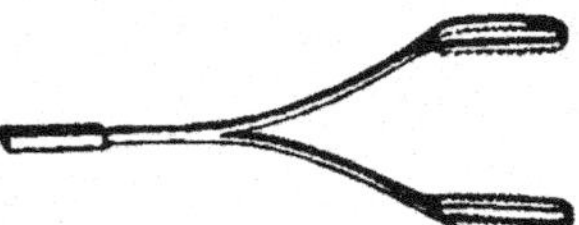

Fig. 32. Killian's "bean forceps" showing the cant of the serrations to prevent slipping which should be on all foreign-body forceps. The fenestra are to lessen the tendency to crush friable bodies like beans.

most instances, however, the plain jaw-forceps with canted serrations shown in Fig. 28, will serve every purpose. Almost equally useful is the side-curved forceps shown in Fig. 29, and if the author were limited to a single forceps, it would be this side-curved form (Fig. 29). The jaws projecting sidewise are easily seen closing. A large proportion of the successful foreign-body extractions by the author have been done with these two forms of jaws. The exceptions to their use are when the foreign body must be turned in order to make the proper points present themselves. In the case of pins and needles, the side-curved forceps can always be used to cause presentation of the foreign body in the proper axis for removal. With irregular objects, however, having one point sharp such as angular pieces of bone, it is very necessary to disengage the foreign body near the point with a forceps that will permit rotation; and for this purpose, the rotation forceps shown in Fig. 33 are ideal, because the points will hold firmly, yet will permit the foreign body to turn in the direction of least resistance. In another class of cases they can be made to throw the point out from the wall and into the mouth of the tube where the point is shielded from doing damage to the tracheal or esophageal wall, as will be explained in connection with the mechanical problems of bronchoscopic and esophagoscopic extraction of foreign bodies. The author has a separate handle for each forceps in order that not a moment may be lost in changing handles at a critical moment, should a different form of jaw be required. The jaws can be adjusted at any angle, but it is the author's practice always to have them open in an up and down direction, and when other directions are needed, the forceps' handles are turned in the proper way; thus a certain co-ordination and nerve-cell habit is established by which the operator always knows in which direction the jaws are opening. This facilitates promptness in the ocular endoscopic recognition of the jaw movement, because the observer knows for what to look. The curved-jaw forceps should always have the curve to the left of the operator, as this is the most convenient position in which to observe the jaws close and to guide their work with the eye. Unfortunately, many instruments were turned out by various manufacturers labeled with the author's name which were heavily constructed, having the jaws of poor temper and without the very essential little thumb nut, Fig. 28. This omission may have been partly due to the fact that it was not shown clearly on the early illustrations. This thumb nut permits the operator to exert great power without any danger of the jaw-stem pulling through. The screws at the side are still used in order to lock the jaw-stem so that it will push forward for opening the jaws. Another misfortune is the fact that many of these instruments are very clumsily manufactured. The author uses two different strengths of forceps, the one reasonably heavy for use through all except the very smallest tubes. For the infant bronchoscopes, very lightly constructed forceps are used because great strength is not necessary. It is necessary to see the forceps close, and for this very slender forceps are required. They are just half the strength and half the size, in all dimensions, of the regular forceps, except that the handle is the regular size. They are 45 cm. in length of cannula.

Occasionally, it is desired to twist a foreign body. The regular forceps will be found to give all the rotatory force that it is safe to use. If excessive twisting movement is to be applied, use may be made of the author's forceps with square cannula, into which the stilette, also squared, works at a good easy fit, yet will not spring.

For cutting in two of pins, wires and the like, Casselberry's forceps, Fig. 34, are excellent. Before using, however, it is well to test them on a pin similar to the one in the patient, because if not correctly made they will not hold the fragments.

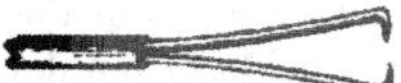

Fig. 33. Pointed jaws for the author's forceps. Useful when it is desired to permit turning of a foreign body to a safer relation for withdrawal, while securely held, as with bones, vulcanite dentures, pin-buttons, safety-pins, etc. The points must meet point to point exactly; the bend must be acute and the length of the point from the bend must be short—not over 2 mm. These forceps are especially valuable for the esophagoscopic removal of open safety-pins by the author's method of pushing them to the stomach, turning and withdrawing as elsewhere herein explained. They are called "rotation forceps."

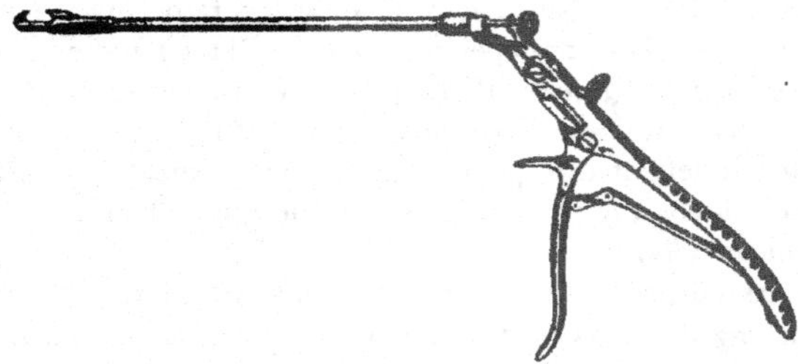

Fig. 34. Casselberry's forceps for endoscopic pin cutting. When correctly made the ends of the pin are held by the forceps so as not to be lost.

Brünings uses an extensible forceps which can be adjusted for different tube lengths.

Tissue forceps. For the removal of specimens from any part of the air or food passages, the author's forceps illustrated in Fig. 35, far surpass anything ever tried by him. The movable jaw will take hold directly on the side wall, and there is no need of a side-acting forceps. Indeed, a side-acting forceps will not work because it cannot be pushed sidewise unless the lateral push is furnished by the movement of the endoscopic tube. With the forceps illustrated in Fig. 35, however, a ready hold is gotten in any kind of tissue without any lateral movement of the endoscopic tube through which the forceps is passed. The jaws can be turned in any direction, though the author's own personal habit, as with foreign body forceps, is to leave the jaws fixed in the up and down direction and to get all movements by placing the handle, during the work, in the desired position, leaving the jaws always in the same position relative to the handle. It is wonderful what facility can be developed by using this

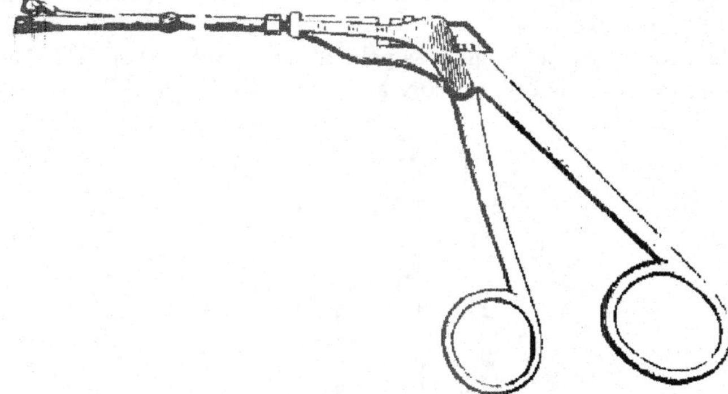

Fig. 35. Author's tissue forceps. The side jaw will bite into a flat lateral wall. The cross forms the bottom of a basket to hold the tissue removed. The action is very delicate, there being no springs. The sense of touch can often make the diagnosis. The best form for removal of a specimen and for endoscopic operations. The actual lengths of the forceps cannulae are 60 cm. and 30 cm., respectively; the latter being for laryngeal use.

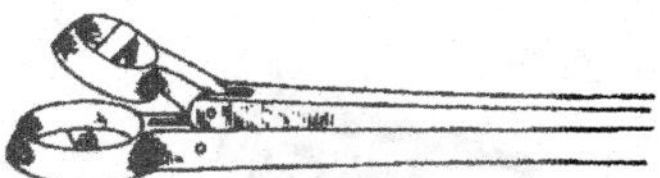

Fig. 36. Author's alligator punch forceps with bar across both upper and lower rings to form a "basket" to hold the excised fragments. These forceps will go through the author's adult laryngoscope, but he finds it advantageous to insert the forceps alongside the laryngoscope, which latter is only used to look through in the ocular guidance of the forceps.

method. Of course, different lengths are required for work in the larynx and in the esophagus, but clinically forceps with a 30 cm. cannula are best for the larynx, and a 60 cm. cannula will cover all other needs. There are no springs to oppose the bite, and it is often possible to distinguish the nature of the tissue bitten by the sensation communicated to the fingers, so delicate are the touch and action of the forceps.

Sliding punch forceps should have the upper ring the smaller one in order that the view of the growth, as the jaws close, shall not be obscured, as would be the case if the nearer ring were the larger. Thus precision may be assured in operating or in the removal of specimen, as the case may be. The author has seen a number of instruments in the shops with his name attached, in which this arrangement of jaws has been neglected (Fig. 37).

With a guillotine attached to the author's tissue forceps, a projecting mass may be amputated without injury to the basal tissue where this is deemed desirable.

Mouth-gag. Wide gagging, as pointed out by the author (Bib. 236), prevents proper laryngeal exposure and may thus defeat efforts at bron-

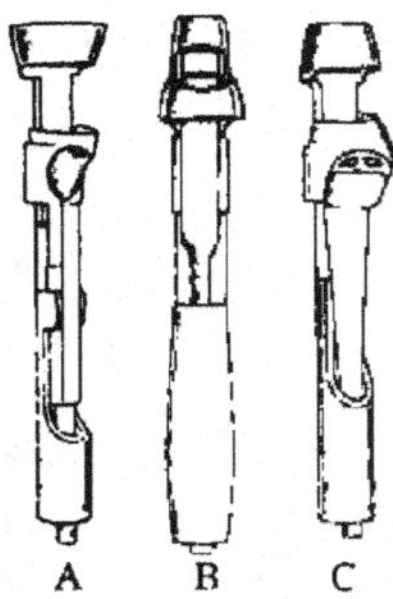

Fig. 37. Correct and incorrect forms of punch forceps. A, correct model. The near jaw is the smaller. B and C incorrect forms. The near jaw is the larger, and, consequently, obscures the view of the cutting edge. B has a swell on the shank which also obscures the view.

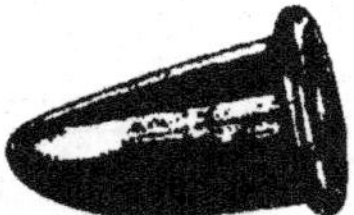

Fig. 38. Boyce thimble bite block, to be used instead of a gag to prevent the patient biting the tube. A gag makes peroral endoscopy difficult by jamming the mandible down on the hyoid bone.

choscopy and esophagoscopy by forcing the mandible down on the hyoid bone. All that is needed in the way of a gag is a bite block to prevent the patient closing his jaws on the delicate tube. For this, Dr. Boyce devised the thimble bite block (Fig. 38) which has recently been modified in shape by Dr. McKee and an ether tube has been added by Drs. McKee and McCready (Fig. 39). Ether is insufflated when needed for esophagoscopy. In bronchoscopy the insufflation is done through the bronchoscope if general anesthesia is used.

Snares. For indirect laryngoscopy the snare has the advantage that it can do no harm as could the forceps if misapplied. For direct laryngoscopy the forceps can be used so accurately that the snare is rarely useful except for large tumors of the laryngopharynx and the upper laryngeal aperture. For these purposes and for the amputation of the cancerous and the tuberculous epiglottis the author has found useful a very heavy snare cannula (Fig. 41) armed with No. 5 steel piano wire and fitted to the

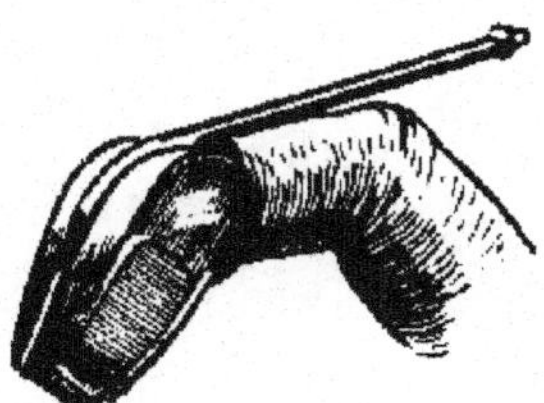

Fig. 39. Thimble bite block (on finger) originally suggested by Boyce and improved by McKee and McCready. Ether is insufflated through the tube, if needed, for esophagoscopy. The tube on the bite block is not used in bronchoscopy.

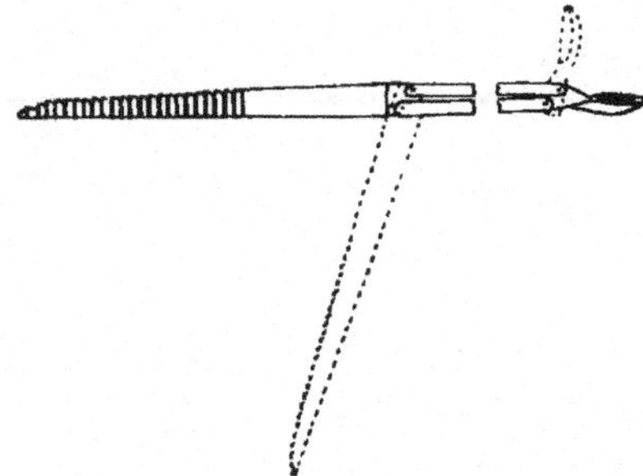

Fig. 40. Author's mechanical spoon for the endoscopic removal of soft friable bodies like beans, peas, meat, and nut kernels. The spoon-shaped extremity is inserted alongside the intruder which is then lifted and drawn into the end of the bronchoscope or esophagoscope by the action of the spoon when the handle is depressed as shown by the dotted line.

massive handles of the Peters tonsil snare. By firm downward pressure on the cannula the loop can be made almost completely to amputate the involved epiglottis *en masse,* as demonstrated by dissection of the removed tissues. The cannula is passed beside the laryngeal speculum, not through its lumen. Bronchoscopic and esophagoscopic snares are occasionally of service in solving the mechanical problems of foreign body extraction. The author on rare occasions uses a very delicate snare

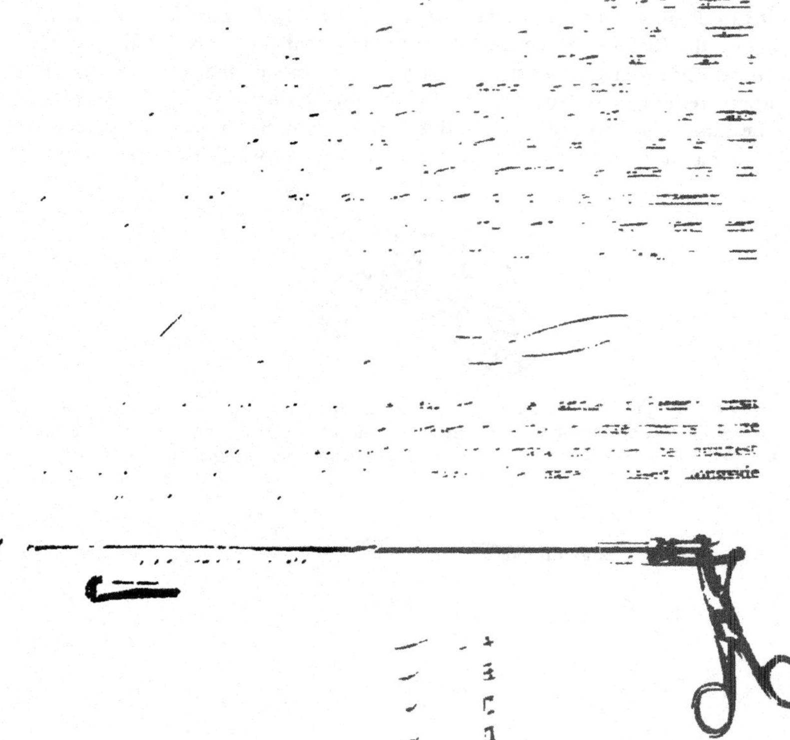

[illegible] author's form of forceps handle. The [illegible] in the lower illustration, are imparted to the snare loop as [illegible] position [illegible] by the particular case.

[illegible] that the [illegible] direction of the hooked end may be [illegible] right. The [illegible] hook and the half-curved [illegible] Killian have done good service. Ingals has de-[illegible] to bring a pin into the center of the lumen.

[illegible] has devised an ingenious screw pointed ex-[illegible] with which he removed a rubber pencil eraser.

[illegible] A most important part of the armamentarium is prop-[illegible] specially devised for the work. If the endoscopist has no [illegible]

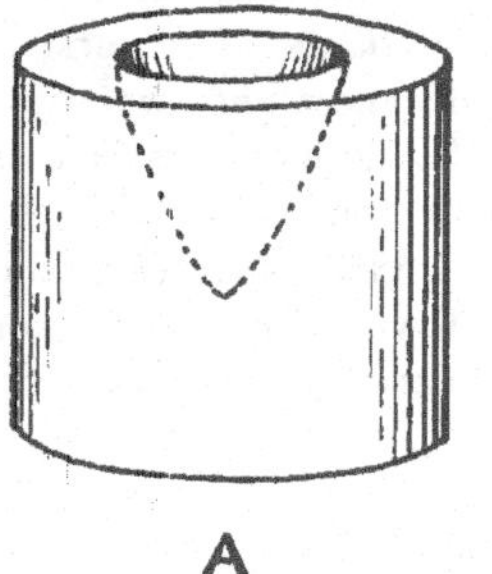

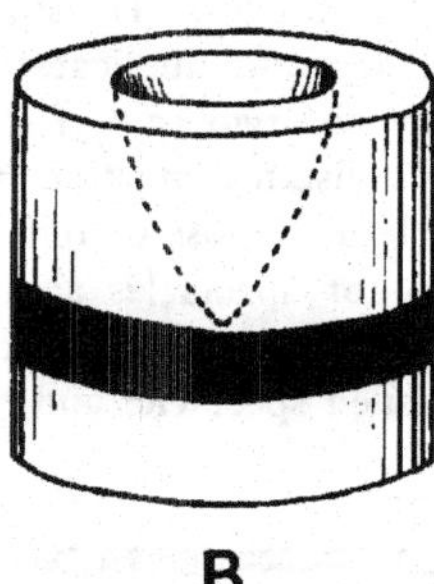

Fig. 43. Cups for anesthetic solutions designed originally by Yankauer for nasal use. Being heavy and broad based, they do not upset readily. The author has had a red band painted on one (B) which is for 20 per cent solution, which is used with great caution.

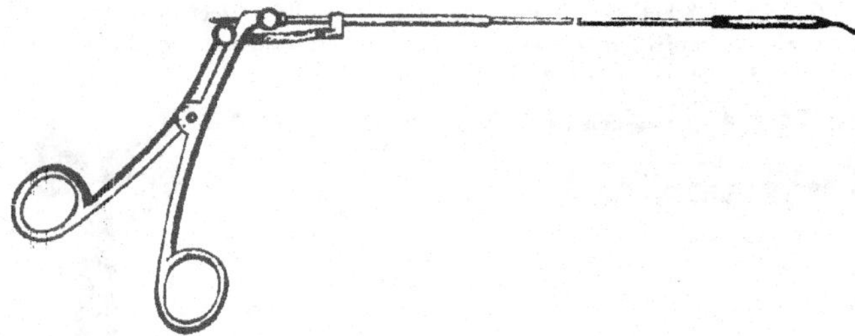

Fig. 44. The author's endoscopic syringe for injection of solutions of radium salts, local anesthetics, and other medicaments. It is made in 60 cm. length for bronchoscopic and esophagoscopic use, 30 cm. for direct laryngoscopic use. The capacity is 25 mgm., though it could be made for larger quantities of solution if desired.

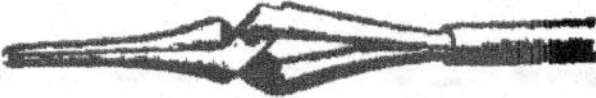

Fig. 45. The author's small dilator for bronchoscopic dilatation of bronchial strictures. The dilator is actuated by the author's universal forceps handle.

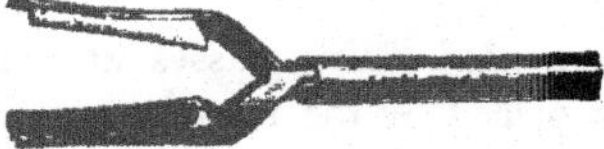

Fig. 46. The author's larger dilating forceps with a channel in each member. so as to furnish a canal when the dilator is closed for insertion. In use, this canal permits the dilator to be pushed down over the presenting point of such bodies as tacks. An enlarged form of this is sometimes used for the larynx.

very large eyes. If astigmatic, hypermetropic or myopic, correction is necessary and duplicate spectacles must be in charge of a nurse. If presbyopic, two pair of spectacles for 40 cm. distances and two pair for 65 cm. distance must be at hand. The reason for duplicates is that there is little or no loss of time in cleaning spattered lenses. One nurse is detailed for spectacles and she keeps them on a gauze-covered basin of warm water on the stand of which hangs a dry towel. The nurse cleanses the soiled spectacles and has them ready for immediate exchange. Hook-

Fig 47. The author's galvanocautery electrode for endoscopic use. It is especially adapted to cauterization of subglottic edema, and subglottic hyperplasia such as follows diphtheria. As with the author's pointed electrode (Bib. 269) the hard rubber is vulcanized onto the conducting wires, assuring cleanliness. Thread wound electrodes become filthy with blood and secretions.

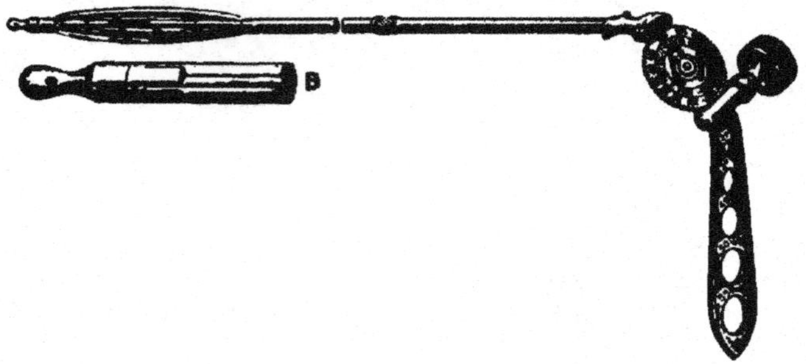

Fig. 48. Mosher's esophageal dilator. B. Actual size of distal end

Fig. 49. Plummer's double olive bougie. The stem between the two olives is vertebrated.

temple frames should be used. Eye-glasses are objectionable because they are not so quickly placed by the nurse when exchanging, and also because they are very apt to become displaced while working. Of course, the operator cannot handle them after he has sterilized his hands.

Endoscopic table. In an emergency any sort of table can be used, but where a special table is to be provided, the best one to be obtained is that of Dr. T. R. French (Fig. 54) designed especially for nasal and throat operations. The ease with which a trained assistant can raise or lower, or change the angle of inclination of the patient is a great convenience. The shortening and lengthening of the head-end of the table enables the operator to have any desired degree of overhang of the shoulders. All of these movements are under perfect control of the wheels manipulated by the second assistant. The table should be covered with a good pad against which a child can be held firmly without discomfort.

Operating room. All peroral endoscopy, except the diagnostic examinations of children suspected of diphtheria, should be done in an

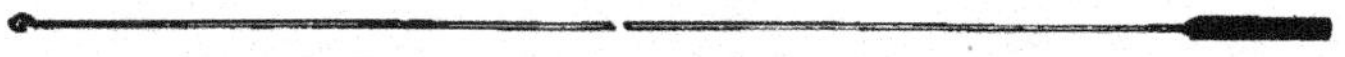

Fig. 50. Author's eyed bougie for esophagoscopic threading over a swallowed braided silk string. Twelve bougies with successive sizes of olives are made. The proximal end of the string is threaded through the esophagoscope. The esophagoscope is passed; then the bougie is threaded and passed along the thread which is held taut.

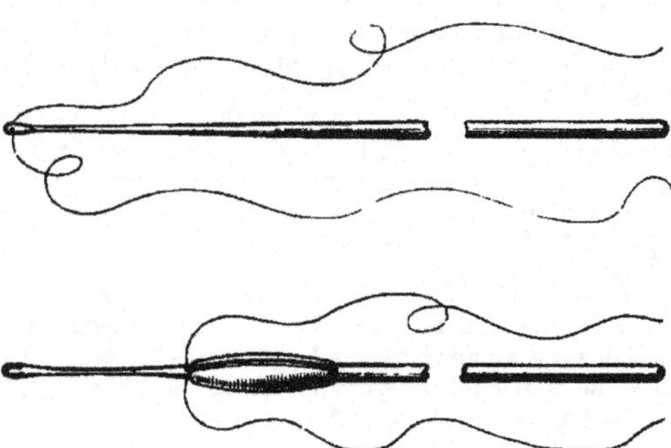

Fig. 51. Upper illustration. Author's eyed-probe for endoscopic use. Lower illustration. Author's string-cutting esophagotome. The braided silk cord works in a protecting groove on one side of the olive, the cutting being done on the other side which is turned toward the cicatrix when the latter is not annular.

operating room. A room which can be darkened is a necessity for endoscopy. Absolute darkness is of course not necessary nor desirable. There should be enough illumination, of a feeble kind, to permit the nurses and assistants to find what is needed on the sterile table. It is quite necessary that whatever windows there are should be at the back of the operator, because a little streak of light leaking in past blinds and shining directly into the eye of the operator, is particularly annoying and an inconvenience. The expert operator will get along with quite a bright light in the room, but when it comes to intricate and difficult work, it is necessary to have a darkened room. All endoscopy should be done with both of the endoscopist's eyes open. Prolonged work with the left eyelid closed is very fatiguing, and interferes with vision of the right. Ignoring of the image of the open left eye is facilitated by a darkened room.

Operating room organization. Once an endoscopic procedure has been started, moments are exceedingly precious. For this reason, every de-

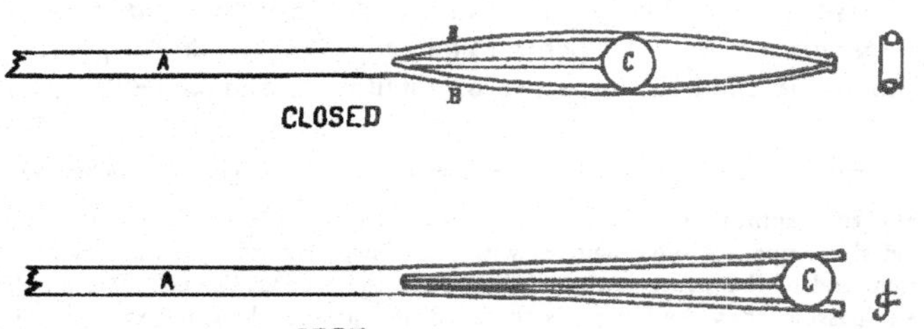

Fig. 52. Author's dilator for endoscopic use in bronchial and esophageal strictures. Invaluable in dilating successively each of a series of strictures, especially when the lumina of the lower ones are eccentric to those above, because it does not need to be inserted far.

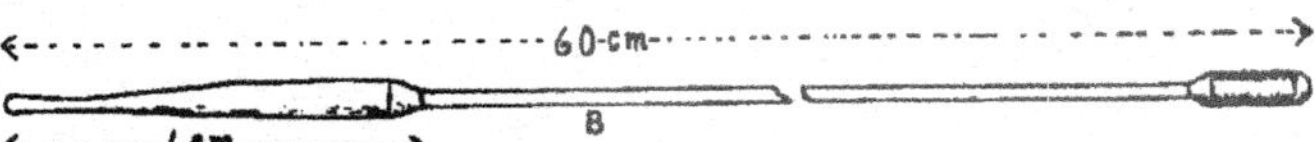

Fig. 53. Filiform bougie for minute cicatricial strictures of the esophagus. The filiform silk woven end, A, is joined securely to a spring steel shaft, B, thus giving all the advantages in safety of a silk woven bougie at the tip with a stiff shank that enables the bougie to be carried down rigidly through the length of the esophagoscope. Twelve sizes are made. The total length of 60 cm, is only necessary in case of a very low stricture in an adult. For use in children, the bougie can be shortened by unscrewing. The great advantage of the steel shaft over any sort of stylet inserted into a hollow filiform is that the small diameter of the steel shank permits of more accurate ocular guidance. These bougies are modeled after those of Guisez.

tail must be carried out including every instrument that would ever be wanted. Instruments not likely to be needed are kept sterile on a separate table, so that the working table will not be encumbered by anything but the regular working-set of instruments. The tubes are all kept with the batteries in the manner shown in Fig. 55, so that the surplus tubes not in use will in no way interfere with the quick handling of forceps and sponge carriers. The arrangement of the instrument table, the assistants, the battery, instrument nurse and anesthetist, as shown on page 46 in the earlier volume, has been proven to be invaluable in expediting careful work. The great advantage of having these regular positions is the avoidance of confusion. Anything needed is always in precisely the same location. The author has been able by this means to do just as good work in one hospital as in another by taking an assistant and a nurse with him. This, however, is not meant to say how good or how bad the work may have been, but such as it was, it represented the best that the author could do under any circumstances.

Oxygen tank and tracheotomy instruments. In all instances, as a matter of routine, instruments for tracheotomy should be on the sterile table ready for immediate use in every case of bronchoscopy or esophagoscopy, or direct laryngoscopy. It is exceedingly rarely, relatively,

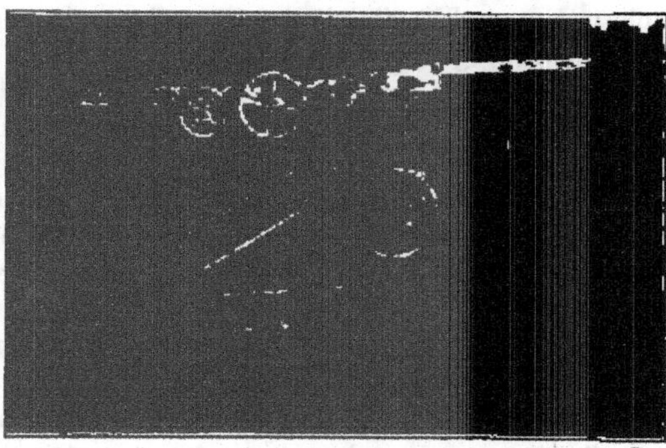

Fig. 54. Dr. T. R. French operating table. All positions are readily obtained by the three control wheels. The head board can be extended or shortened to bring the shoulders of the patient to the best position.

that they will be required, but when needed, they should be immediately at hand, sterile and ready. By having these preparations always part of the sterile table settings, a few lives can be saved that otherwise would be lost by the delay or by sepsis. An oxygen tank in a roller stand (Fig. 56) is most manageable. It should be covered with sterile towels pinned on, over valve-wheel and all, and a length of sterilized rubber tubing should be connected. If this tank should be prepared only in such cases as may seem beforehand likely to need it, the surgeon will find, to his chagrin, that when most wanted it will not be at hand. It is just such little details that make the difference between high and low mortality in any surgical procedure. In respiratory arrest from the pressure of the esophagoscope or of the foreign body, tumor, diverticulum full of food, respiration will not be started again unless a bronchoscope be introduced into the trachea or a tracheotomy be done for oxygen and amyl nitrite insufflation. Amyl nitrite should always be at hand in the form of capsules.

Head cover. The author uses a head cover for the patient, which is simply a muslin bag large enough to go down to the shoulders. A round hole about four inches in diameter is cut at the level of the mouth. This cap enables the operator and the second assistant to hold the head without infecting their hands. It involves a grave risk to handle instruments that go into the lung after handling a patient's head.

Asepsis. The author's early insistence (Bib. 269) upon strictly aseptic operating-room technic in all forms of peroral endoscopy, while much ridiculed at the time, has come to be recognized everywhere as quite essential in a procedure which necessarily frequently comes in contact with tuberculosis, pneumonia, diphtheria, erysipelas, lues and other infectious diseases and pyogenic infections. It is a matter of great gratification to the author that in fifty examinations of swabs used for wiping secretions from the bronchi, in no instance was there found any trace of such epithelial cells or of such forms of bacteria as would prove that the instruments had been in any way contaminated by contact with the mouth. This is worthy of note in connection with the obtaining of inoculation material for the production of autogenous vaccines in cases of chronic bronchitis, etc.

As before pointed out (Bib. 269), it is necessary to remember that though the field cannot be sterilized, yet the patient is more or less immune to the organisms that he, himself, harbors, while he may be extremely susceptible to organisms introduced from another source, even though such newly-introduced organisms may be morphologically the same. Bacteria from the patient's own skin and hair come under the class of foreign organisms when introduced into the lungs or into the blood and lymph channels in operative work. The only way to be certain of avoiding the introduction of pathogenic organisms from a previous patient, or from any other source, is to carry out all the details of aseptic operative technic. Then if a patient gets pneumonia or any other infection the operator has all the comfort of a clear conscience. A mask should always be worn by the operator to protect both the patient and himself from infections that either may unknowingly have. It is not pleasant to have even uninfective secretions coughed in one's face. Large plane protective spectacles should be worn over the operator's eyes it he does not require corrective lenses. The patient should be covered with a sterile gown, and a cap coming down to the shoulders with a hole in it corresponding in position to the mouth, but larger: about 10 cm. in diameter. Assistants, even the one who holds the head, and also the anesthetist, if one is needed, should put their hands through the same process of sterilization as for any surgical operation. All of the sterile team should wear sterile caps. Instruments should be sterilized by boiling, except the lamps, light carriers, knives and scissors. These should be immersed in alcohol. Extra lamps should be sterilized so as to be ready if needed. Conducting cords may be wiped with alcohol, but it must be strong alcohol, because alcohol diluted with water may temporarily impair insulation. Conducting cords should be covered with close-fitting rubber tubing for cleanliness.

LIST OF INSTRUMENTS.

The following list, given as a convenient basis for equipment, has been listed from the author's armamentarium. The essentials for ordinary work are marked with an asterisk. Bougies, dilators and the like are not so marked because they are not emergency instruments; though they are essential to the endoscopist who expects to deal with all kinds of cases. Special instruments may need to be devised for special cases. The instruments listed, unless names are mentioned, are of the author's design. These might not suit others, and it is better for the endoscopist personally to examine and select instruments that appeal to him personally.

Tubes:

*1 direct laryngoscope for children.
*1 direct laryngoscope for adults.
*1 bronchoscope, 4 mm. x 30 cm., for children.
*1 bronchoscope, 5 mm. x 30 cm., for children.
*1 bronchoscope, 7 mm. x 40 cm., for adults and older children.
*1 bronchoscope, 9 mm. x 40 cm., for adults.
1 esophageal speculum for children.
1 esophageal speculum for adults.
*1 esophagoscope, 7 mm. x 45 cm., for children. (Slanted end.)
1 esophagoscope, 8 mm. x 45 cm., for older children.
*1 esophagoscope, 10 mm. x 53 cm., for adults. (Slanted end.)
Extra lamps. (At least 1 dozen.)

Accessories:

*1 bite block, McCready-McKee.
*1 Sajous laryngeal cotton forceps, long, full, curved.
*1 aspirator and tubing for both positive and negative pressure.
*18 sponge holders with long screw collar.
*1 forceps, plain foreign body jaws with handle 45 cm. and 60 cm.
1 forceps, side curved, with handle 45 cm. and 60 cm.

1 forceps, with rotation jaws with handle, 45 cm. and 60 cm.
1 Casselberry's pin-cutting forceps.
*1 laryngeal tissue forceps with basket tip.
*1 Mosher alligator forceps.
1 punch forceps with round and triangular jaws.
1 guillotine forceps.
*1 mechanical spoon.
1 bronchoscopic snare.
1 esophagoscopic snare.
1 Lister hook.
*1 full-curved hook.
1 half-curved hook.
2 bronchoscopic dilators, large and small.
1 safety-pin closer.
*1 steel measuring rule, 20 cm. long.
2 cautery electrodes and cord.
1 bent hook mouth-aspirator.
1 laryngeal dilator, parallel blades.
1 Mosher's esophageal dilator for cardia.
Bougies metal with silk-woven ends.
Bougies, double olive.
Porcelain cups for local anesthesia solutions, 1 with red band.
*Sponges, a good supply would be about 4 dozen of each size.
4 extra battery cords.
*2 dry cell batteries with two circuits each.
2 battery covers.
1 face cap for patient.
Tracheotomy instruments.
Extra spectacles with large lenses to protect operator's eyes.

Care of instruments. Next in importance to having a well-made and carefully selected instrumental equipment, is the keeping of the equipment in proper order. For this purpose the endoscopist should have an instrument nurse in his own employ, or he should look after the care himself, for, unfortunately, the constantly changing working-force in the usual operating room results in the instruments falling into the hands of a new nurse at frequent intervals, and alas too often a pupil-nurse, who, however competent to scrub and polish the instruments of the general surgeon, will work sad havoc with the endoscopist's equipment; and consequently the next time a bronchoscopy is in order the endoscopist will find his work difficult or impossible because of forceps bent or corroded, small parts lost, tubes dinged, canals choked with blood or secretions, adherent to the inner walls and coagulated by boiling. The sooner the endoscopist realizes that he is simply a mechanic and that to do good work a mechanic must have good tools kept in proper order, the better his results will be. Otherwise, he will never obtain the high percentage of successes of the good mechanic who keeps his tools in good order. To keep instruments in the proper condition requires not only good care but very frequent careful inspection, for the frequent cleansings, the taking apart and putting together, the boiling as well as the actual use of the instruments, result in deterioration. This applies especially to forceps, which have the heaviest work to do, and which must necessarily be delicate in construction. The jaws at the end of all forms of tube for-

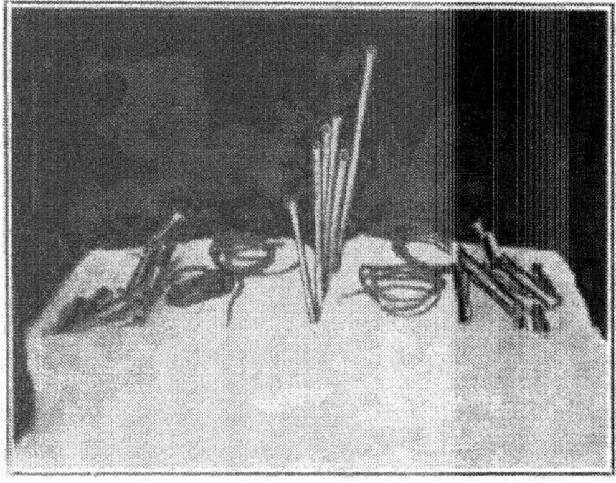

Fig. 55. Manner of arranging sterile instruments and batteries. The battery lids are opened back outward in opposite directions, then each is covered with a special sterile cover. The crevice between is used to hold tubes which are readily identified by their distal ends which are always uppermost. Laryngoscopes are in the battery lids.

ceps are necessarily tempered to a spring temper. If the temper is a little too high, or if slight corrosion has taken place, the forceps are very apt to break. This is an exceedingly embarrassing accident, resulting not only in the loss of the foreign body, but in the introduction of a fresh foreign body in the form of a lost part of the instrument. Consequently after much use it is wise to throw away the stylet jaws of tube forceps and replace them with new ones. This, with careful inspection before each operation, will prevent accidents and failures. After operation the canal for the light carrier, and in the case of the esophagoscope, the drainage canal, should be cleaned first, by forcing cold water through the canal with the aspirating syringe, and then by pushing through a long cotton brush formed on wire, such as used for cleaning the canal in the stem of a tobacco pipe. As usually sold in the tobacco shops it is cut in short lengths, but it can be obtained from the factory in coils. It is stiff enough to be pushed through the canals, provided the canals are always cleaned immediately after operation and the secretions not permitted to stick in the canal, either by coagulation or by boiling. Forceps should be taken apart and the cannula cleaned thoroughly by running cold water through it. The stilette should be cleaned and then polished with a bit of emery paper and carefully oiled before replacing it in the cannula. If the cannulae of forceps are made of spring-tempered brass tubing, they are

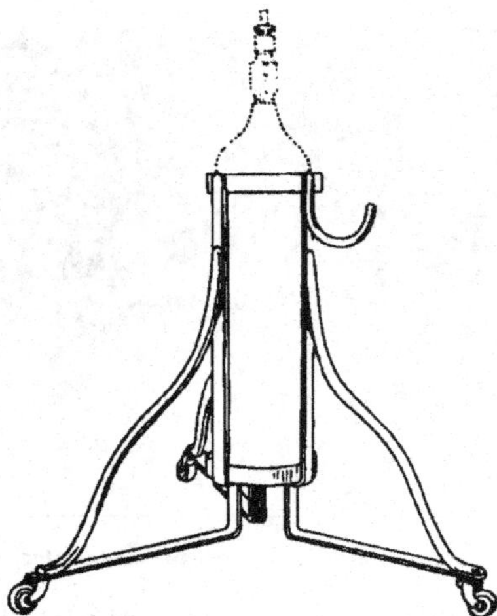

Fig. 56. Oxygen tank stand. Very light and convenient to go under the head of the operating table when needed so as to be out of the way during bronchoscopic oxygen insufflation.

much less subject to corrosion than steel is to rust. It is necessary to see that the sliding edges of the direct laryngoscope are not injured and that the slide works freely and comes away readily, unless as is now done by many the oval laryngoscope is used without the slide. Roughness of tubes is readily detected by passing the finger all over them. The distal ends are particularly prone to get little rough places. Rubbing with the smoothest quality of emery paper will remove roughness. Some of the plating may be thus removed, but the author prefers instruments not plated anyway, for plating is apt to scale off. To keep in order batteries of the form used by the author, it is only necessary to renew the dry cells once every three or four months, whether used or not. If care is taken to see that all connections are screwed up tightly, no one should ever fail for want of current. Before sterilizing, the cords and lamps should be tested, the lamps being allowed to remain in the light carriers which are then immersed in alcohol.

In over three thousand endoscopies neither Dr. Patterson nor the author has ever failed for want of a light. This has not been a matter of luck; but rather a little attention to see that everything is right before starting, and the observance of a rule always to have a duplicate in reserve, precisely as is done in all commercial lighting installations or in the "dual ignition" systems of modern internal combustion motors. This is not boasting. It is too trivial a matter. In fact the matter is so very trivial that few operators will give the electric details any attention. There is no mystery about electric trouble; and he who is master of his instrument and its few and simple details will always have satisfactory light. Violin strings are prone to break; but this does not cancel the virtuoso's concert nor make him resort to wire strings.

CHAPTER II.

Anatomy.

Anatomical knowledge of the kind required for bronchoscopy and esophagoscopy cannot be obtained from a book. The anatomy of the tracheo-bronchial tree and of the esophagus was considered in the author's earlier work. In addition to the notes there given the broncho-esophagoscopist is advised to study the anatomy as given in the standard anatomical works and then to pass the bronchoscope and the esophagoscope repeatedly on the cadaver with the thorax opened to full view in order to get in mind the precise relations of the various surrounding viscera. As the identification of landmarks is very much easier on the cadaver because of the stillness and the absence of renewal of secretions once they are removed, the bronchoscopist should practice the identification of the bifurcation and of the orifices of the upper, middle and the lower lobe bronchi on the right side, and of the upper and lower lobe bronchi on the left side. Variations of the endoscopic appearances in the tracheo-bronchial tree and in the esophagus were considered in the earlier work and will be alluded to still further when writing of the introduction of the bronchoscope and of the esophagoscope. The articles of Ingals, Brown-Kelly, Mosher, and particularly the interesting article of Liebault (Bib. 329) and the very elaborate paper by Mehnert (Bib. 404) are well worthy of careful study. The latter authority distinguishes thirteen physiological constrictions in the esophagus. For endoscopic purposes only four of these need be considered, namely, the cricoidal, the aortal, the bronchial, and the hiatal. To these some authors would add the cardia. Consideration of the endoscopic appearances of the four constrictions mentioned will be alluded to in connection with the introduction of the esophagoscope. The endoscopic anatomy of the larynx will be studied from the new direct view-point under the heading of direct laryngoscopy and elsewhere. The illustrations and even the laryngeal image of the indirect method are quite misleading, and we cannot obtain true direct image simply by inverting a drawing of the indirect image.

CHAPTER III.

Preparation of the Patient for Peroral Endoscopy.

The suggestions of the author in the earlier volume in regard to preparation of the patient, as for any operation by a bath, laxative, etc., and especially by special cleansing of the mouth with 25 per cent alcohol have received general endorsement. Artificial dentures should be removed. Even if no anesthetic is to be used, the patient should be fasted for five hours if possible, even for direct laryngoscopy in order to forestall vomiting. Except in emergency cases every patient should be gone over by an internist for organic disease in any form. If an endolaryngeal operation is needed by a nephritic, preparatory treatment may prevent laryngeal edema or other complications. Hemophilia should be thought of. It is quite common for the first symptom of an aortic aneurysm to be an impaired power to swallow or the lodgment of a bolus of meat or other foreign body. If aneurysm is present and esophagoscopy is necessary, as it always is in foreign body cases, "to be forewarned is to be forearmed." Pulmonary tuberculosis is often unsuspected in very young children. There is great danger from tracheal pressure by an esophageal diverticulum or dilatation distended with food; or the food may be regurgitated and aspirated into the larynx and trachea. Therefore, in all esophageal cases the esophagus should be emptied by regurgitation induced by titillating the fauces with the finger after swallowing a tumblerful of water, pressure on the neck, etc. Aspiration will succeed in some cases. In others it is absolutely necessary to remove the food with the esophagoscope. If the aspirating tube becomes clogged by solid food, the method of swab aspiration mentioned under bronchoscopy will succeed. Of course there is usually no cough to aid, but the involuntary abdominal and thoracic compression helps. Should a patient arrive in a serious state of water-hunger, as explained under "Contraindications to Esophagoscopy," the patient must be given water by hypodermoclysis and enteroclysis, as part of the preparation and if necessary the endoscopy, except in dyspneic cases, must be delayed until the danger of water-starvation is past.

Every patient should be examined by indirect, mirror laryngoscopy as a preliminary to peroral endoscopy for any purpose whatsoever; and it becomes doubly necessary in cases that are to be anesthetized as explained in the beginning of the chapter on direct laryngoscopy.

CHAPTER IV.

Anesthesia for Peroral Endoscopy.

While it is impossible to lay down any hard and fast rules for anesthesia in tube work, yet the time has arrived when we may formulate a few general principles from which deviation can be made to suit the particular case or the operator's personal equation. The herein given rules were submitted by the author for discussion at a meeting of the American Laryngological Association.*

In the very interesting and extensive discussion which followed, the conclusions were endorsed in the main. Particular emphasis was placed upon the statement that the personal equation of the operator and of the particular case should govern the question as to whether general, local, or no anesthetic at all is to be used.

Total abolition of the cough-reflex should only be for short periods. The facile operator will do good work in many cases in spite of a moderate degree of cough. After a short period of tubal contact in bronchoscopy, coughing lessens and often practically ceases, especially in infants. Following the general rule in surgery, an anesthetic should never be used at all unless necessary; never in greater quantity than the needed minimum. In general surgery, anesthesia is required for three purposes: (1) The obtunding of pain (really analgesia); (2) the abolition of reflexes (relaxation), and (3) for psychic effect (mainly abolition of apprehension). For peroral endoscopy, analgesia is not required, for the pain in careful work is exceedingly slight; but anesthesia for the lessening of the reflexes and for the lessening of the apprehension which intensifies the reflexes, is necessary under certain circumstances. These reflexes are manifested by spasmodic action of certain muscular systems, chiefly those of vomiturition and coughing. In so far as these may be excited by mucosal contact they may be controlled by local anesthesia alone; for, of course, local anesthesia is purely and simply mucosal anes-

*Proceedings Amer. Laryngol. Association, 1912, p. 88.

thesia. Muscular contractions, as well as pain, resulting from psychic mechanism, or traction upon tissues remote from the mucosa can only be controlled by deep general anesthesia, or to a less degree, by the control of the patient's mental state by the personality of the operator. The degree of this control varies widely with the personal equation of the operator as well as of the patient. The operator who can keep his patient free from apprehension and who can keep his patient's mind fixed on the task of breathing slowly, deeply, and regularly will get along without any anesthetic and do better work than another operator under profound general anesthesia. As Brünings has pointed out, the operator who is not sufficiently practiced to pass the tubes without general anesthesia is not justified in using general anesthesia to overcome faults in technic.

Anesthesia for esophagoscopy. 1. For foreign bodies, no anesthetic is needed in either adults or children, except in case of very large and sharp foreign bodies, wherein the relaxation of the esophageal musculature, by deep general anesthesia, will obviate the trauma incident to the withdrawal of the intruder through a spasmodically constricted lumen.

2. In case of a sharp foreign body threatening perforation, especially open safety-pins, it is safer to abolish antiperistalsis by deep general anesthesia.

3. In cases of suspected esophagismus and "cardiospasm," the spasmodic element can be entirely eliminated by deep general anesthesia.

4. In case of large foreign bodies, general anesthesia adds enormously to the danger of respiratory arrest from pressure of the foreign body on the trachea and on the peripheral nervous respiratory mechanism.

5. The use of a general anesthetic will greatly lessen the need for skill in the introduction of the esophagoscope; but such use is utterly unjustifiable.

6. Local anesthesia is needless for esophagoscopy. If used at all, it should be applied only to the laryngo-pharynx, never to the esophagus.

Anesthesia for direct laryngoscopy. 1. For diagnosis. In infants and children, no anesthetic whatever in any case. In adults who tolerate indirect laryngoscopy well, no anesthetic, general or local, is needed.

2. Foreign bodies. In infants and children, no anesthesia, general or local.

3. For the removal of foreign bodies from the larynx, both local and general anesthesia should be avoided, lest their application lead to dislodgment of the intruder.

4. For papillomata in children, no anesthetic, general or local, is needed. In adults, local anesthesia is usually necessary for accurate work in removing specimens or entire neoplasms of any kind.

5. In a few adults, intolerant and uncontrollable general excitability, and in some cases of hysteria a general anesthetic may be necessary for accurate work in the removal of laryngeal neoplasms; but such cases are exceedingly rare.

Oral bronchoscopy. 1. For diagnosis, in children, no anesthesia, general or local: in adults, local anesthesia of the trachea and bronchi, as well as of the larynx will be needed.

2. For foreign bodies in the trachea and bronchi of infants and small children no anesthetic, general or local, is needed, except possibly in very complicated removals, such as in case of open safety-pins. Foreign bodies in the trachea and bronchi of adults can often be removed without any anesthesia, general or local; but in most cases local anesthesia is needed. General anesthesia is needed only in complicated cases where there is a stricture to dilate to reach the foreign body, or where the mechanical problem of removal is complex, or where the cough threatens to cause perforation.

3. For the after-treatment of stricture local anesthesia is sufficient, and in some cases none is needed, because tolerance to manipulation becomes established after repeated passage of the instruments.

Tracheotomic bronchoscopy. If lower bronchoscopy is ever justifiable, it is only so in cases with extremely severe dyspnea, and even in such cases the facile operator will slip in a bronchoscope, through which, with the aid of amyl nitrite and oxygen, artificial respiratory aid can be supplied with greater facility than through a tracheotomy wound. Should the bronchoscopist prefer tracheotomy it never need be done under general anesthesia; and in a dyspneic case general anesthesia is utterly unjustfiable because as soon as anesthesia begins, respiration ceases, owing to the loss of the aid of the accessory respiratory musculature. Cocanization of the trachea and bronchi may be used for tracheotomic bronchoscopy in adults; no general anesthetic is necessary.

General rules for local anesthesia. Anesthetic adjuncts, such as adrenalin, antipyrin, and various synthetic compounds, the author has never used; consequently, he cannot formulate any rules, even in a suggestive way, and he is compelled to rely upon Drs. Ingals, Coolidge, Mayer, Mosher, Winslow, Yankauer, Casselberry, and other eminent coworkers to supply the deficiency. Doubtless, adrenalin by the ischemia which it induces, increases anesthesia and also prolongs it by slowing the carrying-away of the cocaine by the blood. Bromides in large doses, some hours beforehand, as suggested to the author by Dr. Frank D. Sanger, of Baltimore, have a marked effect in lessening cough reflex and lessening the amount of cocaine needed. Morphine has this also, but its use is objectionable because of after-nausea; and in cases where repeated sittings are necessary, there is risk of drug habit. Heroin is an adjunct useful in some cases. None of these antibechics should be used in such large doses as to abolish the cough-reflex for a long time because, as the author has frequently pointed out, the cough-reflex is the watchdog of the lungs, quickly ridding the lungs of irritative and infective materials

For esophagoscopy, local anesthesia is needless. If used at all, its application should be limited to the epiglottis and laryngo-pharynx (not hypo-pharynx). The esophagus is insensitive as anyone may determine for himself by swallowing very hot coffee. After the pharynx is passed the burning sensation ceases, though sometimes it is felt again slightly when the stomach is reached.

RULES FOR THE USE OF COCAINE.

(1) Cocaine should never be used in infants or small children.

(2) Its use should be avoided, if possible, in all cases, such as cases of papillomata, in which frequent sittings are necessary.

(3) The patient should never know the name of the drug.

(4) The amount used should be the minimum as to

(a) Strength of solution.

(b) Quantity of solution.

(c) Mucosal area touched.

Hence, only certain highly sensitive areas should be touched with the stronger solutions; the less sensitive areas receiving only the weaker solutions, either by direct application or by the incidental flow over the moist mucosal surface following the application of the stronger solutions to the highly sensitive areas.

(5) Solutions may be applied by

(a) Spray.

(b) Syringe.

(c) Painting syringe (Brünings).

(d) Applicator carrying cotton or gauze saturated, but not dripping, with solution.

Preference should be given to either or both of the last two methods as being more precise. The spray is useful, if the operator desires to use any anesthetic at all in cases of foreign body in the larynx, as a spray is much less liable to displace the intruder than a swab; but for this very reason any form of anesthesia had better be omitted in cases of laryngeally lodged foreign bodies.

(6) The stomach should always be empty, not only because the tendency to vomiturition and vomiting are thus lessened; but because, as proven by Brünings, absorption of cocaine is thus lessened.

The author's technic for local anesthesia. The author has two porcelain jars, thick and heavy, though small, (about 2 c. c.) carried with the instrumentarium. In one, an 8 per cent cocaine solution is freshly prepared, and in the other a 20 per cent solution. The latter is known by a red band around the jar, burned into the porcelain, Fig. 43. This solution is used only with extreme caution and in small quantity. In no case are the jars refilled, hence the total quantity is always limited; and, of course, most of it is thrown away in the swabs and escapes with the secretions, so that only a very small portion of the solutions is absorbed by the patient. Used in this way, the author has never had a serious symptom. This method was adopted after the death of a child in rhythmic, symmetrical convulsions one hour after the removal of a papilloma of the larynx under cocaine anesthesia. He has never, however, used cocaine in children since, and never will. All of his endoscopy on children under seven years of age is done without any anesthetic, general or local, except in a very few cases of complicated foreign-body extractions, such as the closure of safety-pins. The author's method of application for local anesthesia is as follows: With a dossil of cotton held in a Sajous laryngeal forceps, the laryngo-pharynx is swabbed with an 8 per cent solution of cocaine, by sense of touch, without a mirror. After two minutes' wait, the laryngoscope is introduced, and the anterior and posterior surfaces of the epiglottis are painted with a small gauze sponge (Fig. 27) saturated with the 20 per cent cocaine solution and carried in with a sponge holder (Fig. 25). A fresh sponge is saturated and carried through the glottis and down the trachea. After a two minutes' wait, the bronchoscope is introduced if desired and deeper applications made as necessary. The posterior tracheal wall and the neighborhood of the bifurcation are the sources of much reflex-cough, and the bronchus to be entered may need an application; but the skillful operator will often dispense with local anesthesia after the first application, as the cough reflex in many instances soon ceases to be troublesome, and a certain amount of cough need not interfere with work. In case of impacted foreign bodies, it is of advantage to hold the swab in contact with the surrounding tissues for about half a minute.

Technic of general anesthesia. For esophagoscopy and gastroscopy, ether or chloroform may be started by the usual method and continued by dropping upon a folded bit of gauze, several layers thick, laid over the mouth after the tube is introduced. Undoubtedly, there is a remote risk from the inflammability of ether, which is too often forgotten.

For tracheo bronchoscopy, ether or chloroform may be started in the usual way and continued by holding a gauze sponge with a hemostat in front of the tube, though this means frequent interruption of the work as well as of the anesthetic. So far as interruptions of the anesthetic are concerned, they are, in the author's opinion, factors of safety, if care be taken to avoid excessively deepening the anesthesia to prolong the interval. Or, after starting in the usual way, chloroform and ether may be continued by means of the Buchanan attachment (Fig. 17) directly to the bronchoscopic tube, care being taken carefully to time the insufflations properly in relation to inspiration. It is preferable to start with ether and continue with chloroform, which is relatively quite safe after the stimulant effects of ether are established.

ADDITIONAL NOTES ON GENERAL ANESTHESIA FOR PERORAL ENDOSCOPY.

The foregoing is reprinted here exactly as presented and discussed at the meeting mentioned. The following observations may be added and some points may be emphasized.

A serious error has crept into medical literature in regard to anesthesia for direct laryngoscopy, and unfortunately, error in medical literature persists and is handed down from author to author long after men doing the work realize the error. The statement has been repeatedly made that general anesthesia is necessary for direct laryngoscopy in children. Nothing could be farther from the truth, because in children, no anesthetic, general or local, is required in any case for direct laryngoscopy. In certain adults with short, thick necks and of a very muscular type, with engorged irritable throats it requires a high degree of skill to do accurate work by direct laryngoscopy, even with local anesthesia. In such cases there is ample justification for the beginner to use a general anesthetic, provided there is no dyspnea and no obstruction in the larynx. But in children, no one is worthy of the name of direct laryngoscopist if he cannot examine the larynx of any child without any anesthetic, general or local. Children with papillomata are quite likely to die on the table if a general anesthetic be given, unless the operator is exceedingly prompt with a bronchoscopic oxygen insufflation, or a prompt tracheotomy with insufflation of amyl nitrite and oxygen.

In the case of a combative child who is also dyspneic it must be remembered that compelling the child to undergo the anesthetic will be even more than usually dangerous, for dyspnea is always increased by exertion. If a struggle on the part of the patient ends in succumbing to the anesthetic the danger is so great that only quick work will save the child. If on the other hand the struggle had ended with the insertion of a bronchoscope instead of the administration of an anesthetic, the child would be safe at the end of the struggle instead of moribund.

The author has never seen a case of arrested respiration by pressure on, or irritation of, the peripheral nervous respiratory mechanism, such as the so-called "vagus reflex." Such arrest is, in his opinion, always due to occlusion of the air passages, for the following reasons. Respiratory arrest never occurs in work without anesthesia unless the air passages are occluded until the patient asphyxiates. On the other hand, when apnea vera has occurred in the cases that have come to the writer's knowledge, it has always been under deep anesthesia, when, of all times, the patient should be less susceptible to reflex arrest of respiration by presence of the endoscopic tube. Therefore, the author believes that the occasionally given "vagus reflex" as a cause of death in esophagoscopy or "laryngeal reflex" in bronchoscopy, are unwarranted by the facts.

Angiomata, edematous polyps, and a few vascular growths will shrink so completely under cocaine as to render accurate removal impossible. When this is found to be the case a general anesthetic will be necessary.

Small growths projecting from the ventricle in adults may be very readily hidden by the over-riding projection of the ventricular band. This projection is very much more pronounced under even thorough anesthetization by local means, so that unless extremely expert, the operator will require the use of general anesthesia, which has the effect of lessening very much the projection of the ventricular band. Esophagoscopy upon the struggling, resistant patient whose pharyngoesophageal musculature is in a state of spasm, is, in the hands of the less skillful, not without risk unless care is exercised. The skillful esophagoscopist will do it without the slightest danger. The ordinary risks of anesthesia are very much enhanced by risks of respiratory arrest, be this from reflex inhibition or mechanical obstruction of the trachea from the bulk of the tube or of the foreign body or both, or from other causes. Spastic conditions of the hypo-pharyngeal and esophageal musculature, whether from the presence of a foreign body or other causes, are completely relaxed by general anesthesia. For esophagoscopy the author would advise, if any anesthesia is desired, ether insufflation with the Elsberg apparatus (Fig. 57) because it introduces an element of safety which has never pertained to esophagoscopy under general anesthesia before, except in the hands of the most skillful. As elsewhere mentioned, there have been in the practice of various operators a number of deaths on the table from arrest of respiration during esophagoscopy under general anesthesia. This occurred especially in foreign-body cases where the bulk of the tube and the bulk of the foreign body together compressed the trachea when the esophagoscope over-rode the foreign body. The author is not prepared to advocate the Elsberg anesthesia, or any other method, to overcome the faults of technic in esophagoscopy; but it certainly insures safety, so far as respiratory arrest is concerned, to have a silk woven catheter in the trachea insuring the supplying of air to the lungs, and assuring the impossibility of complete obliteration of the tracheal lumen, for enough lumen must exist at both sides of the tube to permit the return-flow of air. The author does not hesitate to say to those who wish to use general anesthesia for esophagoscopy that a death on the table is practically impossible with ether insufflation. Of course, the presence of the catheter in the trachea would render possible trauma by the tube mouth, but only by the grossest technical faultiness.

In many cases of foreign body in the esophagus, the foreign body is prevented from going downward by muscular contractions. Therefore, if a general anesthetic is given, the relaxation of this clonic contraction by the anesthetic permits the foreign body to escape downward. The author believes this to be one of the reasons why it has so rarely

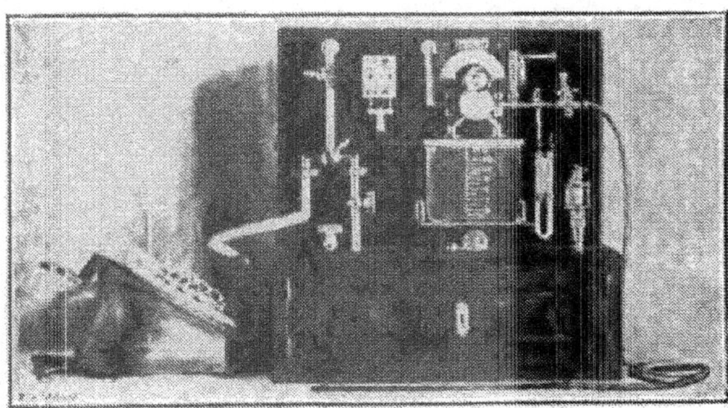

Fig. 57. Elsberg apparatus for intratracheal insufflation ether anesthesia.

happened in the Pittsburgh Clinic that a foreign body has been lost downward. In the absence of anesthesia, the presence of the tube excites still greater spasmodic contractions of the esophageal wall and the foreign body is held all the more tightly, which gives the operator a good chance to approach it with the tube and seize it with the forceps. Out of 206 cases, only 8 went down, and of these, only 3 went down after the commencement of the esophagoscopy. Of the 3, 2 were under general anesthesia, which leaves but a single case where a foreign body escaped downward during esophagoscopy without anesthesia, general or local.

In the last 107 bronchoscopies and esophagoscopies for foreign bodies in children under 6 years of age, done in the Pittsburgh Clinic, no anesthetic, general or local, has been used. A number of adolescent and adult cases have been done also without anesthesia, general or local.

[illegible] children.
[illegible] the respiratory
[illegible] to be given
[illegible] effect cause re-
[illegible] he should be
[illegible] insufflation, for ordi-
[illegible] when the respiratory
[illegible]

after bronchoscopy, which, by the way, always have occurred in cases in which an anesthetic had been given, were probably due to paralysis of the respiratory center by the combined toxic action of the chloroform with morphine or with codein. Atropin counteracts the effect of morphine to some extent in this direction, but it would seem that to give chloroform, codeine, cocaine, adrenalin, morphine and atropine is loading up the organism with a great many drugs. In the case of children it is an utterly needless lot of drugs, as any one will admit who has seen bronchoscopy in children without anesthesia, general or local. In adolescents, morphine may be used in conjunction with ether or the usual

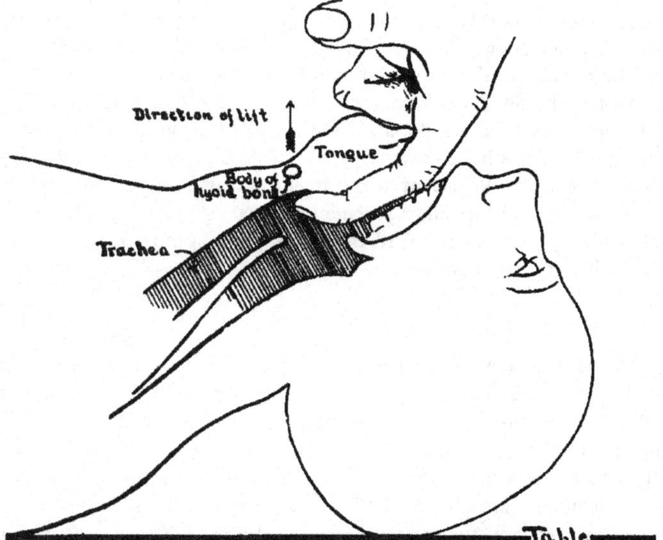

Fig. 58. Schema illustrating the method of hyoid bone elevation to free the air passages during general anesthesia.

morphine and atropine hypodermic combination may be used, though in uncomplicated cases no anesthetic is necessary. In adults this combination is useful especially in difficult foreign-body cases. The use of atropine as advocated by Ingals to lessen secretions during bronchoscopy, not only checks secretions but is a valuable stimulant to both the cardiac and respiratory centers, so that it would seem to be advantageous from a number of points of view. The safety of scopolamine is unproven.

When using general anesthesia and the patient does not take it well, the best thing to do is promptly to insert a silk-woven catheter and proceed with the anesthesia by ether insufflation with the Elsberg or similar apparatus. If for any reason this is considered undesirable or the apparatus is not at hand, the breathing may be promptly cleared by hyoid-bone elevation, using either the direct laryngoscope or the forefinger, Fig. 58, as described by Dr. Ellen J. Patterson (Bib. 429), the head being forced into extreme extension. This extension of itself will usually clear the airway as shown by Hobart A. Hare.

An interesting case of tracheal obstruction by an aneurysmal compression, plus a small mass of mucus is reported by Pratt (Bib. 436). During anesthesia the patient became cyanotic in spite of violent respiratory muscular activity. Insertion of an intratracheal tube gave immediate relief. No case of paralysis of the larynx, even if only monolateral, should be given a general anesthetic except by intratracheal insufflation. If this cannot be arranged, the patient should be tracheotomized. Hence, every adult patient should be examined with the throat mirror before anesthesia, and the necessity becomes doubly imperative before goitre operations. A number of fatalities have occurred from neglect of this precaution.

Davis reports the use of the intra-muscular injection of ether into the buttock of a child primarily rendered unconscious by ethylchlorid.

Joseph A. Stucky and William Stucky have used rectal ether anesthesia with excellent results.

ADDITIONAL NOTES ON LOCAL ANESTHESIA.

If local anesthesia be used in children, the author urges care and gentleness in its application especially to the subglottic region of children. For direct laryngoscopy in adults, some endoscopists have proposed injecting an anesthetic solution with a syringe armed with a hypodermic needle into the laryngeal tissue. This the author believes to be unnecessary as contact anesthesia will suffice for all cases if the patient's eyes are covered and the operator can get the patient to fix his attention on deep breathing. Some very apprehensive patients will anticipate cough at the contact of the instrument and will cough semi-voluntarily in the absence of a true reflex, if they are allowed to see the instrument enter through the speculum. If it is desired to anesthetize locally for esophagoscopy the best method is to make a preliminary application of an 8 per cent solution over the epiglottis and into the laryngopharynx with cotton on the Sajous' applicator. Then either the laryngeal or the esophageal speculum is passed and the right pyriform sinus is swabbed once with a 20 per cent solution on a gauze sponge held in a straight sponge-holder and allowed to remain for about a minute. Examination may begin one minute later. Cocaine tablets may be sterilized by placing a formaldehyde pastille in the bottom of a bottle in which the tablets are kept.

Anesthesia for the use of the esophageal speculum. For the use of the esophageal speculum, local anesthesia is not necessary, but lessens the slight discomfort. General anesthesia is not necessary, but if deep. affords a very much better view of the upper end of the esophagus because it prevents spasm of the inferior constrictor and of the esophageal musculature in general. The author's custom, however, is to use no anesthesia, general or local, in either adults or children. For local anesthetization, the method just given for esophagoscopy may be used.

For gastroscopy, no anesthetic, general or local, is needed to enable the skillful esophagoscopist to put the gastroscope into the stomach; but once there, in the absence of the complete relaxation of general anesthesia, the gastroscope remains fixed because of the muscular activity of the diaphragmatic musculature. To gain full relaxation of this musculature and of the abdominal wall, in order that the gastroscope may be freely movable, profound anesthesia is essential. Intratracheal ether insufflation is most convenient.

ANESTHETIZING A TRACHEOTOMIZED PATIENT.

No hesitation need be felt in giving a general anesthetic to a tracheotomized patient so far as the tracheotomic wound is concerned. Such a patient is far safer than one not tracheotomized and there is no trouble with the tongue or the tissues attached to the hyoid bone falling backward and downward obstructing breathing. They take the anesthetic quietly. It has been necessary many times for Dr. Patterson to remove tonsils from patients under treatment for laryngeal stenosis. In every instance the patient went under ether quietly and was kept fully under until the operation was completed, all vessels twisted and oozing stopped.

The technic is simple. A fold of gauze is laid over the tracheotomy cannula and, if the laryngeal stenosis is not complete, another over the mouth. The ether is dropped upon both pieces so that no matter which way air is taken in, it carries the ether with it. It is necessary to see that a good stout tape is securely attached to the cannula and tied back of the neck in the regular way. One assistant or nurse trained to tracheal work should be stationed to give undivided attention to the cannula and secretions coming from it.

INSUFFLATION ANESTHESIA.

The experiments of Melzer and Auer and the developments by Elsberg, Janeway. Carrel, Quinby, Cotton, Robinson, and others have placed intratracheal insufflation anesthesia on a firm, scientific and practical basis. Thyrotomy can be readily done under local anesthesia by those who fully understand the technic of infiltration. Much time, however, will be saved by insufflation anesthesia; and the strong return-flow keeps the blood and secretions from gaining an entrance to the lower air-passages. This return-flow is in every way more advantageous for the purpose than the use of the tampon cannula, the Trendelenberg position, or even the excellent plan of Moure, using the ordinary cannula with a gauze tampon in place above the cannula. It is surprising how little room the insufflation catheter introduced through the mouth requires in the opened larynx. It lies close along the posterior wall in a region which it is not necessary to invade, because thyrotomy is apt to be unsuccessful in

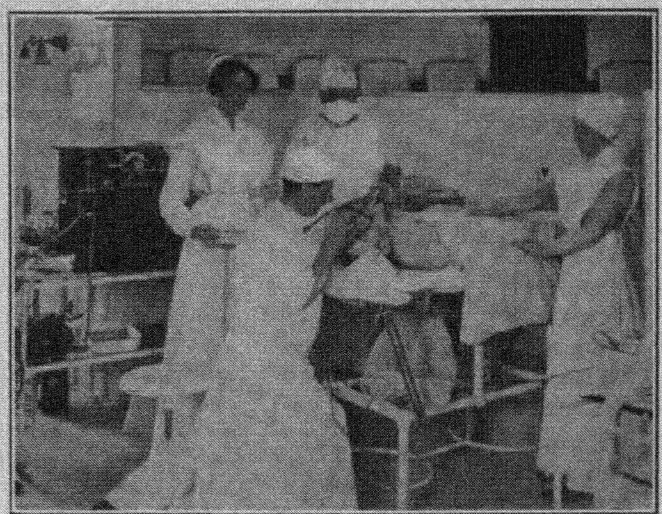

Fig. 50. Insufflation ether anesthesia with the Elsberg apparatus in the clinic of Dr. Otto C. Gaub. The anesthetist, Dr. Wade Elphinstone, has exposed the larynx and is about to introduce the silk woven catheter in a case of head surgery. Note the full extension with the head on the table.

malignancy if the involvement has reached the party wall. Should it be necessary in benign conditions to operate upon this wall, it is very easy to displace the catheter sideways. In malignant cases, if it is found that the growth is not removable by thyrotomy and that a laryngectomy is necessary, it is very easy, after amputating the trachea, to insert the insufflation catheter into the cut-end of the trachea and thus carry out a complete laryngectomy with the anesthetist entirely out of the way and with no loss of time. Dr. Otto C. Gaub and Dr. W. P. Barndollar have demonstrated the great advantage of the intratracheal insufflation method of anesthesia in the extirpation of a nasopharyngeal fibroma, which was so large that it pressed the soft palate forward on the tongue and produced dangerous dyspnea. If to this had been added the free flow of blood usual in such cases, the patient would have been asphyxiated. On the contrary, in this case, from the moment the insufflation was started the patient's color was good. All blood and clots came back out of the mouth and the operation required only a few minutes because it was uninterrupted. The presence of the catheter in the mouth produced no inconvenience whatever. The day of tracheotomy preliminary to the extirpation of nasopharyngeal fibromata is past. In all prolonged, bloody, nasal, pharyngeal, buccal, and laryngeal operations insufflation ether anesthesia diminishes the time of operation at least three-fourths. In aural, ophthalmic, and all forms of general head and neck surgery the distant removal of the anesthetist from the field is not only a time-saving convenience, but it eliminates a serious infective risk. In general surgical operations requiring a prone position of the patient, insufflation anesthesia is ideal. In the short, thick-necked, alcoholic "full-blooded" type of patient that ordinarily behaves so badly under ether by the open method, insufflation anesthesia gives a quiet and perfect anesthesia impossible by any other means.

All the foregoing classes of cases are particularly the sphere of insufflation anesthesia; but it is an ideal method for anesthesia in any sort of case, because of its safety and its precision and minimization of dosage. Meltzer refers to the mouth, pharynx, larynx, and trachea as the "death space," a particularly expressive term, for there can be no doubt whatever that most of the deaths from anesthesia have been due, directly or indirectly, to purely mechanical obstruction in these regions. In resuscitation from respiratory arrest, or collapse, or cardiac failure, it is this "death space" which is hardest to fight because of the difficulty of keeping up artificial respiration in a good and efficient way in the flabby state in which the tongue and all the tissues attached to the hyoid bone are, at such times. Some sort of artificial airway is essential. In insufflation anesthesia the "death space" is entirely eliminated and accidents prevented. In regard to the effect on the mucosa of the air passages, the author is able to state from post-anesthetic laryngoscopy in 80 cases that there is no reaction in the larynx from the presence of the insufflation tube, even in a prolonged anesthesia by insufflation. In quite a number of the cases anesthetized by the ordinary open method there has been quite a great deal of local laryngeal reaction, probably from ether mucus bubbling back and forth in the larynx, so that from an observation of these 80 cases the author is prepared to say that there is less irritation of the larynx from an intra-tracheal insufflation than from an anesthesia of corresponding duration by the open method. In the mucosa of the trachea and bronchi in sixteen cases there was less mucosal reddening, and not nearly as much mucus as is usually seen in patients etherized by the open method. Bronchoscopic observations of the author have proven that the "ether mucus" of the ordinary open method of administration is from the salivary glands and not from the tracheo-bronchial mucosa. True, patients etherized by the open method are found to have their trachea and bronchi full of mucus, but it has been aspirated from above owing to abolition of the cough-reflex. The management of the apparatus varies so much with the form of apparatus, and the apparatus have become so numerous, that the technical management of each cannot be given here. Explicit directions reprinted from the writings of the surgeons who have devised the instruments are supplied by the makers. The dosage is regulated according to the effect on pulse respiration, reflexes, color of skin, etc., as in any other method of administration. The great difference, however, is the quickness of response to increase, diminution, or withdrawal of the ether-content of the insufflated air. The anesthesia can be deepened, shallowed, or the patient brought out with a promptness and precision that seems incredible to those accustomed to the slow response inevitable with other methods in all of which control is befogged by the unknown and unknowable residual ether-content of the air and food passages. With insufflation there is no fluid ether anywhere in the body, except that already absorbed into the blood, and as soon as the ether is shut off, the warmed air-current blows out the ether-vapor from the air passages. The author's first experience with insufflation anesthesia was with the insufflation attachment to the bronchoscope (Fig. 17) suggested to the author by Dr. T. Drysdale Buchanan. (Bib. 229). This was for the insufflation of chloroform during bronchoscopy and was intended simply to carry on anesthesia without interruption of the work through the bronchoscope, for which purpose it is ideal. It was not intended for a method of anesthesia for other procedures.

*Technic of insertion of intratracheal insufflation tubes.** Practically all authorities are now agreed that the larynx should be inspected before the insertion of the insufflation catheter or tube, for the purpose of ascertaining whether or not there is disease present in the larynx, and also to determine the size of the larynx, so that the size of the insufflation tube may be selected accordingly, in order to make sure that there is an ample laryngeal lumen around the tube for the return-flow. Not only

*This section contains liberal quotations from the author's communication to the Clinical Congress of Surgeons of North America, Nov., 1913 (Bib. 266).

do the sizes of the larynges vary in normal individuals, but the laryngeal lumen may be modified by lesions present or past. There is another reason why the larynx should be inspected; namely, throughout the whole category of diseases to which human flesh is heir, it is a frequent thing for patients to date complaints from some particular period, accident, or operation in cases in which the physician or surgeon is absolutely certain that the disease existed long before the incident blamed by the patient. In view of this, it behooves the surgeon to know whether the larynx is diseased or not at the time the insufflation catheter is inserted. One such case has occurred where the patient dated laryngeal trouble from the taking of an anesthetic given by the ordinary open method. The author's own case-records and sketches showed that the larynx had been the seat of an infiltration of tuberculous origin for years before the anesthetic was given, showing that the anesthesia was in no way responsible, and showing, also, the necessity of knowing the state of the larynx beforehand. Only one thing seems to deter anyone from using the method advocated by Elsberg of inspecting the larynx and passing the catheter or tube by sight. This is the lack of confidence in the ability promptly and skillfully to expose the larynx with the laryngeal speculum. No one capable of giving an anesthetic should hesitate for one moment about this procedure, if he will take the trouble to pay attention to a few points.

RULES FOR INSERTION OF INSUFFLATION ANESTHESIA.

1. The patient should be fully under the anesthetic by the open method so as to get full relaxation of the muscles of the neck.

2. The patient's head must be in full extension with the vertex firmly pushed down toward the feet of the patient, so as to throw the neck upward and bring the occiput down as close as possible beneath the cervical vertebrae.

3. No gag should be used, because the patient should be sufficiently anesthetized not to need a gag, and because wide gagging defeats the exposure of the larynx by jamming down the mandible.

4. The epiglottis must be identified before it is passed.

5. The speculum must pass sufficiently far below the tip of the epiglottis so that the latter will not slip.

6. Too deep insertion must be avoided, as in this case the speculum goes posterior to the cricoid, and the cricoid is lifted, exposing the mouth of the esophagus, which is bewildering until sufficient education of the eye enables the operator to recognize the landmarks.

The most important thing of all is the position of the patient, and next to that comes recognition of the epiglottis, and next the proper motion of lifting the hyoid bone to expose the larynx.

The correct position will be understood by reference to the illustrations. In Fig. 60, the patient is placed on a pillow in a natural position. The larynx can readily be examined in this position, if it is desired merely to inspect it, and is useful for laryngeal diagnosis and some endolaryngeal operations; but for the insertion of an insufflation tube, bronchoscope, or other instrument, it is absolutely necessary for any but the most expert to have the head in full extension. It has been customary to draw the head over the table to gain the full extension in the Boyce position, and for bronchoscopy this is needed for the purpose of moving

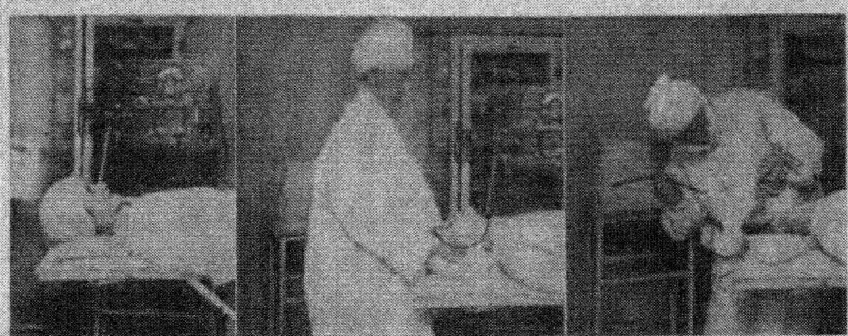

Fig. 60. Fig. 61. Fig. 62.

Fig. 60. Photograph of patient with head upon a pillow, the head flexed. In this position it is easy to examine the larynx with the laryngoscope for diagnosis, but the larynx will not be exposed in a line with the tracheal axis so that this position is not adapted to the passing of tubes through the laryngoscope.

Fig. 61. The pillow is removed, the head is flat on the table and the anesthetist is beginning to force the head into the extended position. The thumbs are on the forehead and the fingers are at the side of the head. The direction of motion is shown by the dart.

Fig. 62. The anesthetist is lifting with the tip of the laryngoscope in the direction of the dart. The laryngoscope is always held in the left hand. The right hand, of which the index has been protecting the upper lip, has now received the catheter from the nurse. The head must be in full extension.

the head and the bronchoscope about so as to enter the particular bronchus desired. But for the insertion of the insufflation tube, it is quite unnecessary to have the head extend beyond the table, and in fact it is undesirable. The author's "elbow rest position," so called because the operator's left elbow can be rested upon the table during long endo-laryngeal operations, is admirably adapted to the introduction of insufflation tubes. All that is necessary to do to the patient is to remove the pillow, place the thumb of each hand (as shown in Fig. 61) on the forehead of the patient with the hands at the sides of the head and then force the forehead vigorously downward and backward, causing an anterior movement of the skull on the atlas and throwing all the cervical vertebrae forward (upward in the recumbent position). The effect of this is to throw the hyoid bone and all the tissues of the neck, including the larynx, high up and to elevate the tongue. The neck and shoulders are arched up away from the table. In a fully relaxed patient, it is not necessary for an assistant to steady the head in this position, while the anesthetist takes the speculum always in the left hand, his right index being used to pull the upper lip of the patient out of the way so that the lip will not be pinched between the speculum and the upper teeth. The spatular end of the speculum is now inserted posteriorly to the tongue over the dorsum of which it is passed until the epiglottis comes into view. The spatular end is made to pass posteriorly to the tip of the epiglottis, and inserting the speculum a distance of, on the average, about 1 cm., the hyoid bone and all of the attached tissues are lifted by a motion which is best expressed as the suspension of the head of the patient on the epiglottis by the tip of the spatular end of the laryngeal speculum. Great care is necessary at this point not to use the upper teeth as a fulcrum upon which to pry upward with the tip. The motion is rather the lifting of the epiglottis and especially the hyoid bone by the tip of the instrument just as if it were desired to lift the patient's neck upward. Hyoid bone elevation opens the laryngeal door. After the larynx is exposed, the right hand releases the upper lip, which is now safe, and the catheter of the desired size is handed to the anesthestist by the nurse and the introduction is simple and easy, because the trachea is in a straight line with the laryngeal speculum. This is the great advantage of the extended position with the head on the table. At first sight, it might be thought that the speculum, as shown in Fig. 62, could not be in line with the axis of the trachea. It seems to be the erroneous conception quite prevalent among the profession that the trachea is perpendicular in the neck and chest. As a matter of fact, it enters the chest in a direction backward as well as downward, as illustrated schematically in Fig. 64, so that in the extended position proper for the exposure of the larynx and the insertion of any sort of tube into the trachea, the axis of the speculum, as shown in Fig. 62, is precisely in line. This must be remembered in placing the patient in position, but for the insertion of the speculum it is well to forget it and remember only that the motion is a strong lifting of the *tip* of the speculum, as shown in Fig. 62. In some patients after the introduction of the catheter there may be a large amount of thick tenacious secretion enter the catheter which may occlude respiration through the catheter, so that the hand held in front of it does not receive the expiratory blast, leading to the impression that the catheter is not in the trachea. If there is any doubt on this point it is better to insert the speculum and to lift the epiglottis and note particularly that the arytenoid eminences are posterior to the catheter. Of course in cases in which the patient is not deeply anesthetized cough will free the catheter but when the cough-reflex is abolished the patient will breathe on each side of the occluded catheter through the lumen of which no air will emerge at ordinary respiratory pressure. If occluded a fresh catheter may be substituted, but in most instances probably no harm whatever would come from inserting the nozzle of the insufflation apparatus and proceeding with the insufflation anesthesia in the regular way, because the catheter will be blown clear by the insufflation pressure and brought out by the return flow. The reason why the expiratory current does not clear it is that there is so much room for expiratory air around the catheter that there is very little pressure on the secretion in the catheter. The author recently insufflated a patient with bilateral laryngeal paralysis. He put in an extra tube for the return-flow but found it quite unnecessary, for, even with the tracheotomic wound closed with the finger, there was ample return-flow between the flaccid cords which flapped in the breeze of the return-current. He had feared that in the absence of the inspiratory abducting excursion there might be some obstruction in the larynx and the tracheotomic wound was obstructed with granulations. For the introduction of insufflation tubes the side-opening laryngoscope (Fig. 15) has some advantages. After the catheter is inserted, the laryngoscope may be removed sideways through the lateral opening. After skill in direct laryngoscopy is acquired, the slide may be left off entirely, but at first one is apt to be troubled by the tongue curling in and obstructing the view. This is prevented by passing the speculum to the right of the tongue, thus leaving the tongue on the closed side of the speculum. The author's personal preference is for the regular laryngoscope, Fig. 14.

Mention is made above of deep anesthesia. Once the knack is acquired no anesthetic whatever, general or local, is needed to expose the larynx in any patient; but to the beginner it simplifies the acquiring of the knack of direct laryngoscopy to abolish the reflexes of vomiturition and coughing, and to abolish entirely the antagonism of certain muscles attached to the hyoid bone. In the author's clinic an anesthetic, general or local, is never used for direct laryngoscopy, bronchoscopy or esophagoscopy in any child under 6 years of age, and rarely in adults, except for a few special procedures; but for insufflation anesthesia, the patient may as well be put completely under by the open method as only partially. To cocainize the larynx for the insertion of an insufflation tube to help along in partial anesthesia is an utterly needless waste of time.

CHAPTER V.

Bronchospic Oxygen Insufflation.

Bronchoscopic oxygen insufflation. Some experiments made upon the dog by Dr. Otto C. Gaub, with the assistance of the author, showed clearly that the lung which ordinarily collapses when the pleural cavity is opened may be inflated with oxygen, deflated or held partially inflated, by the bronchoscopist at the command of the surgeon. Oxygen can be admitted to the unoperated lung and a constant return-flow maintained so that the vital pulmonary hemic changes go on normally and pleural shock is also lessened. Furthermore, the lung on the operated side can be allowed to collapse without danger to the patient, thus allowing the surgeon ample room for work with the hands and instruments within the thorax. Again, independent of inflation and deflation a constant supply of oxygen is kept streaming through the lungs supplying every need, as shown by the pink color of the blood. The usefulness of this procedure so far as thoracotomy is concerned has disappeared since the method of intratracheal insufflation anesthesia has been introduced by Melzer and Auer and developed by Elsberg, Janeway and others; but for the bronchoscopist, the bronchoscopic oxygen insufflation is a life-saving procedure always at immediate command. The method is simple and is shown schematically in Fig. 63. The bronchoscope preferably of small size (7 mm. for adults, 4 mm. for children) is inserted through the glottis. The tube from the oxygen tank is attached to the anesthesia-inlet of the bronchoscope and the oxygen turned on at the tank valve (V). There is no danger from over-pressure because the bronchoscope is open. The operator's thumb (T) must never be placed over the proximal opening of the bronchoscope, because of the danger of over-pressure. The fundamental law which must be constantly before the mind is that of Crile. In brief, the intrapulmonary pressure must not exceed the capillary blood pressure or the compression of the capillaries and consequent ischemia will prove fatal. This cannot occur if the orifice of the bronchoscope is open because there is such an ample return-flow through the bronchoscopic lumen that absolute safety from over-pressure is assured. Of course the lungs cannot be thus forcibly inflated, and the usual arm-motion artificial respiration must be used in addition in this form of bronchoscopic oxygen insufflation. But the bronchoscope establishes an artificial airway which is strongly charged with oxygen and which cannot be obstructed by dropping back of the tongue. A small esophagoscope may be used instead of the bronchoscope, the oxygen tubing from the tank being attached to the drainage outlet. The drainage canal will thus carry oxygen right down to the bifurcation. Nitrite of amyl pearls should be carried in every bronchoscope box as amyl nitrite is the most

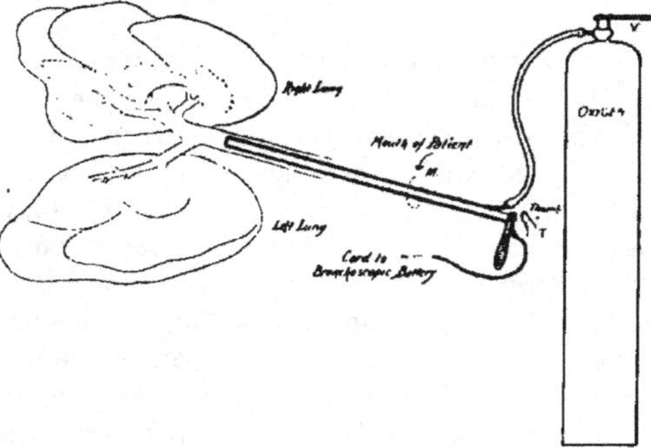

Fig. 63. Schema showing bronchoscopic oxygen insufflation. The bronchoscope is in the trachea. Oxygen enters by the small branch tube and is taken in by natural or artificial respiratory movements. If an esophagoscope is used the oxygen can be blown in through the auxilliary drainage canal to the distal end of the esophagoscope. This is safe. The lungs could be inflated by momentarily closing the escape by putting the thumb, T, over the proximal end of the bronchoscope alternately releasing it, but this would be a very dangerous procedure unless over-pressure be carefully guarded against. If preferred, the independent drainage tube used for aspiration can be inserted through the bronchoscope.

promptly available stimulant in such cases. A pearl may be broken in a tuft of cotton and thrown, cotton and all, into the wash bottle of the oxygen tank. There is only from two to three minutes between the respiratory and the cardiac arrest, so that in cases of serious respiratory arrest in which the operator does not feel confidence in the promptness and certainty of his bronchoscopic introductory technic, it is far safer to do an emergency tracheotomy, dilate the wound, crack an amyl nitrite pearl in cotton, hold the cotton over the wound and blow oxygen past the cotton into the trachea, while an assistant performs artificial respiration. In this case it is necessary for the operator to stand at the head-end of the table facing the patient's feet so as not to interfere with the arm movements. The great drawback to machines for artificial respiration using masks is that the vocal cords, because of their shape, elsewere shown, have a natural tendency to be forced shut by the in-going blast, and because of the pharyngo-laryngo-faucial danger-zone. The latter can be overcome to a great extent, in using the mask, but the laryngeal closure cannot. Both danger-zones are very much increased by the flaccid condition of the parts in impending death from respiratory arrest; but this same flaccidity is a great advantage in the peroral insertion of a bronchoscope because of the associated total absence of spasm. When a tube is inserted into the trachea for the insufflation of oxygen, conditions are ideal because there is no obstruction to the return-flow such as there is to the in-flow. This does not mean that there is no danger from excessive plus pressure, which must be carefully guarded against; nor should any of the foregoing be taken as a criticism of machines of pulmotor type. Such machines are life-savers of the greatest value, because they can be used by anyone with but little instruction, without the training necessary for the insertion of an intratracheal tube. Yet this does not alter the fact that intratracheal oxygen insufflation is ideal and everyone who has to deal with respiratory arrest should be taught the technic of laryngeal exposure for intratracheal insufflation, because the visual method is the only one which is certain under all conditions. For instance, the author, in one of our hospitals was called into an adjoining operating room, where a surgeon and his assistants had tried forced mask respiration, then tracheal intubation by blind method. The mask method had given relief for a time but the patient had gradually become unconscious and cyanotic. The surgeon's assistant was an expert at blind intubation and could not understand his inability to intubate in this instance. The author took with him his laryngoscope and exposure of the larynx revealed occlusion with a grayish mass which proved to be meat. Intratracheal oxygen insufflation after removal of the meat kept the man alive until he could be trusted to do his own breathing. The man was in a state of profound alcoholism when brought in from the gutter in front of the hospital and doubtless the meat had been vomited. That the respirator machine had forced the meat farther into the larynx is no criticism against the machine for the general run of cases; and the surgeon, had a laryngoscopist not been available, would have done a tracheotomy, with, doubtless, an equally happy result; yet this does not lessen the force of the lesson that in cases of respiratory arrest the fundamental requirement is to *see that the larynx is free from obstruction.* If this laryngeal inspection required special aptitude the author would not feel like urging it so strongly; but anyone capable of dealing with respiratory arrest at all can by practice acquire the ability to inspect any case, and the easiest of all cases is the one of respiratory arrest, because of the total absence of spasm. Such a patient is just like a cadaver and practice upon the cadaver is excellent training for this work. There is the same insertion of the direct laryngoscope and the raising and suspension of the limp head on the beak of the spatular end, the operator being in the standing position for a patient on a table, and kneeling on the floor, for a patient recumbent on the floor. Of course the cadaverous limpness and ashy blue-blackness of the mucosa does not conduce to the operator's equanimity, but the confidence in his ability promptly to expose and inspect the larynx and to catheterize the trachea, which comes with practice, will meet the emergency. Life-saving efficiency demands that every well-equipped hospital shall have at least one man trained for this emergency work.

CHAPTER VI.

Position of the Patient for Peroral Endoscopy.

General considerations. The position of the patient varies with the age of the patient, the part to be examined, the purpose of the examination and especially with the personal equation of the operator. Practically all procedures of the laryngologist other than endoscopy are done "face to face" with the patient. When the patient is dorsally recumbent all the interior anatomy seems strangely unfamiliar; and all the more so because the book illustrations, which unconsciously form the basis of mental pictures, have never shown the parts in this position. It is the effort of this book to supply this need as to illustrations, and to encourage others to practice diligently to overcome the preference for the sitting position and for the exceedingly awkward lateral recumbent position. Once the habit of working in the recumbent position has been acquired, better work can be done in both adults and children because of the greater ease with which secretions and foreign bodies are removed unopposed by gravity. In children we have the added reason of greater controllability; not but that a child can be held as is usual (though not necessarily desirable) for laryngeal intubation; but harm may be done if the child is not perfectly controlled. There is no upright control that compares with the fixity of the child held down on a well padded flat table top. In dyspneic cases, should tracheotomy become necessary, the bronchoscope can be inserted for breathing, and then the child is all ready upon the table for tracheotomy.

In children from every point of view, therefore, it is desirable, for every form of peroral endoscopy, to use the dorsally recumbent position, which, if correctly posed, is much easier for both patient and operator than the lateral.

The lateral position for bronchoscopy and esophagoscopy, in either adults or children, has found but little favor in America. Its only real advantage is the facility with which secretions drain from the lowermost corner of the mouth. This can be accomplished almost as well in the dorsal position with a wick of gauze hanging out over from the pharynx, the outer end the longer. If secretions are too thick to drain by capillarity, the gauze is frequently replaced by a fresh piece. An aspirating drainage tube of metal (Fig. 24) connected with the author's esophagoscopic aspirator (Fig. 23) is hooked into the lowermost portion of the patient's mouth in bronchoscopy. This rids the mouth of secretions while the patient is in the dorsal position. One thing that has led some endoscopists to think that the lateral position is easier is that in the lateral position the operator does not so readily make the mistake of extending the cervical spine instead of extending simply the head upon the atlas. If the operator should stand instead of crouch, in doing a peroral endoscopy upon a patient in the dorsal position, he would have the correct head-position of the patient.

In foreign-body cases, whether in adults or children, no matter where the foreign body is located (even in the fauces or nasopharynx), the patient should always be recumbent, never erect, because in the erect position gravity works against the operator, and the foreign body may reach a deeper point in the air passages than it would in the recumbent position. This is particularly true of foreign bodies in the larynx and pharynx, which should never be touched unless the patient is in the Trendelenberg position. Quite a large proportion of the foreign bodies in the bronchi that have been sent in to the author, were originally in the larynx, pharynx, mouth or nasopharynx and fell down when displaced by the attempts of the operator, who first saw the case, to remove the intruder with the patient in the sitting position.

In adults. For the diagnosis of laryngeal disease and for the removal of specimens, or of entire growths, by direct laryngoscopy under local anesthesia the sitting position of both patient and operator is the best. In the few cases in which a general anesthetic is needed for direct laryngoscopy the recumbent position is obligatory as well as advantageous.

For bronchoscopy for diagnosis, which is practically always done under local anesthesia, the adult patient may be sitting. If there is much secretion to be removed this is somewhat of a disadvantage, but with an active cough-reflex the secretion may be gotten rid of without difficulty, even in bronchiectatic and pulmonary abscess cases. The author's personal preference in such cases is for recumbency. For bronchoscopy for foreign bodies in adults, as before mentioned, the recumbent position is always best.

For esophagoscopy for diagnosis and treatment, with or without anesthesia, the author's preference is for the recumbent position. It has great advantages in dealing without interruption with the secretions and food debris, so abundant in many cases, and the patient is much more controllable. When a start is made it is a waste of time to withdraw the tube because the patient has slid off the stool or is strangling with secretions which have overflowed into his larynx.

General principles of all positions. The general principles of all useful positions are the same. The author was the first to call the attention of endoscopists to the fact that the trachea and esophagus are not

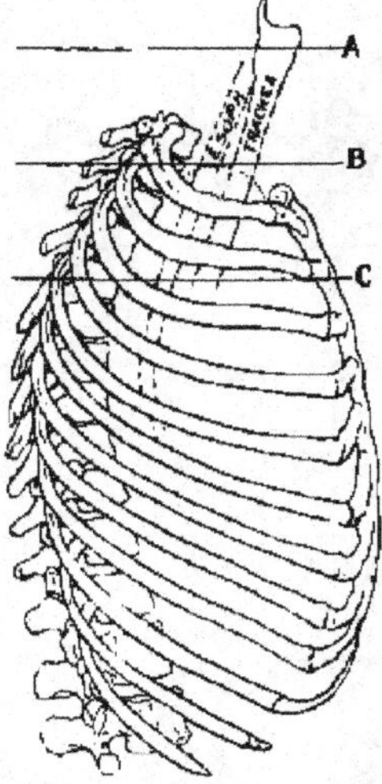

Fig. 64. Schematic illustration of normal position of the intra-thoracic trachea, and also of the entire trachea when the patient is in the correct position for peroral bronchoscopy, such as the original Kirstein position, or that shown in Fig. 70. When the head is thrown backward (as in the usual or in the Rose position) the anterior convexity of the cervical spine is transmitted to the trachea of which the axis is thus deviated. The correct position is produced in the recumbent patient by raising the head. The anterior deviation of the lower third of the esophagus shows the anatomical basis for the author's "high-low" position for esophagoscopy. (Figs. 149 to 152).

perpendicular. Their long axis passes backward as well as downward following the general direction of the thoracic spine (Fig. 64). Therefore, if we throw the patient's head backwards we cause an anterior convexity of the cervical spine, and with it the esophagus and trachea, as shown in the radiograph, Fig. 66. The Rose position and the usual incorrectly applied extended position make this extension throughout the entire cervical spine as shown in Fig. 66, rendering peroral endoscopy

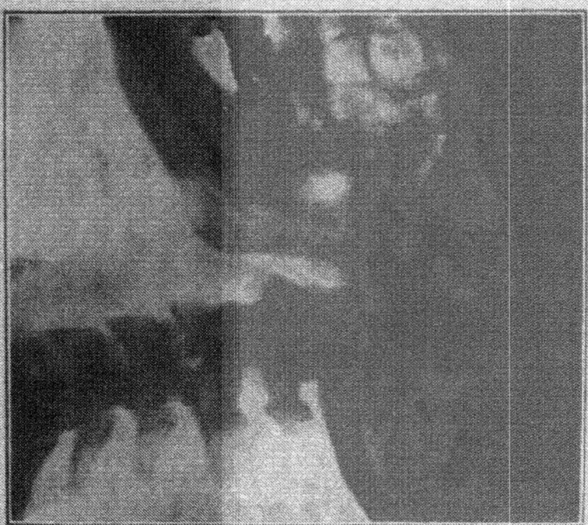

Fig. 65. Correct position of the cervical spine for esophagoscopy and bronchoscopy. (Illustration reproduced from author's article, *Jour. A. M. A.*, Sept. 25, 1909).

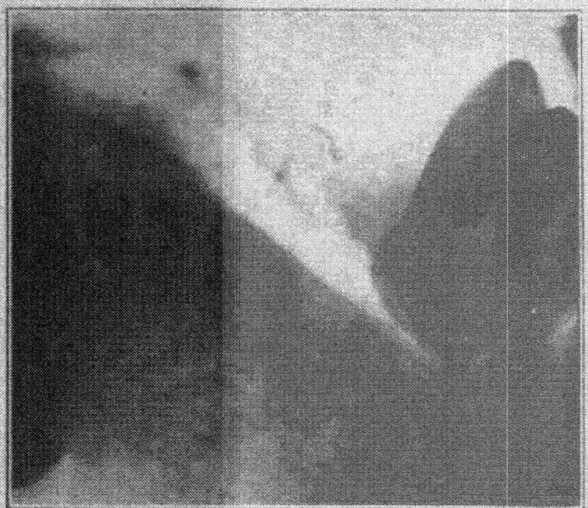

Fig. 66. Curved position of the cervical spine, with anterior convexity, in the Rose position, rendering esophagoscopy and bronchoscopy difficult or impossible. The devious course of the pharynx, larynx and trachea are plainly visible. The extension is incorrectly imparted to the whole cervical spine instead of only to the occipito-atloid joint. This is the usual and very faulty conception of the extended position. (Illustration reproduced from author's article *Jour. A. M. A.* Sept. 25, 1909).

extremely difficult or impossible, as demonstrated by the author years ago (Bib. 236). In the correctly posed extended position the extension is at the occipito-atloid joint, and the cervical spine is strongly inclined forward (upward in the recumbent position as shown in Fig. 65). If it is not desired to extend the head the cervical spine nevertheless remains

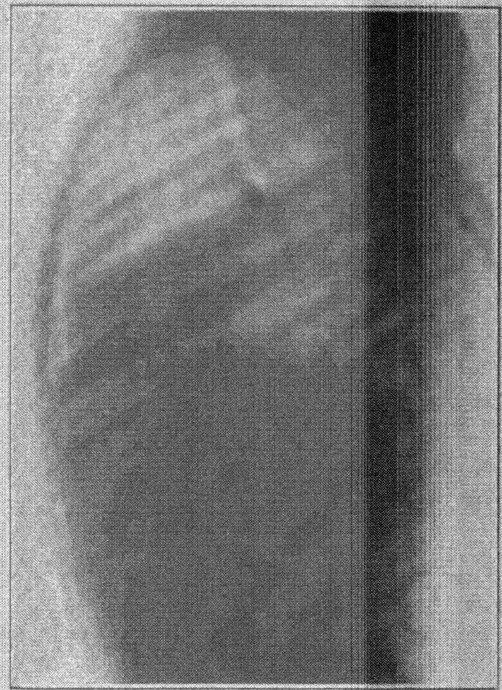

Fig. 67. Lateral radiograph of a child of 4 years, showing the normal direction of the trachea. A pale streak is seen extending backward as well as downward, ending at the foreign body in the right bronchus. There is a narrowing of this streak at the bifurcation, representing a flattening from before backwards. Compare schema, Fig. 64.

the same. Whether the head is flexed or extended or kept midway, the fundamental principle of all positions is the anterior placing of the cervical spine (Fig. 65).

Sitting position of the adult patient for direct laryngoscopy. The original position of Kirstein described by him 20 years ago, when he originated direct laryngoscopy, contained the essentials of the correct position and has been but slightly improved upon. As it seems to have been forgotten, an illustration of it taken from an old instrument catalogue is here reproduced (Fig. 68).

Mouret (Bib. 406) arrives at the necessary forward position of the head by having the patient sit astride of a narrow backed chair facing backwards with the pelvis as far toward the front edge of the chair as possible, the pelvis being tilted forward toward the operator who is back of the chair as will be seen by referring to Fig. 69.

The author's position for direct laryngoscopy upon the sitting patient under local anesthesia will be understood by reference to Fig. 70. This position is also used occasionally for diagnostic bronchoscopies, never for esophagoscopies.

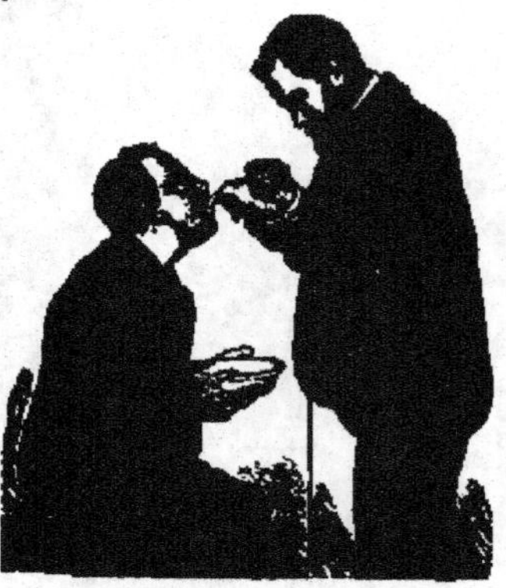

Fig. 68. Kirstein position which contains the essentials of the best position for direct laryngoscopy on the sitting patient. The extreme anterior displacement of the cervical spine with extension only at the occipito-atloid joint and avoidance of instrumental counterpressure on the upper teeth are fundamental. This illustration is reproduced from an old instrument catalogue. (1895) Bib. 323.

The patient should be seated on a stool about 30 cm. high. The operator sits upon a stool rather lower than shown in the illustration. The second assistant sits on a high stool back of the patient keeping the patient's head far forward toward the operator, extended or flexed as desired, usually extended as shown, but always forward. The assistant's knee at the back of the patient prevents the patient moving backward, and, most important, prevents the patient arching his spine backward. This assistant's right index-finger is used when necessary for making counterpressure externally by pulling the thyroid cartilage backward. The operator's knee against the patient's knee holds back the patient's hips. In exposing the larynx by direct laryngoscopy it is absolutely essential for prompt work and especially for prompt recognition of landmarks that the head be held exactly in the anteroposterior vertical plane. In other words, neither the cervical spine nor the head should be permitted to rotate. The head may be in any position desired as to flexion or extension, but the fundamental instruction to the assistant who holds the head should be: "Prevent rotation of the head."

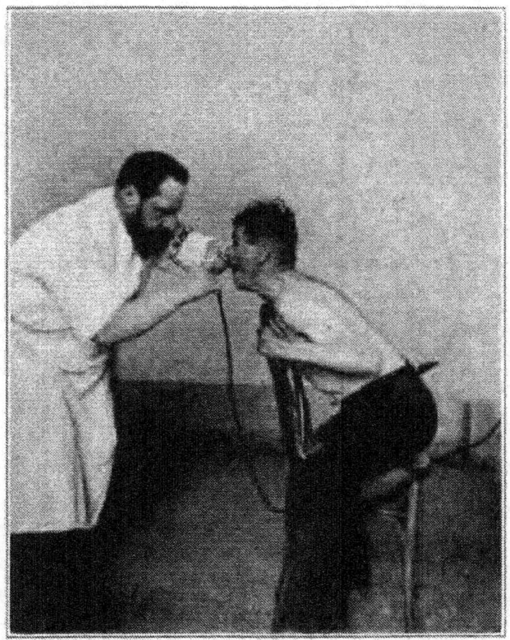

Fig. 69. Position of Mouret. This has the advantage that the patient's body cannot slide forward toward the operator when the head is pulled forward. Prof. Mouret demonstrated that the position of the pelvis and dorsal spine are important.

Recumbent position for direct laryngoscopy, bronchoscopy and esophagoscopy in adult patients. For the last eight years the author has used the Boyce position for bronchoscopy and esophagoscopy and has found it to fulfill every requirement. In the few adult patients requiring general anesthesia for direct laryngoscopy it is also used. A full description written by Dr. Boyce is given in the earlier volume. (Bib. 269, 1907.) Essentially the position (Fig. 72) consists in having the patient's head and upper part of his shoulders out in the air supported by the second assistant's *left* hand, which in turn is supported on the assistant's *left* knee, the *left* foot being upon a stool whose top is about 62 cm. below the top of the table. All the extension and raising of the patient's head is done with the left hand of the assistant whose thumb is on the patient's forehead, the fingers being under the occiput. The motion is as if to tuck the forehead back, down and under, while at the

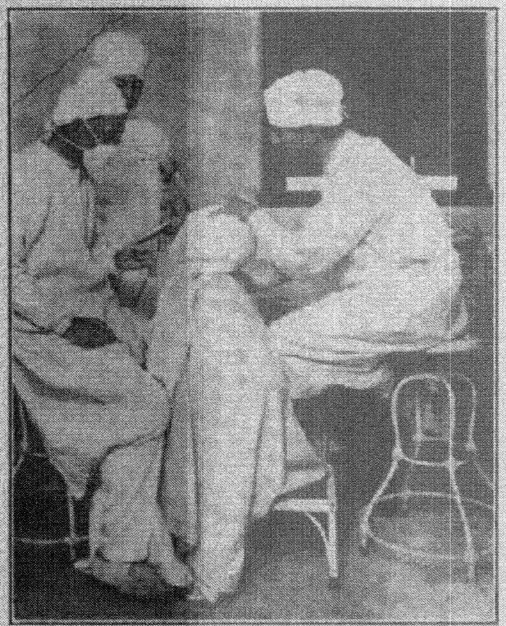

Fig. 70. Showing the author's position of the operator, patient and assistant for direct laryngoscopy on adult patients under local anesthesia. The sitting position of the operator renders laryngeal exposure easy for patient and operator; whereas the usual standing position of the operator throws the patient into a posture that renders laryngeal exposure difficult besides throwing the trachea out of line. The author prefers a lower stool as shown in Fig. 77.

same time the neck, chin and whole head are *raised*. The right hand is passed under to the far side (left) of the patient's mouth, the right index carrying the bite block. The *right* arm, however, usually carries but little weight, most of the extension and the very important prevention of rotation being done by the *left* hand. If the operator and assistant work together frequently they can do bronchoscopies without loss of time and with a precision that cannot be equalled by any other method. This position has nothing to do with the kind of instrument used. There is no instrument made for bronchoscopy or esophagoscopy that will do away with the necessity for a correct position of the patient for best results in quickness and precision. With the patient recumbent on an operating table of the ordinary height the direct laryngoscopist should sit on a stool such as the anesthetist uses. For bronchoscopy (recumbent position), especially after the bronchoscope has been introduced, a lower stool is often required unless the posterior branches are being explored. For the middle lobe bronchus it is necessary for the operator to sit on a footstool. In beginning an esophagoscopy the operator stands. Later he sits on a low stool for the lower third of

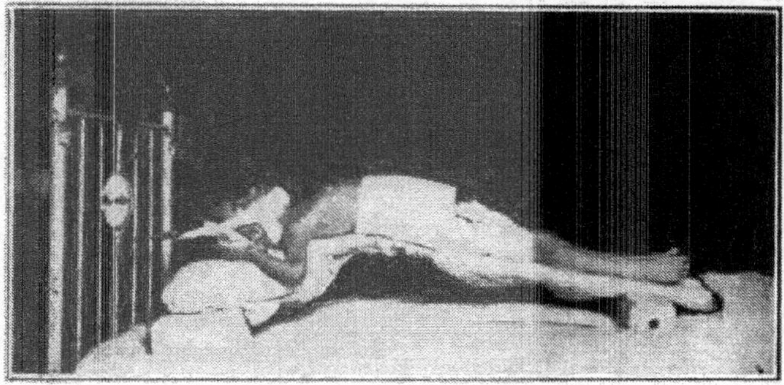

Fig. 71. Child with high dorsal tuberculosis at the Pittsburgh Hospital for Children. The author made a direct laryngoscopic examination, without changing the child's position or removing the apparatus, by standing on the left side of the bed, as demonstrated by Richard H. Johnston, Fig. 11. This child had a flabby upper laryngeal orifice causing an inspiratory stridor.

the esophagus. The necessity for stools of different heights for the operator is lessened in special tables by the elevation or lowering of the entire table, patient and all, by special mechanism. The raising and lowering of the head and the lateral movements will be considered when writing of the introduction of the instruments and of various procedures.

Mosher (Bib. 390) demonstrated the value of flexion of the head in the recumbent position for direct laryngoscopy by a laterally rotating speculum. Richard H. Johnston (Bib. 286) demonstrated the usefulness of *flexing* the head in certain cases for direct laryngoscopy on the recumbent patient, putting a small pillow under the patients' head, the operator standing to the left side of the patient. This flexed position is particularly advantageous where the operator is without a regularly trained assistant with whom he is in the habit of working, because any-one can hold the head on the pillow. The position is not adapted to bronchoscopy, though Johnston uses it to start the tube, and then the head of the patient is brought into the Boyce position. This change requires a well-trained assistant and great care to prevent any traumatism to the trachea in making the change. I have found the Johnston position exceedingly useful in disease of the cervical spine where the children were fixed in an apparatus which I did not need to disturb to get an excellent view of the larynx (Fig. 71).

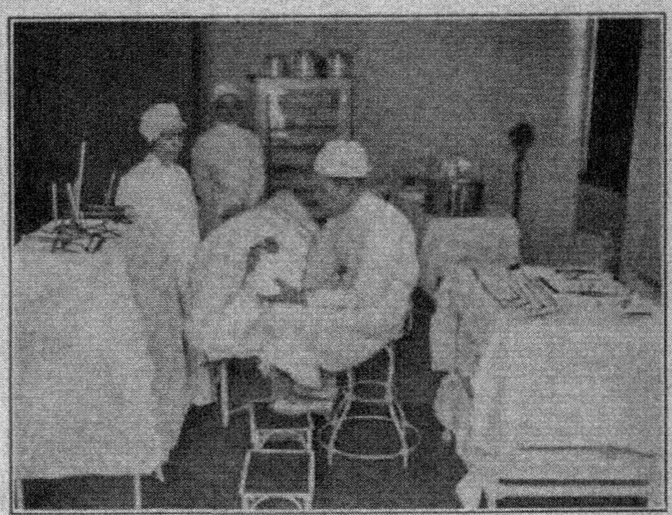

Fig. 72. Position of patient and second assistant in bronchoscopy and esophagoscopy (Boyce position). The left hand is supported on the left knee, the left foot being elevated on a stool. The right forearm is under the patient's neck, the right index carrying the bite block. The right forearm carries little weight, most of the extension being done with the left hand.

Position of the patient. Children. Children are always best examined in the recumbent position, and there being no anesthetic, general or local, it is usually required that they be held. The method of doing this is as follows: The child is placed in the correct position on the table with reference to the end of the table so that the head will be out in the air for the second assistant to hold. Both knees are held down by a nurse who stands at the foot of the table. Both hands are held down, one at each side of the patient either by a nurse or by a physician who is watching the pulse. This same person can also prevent the child from throwing the chest upward, as some children do. Upward movement of the chest is to be avoided because it has relatively the same effect as depressing the head. The position of each of the three persons required will be understood by reference to Fig. 73.

This holding is only required with a terrified child especially the first few times. Most children soon lose all fear and where necessary

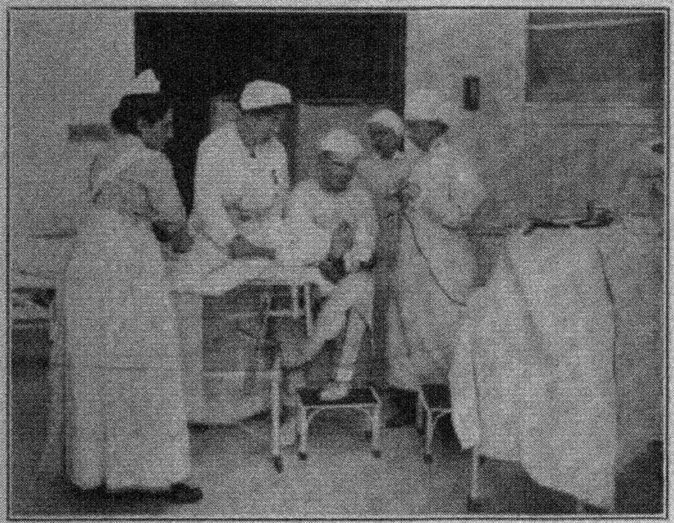

Fig. 73. Position of patient, assistant and two nurses to hold a child for direct laryngoscopy, bronchoscopy and esophagoscopy. The assistant holds the head in the Boyce position. The nurse on the patient's right holds the patient's wrists down on the table. The nurse on the left side of the patient holds down the patient's knees. The operator is holding the direct laryngoscope. As soon as it is introduced the patient's head is raised above the level of the table.

to have repeated endoscopies they soon learn that the procedure is not painful and submit without being held.

The author often has children of 3 and 4 years lie down on the table, open their mouths and wait for a speculum to be inserted and papillomata removed, time after time, without any holding whatever except the support of the head by the second assistant.

As in the sitting position of the patient, one of the most important things is strongly to impress upon the mind of the assistant who holds the head that never, under any circumstances is he to permit the head to rotate. The head must yield freely and follow the operator in the lateral or vertical plane, but it must never rotate on the axial bone or the cervical spine. Such rotation distorts the endo-anatomical landmarks and renders difficult the otherwise easy task of finding the larynx or pyriform sinuses, as the case may be.

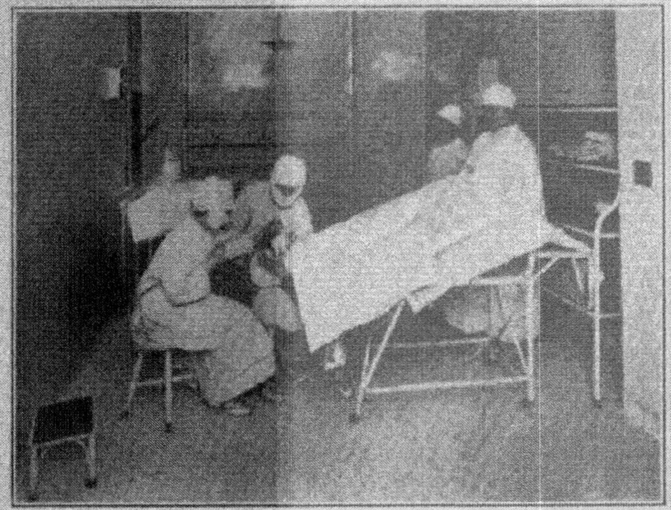

Fig. 73A. Author's position of the patient for the removal of foreign bodies from the larynx or from any of the upper air or food passages. If dislodged, the intruder will not be aided by gravity to reach a deeper lodgement.

For the use of the esophageal speculum the patient may be placed either in the sitting position as for laryngoscopy (Fig. 70), or in the recumbent position as for starting the introduction of the esophagoscope (Fig. 73). The author prefers the latter.

CHAPTER VII.

Direct Laryngoscopy.

General considerations. Enthusiastic as he is in regard to the usefulness of the direct method, for both diagnosis and treatment, the author wishes to state at the outset that he examines every case by the indirect method first, if it is possible to make such an examination. The exceptions are in infants and small children who cannot be examined by the mirror unless they are under a general anesthetic, and also an occasional case of great urgency in adults. The field of the two methods is entirely different. The presence of the tube excites reflexes which interfere with the detection of slight variations in mobility, unless anesthesia is profound, and then only respiratory movements could be present. Of course, great facility enables one to overcome this drawback to some extent and also the disadvantage which comes from the increased tendency to distortion, owing to very slight lateral displacement of the tube or the tissues. Nevertheless it may be stated as a general rule that the direct method is not adapted to accurate determination of motile defects. One great advantage of the use of both methods in the same case, whereever possible, is that the view-point is entirely different, the one supplementing the other. The view obtained in the mirror, M, Fig. 74, is as if the observer's eye were at the vertex of the patient's head, represented by A In contrast to this, in the direct examination, the observer's eye is at D. Were the tissues to be examined a plane horizontal surface, there would be practically no difference, but in examining a more or less funnel-shaped cavity, like the larynx, the difference of the point of view becomes very great, especially as to the position of growths down within the funnel (as for instance at the cord) in their relation to the upper laryngeal orifice. It will be easily understood from the schema, Fig. 74, that growths on the cords always give the appearance of being located nearer the posterior commissure than they actually are, and very much nearer than they seem to be by the direct method. Another great difference is that the direct method gives a better view of the anterior aspect of the posterior wall, H, of the larynx because the visual axis is more nearly perpendicular to the surface. The indirect view of the posterior surface of the posterior wall can, of course, be very much increased by von Eicken's method of drawing the larynx forward so as to see the hypopharynx by

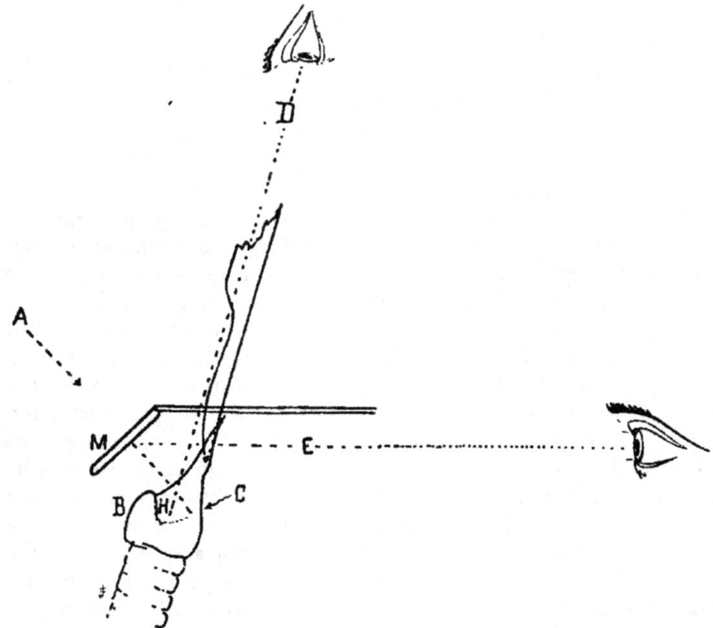

Fig. 74.—Schema illustrating the difference between the views obtained by direct and by indirect laryngoscopy. The observer's visual axis at E, looking into the mirror, M, gets an image as if he were looking from a point back of the patient's head, A. Looking thus, the image of a growth on the cord at C is seen just over the top of the arytenoid eminence to which it seems very close, because almost in line. This schema also shows how the anterior surface of the posterior wall at H, is in the line of vision by direct laryngoscopy and more or less hidden in some cases during indirect examination, by an apparent forward overhang of the border of the arytenoid eminence and the aryepiglottic fold.

hypopharyngoscopy. The hypopharynx can also be viewed by putting the direct laryngoscope down back of the posterior wall at H, and drawing the entire larynx forward. It is also worthy of note that the anterior surface of the posterior wall can often be observed by the Killian method of using the laryngeal mirror with the patient standing and the observer kneeling, the patients' head being bent forward and downward toward the observer.

It may seem strange at this late day for anyone to advocate the more frequent use of the indirect, mirror laryngoscopy, and yet it is neglected in routine surgical work. The author believes that general anesthesia for any purpose should always be preceded by a preliminary examination of the larynx by the indirect method, provided the patient can be so examined; and this statement applies to any and all cases, surgical or otherwise, for which an anesthetic is desired to be given. It is incomprehensible why it is so generally neglected before goitre operations. If this rule were observed, there would not be as many mysterious deaths on the table and shortly after operation to be accounted for by such highly hypothetical diagnoses as hyperthymization, cardiac failure, etc. The author knows of a number of deaths on the table where paralysis of the larynx had existed unknown to the surgeon; and a perusal of surgical literature reveals cases strongly suggestive of unsuspected laryngeal paralysis.

When it comes to operations, however, the indirect method has no place in the author's technic. In making this statement, the author wishes to qualify it by saying that he does not pretend to have the facility in indirect operating that is possessed by many of the laryngologists, who, by a lifetime of training, have acquired wonderful skill in working by the aid of the reversed image seen in the mirror. The skill of such men as Delavan, Semon, St. Clair Thomson, Bryan, French, Curtis, McKernon, Simpson, Tilley, Dundas Grant, Moritz Schmidt and others in overcoming the disadvantage of being compelled to move a forceps backward when it is desired to bring it forward, and to make a diagonal movement by combining a reversed antero-posterior and a true lateral movement, is marvelous and probably will not be equalled by any future generation of laryngologists because there is not now the incentive to spend the lifetime at practice necessary to acquire the skill to work under the peculiar circumstances of having the antero-posterior movement reversed while the lateral movements are unchanged. This must not be taken, however, to mean that good work can be done by the direct method without a large amount of practice, nor that a superlative degree of skill cannot be acquired in the direct method. The same amount of work will produce equally marvelous results with the direct method as were accomplished by the indirect, and the results will be vastly greater because of the greater possibilities of the direct procedure.

Very young children, because of their being intractable and terrified, are difficult cases for the mirror-method of indirect laryngoscopy, but in addition, as shown by Swain (Bib. 508), the epiglottis adds greatly to the difficulty as compared to the adult epiglottis. Moreover, the child's epiglottis is prone to curl. In the direct method, on the other hand, we have a method by which the larynx of any infant or older child can be examined without any anesthesia, general or local. The erroneous statement that anesthesia is required has crept into the literature, and has prevented the widest use of direct laryngoscopy for the diagnosis of the various causes of croupy cough in children too young for mirror inspection. Nearly all cases of papilloma and of unsuspected foreign body in the larynx have had diphtheria antitoxin given because it was supposed that the larynx could not be examined without anesthesia. Worse still, are the deaths from attempts to administer an altogether unnecessary general anesthetic to a child with a stenosed larynx.

In dyspneic cases, the possibility of retropharyngeal abscess must be borne in mind, and the posterior pharyngeal wall should always be carefully inspected before bronchoscopy. Of course, this can be done with the fingers by palpation, but the most ready way is just habitually to note the condition of the posterior pharyngeal wall when introducing the direct laryngoscope.

Contraindications to direct laryngoscopy. The author can recall no absolute contraindications to direct laryngoscopy in any cases where direct laryngoscopy is really needed for either diagnosis or treatment. In extremely dyspneic cases if the operator is not prompt and certain in his introduction of a bronchoscope it may be wise to do a tracheotomy first.

The direct laryngoscopic appearances. The illustrations in this book may seem a little queer to those accustomed to the old indirect illustration. The views in the sitting patient seem "upside down." Yet simply to reverse an indirect view will not give a direct picture because the view point is different as already explained. The epiglottis does not show because it is hidden by the direct laryngoscope. If the glottis is widely open, the observer looks directly into the trachea in the direction of its long axis; and therefore does not see one tracheal wall any more than the other, if the head and neck of the patient are placed in the proper position. All the indirect illustrations represent the rings of the trachea showing below the glottis. If the patient gets his head too far backward (in the sitting position), the anterior wall may possibly be thus seen, because in such a position the observer's eye is back of the larynx and is in almost the same position with reference to the larynx as is the mirror in indirect laryngoscopy. This will be understood by referring to Fig. 74. But this is a very wrong position for direct laryngoscopy, as elsewhere herein explained. When the patient is in the position shown in Fig. 70, the posterior wall of the trachea is more easily seen than the anterior, though if the position is exactly correct, neither will be more conspicuous than the other, because the operator will be looking directly down in the tracheal axis. If the posterior wall is viewed, no rings will show because the posterior wall of the trachea is devoid of cartilage below the cricoid.

Illustrations of the laryngeal image on mirror view have always been misleading. They are semidiagrammatic and lack depth. This is one of the things that contributes most to the disappointment of the beginner in direct laryngoscopy. He never knew that the vocal cords were so deep. They are, in the adult, nearly 3 cm. below the aryepiglottic folds, and not almost on a level with them as illustrations of indirect views have usually pictured them. When the beginner in endoscopy examines them directly, and still more when he first attempts to operate upon them, they seem almost hopelessly far away; and to make matters worse they are quite likely to be obscured from time to time by spasmodic narrowings of the lumen by the false bands and even by the upper orifice of the larynx posteriorly. The illustration, Fig. 9, Plate 1, gives some idea of the depth of the larynx because the hand stretches across near the level of the top of the false bands. The reasons for the misconceptions as to the real depth of the cords are four: 1. Illustrations of the larynx are made from memory and are always more or less diagrammatic. 2. The cords are the central point of interest and are unconsciously always strongly represented in the illustrations with a glistening whiteness that brings them right up to the nearest plane in the laryngoscopic picture. 3. Text-book tradition has called them white so that white they are painted, it matters not whether they are gray, pearly, dark greenish gray, bituminous, yellowish pink, bluish pink, bright pink, or tinged by reflected light. The artist giving them their true color value would make them stand back at their true depth. But it takes a lifetime to train the artist's eye to see values, and it takes another lifetime to train the laryngologist to see larynges. Consequently there are no artist-laryngologists. 4. There is, owing to well-known optical laws, an actual foreshortening of the laryngeal image as seen in the laryngeal mirror. If anyone doubts the author's statement that the cords are rarely really white, let the doubter compare the whiteness of some cases of papilloma or of the white, grass-like projections sometimes seen in certain cases of malignancy. A good demonstration of the foreshortening affect of the mirror is apparent in comparing the flat ribbon-like appearance of the cords, with their actual appearance. This ribbon-like appearance is not so much in evidence with the direct method, and when the larynx is opened by thyrotomy it is seen to have been an illusion. (See Figs. 81 and 488).

In studying the direct laryngoscopic image it must be remembered that the larynx, like the face, is full of muscles and is changing its expression every moment. The laryngologist who sketches as accurately as he can will notice that no two sketches are exactly alike. The author has been criticised, by students who did not understand this, for representing the same epiglottis or the same larynx differently at different times. It is only under the most profound anesthesia with abolition of all except the deep reflexes that we see the glottic chink enlarge and diminish in perfect rhythm with the respiratory movement without accessory movements in any part. And even then symmetry may be interfered with by distortive instrumental traction. Without anesthesia there is usually more or less spasmodic traction of the arytenoids, and the ventricular bands are very apt to close over the cords and to narrow

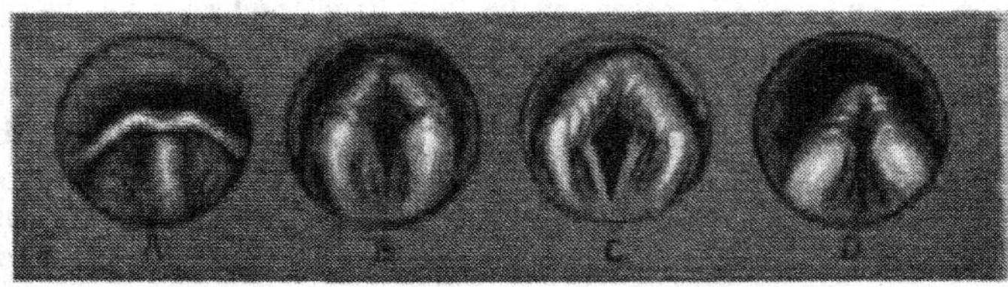

Fig. 75.—Direct laryngoscopic views local, partial or no anesthesia. A, epiglottis. (It is often more curled than this.) First stage of direct laryngeal exposure. B, larynx exposed but orifice is narrowed by spasm. C, a moment later when orifice widens and glottis opens on deep inspiration. D, posterior part of larynx as usually seen at beginning of third stage. This is more frequently seen than B. If the larynx should open it would be seen that a much larger portion of the glottis is visible than anticipated.

the upper laryngeal orifice, so that no cords are visible. This pertains, to some extent, even under quite perfect local anesthesia. The picture is very apt to be as shown at D in Fig. 75, consisting of two rounded masses posteriorally with more or less showing of the rounded masses anteriorally, corresponding to the ventricular bands. If, however, the patient is commanded to keep on breathing and not to hold his breath, the first deep inspiration will open up the glottis and then the view should be as at C in Fig. 75, except that it is not often that the beginner will be able to expose the anterior commissure as there shown.

The field of vision at any particular moment appears much larger than the diameter of the tube, and the author has so drawn and painted it in the illustrations. The field actually is larger, the degree being dependent upon the distance of the object viewed from the distal end of the tube mouth as will be understood by reference to Fig. 76; but this factor, of course, in a long tube of small lumen, is very slight unless the object be very far from the distal tube-mouth. What contributes more to the apparently larger size of the field as compared to the tubal diameter is the general law of optics which explains why the farther away an object is from the eye, the smaller the image, and consequently the greater the area visible. Perspective contributes also the additional fact that the nearer the plane of a receding surface approaches the visual axis the greater the foreshortening, and the greater the foreshortening the greater the area visible. In plain language the nearer a surface approaches to being seen on edge, the greater the area visible through an aperture of a certain size placed at a certain distance from the eye. Hence, in endoscopically viewed surfaces close against the tube-mouth, and vertical to the axis of the tube, we see an area equivalent to that of the lumen of the tube mouth, whereas in viewing surfaces receding in

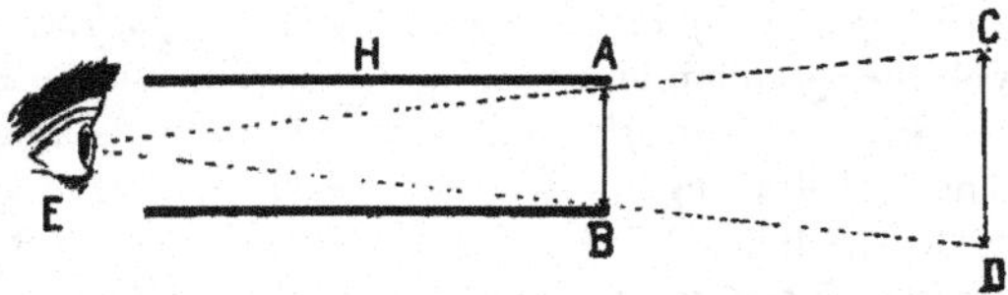

FIG. 76.—Schema showing one of the reasons why the endoscopic image always seems larger than the actual diameter of the tube through which it is seen. This is most apparent with the direct laryngoscope. The field of vision is larger in proportion as the distance between the tube-mouth, A B, and the farther limit of the visible field, C D, increases.

planes more or less approaching parallelism with the tubal axis we see areas equivalent to many times the area of tubal aperture.

Instructions to patients. Before beginning endoscopy the patient should be told that he will feel a very disagreeable pressure on his neck and that he may feel as if he were about to choke, and that he cannot get his breath. He must be gently but firmly made to understand: (1) that while the procedure is alarming that it is absolutely free from danger: (2) and that you know just how it feels; (3) and that you will not allow his breath to be shut off completely; (4) that he can help you very greatly as well as make the procedure very much easier for himself by paying close attention to breathing very deeply and regularly, in and out; (5) that he must not draw himself up rigidly as if he were "walking on ice," but must be easy and relax. It will contribute very much to this end if the operator will be particularly gentle and careful about the early manipulations of applying the local anesthetic and the like; and will tell the patient, after the epiglottis is exposed and the application of the local anesthetic made to it, that there will be nothing worse to be gone through with. Some endoscopists advocate telling the patient to put up his hand if the procedure is too severe. The author prefers not to do this because it leads the patient to think that he is about to go through a severe ordeal which he may not be able to survive, and that he must give notice of impending death. Moreover, he is apt to raise his hand and grasp the instrument or the operator's hand. It is better to have the patient's hands held down by a nurse. However, each operator will develop his own method of controlling the patient and the author does not care to urge his own method too strongly. A suggestion of Mr. Waggette (Bib. 567) is particularly good: Namely that a special signal be arranged by which the patient may inform the operator that the lips or teeth are being painfully pressed upon. The operator interested in his deeper work may otherwise overlook this little detail which is often, needlessly the painful part of the procedure.

Technic of exposure of the larynx in the sitting patient. Exposing the larynx with the speculum in the sitting position should be approached from the standpoint of depressing the tongue to find the epiglottis and then depressing and drawing forward the epiglottis, tongue and all tissues attached to the hyoid bone. By keeping this constantly in mind, two of the greatest difficulties and errors will be prevented; namely, (1) the tendency on the part of the patient to throw his head far back as if he were about to have his neck shaved, and (2) the tendency on the part of the operator to follow the patient and thus to get his elbow higher and higher, his own head farther back and to use the patient's upper teeth as a fulcrum in an effort to pry open the larynx, a movement that defeats its own object. To avoid this, the author sits on a stool in front of the patient precisely as if he were about to use a tongue depressor to examine the pharynx. The position of the operator shown in Fig. 70 is the highest that should be attained at the complete exposure of the larynx when the operator is looking directly into the trachea. In beginning to introduce the laryngoscope the operator should stoop much lower, having his head about level with that of the patient. (Fig. 77). The introduction of the instrument should be considered in three stages.

1. Exposure and identification of the epiglottis.
2. Placing the spatular tip back of the epiglottis.
3. Anterior downward traction on the epiglottis and all the tissues attached to the hyoid bone.

First stage. The patient's head being covered with a sterile cap, the second assistant pushes the patient's head and neck forward as shown in Fig. 70. The operator holds the laryngoscope in his *left* hand (Fig.

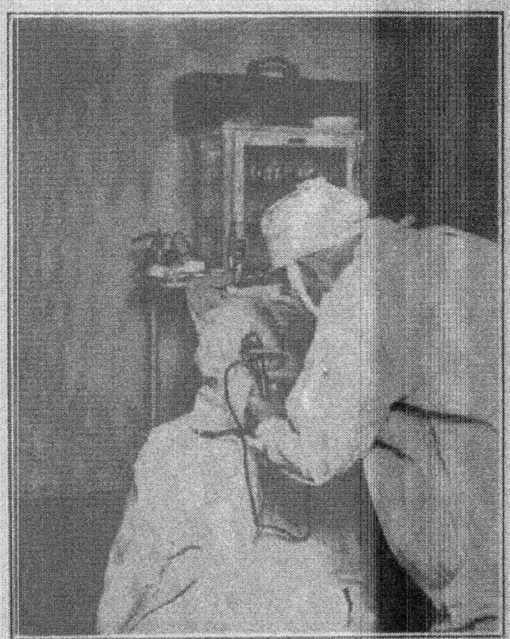

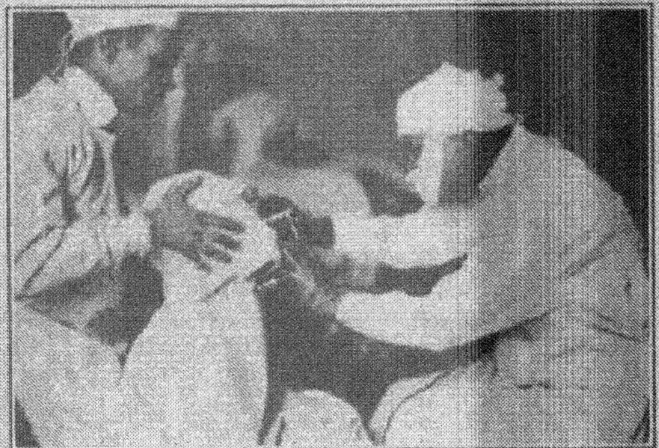

FIG. 77.—The upper illustration shows the first stage of direct laryngoscopy. The operator is inserting the laryngoscope with his *left* hand while he holds the patient's upper lip out of the way with the *right* index finger. In order to show the instrument and the operator's hands the operator is standing to one side of the patient. In actual work the operator sits squarely in front of the patient as shown in the lower illustration.

77) while with his *right* index he raises the patient's upper lip so that it cannot be pinched between the laryngoscope and the teeth. The distal end of the laryngoscope is passed backward over the median line of the dorsum of the tongue, and, depressing the tongue, in the direction of the

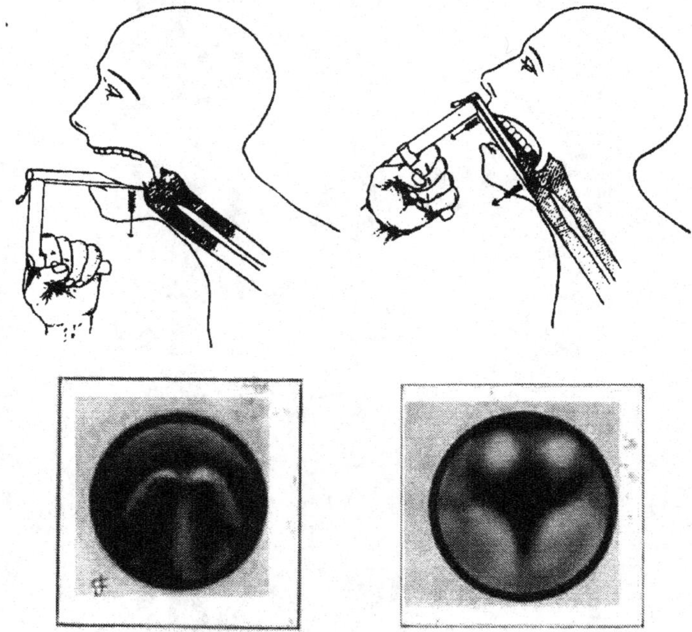

FIG. 78.—Schema showing the first and third stages in exposing the larynx in direct laryngoscopy. At the left the tongue is being depressed as indicated by the dart, causing the epiglottis to project into the line of vision as shown in the lower illustration. Then the laryngoscope is inserted deeper constituting the second stage. At the right is shown the third stage, the drawing forward of the epiglottis and all of the tissues attached to the hyoid bone with the *tip* of spatular end, thus exposing the spasmodically closed larynx as shown in the lower right hand illustration. At the next inspiration the larynx will open, exposing the cords and glottis as shown in Fig. 75. (See Fig. 70 for photograph of the positions at the third stage.)

dart in the left half of Fig. 78, the upper edge of the epiglottis will come into view, as shown in the circle. The tongue is depressed until the epiglottis stands up rather prominently like the spout of a pitcher, and shows a goodly portion of its anterior surface. Absolutely no effort should be made to see the larynx until the first stage is accomplished, namely, the identification of the epiglottis. If it fail to come into view, it must be searched for a little more to the right or to the left; but deep insertion must be strictly avoided. Failure to find the epiglottis nearly always means too deep insertion: because, if the first step is properly taken, namely, to depress the dorsum of the tongue slightly until the epiglottis comes up into view, and if the speculum is exactly in the median line, the epiglottis will promptly project upward right in the line of vision, with the lingual surface of the epiglottis toward the operator, as shown in A, Fig. 75, and in the left hand circle in Fig. 78.

Second stage. Having identified the epiglottis in the manner just described, the next step is to pass the spatular end of the speculum posteriorally to the epiglottis for a distance of about 1 cm. or 1.5 cm. (slightly less than 1 cm. in a child). The depth of insertion cannot be gauged by arbitrary measurements. Nothing but experience will enable the operator to get it exactly right for the particular case, since the necessary distance is subject to wide individual variations. If the depth is not correctly gauged the error will be revealed in the third stage.

Third stage. Without permitting the laryngoscope to go deeper, the larynx is exposed by a movement of the spatular end of the laryngoscope in the direction of the dart in the right half of Fig. 78. This movement is fundamental in exposure of the larynx. It is, perhaps, best described as an effort to pull the epiglottis and hyoid bone downward, outward and forward toward the operator with the tip of the spatular end. The patient's whole head should be pulled forward by the power exerted. If this is kept in mind there will be no danger of falling into the error of trying to pry open the larynx using the upper teeth as a fulcrum. If the operator expects now to see the larynx as in the laryngeal mirror, he will, in most instances, be disappointed for reasons already given. Usually a spasm of the larynx hides the cords from view and all that is seen is the two rounded eminences over the arytenoids. The patient must be encouraged and pacified if alarmed, and must be frequently admonished to breathe deeply. At the first inspiration the cords will be seen more or less hidden by the overhanging ventricular bands, if the laryngoscope is properly placed and the effort of the operator's left hand is properly exerted. It requires considerable strength and endurance in the wrist to hold out of the way the tissues of a muscular patient with a short thick neck. If the cords are seen, then it is known that the laryngoscope is properly placed and that no harm can be done by firm pulling in the proper direction, provided the instrument is in the middle line. If in executing the third stage the epiglottis slips away downward, the insertion of the second stage has not been deep enough, and the epiglottis must be very carefully identified again and the insertion made slightly deeper. If a hasty movement is made to catch the epiglottis the aryepiglottic fold may be mistaken for the epiglottis and then forward traction will expose the corresponding pyriform sinus; which is bewildering to the beginner who concludes that the larynx is hard to find. If, on the other hand, in executing the second stage the laryngoscope is inserted too deeply, the hypo-pharynx will be entered and the third stage will fail to expose the larynx and very strong muscular effort will result in exposing the pyriform sinuses or even the mouth of the esophagus.

Difficulties. If careful attention has been given to all the instructions as to position of patient and operator and to the successive execution of each of the three stages, there should be no great difficulty in succeeding in an average case after a few trials. But it is by no means easy to execute every detail correctly, especially without a trained assistant. If the head of the patient has been allowed to rotate or to deviate laterally, the larynx will not seem to be where it ought to be—in the median line. If the laryngoscope has not been held firmly in the middle line, the same "lost larynx" may result from the distortion due to the slipping sidewise of the tongue and its attachments. If the laryngeal aperture cannot be found the patient should be allowed a moment's rest during which he can expectorate secretions. Each time the instrument is removed it should be wiped clean with a square of gauze, because a patient does not like even his own saliva put back in his mouth. The same movement wipes the lamp. Then a fresh start should be made. If the larynx still fails to be revealed the endoscopist should ask himself which of the hereinafter given "rules" he has violated. If the larynx is correctly exposed squarely before the laryngoscope, but only the posterior commissure is visible even on deep inspiration, the pulling with the tip of the spatular end should be increased and the patient's head should be brought further forward toward the operator, and extension lessened rather than increased. If the anterior commissure still fails to appear the second assistant who holds the head should, with his right index finger externally on the neck, pull the thyroid cartilage backward. If properly done, this will expose the anterior commissure in any case, and this is often necessary, in order to counteract the forward traction of the larynx by its attachments to the hyoid bone. Like all purely manual procedures, practice is required to render direct laryngoscopy easy and smooth in its execution, which is a matter entirely separate from *knowing how* to do it.

RULES FOR DIRECT LARYNGOSCOPY.

1. The laryngoscope must always be held in the *left* hand, never in the right.

2. The operator's right index finger (never the left) should be used to elevate the patient's upper lip so that there is no danger of pinching the lip between the instrument and the teeth.

3. The patient's head must always be exactly in the middle line, not rotated to the right or left nor bent over sidewise, and the entire head must be *forward* with extension at the occipito-atloid joint only. (Fig. 65).

4. The laryngoscope must always be passed over the dorsum of the tongue exactly in the middle line (until the endoscopist is sufficiently skilled to try the oblique position).

5. The epiglottis must always be identified before any attempt is made to expose the larynx.

6. When first inserting the laryngoscope to find the epiglottis, great care should be taken not to insert too deeply lest the epiglottis be overridden and thus hidden

7. After identification of the epiglottis, too deep insertion of the laryngoscope must be carefully avoided lest the spatula be inserted back of the arytenoids into the hypo-pharynx.

8. Exposure of the larynx is accomplished by pulling forward the epiglottis and the tissues attached to the hyoid bone, and not by prying these tissues forward with the upper teeth as a fulcrum.

9. Care must be taken to avoid mistaking the ary-epiglottic fold for the epiglottis itself. (Most likely to occur from rotation of the patient's head.)

10. The tube should not be retained too long in place, but should be removed and the patient permitted to swallow the accumulated saliva, which, if the laryngoscope is too long in place, will trickle down into the trachea and cause cough. (Swallowing is almost impossible while the laryngoscope is in position).

11. The patient must be instructed to breathe deeply and quietly without making a sound.

12. In the sitting position of the patient, the operator should also be sitting.

Direct laryngoscopy by lateral and oblique methods. In the foregoing description of the technic of direct laryngoscopy, it is stated that the instruments should be passed exactly in the middle line over the dorsum of the tongue. This is intended to render orientation easy. After facility is acquired and the faculty of readily recognizing various landmarks is developed, it will be found a great advantage in exposing the larynx to pass the laryngoscope at the side of the tongue from the corner of the mouth, the head being turned very slightly toward the opposite side. Otherwise the position is the same as by the regular method.

As the exposure is oblique, the larynx will look somewhat asymmetrical and more will be seen of one wall than of the other. This, however, is of very great advantage when it is desired to inspect the ventricle, the laryngoscope being passed from the corner of the mouth opposite to the ventricle to be examined; that is, through the right corner of the mouth when the left ventricle is to be examined, and vice versa. The oblique method also is of very great advantage in the removal of tumors from the ventricle and from the subglottic regions, and very often from the cords themselves, the speculum being passed from the corner of the mouth opposite to the side of the larynx on which it is intended to operate. A narrow tube laryngoscope such as shown in Fig. 21 (child's size) is best adapted to laryngoscopy at the side of the tongue. The author cannot understand Brünings' objections to the lateral route.

In using lateral opening specula such as the one shown in Fig. 15, with the slide off, it is best to pass the instrument to one side of the tongue, selecting the side that will leave the tongue on the side of the instrument that has no opening. If the tongue is on the side of the opening the tongue will crowd into the opening, and obstruct the view. These lateral opening specula, however, are not especially intended for lateral use. They are useful only for regular dorso-lingual passage under general anesthesia. They are too wide for use under local anesthesia.

Exposure of the larynx with the instruments of Brünings, or of Kahler, and with all modifications of these and of the author's laryngoscope, is precisely the same as described in the foregoing. The technical illustrations show the author's instrument but the movements are identical with all other instruments of the same position of handle, which has come to be universally employed for the sitting position. The simple L-shaped laryngoscope has been generally abandoned for laryngoscopy upon the sitting patient. The only difference in the use of the various laryngoscopes for this purpose is in the management of the illumination, proximal, distal or headband types. Killian uses an improved form of Kirstein headlamp for all direct laryngoscopic procedures except for demonstration, for which he uses the handlamp at the proximal end of the tube.

Subglottic laryngoscopy. For examining the subglottic region in adults the child's size of the esophageal speculum, Fig. 21, is very satisfactory. It is used instead of the laryngoscope to expose the larynx, and then it is gently slid down into the glottis while carefully keeping in view the two arytenoid eminences as the tip of the speculum enters the glottis. In children, however, the author prefers to insert one of his regular bronchoscopes, Fig. 16, because the instrument is extremely light and delicate, therefore there is no danger of causing subglottic edema. The Brünings and Kahler bronchoscopes may be used for either adults or children in the way just described for the child's esophageal speculum. Great care should be used in thus examining the subglottic region of children, for the reason given.

THE TECHNIC OF DIRECT LARYNGEAL OPERATING.

The preparation of the patient, local as well as general, should be carried out as elsewhere herein suggested. Particular attention should be given to oral antisepsis, however trivial the growth and its removal may seem to be; and the general examination should never be omitted except in great emergency.

Anesthesia has been elsewhere considered in detail. For direct laryngoscopy upon the sitting adult patient it is usually local, never general. The more thoroughly it is carried out the easier will be the operation, because of the lessening of the reflex spasm, not because of need of analgesia.*

Left-hand exposure. The prime essential of direct laryngeal operating is perfect mastery of continuous left-handed laryngeal exposure. The left hand must be able, unaided, not only to expose the larynx but to maintain the exposure for at least a minute. Many operative procedures can be completed in this time if a proper plan of working has been devised. Those that require a longer period can be completed by removal and reinsertion of the laryngoscope. The author personally finds no difficulty in holding the larynx open for ten to fifteen minutes if need be, and Dr. Ellen J. Patterson has frequently held the larynx exposed for a twenty-five minute radium application. Yet most operators find prolonged exposure tiresome; and there is no objection to intermittent exposure, with intervals for expectoration, provided the exposure is steady and efficient with the left hand only. This is not at all difficult to acquire if the student will begin right, as previously explained, and follow precisely the directions herein given for direct laryngeal exposure, always with the left hand only. Like all purely manual procedures, especially bimanual procedures, such as the playing of musical instruments, what seems at first difficult becomes easy with practice to those who are not discouraged by early difficulties.

Endoscopic use of laryngeal forceps. Having mastered direct laryngeal left-hand exposure the next step is to learn the use of for-

*The reflex spasm here referred to is the ordinary glottic movement. The statement of some authors that the interior of the larynx should be cocainized to prevent respiratory arrest from "vagus reflexes" can only refer to patients under general anesthesia, possibly partially under. In over one thousand direct laryngeal operations and bronchoscopies by Dr. Patterson and the author there has never been an arrest of respiration when no anesthetic, general or local, was used.

ceps. A multiplicity of forceps for the removal of growth is quite unnecessary and is really a great hindrance to good work. It is far better to rely upon one forceps such as that shown in Fig. 35, and by cultivating dexterity with this instrument all the different forms and positions of growths as shown in Fig. 79 can be removed with far greater precision than if all different forms and angles of jaws, guillotines, etc., are tried first and found wanting. When the one forceps is mastered, others may be added as found desirable. It is the author's custom to have the jaws always set to open the one way—up and down. If any other angle may seem desirable, the forceps are turned in the hand even to complete reversal, the thumb and finger exchanging rings. This may not appeal to many, and the author would not urge it; but he does espe-

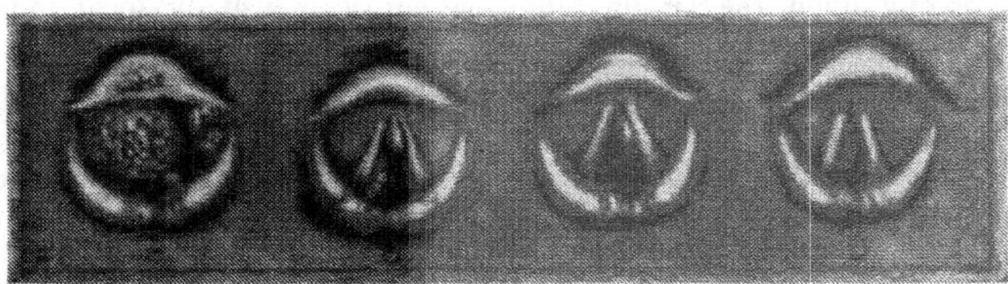

FIG. 79.—Indirect views of different types of laryngeal growths. A. Multiple papillomata in a woman of 25 years, requiring tracheotomy. Cured by repeated direct laryngoscopic operations. B. Multiple infra-glottic fibro-papillomata in a woman of 54 years, cured by direct operations. C. Fibroma attached to the under surface of right cord at the anterior commissure in a man of 39 years. Cured by a single removal. D. Subglottic angioma in a man of 42 years. All of these different types of tumor were removed with the one form of tissue forceps (Fig. 35) illustrating the needlessness of a large variety of forceps.

cially urge that all early practice work be done with the one forceps and with the jaws opening only one way until the eye is trained to watch the forceps open and close.

The gauging of depth by the use of one eye only is at all times difficult except by prolonged practice. It is more than usually difficult in direct laryngeal operating because of the misconception as to the real depth of the larynx, as before mentioned. These two factors contribute to such accidents as shown at B, in Fig. 80, where, in the attempt to reach a growth of the cord, miscalculation as to the real depth of the growth and of the cord from which it sprung caused the operator, who was a very skillful man by the indirect method, to punch out a section of the ventricular band leaving the floor of the ventricle exposed to view. While this is not a very grave accident, if not too far posteriorly, it is one to be avoided on the general principle that all unnecessary laryngeal trauma is always to be avoided with the utmost care, because only by so doing can we hope for the highest percentage of good results. Serious vocal impairment may result from such an accident if relatively deep down posteriorly. A still more serious accident is seen at C, where a large part of the left cord was afterward discovered at indirect laryngoscopy to have been punched away leaving the fibroma unharmed. Worse yet is the accident shown at D, where a large part of the arytenoid cartilage has been removed and the arytenoid movements permanently impaired. As shown by the author the chief factor in the production of an efficient adventitious vocal cord is the traction of an unimpaired arytenoid. Unfortunately misdirected excisions are especially liable to be located posteriorly. Only by practice can the

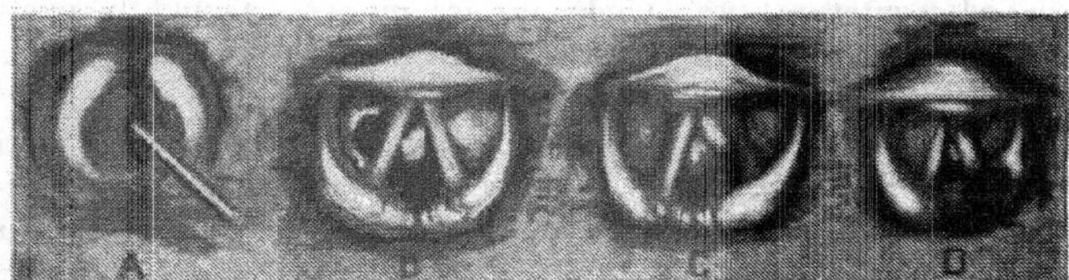

FIG. 80.—A direct view showing hiding of the end of the forceps by spasmodic closure of the ventricular bands. At the same moment the upper orifice of the larynx closes somewhat also, though this is not shown in order to illustrate the spasmodic closure of the bands. The operator thinking his forceps correctly placed, closes them, and, later at indirect laryngoscopy, is surprised to find the ventricular band cut away and the growth below unharmed, (B). A worse accident is shown at C where the posterior half of the cord is removed leaving the fibroma unharmed. Still more serious is the accident at D, where a large part of the left arytenoid was removed. (B, C, and D were sketched by the author from cases seen in consultation immediately after the accident.)

faculty of gauging depth be acquired, and especially by practice which enables the operator to work with both eyes open, ignoring the image of the left eye. A darkened room assists in acquiring this faculty. If the habit of holding the left eye closed is formed, the vision of the right eye is, for the time being, impaired and the operator is needlessly fatigued, as pointed out by the author many years ago. Another factor in the avoidance of the accidents above referred to is to make it a rule to work only by sight. The jaws must be seen to close properly on the growth, otherwise they must not be closed. In the event of a spasmodic contraction of the larynx, grasping the forceps as shown at A, in Fig 80, the forceps should be withdrawn and if working under a local anesthetic more of the anesthetic solution should be applied. If working under a general anesthetic, (recumbent patient) the depth of the anesthesia should be increased. If working without an anesthetic an opportunity must be awaited when the larynx is free from spasm. A child will clean its throat by swallowing or the secretions will drain out if the child is turned over. If the field is covered with blood or secretions, rendering accurate guidance of the forceps impossible, the laryngoscope and forceps must be removed and the patient told to "clear his throat." If a growth at the anterior commissure fails to come into view, the assistant holding the head uses his index finger to press backward the thyroid cartilage, at the same time steadying it, and this counterpressure, when properly exerted will bring into view the anterior commissure in any case where the endoscopist is holding his speculum properly. Either lateral wall above or below the commissure can be rendered prominent by skilled counterpressure. Under no circumstances should the operator attempt to reach a growth anteriorly that he cannot see, simply from his memory of its location at previous indirect laryngoscopy.

In the removal of small tumors, either on the cords or below, it is often a very great advantage to introduce the speculum and to work from the opposite side; therefore, in rightsided tumors, the speculum is put in the left side of the mouth and on the left side of the patient's tongue. Then by moving the patient's head to the right, we get a good view of the right wall of the larynx. In very sensitive adult patients, it may be wise to make an application of 8 per cent cocaine solution along the side of the tongue at the back, on the side through which the speculum is to be passed. To those who try this method for the first time, there may be some trouble with the tongue rolling over the open portion of the speculum and obstructing the view, but the operator soon learns to control this. In tumors below a cord (as at D, Fig. 79) there is a great temptation to use a sliding punch forceps, which, however, is almost certain to remove the cord and muscular tissue. A better method is to tilt the cord over sidewise with the spatular end of the laryngoscope and the growth thus can be presented fairly in front of the spatula by extreme lateral movement, as shown in Fig. 83, and by pushing firmly on the laryngoscope. Then the tissue forceps (Fig. 35) can be accurately placed without the growth slipping away. When the patient coughs up much blood the lamp may become somewhat obscured. Conditions here are very different from work in the tracheo-bronchial tree and in the esophagus because in the latter two regions the tube, when introduced, is allowed to remain throughout the entire procedure, and the swabs with which the field is wiped also at the same time, without any effort, wipe the lamp. In the larynx, however, working as is almost invariably the case, with local anesthesia or with none at all, the direct laryngoscope is frequently withdrawn, and then reintroduced after the patient has been permitted to expectorate the blood and mucus. At these intervals the spatular end of the direct laryngoscope is wiped by the operator with a square of gauze without removal of the light carrier. This wiping cleanses the portion of the lamp which emits the light needed. There is no need to cleanse the back of the lamp nor the socket, nor the little pocket in which the lamp lies. In working with the hand lamp the mirror is cleansed of the spattered coughed-out secretions at these removals. With the head lamp the lens front and mirror are to be similarly cleansed and readjusted in the visual axis. With the Claar reflector the mirror and lamp both are cleansed and readjusted to position before the eye. With any of these forehead forms of illumination a nurse should be instructed as to this cleansing so as to minimize the loss of time.

In the foregoing the author has referred only to the one kind of forceps. By this he does not wish to disapprove of sliding-punch forceps. On the contrary, punch forceps are very useful at times, but their use should not be attempted until the operator is quite familiar with direct laryngeal operating, because of the greater liability to such accidents as shown at B and C in Fig. 80.

Taking of a laryngeal specimen for diagnosis. This work is not concerned with diagnosis, yet, it may be said in passing that the diagnosis of carcinoma rests largely upon the histologic examination. The diagnosis of sarcoma rests largely on the exclusion of laryngeal tuberculosis by histologic and bacillary tissue examinations, animal injections of tissue, emulsions, etc.; and on the exclusion of lues by the therapeutic, the Wassermann and the luetin tests. But for biopsy to be of any value either positively or negatively, it is essential to have an ample specimen. In the old days the minute fragment from an uncertain location was a disgrace to the laryngologist, an enormity of injustice to the microscopist and, worst of all, to the patient. Too often the so-called "specimen" was, as aptly described by Jonathan Wright (Bib. 582) "A tiny bit of tissue chipped off the surface of a laryngeal growth with a pair of forceps, nay, not even surely off the growth, but perhaps from some other part of the endo-laryngeal surface in the neighborhood of the growth, with the assertion from the operator that it *did* come from the growth." Direct laryngoscopy for the removal of a specimen has changed all this.

The best plan for the removal of the specimen depends upon the topography of the laryngeal lesion. If a small growth, it should be removed entirely with a goodly portion of the normal basal tissues. If a large growth, and there are objections to entire removal, the edge of the growth including apparently normal as well as neoplastic tissue is necessary. If the larynx is the seat of a diffuse infiltrative process pervad-

[illegible]

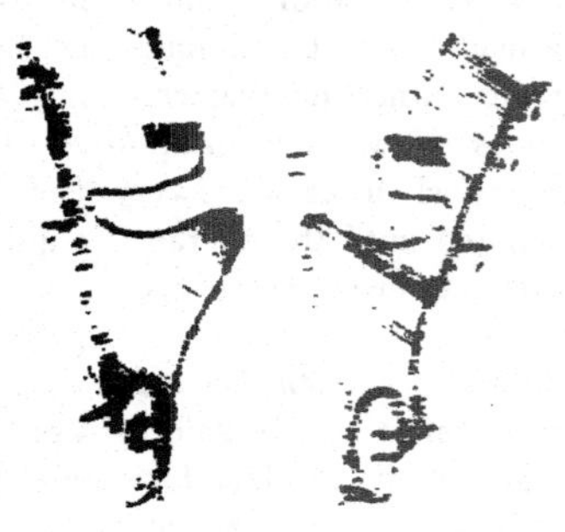

[illegible] ... and V. E. must [illegible]

of a specimen the patient should be watched for a few days, lest undue reaction supervene from mixed infections getting into the wound, and especially if potassium iodid, which especially predisposes to acute edema, has been given. In possibly luetic cases a prompt report must be urged because of the necessity of immediate institution of treatment. In malignancy promptness is also needed. As Sir Felix Semon (Bib. 494) has so ably pointed out not only should operation closely follow the taking of the specimen but if the patient should not agree beforehand to radical operation in the event of histologic examination showing malignancy no specimen at all should be taken in cases which clinically seem quite certain to be malignant. Should the since-discovered effect of radium in controlling malignancy fulfill early promises, this latter advice, sound in its day, may require modification.

Removal of growths from the laryngeal ventricle. Growths in the ventricle, especially when of small size, may be rendered exceedingly difficult of removal by the overhanging projection of the ventricular bands, which, for the time being, exaggerates very much the outward depth of the ventricle. In such cases, general anesthesia may be required and it is perfectly justifiable, provided there is no stenosis whatever, and not the slightest dyspnea. With thorough cocainization, however, it is always possible to get these growths by the lateral method of operating. The degree of overhang of the ventricular band especially when in a state of spasm is seldom realized (Fig. 81). Where a growth involving the cord probably extends far back into the ventricle, or where a

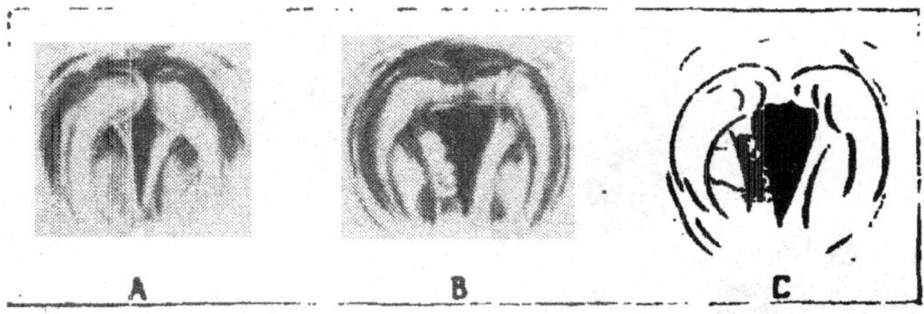

FIG. 82.—Pencil sketch of direct laryngoscopic view, sitting patient, showing, at B, a growth springing from the outermost depth of the right ventricle. At A, the growth is hidden by the overhang of the ventricular band. At C, the dotted line indicates the growth under the overhanging ventricular band.

growth springs from the ventricle itself and is hidden by the ventricular band as in Fig. 82, it is not necessary to punch out the ventricular band (as shown to have been accidentally done in Fig. 80) in order to expose the floor of the ventricle and thus render more accurate the tumor removal.

In such a case as that shown in Fig. 82 the head of the patient is carried far over to one side after the larynx is exposed (Fig. 83). If the tube, E, has not been passed at the side of the tongue it is now slipped over to the lower corner of the mouth, B, and the patient's head is tilted over to the same side while the observer watches through the tube. The second assistant must keep the larynx fixed and in the vertical position. The tube is advanced until the ventricular band is flattened and the growth can be removed from the ventricle.

Removal of large benign tumors of the larynx above the cords. The author often uses for this class of case the alligator punch forceps, Fig. 36. They can be inserted through the author's laryngoscope, but the best way is by the author's "ex-tubal" method. The forceps are inserted alongside the laryngoscope, which is used only to look through for the accurate ocular guidance of the forceps as shown in the schema Fig. 84. The jaws can be placed and the bite made with great accuracy. The side-slide laryngoscope (Fig. 15) because of its oval lumen is pre-

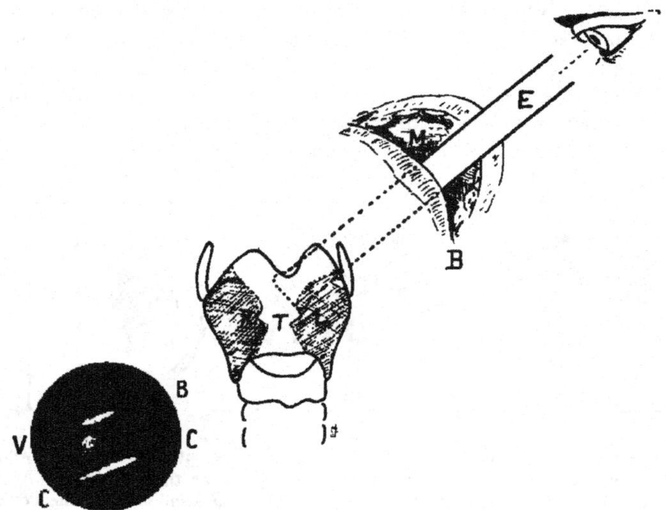

Fig. 83.—Schema illustrating the lateral method of exposing a growth in the ventricle of Morgani, by bending the patient's head to the opposite side while the second assistant externally fixes the larynx with his hand. M, patient's mouth. T, thyroid cartilage. R, right side, L, left. V, B, ventricular band. C, C, vocal cord. The circular drawing indicates the endoscopic view obtainable by this method. The tube, E, is dropped to the corner of the mouth, B, and the tube is inserted down to R.

ferred by many operators some of whom leave the slide off. In case of still larger tumors with more or less pedunculated base the heavy snare, Fig. 41, may be used to excellent advantage by the "ex-tubal" method. In some of the author's cases tumors the size of a hen's egg have been thus removed. Sessile growths may be removed by the galvano-cautery snare, but the author prefers forceps. Of course, there could be no hope of thorough removal of malignancy by such means; and incomplete removal is rarely if ever justifiable.

Amputation of the epiglottis for palliation of dysphagia in tuberculosis or malignant disease is an operation easily performed and of benefit where the dysphagia is due to ulceration of the epiglottis. It is possible that very early malignancy of the extreme tip can be cured by such means, and the author has had such a successful result in two instances. Closure of the air passages to the entrance of food during swallowing seems to be a three-fold process. The tilting of the larynx and especially of the arytenoids and the arytenoid approximation are prob-

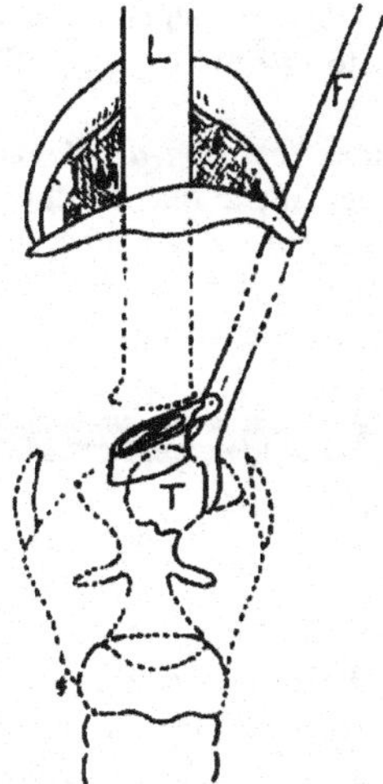

FIG. 84.—Schema illustrating removal of a tumor from the upper part of the larynx by the author's "ex-tubal" method for *large* tumors. The large alligator basket punch forceps, F, is inserted from the right corner of the mouth, and the jaws are placed over the tumor, T, under guidance of the eye looking through the laryngoscope, L. This method is not used for small tumors. It is excellent for amputation of the epiglottis with these same punch forceps (Fig. 36) or with the heavy snare. (Fig. 41.)

ably the chief factors. In addition to this, however, there is the closure of the ventricular bands below and the capping by the epiglottis above. The least important of the three seems to be the epiglottis and it can very readily be dispensed with if necessary to relieve pain or cure disease. Probably its chief function is to act as a snow plow in splitting the food bolus and drifting the two portions laterally into the pyriform sinuses thus directing the food bolus past the aditus laryngis. Mr. Walter G. Howarth states that the epiglottis has nothing whatever to do with laryngeal closure during swallowing. As a clinical fact we know that amputation of the epiglottis is not often followed by serious symptoms and results in the relief of pain are excellent. Lockard (Bib. 346) has collected statistics on the results in tuberculosis. It would not be easy to get out more than the projecting part of the normal epiglottis, but it is not difficult to remove all of the involved portions. The projecting part may be amputated with the heavy snare shown in Fig. 41, and this is the better way in those rare cases of disease limited to the tip because of the *en masse* removal. In more general involvement either the snare or the large basket alligator punch forceps may be used. With either instrument it is best to operate by the author's "ex-tubal" method shown in the schema, Fig. 84.

Endolaryngeal operations favoring development of adventitious vocal cords. In some instances liberation of adhesions will favor the formation of adventitious vocal cords. In other instances where there is tension from contraction of cicatricial tissue hampering mobility of the arytenoids an incision designed to relieve the tension and supply a re-

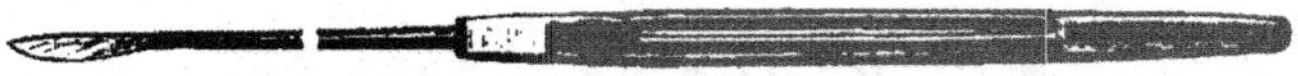

FIG. 85.—Author's laryngeal knife, 30 cm. long. Illustration reproduced from the earlier volume.

dundancy of tissue for later absorption will bring back the voice as illustrated in the case cited in the section of this work that deals with papilloma. For such incisions the author's laryngeal knife, Fig. 85, is excellent. The sharp anterior commissure is essential to good phonation. In Fig. 15, Plate 1, is illustrated a case in which the action of the laryngeal musculature was unable to approximate and draw tense the adventitious vocal bands. The patient, a man of thirty years, when convalescent from a very severe attack of typhoid fever became dyspneic and was tracheotomized by Dr. James W. McFarlane. When the perichondritis had subsided the larynx remained stenosed by cicatricial tissue, and the case was transferred to the author's service at the Western Pennsylvania Hospital for decannulation. The stenosis was cured by laryngostomy by the author's method as described in a later chapter. After decannulation and plastic closure the patient could not speak louder than a whisper because of inability of the laryngeal musculature to approximate and draw tense the cicatricial adventitious vocal bands (Fig. 15, Plate 1). With a sliding punch forceps the author cleared the anterior commissure of all tissue out to the perichondrium, as shown by the dotted line, with excellent vocal results. In this kind of case, it is absolutely necessary to remove the tissue anteriorly very radically but to harm the tissue at the sides as little as possible. There was a thick redundancy of tissue not under tension. With a thin band-like web under tension it is usually better to incise with the knife as in the case referred to under "Papilloma."

Endoscopic evisceration of the larynx is a procedure which will cure a few cases of cicatricial laryngeal stenosis especially those where the cicatrices are thin and web-like. Illustrative cases are shown in Plate 1. Fig. 1 shows a post-diphtheritic stenosis in a boy of fourteen years admitted to the Western Pennsylvania Hospital for decannulation. An incision was made in the plane of the glottis, so that the slide punch-forceps could be inserted. All of the endolaryngeal tissue that could be removed without injury to the arytenoid cartilage was extirpated, the effort being made to lay bare the perichondrium of the laryngeal wall, as shown schematically in Fig. 86. Healing was prompt but left a slight recurrence of the cicatricial tissue in the anterior commissure. Thorough removal of this with a pointed slide-forceps was followed by an excellent result (Fig. 5, Plate 1) both as to voice and cure of stenosis. He was seen two years after decannulation and was learning a trade in a mill. A similar case was that of a man, aged 40 years, who applied to the Eye and Ear Hospital Dispensary for decannulation. He had been tracheotomized during typhoid fever about a year before. The larynx was occluded by a thin membranous cicatrix which left only a small opening posteriorly (Fig. 4, Plate 1). There was slight arytenoid movement on both sides. The larynx was eviscerated as in the previous case, but required two subsequent removals of tissue to clear the anterior commissure. An excellent result was ultimately obtained (Fig. 8, Plate 1) and the patient was decannulated after two months' watching. The voice was loud, though rough, and there was no recurrence of the dyspnea when seen two years later. In three other cases the same method was not sufficiently successful to permit decannulation but the method is well worthy of trial before resorting to laryngostomy. A simple punching out of the occluding membrane is not sufficient. An effort should be made to remove all of the tissue in the larynx clear out to the perichondrium, but without removing any part of either arytenoid cartilage, in non-paralytic cases. In cases of posticus paralysis the excision may be carried farther back, excising a portion of the processus vocalis of the arytenoids.

Vocal results. Two classes of cases must be considered.

1. In cases of laryngeal stenosis in which no air is going through the larynx on expiration with the cannula temporarily occluded with the finger, the patient of course has no voice except the "buccal voice" like

that developed by the laryngectomized patient. These patients can be promised a good whispered voice immediately after operation. Phonation will depend on the conditions mentioned below in the next class of cases.

2. In cases of laryngeal stenosis in which any expiratory air at all is going through the larynx when the tube is temporarily occluded with the finger, the voice is usually fairly good. Therefore, one of the first questions to be considered is in regard to the voice after operation. The author has demonstrated that the most important factor in the production of an adventitious cord, after operative or morbid loss of the true cord, is the traction of the arytenoid. The thousands of pulls daily end in a band which more or less perfectly in appearance and function replaces the lost cord. So close is the resemblance in some cases that ex-

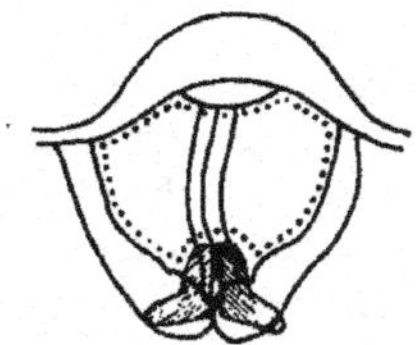

Fig. 86.—Schema showing endoscopic evisceration of the larynx for posticus paralysis. The attempt is made with the sliding punch forceps (Fig. 37) to eviscerate all of the laryngeal tissue inside of the dotted line. It is practically an impossibility to remove all of the tissue but the attempt will relieve the stenosis in some instances. In non-paralytic conditions it is very necessary to avoid injuring the arytenoid cartilages; for in these cases good arytenoid mobility will assist in the formation of an adventitious cord.

pert laryngologists are unable to say whether a cord is original or adventitious. To get such results, however, it is absolutely necessary that there shall be mobility of the cricoarytenoid joint. Of course the whispered voice will never be lost so long as the respiratory air passes through the larynx. The "stage whisper," for which no cord is necessary, may to be very loud, and in some instances the ventricular bands will approximate and phonate, but to phonate effectively requires a cord, natural or adventitious. The voice of the ventricular band is deep and rough, and lacks flexibility. The ventricular band, however, is mostly removed in endolaryngeal evisceration. From his results with endolaryngeal evisceration, the author believes that, in all forms of non-malignant chronic laryngeal stenosis a good chance of a cure of the stenosis may be promised in any case in which there is not too much loss of the cartilage which maintains the patulence of the laryngeal box. An ultimate good voice can be promised in all cases in which there remains good arytenoid mobility. A fairly loud, though rough and inflexible voice, can be promised in any case without mobility. Endolaryngeal evisceration should be tried before resorting to laryngostomy.

Galvano-cauterization for chronic hypertrophic laryngeal stenosis. The author has had excellent results from the galvano-cauterization of chronic subglottic edema or hyperplasia seen in children after diphtheria. In some instances the children had been intubated in others tracheotomized for dyspnea during the height of the diphtheritic process. An illustrative case is shown in Fig. 87, referred to the author by Dr. Torian for extubation. A boy of two years, after laryngeal diphtheria requiring intubation, could not be extubated because of a recurrence of dyspnea within a few minutes of the removal of the intubation tube. A number of attempts had been made during two months. In the recumbent position the author removed the intubation tube through the direct laryngo-

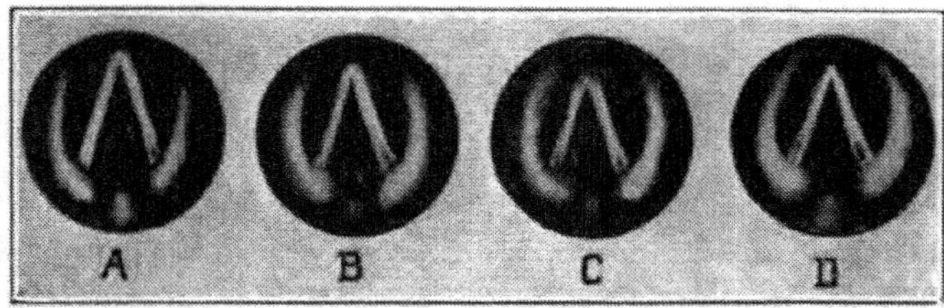

Fig. 87.—Direct view. Recumbent position. Illustration of the effectiveness of galvano-cauterization of post-diphtheritic subglottic stenosis. A, shows the larynx immediately after the removal of the intubation tube. B, five minutes later the hypertrophic subglottic masses on each side are seen to have closed in like intumescent turbinals. C, the left mass has been cauterized and is bound down by a linear cicatrix parallel with the long axis of the trachea. D, shows the larynx after cure by repeated cauterizations.

scope. A subglottic mass could be seen on each side, but an ample chink was left for breathing, as shown at A, Fig. 87. At the end of five minutes the masses had swollen until they almost met in the median line and the child became intensely cyanotic. A bronchoscope was inserted and left in the trachea while a tracheotomy was done. Later the galvanocautery knife was used to incise the hypertrophic masses, one such incision being shown at C. A perfect cure resulted and the child was reported well six months later. Another case, that of a young child tracheotomized for diphtheria three months previously, was referred to the author for decannulation by Dr. J. W. Murphy. Galvano-cauterization of the subglottic hypertrophies, as in the previously mentioned case, resulted in a complete and permanent cure. It was still well a year and a half later. In one case admitted to the Western Pennsylvania Hospital subglottic edema followed an influenzal tracheitis for which tracheotomy had been done. The same method resulted in perfect cure that has borne the test of time. The method is ideal for hypertrophic conditions, but is not so well adapted to cicatricial stenoses, though the author had a partial result in one case.

Galvano-cautery puncture has superseded all caustics for laryngeal use. The excellent results achieved by Heryng, Hajek and Mermod (Bib. 407) in the galvano-caustic treatment of tuberculosis, led the author to develop the endoscopic technic and his results have been very satisfactory. This plan of treatment has also been advocated in an excellent monograph (Bib. 20) by Prof. Louis Bar of Nice. The use of the curette

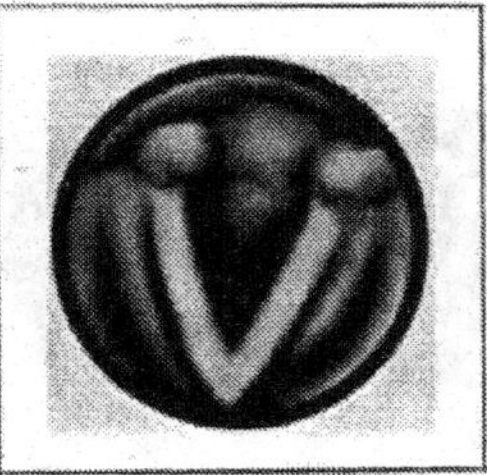

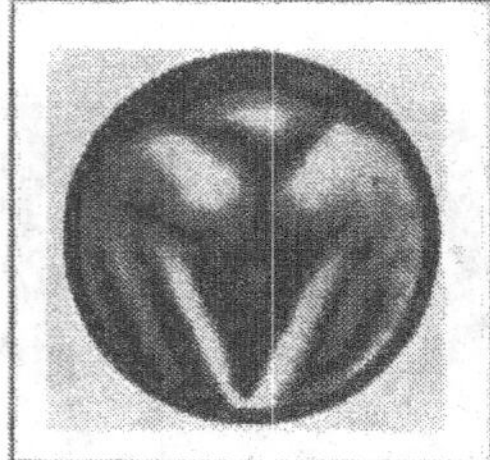

Fig. 88.—Direct view (sitting position) of a tuberculous larynx, in a girl of 17 years. The large club-shaped infiltrations in the right hand view were reduced by three cauterizations at three weeks' intervals to the size shown on the left hand. Slight sloughing occurred near the right arytenoid (upper left quadrant of the left circle). This is a rare sequel, and it did no harm.

and of lactic acid have been quite generally abandoned since such abundant evidence has been forthcoming, proving the great usefulness of the galvano-cautery in the treatment of tuberculous infiltrations in the larynx and all of the laryngologists who have used the direct methods for these applications are enthusiastic as to the precision with which the caustic point can be applied. The direct method exposes to view the anterior surface of the posterior wall of the arytenoid masses, and thus the point can be applied practically perpendicularly to the surface, which is in great contrast to the indirect method by which a more or less lateral application of the point renders accurate puncture more difficult, and sometimes impossible. Furthermore, it matters little how intolerant the patient may be to the laryngoscopic mirror; he cannot in any case whatsoever prevent the skillful operator from making an accurate application. Direct laryngoscopy has opened up a new field in the local treatment of tuberculous lesions. It seems equally well adapted to ulcerative and non-ulcerated infiltrations. Of course, it is subject to the same general and local contraindications that apply to any surgical treatment of laryngeal tuberculosis, especially the inadvisability in cases with advanced pulmonary disease. In severely stenosed larynges a tracheotomy should first be done, for though the reaction is slight, it might be sufficient to close the narrowed glottis. Application of the galvano-cautery to tuberculous lesions below the larynx has been unsatisfactory in the author's hands. The technic is simple. The author uses the electrode illustrated in his earlier work (Bib. 269) with hard rubber insulation vulcanized onto the copper conductors insuring cleanliness. In a few instances a right-angled point is useful but usually the straight point is better. The larynx is anesthetized locally and exposed with the direct laryngoscope, the patient sitting. The rheostat having been previously adjusted to heat the electrode to a very nearly white heat, the circuit is broken and the electrode is introduced cold. When the point is in contact with the desired location the current is turned on and the point thrust in as deeply as desired. Usually it should penetrate until a firm resistance is felt; but care must be used not to damage the cricoarytenoid joint. The circuit is broken at the instant of withdrawal. Punctures should be made as nearly perpendicular to the surface as possible, so as to minimize the destruction of epithelium, and to minimize the reaction which is greater after a broad superficial cauterization. The reaction is usually slight, a gray fibrinous slough detaching itself in a few days. In one case the author had rather extensive sloughing, but it left no bad result. No after-treatment is needed. Cautery-punctures should be repeated every two or three weeks selecting a new location each time until the desired result is obtained.

After-care. After any endolaryngeal operation, cleanliness of the mouth must be insured by brushing the teeth after taking food, and by the rinsing of the mouth with alcohol 1 part to 5 of water. If the operative wound extends out of the interior of the larynx, sterile water and sterile liquid food should be given for four days. No local applications are needed. Complications should, of course, be watched for. In all cases, whether tracheotomized or not, the patient should be watched by a special tracheal nurse. In cases not tracheotomized, the possibility of laryngeal dyspnea should be in the mind of the surgeon and the nurse. Inspiratory indrawing around the clavicles, inspiratory indrawing above the sternum and at the epigastrium, and a forward movement of the chin at each inspiration are the danger signs demanding immediate tracheotomy. Cyanosis should not be waited for.

Complications during endolaryngeal operation are very rare. Dyspnea may increase if the larynx is stenotic before operation, and tracheotomy may be required in such cases. Idiosyncracy to cocaine may induce toxic symptoms. The sight and taste of blood may nauseate the patient, causing syncope. Serious hemorrhage could occur only in a hemophile, and it would be long after the operation before the loss of blood would be serious. Injury to an incisor tooth can only come from misdirected effort in a false position. The bite-block, however, unless carefully handled might damage a frail tooth, "bridge-work," a capped tooth, or other dental fixture. The loss of a portion of an instrument down into the air passage is a complication to be avoided by having well made instruments and especially by careful inspection from time to time.

Complications after endolaryngeal operations are unusual, yet all patients should be watched closely. Inflammatory reaction is rarely severe if the aseptic technic has been without a slip. Cervical cellulitis has been known to follow carelessness in this respect. Edema of the larynx occasionally occurs and in rare instances necessitates tracheotomy. Emphysema of the neck occurs very rarely. It does not require treatment ordinarily; but may be treated in the usual way if desired. Hemorrhage sufficient to require attention, either at operation or subsequently, is very rare, except in hemophiles. Hemorrhage within the larynx of a hemophile can be stopped by packing a roll of gauze tightly down into the larynx from above, if the patient is tracheotomized; and if not, tracheotomy should be done. This was required in one case of the author, that of a hemophile. Styptics are very objectionable for laryngeal use, and have been known to set up serious lung complications. Mermod (Bib. 384) advises morphine subcutaneously.

DIRECT LARYNGOSCOPY, ADULT PATIENT, RECUMBENT.

Exposure of the larynx in the recumbent patient is precisely the same as in the sitting patient so far as the relation of the instrument to the patient is concerned, and so far as the position of the head and neck of the patient relatively to the patient's body is concerned. The manner of grasping the handle of the direct laryngoscope, however, varies, and the endoscopic image is reversed with reference to the operator's eye both in the vertical and the horizontal direction. What was to the operator the left side of the image now is the right, and the anterior commissure which before was at the bottom of the circular endoscopic picture, is now at the top of the circle. For this reason, practice in the sitting position is of but little avail and a large amount of practice is required in the recumbent position, because much of the endoscopic work, and practically all of the foreign body work in the larynx and the tracheo-bronchial tree is, or should be, done in the recumbent position. The best position for the recumbent patient is that of Boyce, as described in a previous chapter and shown in Fig. 72 with the head raised high and fully extended. Under no circumstances during direct

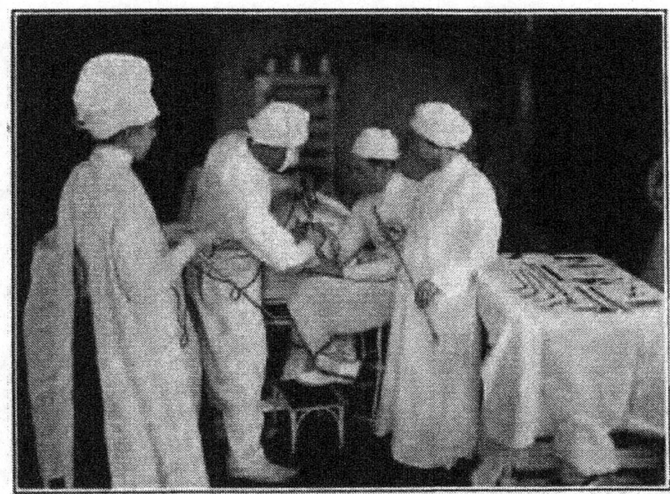

Fig. 89.—Direct laryngoscopy, recumbent patient. The second assistant is sitting holding the head in the Boyce position, his *left* forearm on his *left* thigh, his *left* foot on a stool whose top is 65 cm. lower than the table-top. His *left* hand is on the patient's sterile-covered scalp, the thumb on the forehead, the fingers under the occiput, making forced extension. The *right* forearm passes under the neck of the patient, so that the index finger of the *right* hand holds the bite block in the *left* corner of the patient's mouth. The operator stands, but may sit on a stool of the same height as that on which the second assistant is sitting. An enlarged view of the operator's hands is shown in Fig. 90.

laryngoscopy should the head be allowed to hang over the end of the table in the Rose position.

Before a start is made, every detail mentioned under the head of operating room organization should have been carried out. Every instrument that might possibly be needed should be sterile and ready, sponge holders armed, assistants in position, including those who are to hold the patient's arms and legs, as well as the one who holds the head and the other who passes the needed instruments. The second assistant who holds the head, then takes the sterile cap, slips it over the patient's head until the opening comes opposite the mouth of the patient. Then he grasps the patient's head and elevates it while the unsterile nurse drops the head-board or shortens down the back-board of the Dr. French table, as the case may be, leaving the patient's shoulders as far as the ridge of the scapula, as well as the head and neck of the patient, out in the air supported by the second assistant, who now raises the head

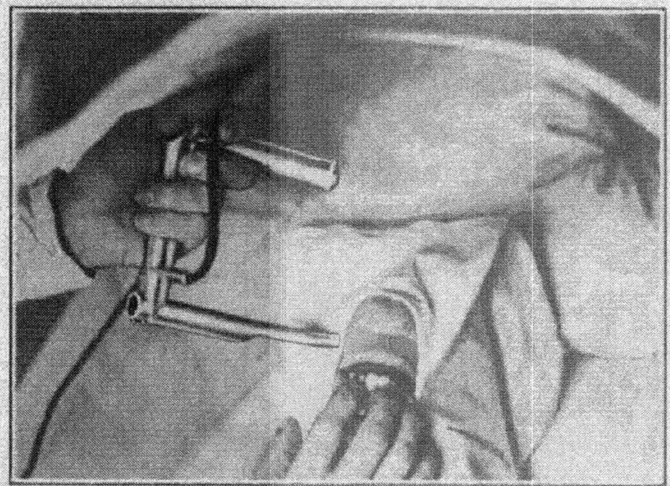

FIG. 90.—Direct laryngoscopy, recumbent patient. The laryngoscope is held in the *left* hand. The first, second and third fingers of the *right* hand are used to pull down the upper lip of the patient to prevent pinching the lip between the laryngoscope and the teeth. The camera being above the patient gives a false impression of the position of the head and chest. The chest is really very much lower than the head.

with the left hand, his thumb being on the patient's forehead, while the right hand is passed below the patient's neck so that the thimble gag on his first finger can be inserted between the teeth at the left side of the patient's mouth, the second assistant being on the right hand side of the patient (Fig. 89). The most important part of the procedure at this point is the high elevation of the patient's head. Under no circumstances must it at this stage be permitted to fall until the vertex is lower than the table top.

The introduction of the direct laryngoscope and the exposure of the larynx may best, for clearness of description as well as for promptness and effectiveness of execution, be divided into two stages.

1. Exposure and identification of the epiglottis.

2. Elevation of the epiglottis and all the tissues attached to the hyoid bone so as to expose the larynx to direct view.

The tongue of the patient need not be held out. The patient is simply told to open his mouth, or, in the case of general anesthesia, the mouth is opened and the bite-block, Fig. 39, is inserted. The direct laryngoscope is grasped, as shown in Fig. 90, which is perferable to that shown in Fig. 59. Absolutely always and invariably the left hand must be used to grasp the laryngoscope. If this be not done, the operator will be seriously handicapped when it comes to passing a bronchoscope, or to

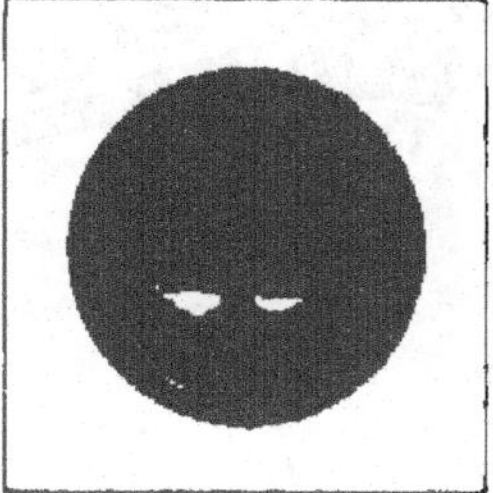

Fig. 91.—End of first stage of direct laryngoscopy, recumbent adult patient. The epiglottis is exposed by a strong lifting movement of the spatula tip on the tongue anterior to the epiglottis.

operate on the larynx, because the right hand should be free just as soon as it is through with its very important duty of drawing the upper lip toward the nose of the patient in order to prevent the lip getting pinched between the laryngoscope and the upper teeth. The laryngoscope is passed into the patient's mouth posterior to the dorsum of the tongue, exactly in the middle line, particular note being taken that the patient's head is exactly square with the body; that is, not deviated to either side. nor rotated. The dorsum of the tongue is now pressed anteriorly, in other words, lifted, in the recumbent position of the patient, until the epiglottis comes into view. Great care must be taken not to pass the spatular tip beyond the epiglottis in this first stage; and it is better to elevate the dorsum of the tongue from time to time in order that there shall be no danger of the epiglottis being overridden. When the epiglottis is seen to project into the endoscopic field, as shown in Fig. 91. the first stage is completed.

Second stage. The spatular end of the direct laryngoscope is inserted to a distance of, on the average, about 1 cm. and then the larynx is exposed by a motion that is best described as a suspension of the head and neck of the patient on the tip of the spatular end of the laryngoscope Fig. 92. In other words we try to lift the patient's head with

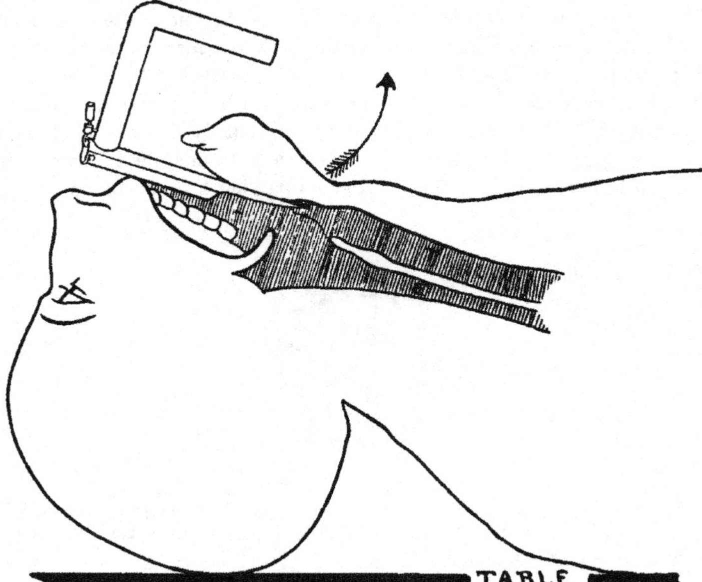

FIG. 92.—Schema illustrating the technic of direct laryngoscopy on the recumbent patient. The motion is imparted to the tip of the laryngoscope as if to lift the patient by his hyoid bone. The portion of the table to the left of the word "TABLE" may be dropped or not, but the back of the head must never go lower than here shown, for direct laryngoscopy. The table may be used as a rest for the operator's left elbow to take the weight of the head. The author prefers head section of the table dropped. (Note that in bronchoscopy and esophagoscopy the head section of the table *must* be dropped, so as to leave the head and neck of the patient out in the air, supported by the second assistant.)

the tip of the speculum. The assistant, consequently, must not take *all* the weight of the head. Particular care must be taken at this stage not to pry upon the upper teeth; but rather to impart a lifting motion with the tip of the speculum without depressing the proximal tubular orifice. If the teeth are used as a fulcrum, there will be a tendency to pry the head downward, which is a distinct disadvantage; because the head should be kept high as well as extended. The view first obtained of the larynx is, to the beginner, often unsatisfactory, because the larynx is in a state of spasm; and usually but little is to be seen but two rounded masses, and anterior to them the ventricular bands in more or less close apposition hiding the cords (Fig. 93). Of course in deep anesthesia, or often even in the very thoroughly locally anesthetized larynx, this spasm does not occur, and the second stage at once reveals the cords moving rhythmically with inspiration and expiration. It is customary with some endoscopists to ask the patient to phonate continuously in order to render more easy the identification of the glottic chink and vocal cords. It is very much better, however, in the author's opinion, to insist upon the patient breathing steadily and deeply; but the begin-

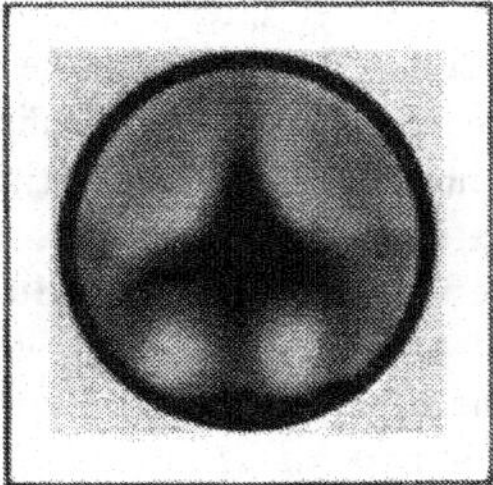

FIG. 93.—Endoscopic view at the end of the second stage of direct laryngoscopy. Recumbent patient. Larynx exposed. Waiting for larynx to relax its spasmodic contraction. A deep inspiration will then show the cords beautifully exposed. In the full relaxation of deep anesthesia this spasmodic closure does not exist and the second stage reveals the cords opening and closing rhythmically with inspiration and expiration.

ner should try both ways. If his attention is fixed upon this beforehand, almost any adult will keep on breathing if the command is repeated frequently.

Difficulties of direct laryngoscopy. The difficulties may be classified under two heads: Those that pertain to the patient and those that pertain to the operator.

The ease of exposure of the larynx varies within very wide limits in adult patients. There is very little difference in children. A very muscular, stout adult with a short, thick neck and a full row of upper teeth will usually be very much more difficult than will a flaccid, slender patient with a long neck and upper teeth absent. But it must be remembered that there is absolutely no patient whatever, whose larynx cannot be exposed to direct view with the sole exception of a patient with ankylosed jaws, preventing the opening of the mouth, so that while the ease of exposure may vary within wide limits, there is none in whom direct laryngoscopy is impossible.

Failure to expose the epiglottis is usually due to too great haste to enter the speculum all the way down. The efforts should be rather to lift the tongue at its dorsum and gradually to slide the spatula downward so as to get into the glossoepiglottic fossa. When this is done, the epiglottis will loom large. In some cases the anterior one-third of the larynx does not readily come into view, because it is drawn upon by the elevation of the hyoid bone. To expose this anterior one-third all the way to the anterior commissure, it is in some cases necessary for an assistant other than the one who holds the head to make counterpressure on the thyroid cartilage externally, pushing the larynx backward (downward in the recumbent patient). Either lateral wall can be made prominent, and the whole larynx can be fixed. To get the best results from counterpressure, it is necessary to be careful that the direct laryngoscope is not too deeply inserted. It should not be deeper than is necessary to hold the epiglottis. In various laryngeal operations, this counterpressure by an assistant trained to the work, is of great help to the operator by fixing the larynx, turning it to one side or to the other, as required, to bring into view one or the other side of the larynx. Practice together on the part of the operator and his assistant, in this respect as in every other, will produce results by "team work" unobtainable in any other way. In most instances the best results are obtained by having the assistant fix the thyroid cartilage in a vertical position, while the head, only, of the patient is turned over to the side opposite to that on which the growth is located. This side method of operating is shown for the sitting position in Fig. 83. It is relatively the same in the recumbent patient. After learning how, passing the tube at the side instead of over the dorsum of the tongue will render the most difficult case easy.

The difficulties that pertain to the operator himself, are chiefly due to lack of practice. Absolutely nothing will dispense with the necessity of continued practice, and while much may be done, as mentioned under the head of acquiring skill, nothing will take the place of frequent work upon the patient in the recumbent position. As one of the greatest difficulties is caused by the spasmodic contractions, not only of the laryngeal muscles, but also of the muscles of the neck, and especially all of the muscles attached to the hyoid bone, it will be of great assistance if the operator can have the advantage of acquiring the knack of exposure of the larynx first in patients deeply generally anesthetized.

One of the greatest difficulties of the beginner is in recognizing the landmarks. We are so accustomed to seeing classical pictures of the larynx during inspiration, expiration and phonation, that we are quite confused and discouraged when we do not see such a picture by the direct method. It must be remembered, however. that in proceeding by the old indirect method, observation is usually terminated when the patient has very much of spasmodic contraction about the pharynx and larynx, while in direct laryngoscopy these spasmodic contractions are no bar to a continuation of the examination; and we must learn to recognize the landmarks in the state of a high degree of spasm. This, of course, is especially necessary in working without any anesthetic, general or local, as in the case of children. We must therefore fix in our minds the previously mentioned landmarks, namely, the two rounded eminences, corresponding to the arytenoids. It is only on deep inspiration that anything like a typical picture of the larynx will be seen. Therefore, we must terminate our search upon the identification of the two rounded masses and wait for the inspiratory opening to get a view of the interior of the larynx. Herein consists one of the great advantages of working with local anesthesia. Should the patient be anesthetized, though not quite deeply enough to abolish the reflexes about the pharynx and larynx, and especially if the patient has been given chloroform along with any of the opium derivatives, it is a very serious risk to wait very long for the glottis to open, because of the paralyzing effect of choloroform and the opium derivatives upon the respiratory center. On the other hand, when a local anesthetic alone is being used, we can safely wait indefinitely for the patient to breathe, meanwhile telling him to take a deep breath and not to hold it, and reassuring him that he can get his breath perfectly well if he only will. It is only in infants and very young children that the injunction "keep on breathing" will not be followed promptly by an inspiration, but as these are examined without any anesthetic, general or local, we can wait indefinitely for the opening inspiration, except in very dyspneic cases.

Elbow-rest position. If the operator is not strong in the wrist and forearm he may experience fatigue in holding the larynx of the recumbent patient exposed for any length of time. By this it is not meant that great strength is required. Like most similar procedures there is more in the knack than brute strength. If endurance is being taxed the author's elbow-rest position will enable the operator to work for any length of time that could possibly be needed for an endolaryngeal procedure. The head board of the table is not dropped for this position. If already dropped the head board is raised to a level position. The operator's left elbow rests on the table beside the patient's head, the head being suspended on the tip of the laryngoscope. The operator sits on a stool at the head of the table facing towards the patient's feet.

Suspension laryngoscopy devised by Prof. Killian to render direct laryngoscopy in the recumbent position easier, will be treated in a separate chapter by the great master himself.

DIRECT LARYNGOSCOPY IN CHILDREN.

For those who have practiced it, direct laryngoscopy in children, for diagnosis, is a simple, easy matter requiring but a minute or less, without anesthesia, general or local. On the other hand, for the beginner it may require twenty minutes at the end of which time he may not have had a good view of the larynx. The procedure is easily learned and for five reasons it is an absolute necessity that every laryngologist be able to make the examination without any anesthesia:

1. Anesthesia is unnecessary.
2. It is extremely dangerous in dyspneic patients.
3. It is inadmissable in a case which may prove to be diphtheria.
4. If anesthesia is to be used, direct laryngoscopy will never reach its full degree of usefulness, because anesthesia makes a major procedure out of a minor.
5. There is no more reason for anesthetizing a child to look at its larynx than to anesthetize it to feel for adenoids with the finger.

Whatever may be said on the subject of anesthesia for bronchoscopy and esophagoscopy in children, no one can deny that the larynx of any child can be examined quickly, painlessly and satisfactorily without anesthesia, general or local. By this it is not meant that a diagnosis can always be reached, but the nature of dyspnea or croupy cough can almost always be determined. Seeing the larynx of an adult by the indirect method does not always mean a diagnosis. Cocaine in children is dangerous and its application is more of an annoyance than the examination. This matter has been more fully dealt with in the chapter on anesthesia. The brief mention here is to emphasize a matter in which there has been much misunderstanding and many misleading statements.

In leaving the subject, the author wishes to state that any operator who uses a general anesthetic on dyspneic children will some day regret it, because of the death of a child from a needless procedure. If the operator must have a general anesthetic, he should do a preliminary tracheotomy.

Instruments. For a diagnostic direct laryngoscopy in children the following are needed:

1 child's direct laryngoscope.

1 double bronchoscopic battery.

1 laryngeal alligator forceps, (Mosher's).
1 bite block.
Tracheotomy instruments.

These are the bare necessities. The author prefers to prepare for a bronchoscopy also, with sponge holders, sponges and bronchoscopic forceps complete, as will be given on a future page; because very often the cause of the trouble may not be found in the larynx and not to investigate the trachea leaves a doubt. If children be examined in the recumbent position and fasting there will be little trouble with secretions, consequently swabs and aspirators will not be absolutely necessary for mere diagnostic examinations of the larynx only. On the other hand, if the child has had food or water within four hours, fluid from the stomach will be plentiful. If examined in the sitting position, which is always inadvisable in children, there may be much trouble from fluids overflowing into the larynx. Under no circumstances should the endoscopist start to examine a case of supposed foreign body in the larynx with only a laryngoscopic outfit. Everything needed for a direct laryngoscopy, bronchoscopy and esophagoscopy should be ready in order to get the intruder wherever it may be.

For operative work on the child's larynx, such as the removal of papillomata, we must add to the above list:

4 sponge holders.
2 dozen of 9 mm. sponges.
Tissue forceps.

Tracheotomy instruments are listed and should always be sterile and ready. Not that the procedure itself would ever, in any normal child, render tracheotomy necessary; but so many of the diseases for which a child is laryngoscoped diagnostically are stenotic in character that the endoscopist should be prepared for a tracheotomy.

Direct laryngoscopy of children as compared to direct laryngoscopy of adults. A child is more difficult to examine without anesthesia than the easiest of adults with local anesthesia; but there is little difference between one child and another, and any child is easier without anesthesia than the more difficult adults with good local anesthesia. Any human being, however, can be satisfactorily laryngoscoped directly if his mouth can be opened. In children, the difficulties of direct laryngoscopy are not increased by smallness of the tube, for the lumen of the child's laryngoscope of the author's design, is plenty large (1 cm.). The difficulties lie rather in the very flexible epiglottis of children, and the fact that the entire larynx, though relatively higher than in the adult, is more movable and has a greater tendency to retreat downward during ex

sels. Notwithstanding the reddishness due to engorgement, individual vessels are much less noticeable than in the adult, part of the difference being anatomic and part being due, probably, to the reflex engorgement during examination.

The size and especially the shape of the child's epiglottis vary very extensively. As the larynx is higher, depressing (elevating in the recumbent patient) the tongue strongly will sometimes cause it to project upward in full view (Fig. 1, Plate II). Often it retreats quickly and looks more like Fig. 95. It is usually more curved laterally than in the adult and the lateral margins may curl backward until they meet forming a cylinder.

In children the first view that one gets of the larynx is often similar to A, Fig. 94, where the epiglottis is seen curled up and below it

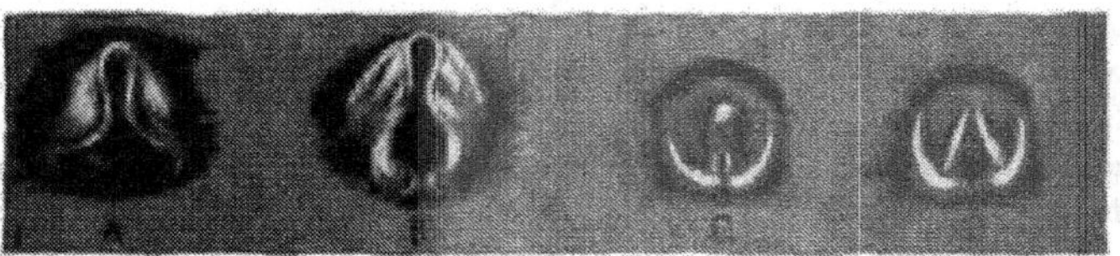

FIG. 94.—Direct laryngoscopic views in children. Recumbent position. A. Larynx exposed by elevation with the spatular tip in the glossoepiglottic fossa, anterior to the tongue. The curled epiglottis hides all but the two arytenoid eminences and the glottis is spasmodically closed. B. Same position glottis open. C. Congenital laryngeal web in a child simulating a neoplasm when glottis is spasmodically closed. D. Same patient, deep inspiration.

are seen the arytenoid eminences. Nothing can be seen of the cords because the larynx is in a state of spasm. The normal infantile epiglottis will curl up fully as much as seen in this drawing. Stronger traction upward on the base of the tongue will often expose the aryepiglottic folds continuous with the arytenoid eminence posteriorly and with the edge of the epiglottis anteriorly (B, Fig. 94). Under these circumstances, also, the cords may not be seen because they are covered by the spasmodic closure of the upper orifice of the larynx especially the ventricular band. At the next inspiration, however, the cords will separate and a good view down the trachea can often be obtained in this way, elevating the larynx with the spatular end in the glossoepiglottic fossa *anterior* to the epiglottis. As a rule, however, this examination is not so satisfactory, and it is better to proceed at once, as in the adult, after identifying the epiglottis, as at A, Fig. 95, to insert the laryngoscope sufficiently deeper to go posterior to the epiglottis and lift it (in the recumbent position) strongly as if to suspend the child by the hyoid bone, using only the *tip* of the spatular end on the posterior surface of the epiglottis. If the epiglottis slip away, the speculum must be inserted slightly deeper, but only enough to catch the epiglottis, and great care should be taken not to insert *too deeply*, as in that case the mouth of the esophagus will be entered and no amount of lifting with the tip will expose the larynx, as before explained. When properly exposed the child's larynx will look very much elongated antero-posteriorly and the arytenoid eminences will project upward and outward like the arms of a thick V. From the top of the arms of the V, the aryepiglottic folds extend forward. The cords are very much deeper down and are only visible on inspiration. (C, Fig. 95 which also shows subglottic papillomata.) If the larynx is lifted away from the posterior pharyngeal

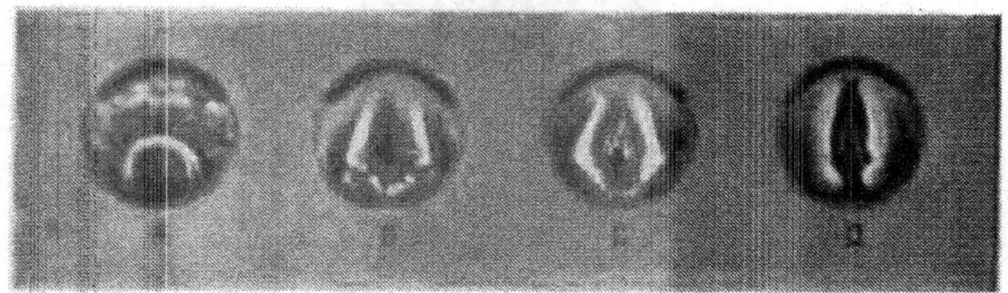

Fig. 95. Direct laryngoscopic views in children. A. Epiglottis. B. Glottis on [illegible] prevented from a wide inspiratory excursion by normal spasm at the [illegible] of the instrument in an examination without anesthesia. A few moments later [illegible] widely, and subglottic papillomata are visible as shown at C. D. Infolding of the upper laryngeal aperture in a moderate case of congenital [illegible] in an infant of [illegible] months.

[illegible] may become a thick based Y. This flaring shape of the up[illegible] the posterior commissure is best understood by contrasting [illegible] the infolded laryngeal aperture seen in congenital laryngeal [illegible] Plate II gives excellent views of the child's larynx [illegible] [illegible] glottic region can be seen well enough [illegible] [illegible] method described in this chapter. It, however [illegible] an excellent [illegible] without pass- [illegible] trachea, as for instance in a case in which [illegible] [illegible] tracheoscopy [illegible] tracheoscopy [illegible] bronchoscopy [illegible] through the glottis. When the mouth of such a tube is inserted in the upper orifice of the larynx (being introduced through the laryngoscope precisely as if doing a bronchoscopy) it will hold the vocal cords, exposing to view the entire length of the trachea, the vocal cords showing slightly at the edge of the endoscopic picture. (Fig. 96). It is necessary to make slight pressure on the tracheoscope, which must be too large to go through. This was discovered in one of the author's earliest cases of foreign body, before he had perfected his equipment, and the only instrument available in a distant city was a short tracheoscope of 8 mm. internal diameter. A safety-pin was thus removed with a hook from the trachea of a twelve months old infant (Bib. 264). To realize the mechanism of supraglottic tracheoscopy it is necessary to understand

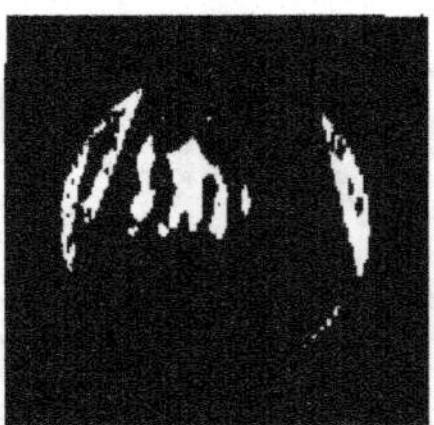

FIG. 96.—Endoscopic image obtained by supraglottic tracheoscopy. A tracheoscope or esophagoscope or bronchoscope whose distal end is not slanted and whose diameter is too great to go through the glottis of the child is inserted in the upper orifice of the larynx which is thus propped open. The widely spread cords are shown at the sides. This patient was suspected of having subglottic hypertrophy but on tracheoscopy was found to have a thymic compression stenosis. A lateral thymic compression as here shown is exceedingly rare. Usually this form of compression is anteroposterior.

the usually overlooked depth of the larynx above the cords. It is into this funnel that the tube-mouth is inserted. Supraglottic tracheoscopy could be used for the cauterization of subglottic hypertrophies but direct laryngoscopy, as elsewhere explained, gives more lateral room in which to work. Supraglottic tracheoscopy is useful in the removal of long-pedicled subglottic growths that flop above and below the rima glottidis.

*Indirect laryngoscopy with the Hays pharyngoscope.** The Hays pharyngoscope is an instrument which can be used either for the examination of the naso-pharynx or the larynx. It is composed of a small telescope (similar to the cystoscope) which is enclosed in a flat metal

*Written by Harold M. Hays, M. D. For further details the reader is referred to the interesting articles of Hays, Beck, Friedenwald and others.

sheath, in which run wires which connect with small electric bulbs situated at the distal end on either side of the prismatic lens. At right angles to this flat piece is a handle which connects with the rheostat.

The instrument is used like a tongue depressor and for the examination of the larynx may be employed in one of three ways.

(1) The distal end is inserted behind the soft palate with the lens turned up. The patient is then told to close the teeth and lips over the instrument and relax the muscles of the throat. One thus obtains a view of the naso-pharynx. If the lens is then turned either to the right or left through a half circle a view of the larynx can be obtained.

(2) The lens is turned down instead of up and the instrument inserted until the distal end almost touches the pharyngeal wall. The mouth is then closed as in the first instance.

(3) In many instances a larger and better view of the larynx can be obtained if the tongue is held by the examiner in the same way as if the laryngeal mirror was going to be used. The instrument is then dipped down towards the larynx until it is just over and behind the epiglottis. An excellent view of the larynx may be obtained in this way.

Operations on the larynx can often be performed by the indirect method, using the pharyngoscope instead of the mirror. The chief advantage of this method is that the operator does not have to work at right angles to his line of vision. In operating in this way the pharyngoscope should be inserted laterally as in method three, and the operative instruments from the opposite side of the mouth. [As the instrument is of fixed focus, the observer should wear his reading glasses.—Author.]

CHAPTER VIII.

Suspension Laryngoscopy.

A—HISTORICAL.

Over the portals of the Anatomical Institute at Freiburg in Breisgau is written in golden letters: "Mortui vivos docent"—the dead are the teachers of the living. This expression may likewise be applied to suspension-laryngoscopy, which originated in the Freiburg Anatomical Institute as a result of observations on the cadaver.

In the winter of 1909-10 I had my artist there produce the picture obtained by direct laryngoscopy upon the cadaver. I utilized the old broad Kirstein spatula on an electric handle and introduced it with the head pendant. As I did not have the time to hold the instrument until the artist had completed his picture I improvised a fixation-apparatus with several iron rods which were attached to the dissecting table. I attached the handle to the rods. Thus the head of the cadaver hung suspended from the mouth-spatula. The mouth was forced widely open. The teeth of the upper jaw were missing. I had a comprehensive view into the depths and was astonished at the excellent birds-eye view of the entire topographical relationship of the mouth and pharyngeal cavity, as well as of the larynx obtained at one glance. I was even able to see into the hypopharynx and, as the larynx was raised from the vertebral column, through the esophageal opening into the esophagus. The situation was about as discernible as in Fig. 97. Laterally from the broad tongue-spatula the tongue arches. We recognize the posterior pharyngeal wall from the uvula to the esophageal opening in its entire length and breadth. In the depth the large cornua of the hyoid bone project on the right and left. The posterior surface of the larynx is visible in its entire area. Of the laryngeal cavity the posterior surface is particularly well seen. Only the anterior sections of the vocal cords are invisible.

*Especially written by Prof. Killian for this book. Translated by J. A. Hageman, M. D.

This experience set me to thinking. It showed me how one must proceed to obtain a broad entry to the depths of the neck. It pointed a way to the fulfillment of a wish I had long harbored—to find a broad entrance to the laryngeal cavity in order to operate there as gynecologists do in their field. But there was still a long journey to the successful consummation of the procedure upon the living. At first I deemed profound narcosis absolutely essential in order to relax the parts as thoroughly as in the cadaver. As sufficient opportunity to narcotize patients for such purpose was not afforded, I made no progress. During

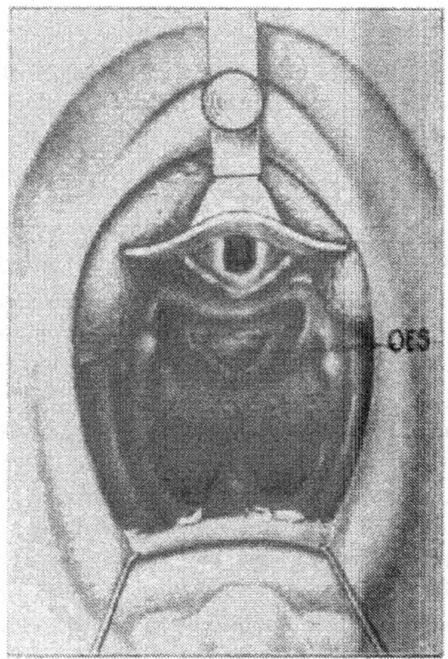

Fig. 97.

the following winter I therefore proceeded to practice upon two clinic patients using only cocaine. These experiments gave me opportunity to construct a fitting instrumentarium, thereby consuming much time. Not until the fall of 1911 had I made sufficient progress to enable me to issue a statement at the International Laryngological Congress in Berlin concerning suspension-laryngoscopy.

The time was very opportune for the further elaboration of the method because of my appointment as Director of the Berlin Laryngological Polyclinic. There I had sufficient material at my disposal to elaborate the new procedure practically in all its minutiae. New instruments were constantly constructed, altered or abandoned. Now I have finally reached the point where I can regard the method as matured.

Since then I have spoken and written about suspension-laryngoscopy. and have often demonstrated it. The procedure has been used by my pupils, Albrecht and Hoelscher, and also by Brieger and Seiffert, Wolff, Hinsberg and Kleestadt, Gerber and Henke, Lautenschlaeger, Storat, Kahler, Katzenstein, Hopmann and Froning, Chiari, Steiner, Pollatscheck, Simoleki, Davis and Howarth, Freudenthal, Iglauer. Through their collaboration the method has attained great clinical importance.

B—INSTRUMENTS.

Whoever desires to familiarize himself with suspension-laryngoscopy must primarily know the instrumentarium thoroughly. I therefore begin with a description of them.

1—THE OPERATING TABLE.

As this method is frequently used, it is desirable to have an operating table particularly suited to this purpose. It should have qualities which make it most practical for the execution of direct examination, and if possible, should be convenient for the numerous operations nowadays performed in laryngology and rhinology. I have, therefore, constructed a new table.*

It seems desirable that the operator should be able to adjust the table itself or at least to change its position. For this reason all cranks were affixed to the head-end of the table. I have always found it very uncomfortable to sit on a stool or kneel and assume a stooped position while using the ordinary operating-table. It is very exhausting. Direct examination should be made while sitting on a chair, or while standing. Therefore the operating-table should be so constructed that it can be sufficiently elevated by means of a screw. Kahler has already built such a table for the Vienna Laryngological Clinic. Mine is somewhat simpler; by means of a screw one can elevate it as much as desired. Besides, it is so arranged that one can securely attach the suspension-appliance. I have likewise attached a separate supporting-apparatus for the head. Further particulars may be gleaned from Figs. 98, 99 and 100. Fig. 98 shows the table in ordinary position, Fig. 99 in high position. In Fig. 100 one sees it from the head-end together with the various screws by means of which the changes of position are made. I need not dilate upon the minutiae of construction. These are based upon simple principles and are evident in practical use.

*All the instruments here minutely described may be obtained from the firms Windler, in Berlin, and Fischer, in Freiburg I. Br.

2—THE GALLOWS.

The gallows is intended to provide a suitable suspension-point. I have used it as it stands now, for two years without altering it in any way. It essentially consists of a column (Fig. G) bearing a horizontal arm (a). The arm extends to the middle of the operating-table. It may be fixed higher or lower, forward or backward. The elevation is chiefly adjusted by transposing the column. In addition the horizontal arm may be changed 20 cm. within the column. The forward and back-

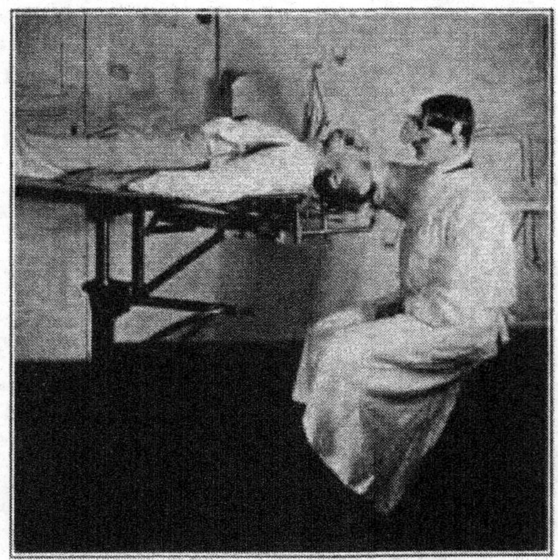

Fig. 98.

ward motion of the entire contrivance is accomplished by means of a screw (b) (compare Figs. 101 and 102). The gallows is screwed to the operating-table on the right in the manner shown in Figs. 99 and 116.

3—THE SUSPENSION-HOOK.

The suspension-hook was formerly more simple in form. It consisted of a straight rod which was curved at the upper end in the form of a hook. (Fig. 103 and 104). Compare my essay in "*Archiv für Laryngologie,*" Vol. 26, 1912. According to Albrecht's investigations, however, it was found necessary to put a joint in the rod (compare Fig. 104a). Within this joint a backward turning of the hook takes place about a horizontal axis (compare Fig. 106). This movement is accomplished when one turns the thumb-screw clockwise. In this manner the hook may be turned almost to a horizontal position. The mechanism is based upon the principle of the endless screw. The portion below the joint shows several peculiarities. The rectangular cavity (e) contains the screw. (Fig. 105f). The tongue-spatulas are attached to the pegs (g). The screw (h) holds the epiglottis-spatula. An attachment which holds the mouth open, a sort of mouth-gag also is supplementary to the suspension-hook (compare Fig. 105). It is provided with a tooth-plate (k) which rests against the upper incisors. This tooth-plate is so

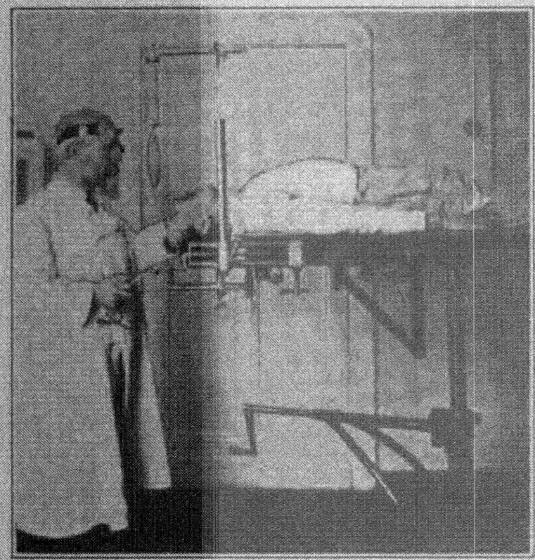

Fig. 99.

arranged, (Lautenschlaeger), that it may be extended or shortened. This is accomplished by means of the screw (h). The screw-end of the handle is inserted into the part (d) of the hook-spatula, and is securely fixed there by means of the screw (f) as shown in Fig. 106. By turning the screw (f) the handle (i) may be variously placed. In this manner the patient's mouth may be opened as wide as seems desirable.

4—THE TONGUE-SPATULA.

The tongue-spatula has in the course of time undergone many modifications, but we now possess a model which meets all demands. In its construction I have adopted the alterations which Albrecht proposed.

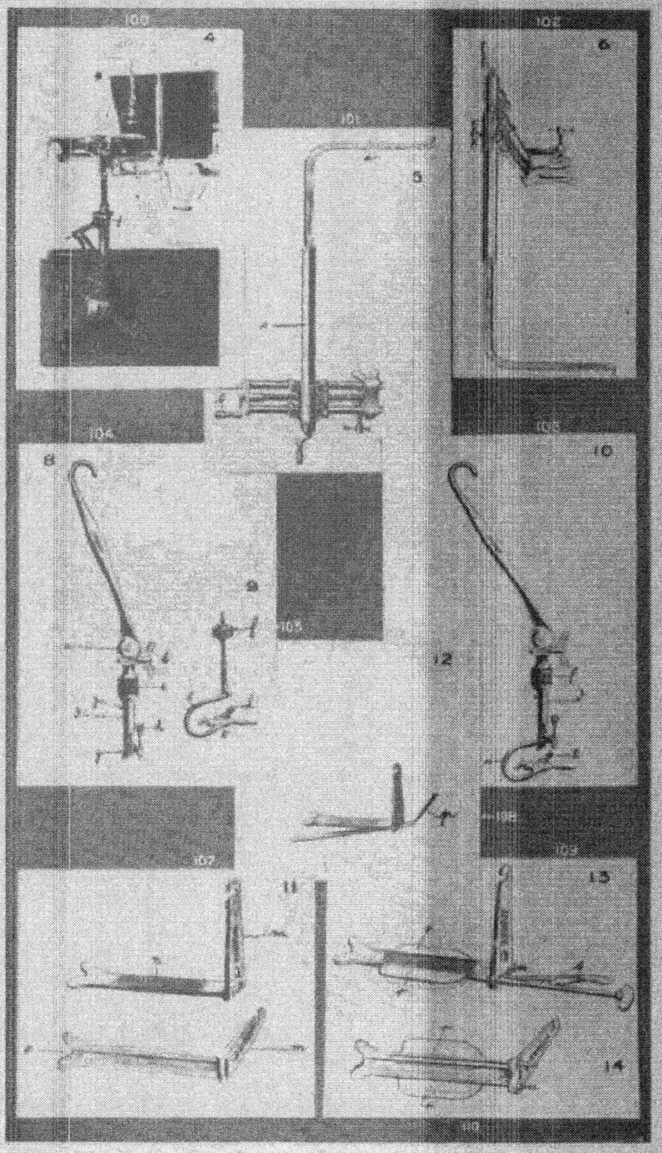

Figs. 100, 101, 102, 104, 105, 106, 107, 108, 109, 110.

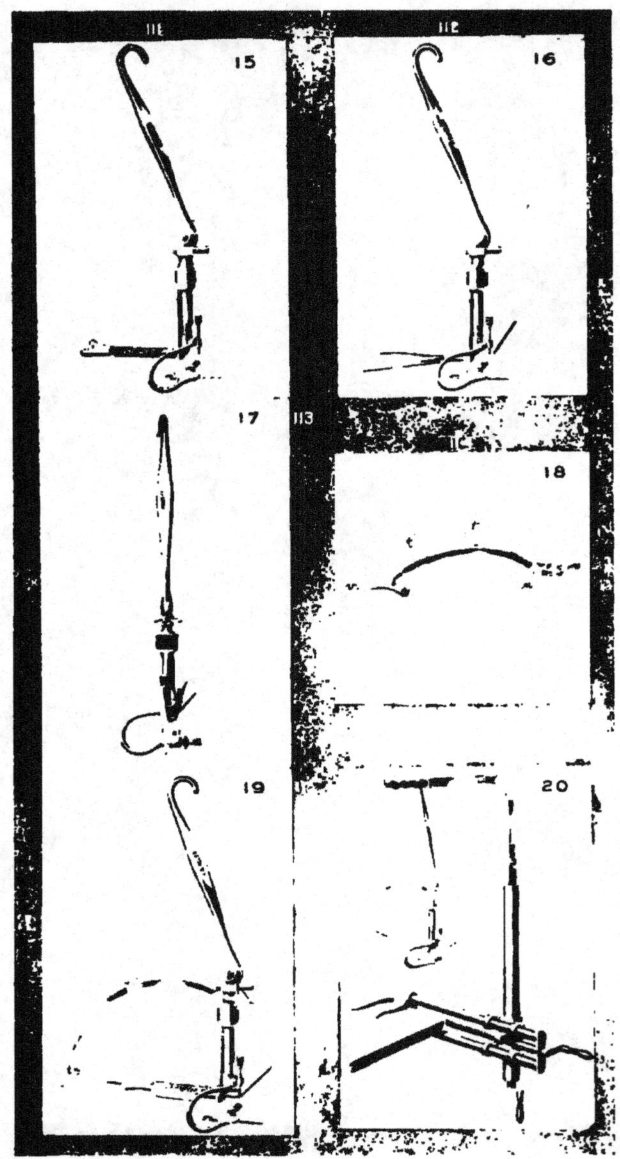

Figs. 111 to 116.

Of late a series of details were added. The tongue-spatula must be a simple instrument which has a peculiarly formed handle for attachment to the suspension-hook, (m) Fig. 107; the upper surface which is directed toward the tongue is rough (Fig. 107n), so that the spatula will not slip off. Its anterior end is heart-shaped after the model of the Reichert hook for raising the epiglottis (Fig. 119). On the free surface of the tongue-spatula one observes a gutter (o). Into this gutter

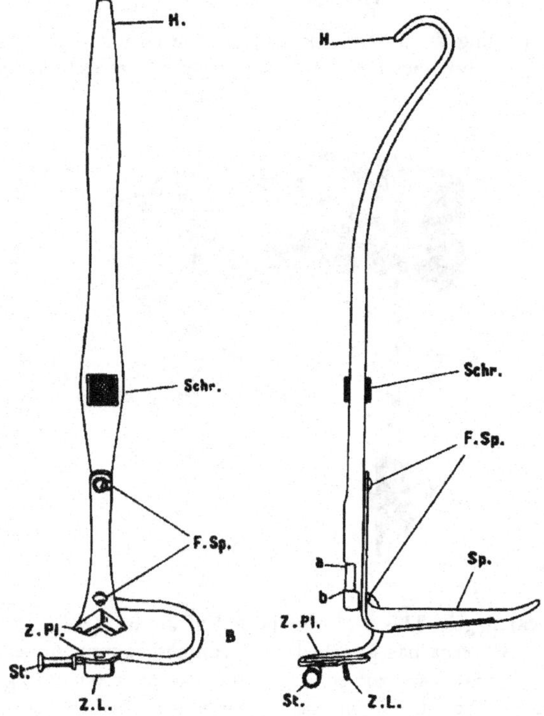

Fig. 103.

is placed a second smaller spatula, by means of which the epiglottis is raised, the epiglottis-spatula (p) Fig. 108. It is inserted through a groove, Fig. 108. If the patient's tongue wells up to the right and left of the spatula, it hinders vision into the depths of the neck. I therefore have recently had two movable lateral wings attached to the tongue-spatula (r) (Fig. 109 and Fig. 110). These wings may be turned by means of a key (Fig. 109r) and (Fig. 109 and Fig. 110) fixed in any position. The key (s) is removed after the fixation of the plates. In Fig. 108 we see the tongue-spatula in connection with the epiglottis-spatula. In Fig. 111 the tongue-spatula is attached to the suspension-hook. In Fig. 112 we see the tongue-spatula on the suspension-hook with the epiglottis-spatula as seen from the side. Fig. 113 shows a front view of the same.

5—THE COUNTER-PRESSOR.

In order to bring the anterior portions of the larynx within the range of vision it often becomes necessary to exert pressure externally against

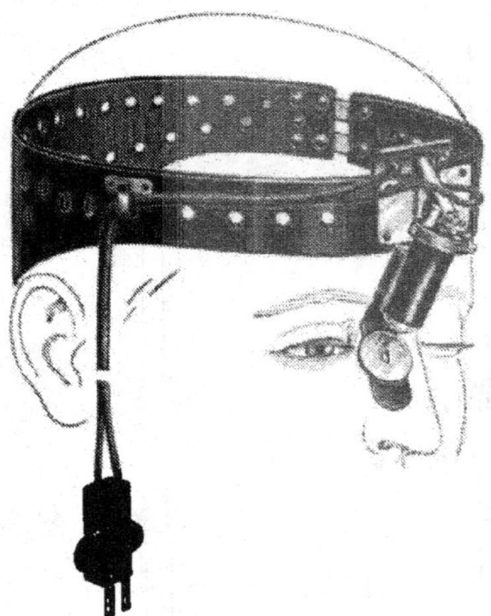

Fig. 117.

the cricoid cartilage. This requires the aid of an assistant. In order to obviate this, Albrecht has attached the Brünings counter-pressor to his instrument. I have constructed a counter-pressor upon new principles (Fig. 114). It consists of two parts, t and t, which can be telescoped into each other, and may thus be lengthened or shortened. It may also be turned upon a horizontal axis at u. It is attached to the portion of the suspension-hook directly over the screw (Fig 115). After the suspension-hook is connected with all its supplementary instruments it is suspended from the gallows as shown in Fig. 116. In this position it is used during suspension-laryngoscopy. Whoever desires to make the examination successfully must first familiarize himself with the minutiae of my construction. Only in this manner is it possible to utilize all its advantages. The whole arrangement may appear somewhat complicated.

These complications, however, are necessary to ensure the best conditions for the prompt engagement of the larynx.

6—THE ILLUMINATION.

In laryngoscopical work the mouth and pharyngeal cavity are illuminated in the usual manner. One may use the head-mirror in connection with a good electric or gas lamp. I usually use the Kirstein head-lamp (Fig. 117). For demonstration purposes it is found very satisfactory to use a diminutive electric lamp whose light is concentrated by means of a lens attaching the light to the tooth-plate of the suspension-hook by means of a clamp. (Compare Figs. 122 and 123, Plate IV).

7—THE PERFORMING OF SUSPENSION-LARYNGOSCOPY.

Not every patient is adapted for the performance of suspension-laryngoscopy. All patients presenting difficulties during the use of the direct method are difficult to examine in the herein described manner, and it may prove impossible to do so at all. Generally speaking the number of such cases is small. In children one practically never meets with difficulties. In order to ascertain in advance if the patient can be comfortably examined, it is advisable to attempt a direct examination of the larynx with the simple Kirstein spatula. By this means one recognizes how far the tongue may be suppressed and the larynx engaged.

PREPARATION OF THE PATIENT.

Adults who are adaptable for the direct examination can be examined by means of suspension-laryngoscopy, using cocaine solely, although as a rule it is wise to administer a morphine injection (0.01-0.015) half an hour previously.

If one contemplates doing an operation which may consume more time and may possibly cause pain, it is better to make use of the morphine-scopolamine narcosis. Scopolamine is lately furnished by the firm Hoffmann-La Roche & Co., in Grenzach (Baden) in permanent form under the name "skopolamine haltbar, Roche." Three decimilligrams are hermetically enclosed in a small glass ampoule. This is the most suitable dose for our purposes.

The best procedure is to administer to the patient two hours before the suspension-laryngoscopy 0.01 gm. morphine and .0003 dcmgm. scopolamine hypodermically. One hour later the same quantity of both substances is again administered. The patient must recline in a quiet place, so that he will go to sleep. In most cases the numbing is only incomplete. But the patient is in such condition that he undergoes the examination without resistance and also bears it longer. It is necessary, too, to pencil the larynx with cocaine before using the spatula. The reflex-irritability of the pharyngeal and laryngeal mucous membrane is not entirely eliminated by the morphine and scopolamine.

Children and young persons must not receive any morphine-scopolamine. In childhood it is best to use ether or chloroform narcosis or a mixture of both. It is preferable to use the Braun insufflation-apparatus, because with it one more rapidly attains a sufficiently profound narcosis, and above all, because the narcosis can easily be maintained sufficiently profound during the manipulation in the neck. (Fig. 119). To hold a mask before the face from time to time during the examination causes

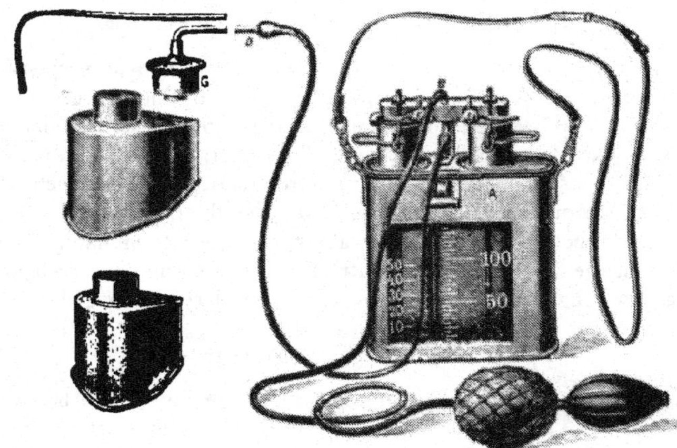

Fig. 118

too much interruption. But when one forces the ether or chloroform into the depths with the insufflator as much will be inhaled as is required to maintain an equable, deep narcosis.

In children, too, it is to be recommended to pencil the larynx with cocaine. By cocainizing, one avoids the reflex interference with breathing which occurs in some cases when one touches the interior of the larynx with an instrument. I generally use the laryngeal mirror and the Kirstein head-lamp when penciling the larynx in adults and children. If the larynx cannot readily be approached the lower jaw is pulled forward or the Reichert hook is inserted at the lingual base and the base of the tongue and the larynx are pulled forward by this means. (Fig. 119).

THE PREPARATION OF THE SUSPENSION-HOOK.

Preceding the introduction a tongue-spatula of suitable length must be selected—Kahler determines the length by means of a graduated Kirstein spatula (Fig. 120)—and connected with the suspension-hook. The handle with the tooth-plate is inserted in such manner that the mouth is forced open only slightly. The counter-pressor is folded upward. In addition it is necessary to move the hook so far backwards by means of the thumb-screw that its end comes to lie perpendicularly above the end of the tongue-spatula. In this form the instrument is introduced.

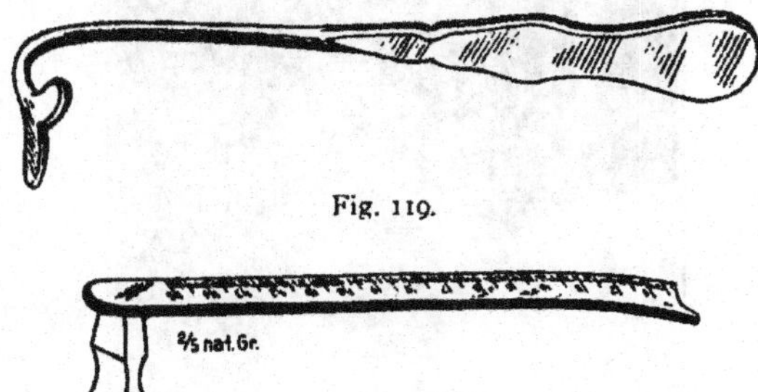

Fig. 119.

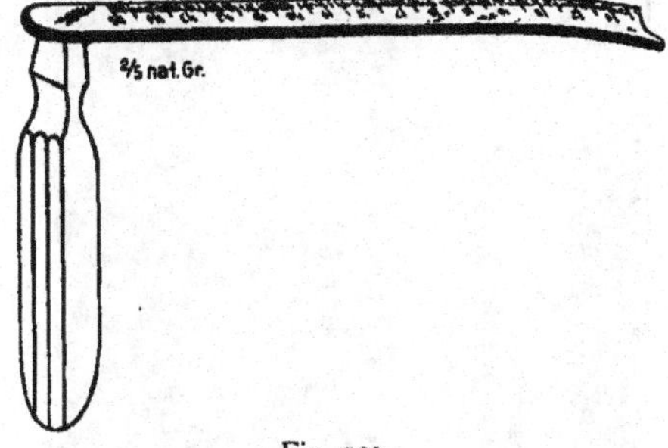

Fig. 120.

Before introducing the tongue-spatula the patient must be put in the proper position. The body is drawn so far upward that the head extends freely above the edge of the operating-table and can readily be lowered. At the same time an assistant holds the head in a slightly lowered position.

INTRODUCTION OF THE TONGUE-SPATULA.

Formerly I always used a special mouth-gag and had the tongue held with a forceps. Lately I avoid both whenever possible. As Seifert has demonstrated the mouth-gag or tongue-forceps is not essential. It is, however, advisable when introducing the spatula to some depth to have the tip of the tongue held, so that the spatula may not push the tongue too far into the depths.

Under illumination with the Kirstein head-lamp the spatula is introduced against the posterior pharyngeal wall and then downward along this wall between epiglottis and base of tongue. The base of the tongue is forced upward as much as possible, and the gallows is now so installed that the hook can be suspended from it. If one has been successful in this, the assistant gradually releases the patient's head, so that its whole weight presses upon the tongue-spatula.

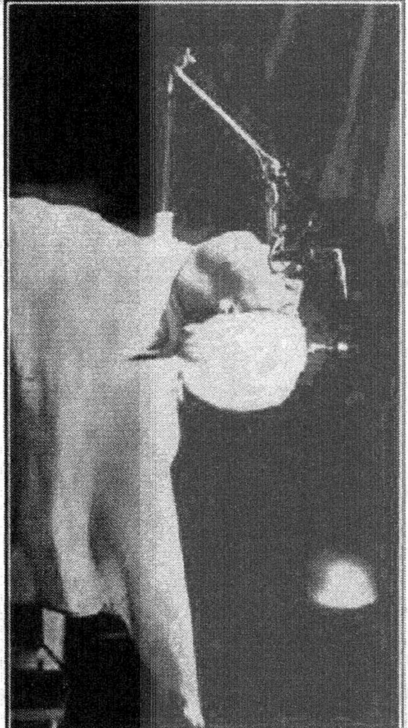

Fig. 121.

In most cases the interior of the larynx does not yet become visible in this position, the epiglottis covers it almost entirely. To elevate this the epiglottis-spatula is required.

As already stated above, the epiglottis-spatula is inserted through the groove in the tongue-spatula, and pushed into the depths under the epiglottis as far as possible. Then one elevates the epiglottis with it and secures the epiglottis-spatula with the screw. After this procedure the arytenoid region and the posterior laryngeal wall ordinarily come into view. It now becomes essential to accomplish the finer adjustment, so that the anterior portion of the larynx may also be seen. For this purpose we turn the thumb-screw clockwise, so that the hook drops even lower. Should this not prove sufficient one may press upon the cricoid cartilage with a finger, or accomplish this pressure with the counter-pressor by adjusting and fixing it at the proper spot. Now it is also time to remove the handle with the tooth-plate somewhat farther from the tongue-spatula and thereby force the mouth open as wide as possible. This is accomplished by turning the large screw (f) (Fig. 106).

If one has been successful in this manipulation the interior of the pharyngeal cavity must, with good illumination, lie in full view. The patient is then in a position as shown in Fig. 121. The head hangs freely suspended from the tongue-spatula; the mouth is held open by the handle with the tooth-plate. The portion of the hook bearing the screw extends approximately in a perpendicular position. The hook itself is turned sharply backward and so is suspended from the gallows. One sees the larynx as in Figs. 122 and 123, Plate IV.

D—DEMONSTRATION IN SUSPENSION LARYNGOSCOPY.

The new method is particularly adapted for demonstration. If the pharynx and larynx are engaged the demonstrator has nothing to do but make the necessary explanations. The pupil readily grasps the subject because he sees the parts directly before him. As above mentioned, it is best for such demonstrations to use a miniature electric lamp attached to the toothplate of the instrument. When the larynx is engaged during suspension laryngoscopy it is very easy to manipulate its interior. One can demonstrate this to the pupil by putting a probe in his hand and having him touch designated points.

Minor operations, for instance the removal of a polyp, can be demonstrated without much trouble. If the patient is under skopolamine-morphine "twilight sleep," the demonstration may be made, without hesitation to a very great number of physicians and students.

E—CLINICAL EXPERIENCES WITH SUSPENSION-LARYNGOSCOPY.

Suspension-laryngoscopy has been successfully applied in practice both in diagnostic and therapeutic respect by my pupils and by me as well as by a list of authors. It is used diagnostically especially in childhood and particularly in all those cases where we are compelled to resort to direct examinations. Its execution is so simple that I believe it will soon replace direct laryngoscopy. We often have occasion to make minute examination under narcosis in vocal and respiratory disturbances in children. One must determine if there exist a simple acute catarrh, a sub-glottic swelling, a croupous or diphtheritic process with formation of pseudo-membrane, a perichondritis, or if there be a foreign body present whether there be a chronic laryngitis, formation of nodules on the vocal cords, papillomata, tuberculosis or syphilis. Even cases of

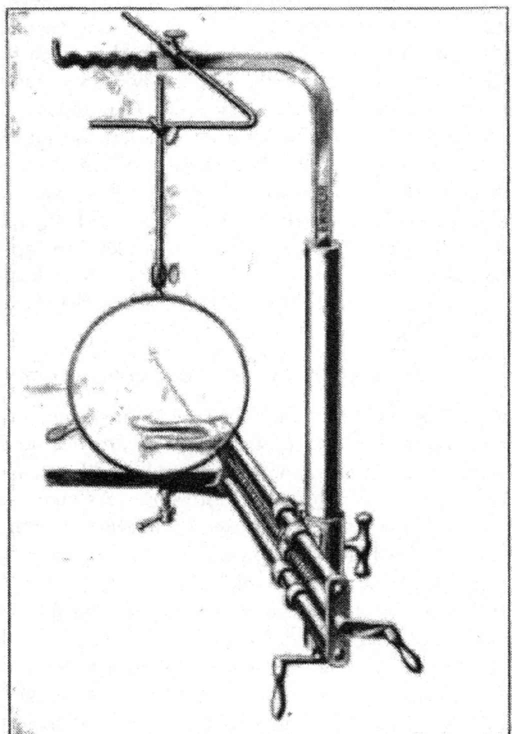

Fig. 124.

difficult decanulement or congenital changes in the larynx may be conveniently examined in suspension. I should like even at this stage, to recommend this procedure as a preparatory step for bronchoscopy and esophagoscopy in small children. With suspension-laryngoscopy one engages the larynx and then inserts the bronchoscopic or esophagoscopic tube into the depths. Narcosis can be maintained without special danger. Seiffert has shown that artificial respiration may be accomplished with the horizontal suspension-hook. One must never neglect to cocainize the larynx before inserting the instruments in order to eliminate the vagus-reflexes emanating from the laryngeal mucous membrane. With the introduction of a cold instrument into the uncocainized larynx temporary discontinuance of respiration may very readily occur.

THERAPEUTIC APPLICATION OF SUSPENSION-LARYNGOSCOPY IN CHILDHOOD.

a. *Foreign Bodies.*

Davis removed a safety-pin from the pharynx of an eleven-months-old child under suspension-laryngoscopy. My pupil, Weingaertner, recently succeeded in extracting a piece of bone which was lodged partly in

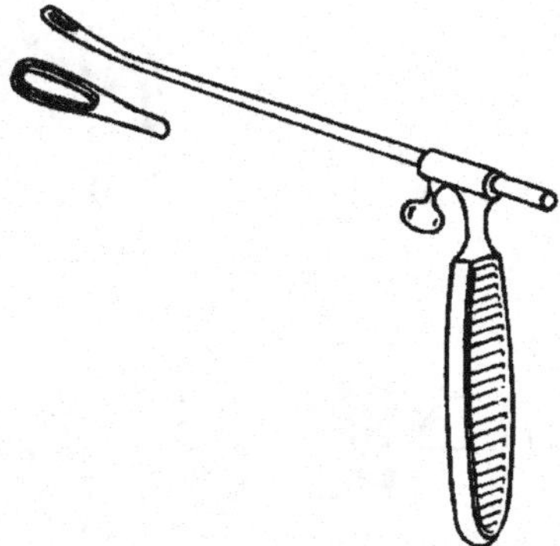

Fig. 125.

the pharynx and partly in the entrance to the larynx of a child one and one-half years old. Seiffert reports the removal of a flat bone from the sub-glottic space in a child of five years. Iglauer removed a piece of safety-pin which had been lodged in the larynx of a child for five months. All observers state that the location and extraction of foreign bodies offer no special difficulties. The condition is probably the same with deep-seated foreign bodies whether lodged in the esophagus or in the larynx or bronchus. A tube is projected into these organs—a very simple procedure during suspension-laryngoscopy. By means of suspension-laryngoscopy I succeeded in locating in and extracting from the right bronchus a metallic capsule. In the same manner I removed a nail which had been lodged for a year in the left bronchus of a two-year-old child. Both cases impressed upon me that this sort of bronchoscopy is easier and better.

LARYNGEAL PAPILLOMATA IN CHILDREN.

In my clinic we were able to gather extensive data bearing on this affection and its treatment. Albrecht has frequently and minutely reported on it. The new method not only permits a certain diagnosis but also a radical removal. Even if the larynx is entirely filled with papillomata, one can remove everything at one sitting. If the children are already dyspnoeic, suspension-laryngoscopy may still be carried out. Obviously the tracheotomy instruments must be in readiness. If one has succeeded in applying the suspension-hook one need no longer fear

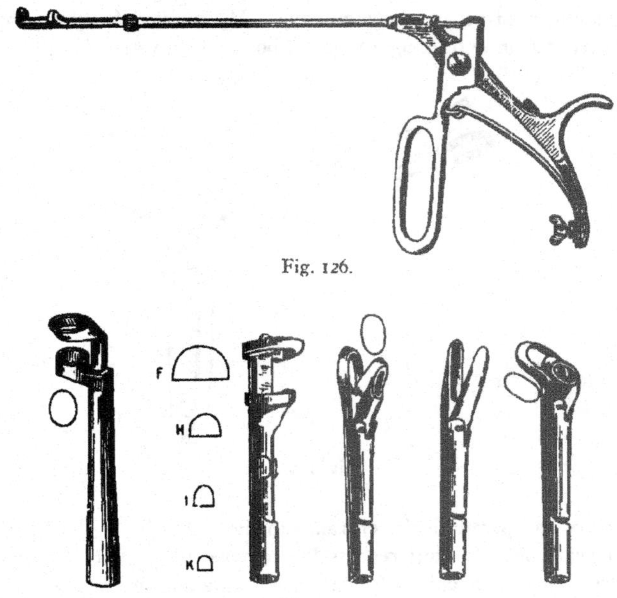

Fig. 126.

Fig. 127.

asphyxiation, for one can without further ado insert a bronchoscopic tube through the larynx and wait until respiration is again in progress. The larynx is always readily accessible in suspension. Obviously one must use narcosis. There is no contra-indication to repeat such sittings. As the papillomata readily recur, many cases require numerous sittings, sometimes even a long series of such. Sometimes one succeeds by means of internal remedies, such as iodide of potassium or arsenic, to prevent recurrences. Penciling with 10 per cent salicyl-alcohol has also been recommended. The mesothorium-treatment as a remedy against recur-

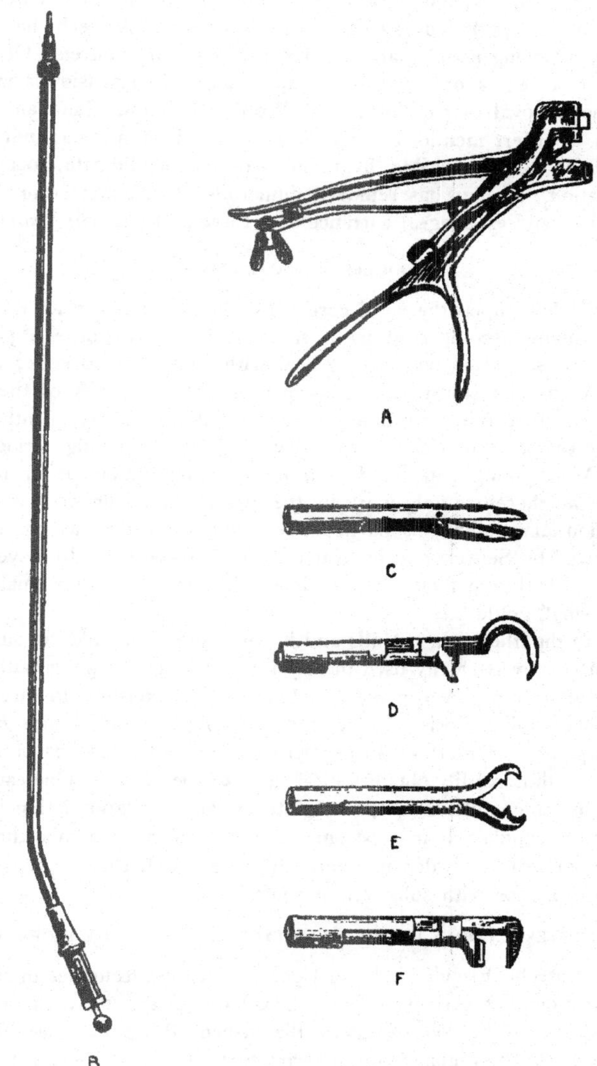

Fig. 128.

rences appears to me to be one of the most promising. However, we have not yet gathered any particular experience. Albrecht has succeeded in removing papillomata in a large number of children. Others, too, have reported favorably upon the application of suspension-laryngoscopy to the removal of papillomata, as Wolff, Kleestadt, Mann and Katzenstein. Seiffert mentions a case in which tracheotomy was indicated but in which it was possible, by removal of the papillomata, to avoid that operation. Kahler has removed numerous papillomata from the hypopharynx and esophageal entrance of a three and one-half year old child.

NODULES OF VOCAL CORDS.

Nodules upon the vocal cords of children are not at all rare. They are usually accompanied by a slight catarrh and cause a permanent hoarseness. Often we have to deal with children who suffer from imperfect nasal respiration in consequence of hypertrophy of the pharyngeal tonsils, turbinal swelling and septal deflections. Frequently one can prove that the children have cried very much for a long period.

Most young patients do not permit interventions in their larynx. One can therefore only work by the direct method under narcosis. Suspension-laryngoscopy is particularly adapted for this, as has been emphasized by Seiffert and by Katzenstein. My best results have likewise been with this method. The nodules are removed with a small forceps or a small guillotine.

In diphtheria, in syphilis and in tuberculosis in children, suspension-laryngoscopy is chiefly used merely for diagnostic purposes, although we have already begun to make curettements and excisions in rare cases of laryngeal tuberculosis. Difficult decanulement should more frequently prompt us to undertake suspension-laryngoscopy. As has been proved one can thus readily obtain a clear view of the larynx. One can also ascertain the conditions in the subglottic region and granulation-formation over the canula. It may become necessary to insert a tube through the rima glottidis in order to approach these granulations. Even Seiffert reports a case with subglottic granulations.

INTERVENTIONS IN THE ORO-PHARYNX AND IN THE ESOPHAGUS.

Albrecht, Freudenthal and I performed tonsillectomies in small children under narcosis by use of a broad tongue-spatula with the suspension-hook. When one works on the suspended head one sees the tonsils reversed. Their upper pole appears to be below. One must therefore accordingly change the technique. It is very convenient that hemorrhage causes no great trouble. The blood flows into the naso-pharynx and can be drawn by suction from there through the nose.

SUSPENSION-LARYNGOSCOPY IN ADULTS.

In the adult suspension-laryngoscopy is chiefly used in tuberculosis of the larynx, especially when one contemplates curetting a diseased portion. One will decide in favor of this method, especially in the cases of advanced laryngeal tuberculosis, for it puts us in position to undertake extensive work at one sitting, to curette, to nip off or even to make one or two deep galvanic punctures. It is very important that phthisic patients who are to enter a sanitarium be relieved of the most pronounced changes in the larynx.

Suspension-laryngoscopy can be carried out under local anaesthesia in such cases following administration of one morphine injection. In order to reduce the great reflex irritability of the tuberculous larynx, how-

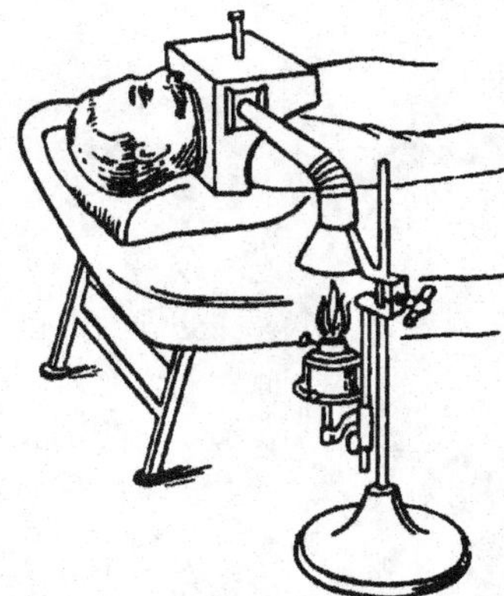

Fig. 129.

ever, it is advisable in just such cases to make use of the skopolamin-morphine "twilight sleep." We have never seen serious disadvantages from it. On the other hand, narcosis does not seem to be especially well borne by some tuberculars.

When a tuberculous larynx has been engaged with the suspension-hook, it is advisable to attach a glass shield to the gallows before beginning the currettement so that tuberculous material may not be coughed into one's face (compare Fig. 124).

For curettement I have had a reversible curette constructed (Fig. 125). The nipping off of infiltrations and granulations is done with the ordinary double-curette for direct operations (compare Fig. 126 and 127). In cases of hemorrhage, clamps may be applied (Fig. 128).

The galvano-caustic deep puncture may be executed with great security. An ordinary pointed cautery electrode which must be at least

20 cm. in length is used for this purpose. Then the larynx is painted with hydrogen peroxide and insufflated with vioform or anesthesin.

The subsequent manipulation in the larynx must be under guidance of the laryngeal mirror. After major incursions oedema may readily

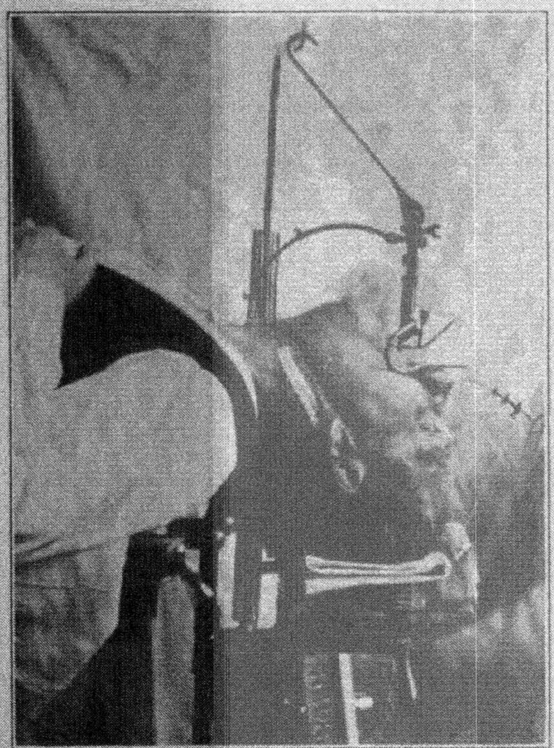

Fig. 130.

occur. For successfully combating such incidents we now have an excellent remedy in the hot-air-chest of Albrecht which can be used again the same day if necessary. (Fig. 129). Temperatures up to 110 degrees Celcius can be applied. The skin of the neck bears this dry heat very well if the chest is well lined with asbestos-fibre. A strongly active hyperaemia results and the oedemas are re-absorbed. The procedure has an anodyne effect. Of course the patient always complains of pain during the first few days. This is caused not alone by the wounds in the larynx, but also by the pressure-effect of the lingual and laryngeal spatulas. One also frequently observes temperature-elevations of minor or greater degree, which very readily occur from various causes in tubercular patients. They soon subside. I prefer in the after-treatment, to give iodine internally and peroxide of hydrogen locally. It is also advantageous to continue treating the cleansed wounds of the larynx with lactic acid.

Obviously the result of such operative treatment depends upon the state of the lungs and the general condition. Patients who can immediately receive sanatorium treatment have good chances of cure if the larynx be primarily affected.

By adopting radical measures in the larynx, tracheotomy has often been obviated (Holscher, Seiffert, Freudenthal). Exposure of the tuberculous larynx to Roentgen-rays through the lumen has also been successfully accomplished in suspension-laryngoscopy by Brieger and his pupil, Seiffert.

In difficult cases of polyps of the vocal cords, especially when the polyps were located far anteriorly, Hoelscher and Steiner used suspension-laryngoscopy with the best results. E. Mayer has successfully removed a carcinoma of the epiglottis under suspension-laryngoscopy. It has further been applied in scleroma, and even in hysterical aphonia.

A new field has arisen for it in mesothorium treatment of laryngeal-carcinoma, about which I have recently made a report. By means of suspension-laryngoscopy not only can the small mesothorium-capsule be applied to the diseased spot introduced into the carcinoma under skopolamine-morphine narcosis, but especially the sitting may be extended sufficiently long. The patient may be left in suspension one hour, or even one and one-half hours (probably even longer) without compunction (Fig. 130).

The mesothorium-capsule is provided with an aluminum-filter attached to a cord and inserted into the larynx with an ordinary claw-forceps. The instrument is secured with cords or clamps. Thus it will remain quietly in position the entire time. During the first days there is generally a light inflammatory reaction, but the improvement in the carcinomatous condition is soon apparent.

Suspension-laryngoscopy is peculiarly adapted for examining and treating operatively changes in the lower pharynx. True, one ordinarily requires the additional help of a dilator to separate the larynx from the spinal-column. Seiffert has reported more in detail regarding this aspect. I am not able, at this time, to state how extensively esophagoscopy may be used in the adult in suspension. Apparently this procedure is of great advantage in the removal of voluminous foreign bodies which are wedged within range of the esophageal opening or immediately below it (Brieger). Seiffert reports the removal of a coin from the hypopharynx in two small children. He also was successful in the removal of a lipoma from the hypopharynx during suspension.

CHAPTER IX.

Introduction of the Bronchoscope.

The description of the introduction of the bronchoscope given in some of the text-books would lead one to suppose that the procedure is difficult and some books even go so far as to say that, if after fifteen minutes' trial the operator fails to introduce the instrument, a tracheotomy should be done for introduction. This state of affairs is almost inconceivable. No one should do bronchoscopy until he is able laryngoscopically to expose the glottis with the left hand in not more than one minute, and having learned this, it ought not to require over one minute more to introduce the bronchoscope into the trachea. The usual time should be from fifteen to thirty seconds, depending on how long the patient holds his breath (if not anesthetized), before taking a deep inspiration. This length of time applies to infants as well as adults. Whatever may be said of the difficulties of bronchoscopy in infants, because of the smallness of the tube, it does not apply to the introduction of the bronchoscope by the author's method, because of the large diameter of the author's laryngoscope for infants (12 mm.). This size is possible because the laryngoscope by the author's method does not go ***through*** the larynx—simply exposes its upper orifice to view. Once the larynx is properly exposed there should be no difficulty in introducing even the 4 mm. tube. This is not mentioned boastfully nor as urging hasty procedure: but rather to urge the necessity of abundant practice in left-handed laryngoscopic exposure of the glottis.

INTRODUCTION OF THE BRONCHOSCOPE, PATIENT SITTING.

For the introduction of the bronchoscope in the sitting position, the patient is usually locally anesthetized, the details for which are given in a separate chapter. This position is advisable only in adults and only for diagnosis. The position of operator, patient and assistants is pre-

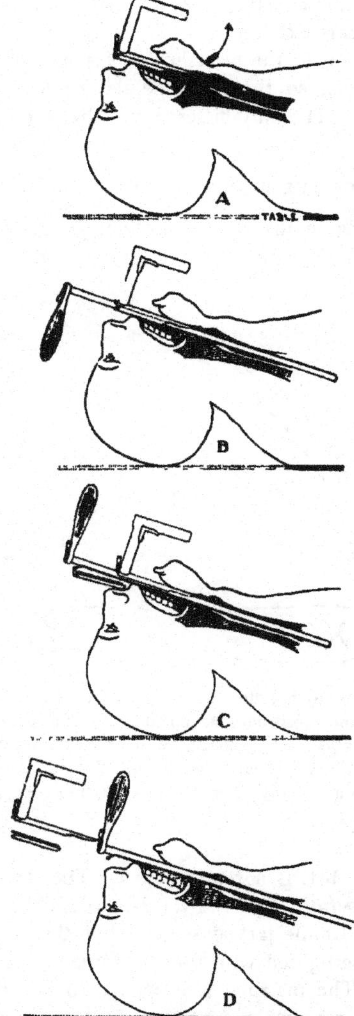

FIG. 131.—Schema illustrating oral bronchoscopy. The portion of the table here shown under the head is, in actual work, dropped all the way down perpendicularly. It appears in these drawings as a dotted line to emphasize the fact that the head must be above the level of the table during introduction of the bronchoscope into the trachea. A, exposure of larynx. B, bronchoscope introduced. C, slide removed. D, laryngoscope removed leaving bronchoscope alone in position. The handle of the laryngoscope in C and D should be shown as rotated down to the left as shown in Fig. 131a.

cisely the same as for direct laryngoscopy, as shown in Fig. 70 and described in the adjacent text. After the larynx is exposed as there described the introduction of the bronchoscope is precisely the same as in the recumbent position, so that the one description of the procedure will answer for both. The only difference is that the laryngeal image is sagitally reversed.

INTRODUCTION OF THE BRONCHOSCOPE. RECUMBENT PATIENT.

The patient being in the Boyce position, as illustrated in Figs. 72 and 73, the glottis is exposed with the laryngoscope as shown in Fig.

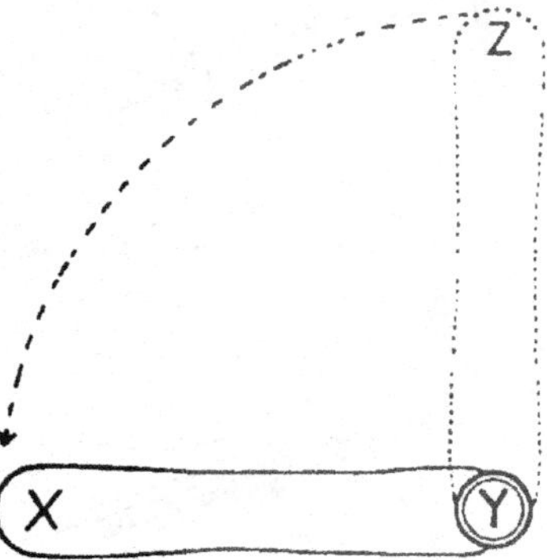

FIG. 131a.—Before removing the slide the handle of the laryngoscope should be moved to the left from position Z to position X, rotating the laryngoscope 90 degrees on its tubular axis (Y). This movement clears the slide of all contact so that it comes off quickly. Used thus, the regular laryngoscope (Fig. 14) is preferable to the side-slide or any form of open laryngoscope for the introduction of bronchoscopes.

92, of which A, Fig. 131, is a reproduction. The same thing is shown in Fig. 132. The operator watches the larynx which is brilliantly illuminated by the light of the laryngoscope, while the first assistant hands him the bronchoscope lighted with its own lamp. (No warming or oiling is necessary). The instrument is passed to the operator, properly pointed toward the proximal end of the speculum so that the operator has but to reach up his right hand, grasp the bronchoscope and start it in, catching the handle of the bronchoscope that is passed to him by the assistant. The bronchoscope is inserted with the handle horizontally to the right (Fig. 133). The eye is now transferred from the laryngoscope to the bronchoscope, and the bronchoscope is advanced until the

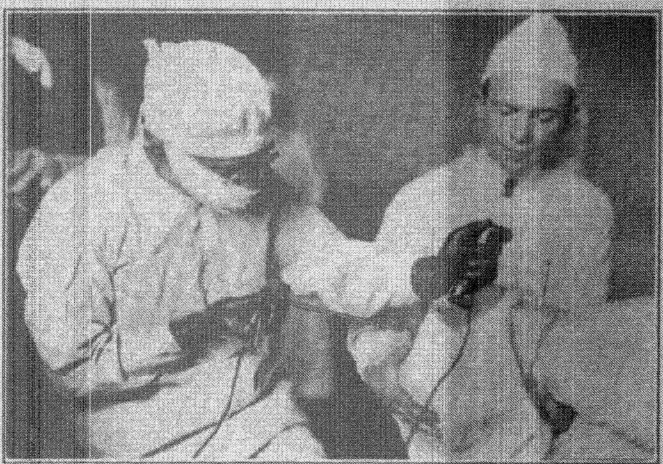

Fig. 132.—Exposure of the larynx of the recumbent patient. The operator is lifting strongly in the direction of the dart.

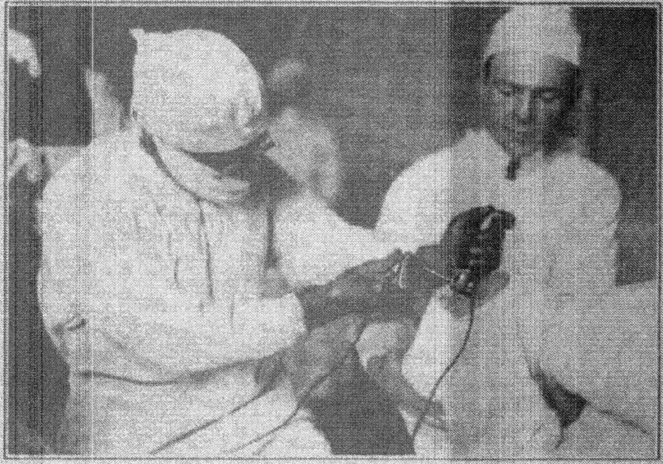

Fig. 133.—Insertion of the bronchoscope. Note direction of the trachea as indicated by the bronchoscope. Note that the patient's head is held above the level of the table. The assistant's left hand should be at the patient's mouth holding the bite-block. This is removed and the assistant is on the wrong side of the table in the illustration in order not to hide the position of the operator's hands. Note the handle of the bronchoscope is to the right.

inner end approaches quite closely to the glottis. If no anesthesia is used, it is to be preferred that the distal end of the bronchoscope does not touch the larynx lest an excess of spasm be excited, which would delay the insertion. The handle of the bronchoscope is now moved slightly to the right so as to throw the lip of the slanted end over into the median line of the glottic chink, as will be understood from Fig. 134. This

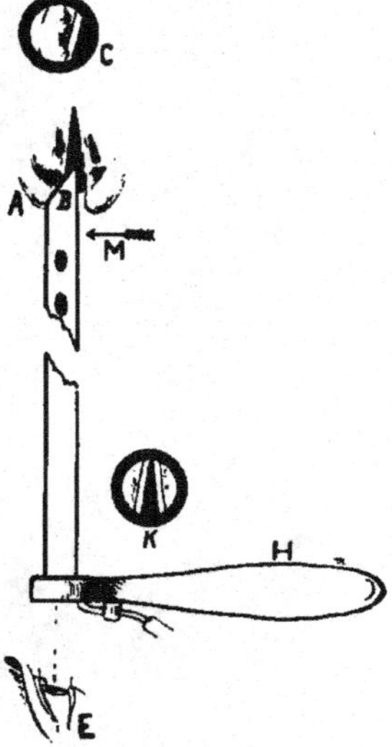

FIG. 134.—Schema illustrating the introduction of the bronchoscope through the glottis, recumbent patient. The handle, H, is always horizontally to the right. When the glottis is first seen through the tube it should be centrally located as at K. At the next inspiration the end, B, is moved horizontally to the left as shown by the dart, M, until the glottis shows at the right edge of the field, C. This means that the point of the lip, B, is at the median line and it is then quickly (not violently) pushed through into the trachea. At this same moment or the instant before, the hyoid bone is given a quick additional lift with the tip of the laryngoscope as shown by the dart (Fig. 132) and at A in Fig. 131. In the sitting patient everything is the same except that the laryngeal image is reversed sagittally and laterally.

sliding over should preferably be done at the moment that an inspiration starts, so that the bronchoscope can be, at the same time, inserted through the glottis. Herein lies a great advantage in the slanted end, because it is very much easier to insinuate the lip of the slanted end through the chink, than to insert the end of a tube which is squarely cut off. Care should be taken not to allow the tube to become hooked over the arytenoid, though there is less likelihood of this in bronchoscopy than there is in esophagoscopy. No great force should be used, because if the bronchoscope does not go through readily either the tube is too large in size or it is not correctly placed. On the other hand, the tube does not normally go through without slight resistance, and the laryngologist or rhinologist who has been trained to manipulative procedures, will very readily determine by his sense of touch the degree of pressure necessary, and will not use a degree that will inflict trauma. If the attempt is made to insert a 5 mm. tube through the glottis of an infant under one year, there may be considerable resistance, and if so, subglottic edma is quite likely to follow forcible introduction. On the other hand, a 4 mm. tube should go through with practically no resistance, if properly placed. Once through the glottis (B, Fig. 131) the direct laryngoscope should be removed as shown schematically at C, Fig. 131. The laryngoscope is turned sidewise just before removal (Fig. 131a) so that the slide will not impinge on the upper teeth. Care must be taken that the bronchoscope is not allowed to be coughed out during the removal of the speculum. The bronchoscope is most easily held in place by the thumb of the left hand of the operator, while the thumb and finger of the right hand are used to remove the slide. At the moment of insertion of the bronchoscope through the glottis, an especially strong upward lift with the beak of the spatula is usually necessary in order to permit the bronchoscope to be given also a forward tilt into the glottis This prevents the bronchoscope reaching the posterior slant of the party wall which would drift it off into the esophagus. The distance of insertion of the bronchoscope into the trachea before removal of the speculum is to be determined by experience. Usually if it has passed two or three tracheal rings it will be found sufficiently deep. In case a foreign body is expected to be located in the trachea, it is better not to exceed this, lest the foreign body be dislodged and move downward. For the same reason, the trachea should always be carefully inspected with the direct laryngoscope before attempting to insert the bronchoscope. unless there is very serious dyspnea. It is very necessary to be certain that the axis of the bronchoscope corresponds with the axis of the trachea, before, as well as after, the bronchoscope is inserted, otherwise the distal end of the bronchoscope will impinge on the tracheal mucosa, inflicting trauma which is one of the factors in the production of subglottic edema. In this connection it must be repeated here that the direction of the trachea is not perpendicular to the long axis of the body, but that it follows the thoracic spine backward as well as downward, as seen in the schema, Fig. 64. To get this direction, in the recumbent patient, the patient's head must be elevated, and at the same time it must be closely observed that the patient's head is neither rotated nor bent to one side or the other. The accurate placing of the head will be watched carefully by a trained assistant, but the operator should also, without direct looking, be able to determine, in a general way, the position of the patient's head and neck. The better the second assistant and the longer he and the operator have worked together, the better the work they will do and the more the operator will come, unconsciously, to depend upon the assistant to keep the head in position.

Difficulties in the introduction of the bronchoscope. The foregoing is a description of how to introduce the bronchoscope, and if closely followed, no one after a little practice should have any difficulty in the introduction in a patient fully relaxed by a general anesthetic. If any serious difficulties are met with, some of the details have been overlooked, such as full extension of the head, elevation of the head, lifting strongly with the *tip* only of the laryngoscope at the moment of insertion of the bronchoscope in the glottis.

The beginner will occasionally enter the esophagus instead of entering the trachea. This is a very dangerous accident, in dyspneic cases, not only by default in not entering the trachea, but directly by compression of the trachea through the bulk of the esophagoscope in the esophagus. Under normal conditions, if properly passed, an esophagoscope does not compress the trachea to any appreciable extent, as the author has previously demonstrated by inserting, at the same time, the bronchoscope in the trachea and an esophagoscope in the esophagus; but in dyspneic cases, it takes but very little displacement of the esophagus to increase the dyspnea to the point where respiration will be arrested. For another reason it is essential to avoid putting the bronchoscope into the esophagus accidentally first before introducing it into the larynx, because, if properly done, the bronchoscope can be introduced through the laryngoscope without coming in contact with the secretions contaminated from the mouth. The trachea is not a septic canal, while the esophagus swarms with bacteria. Getting into the esophagus is simply due to the neglect of some of the details just mentioned, especially insufficient glottic exposure and defective position with failure to lift strongly with the spatular tip at the moment of passing the glottis. It is not always as easy as might be supposed to detect the entrance of the bronchoscope into the esophagus. There is a very distinct respiratory movement to the esophagus, but it is in no way equal to the expiratory tracheal blast and the pink, smooth, collapsing walls of the esophagus are in marked contrast to the normal trachea in which the rings of slightly deeper color contrast with those of the almost white mucosa covering the cartilaginous rings. In a state of disease, however, the tracheal mucosa may be so swollen and edematous that the rings are obliterated, and in children there is more or less collapse of the tracheal wall during expiration, especially the forced expiration of cough, as illustrated in the section on the normal bronchoscopic image. In the esophagus there will usually be a free flow of secretion in the distal end of the tube, which obscures the field; and the secretion usually flows also through the lateral opening of the bronchoscope. There may be secretions in the trachea, but it is seldom the free flow that is seen in the esophagus. The main point of distinction, however, is the tracheal blast, if the patient be breathing or coughing. In cases of respiratory arrest, there is usually no spasm whatever, and the freely open trachea is readily recognized. In such cases, however, the error of inserting the bronchoscope into the esophagus may prove fatal to the patient; not only by default in not getting prompt aeration and oxygen insufflation, but also by the bulk of the bronchoscope in the esophagus compressing the lumen of the trachea. In working without an anesthetic, general or local, this danger is practically nil.

If the patient is profoundly anesthetized, there is no halting of the rhythmic respiratory excursion, and the bronchoscope is very readily introduced through the glottis without the slightest resistance. If, however, the patient is insufficiently anesthetized, either locally or generally, and especially if unanesthetized as in children, the glottis may remain closed for a considerable length of time. In tracheotomized cases the glottis may remain closed indefinitely, and the bronchoscope should be insinuated through without waiting; but in untracheotomized cases, if not dyspneic, it is better to wait for the relaxation of the spasm and opening of the glottis that comes with the first deep inspiration. In older children, or in locally anesthetized adults, the command to take a deep breath will usually be obeyed, especially if the necessity for deep breathing has been repeatedly urged from the beginning. It is not advisable with an incompletely anesthetized patient, especially if chloroform has been used, and still more especially if both chloroform and morphine have been used, to wait too long for the glottis to open, as the respiration may cease. In these cases it is better to push the bronchoscope through. In all dyspneic cases the opening of the glottis should not be awaited for more than a few seconds. The bronchoscope should be pushed through, not violently or roughly, but with the firmness and precision gained from the knowledge that the tube is the right size for the patient, that it is properly placed, and that the patient is in the correct position.

Very often I have found that the difficulties which beginners have encountered in inserting the bronchoscope have been due to the use of a gag. Very wide gagging will render the insertion of a bronchoscope, or even the exposure of the larynx, difficult if not impossible. There is no need for a gag for any other purpose than simply to prevent the patient biting the tube, and for this the bite block, shown in Fig. 39 is ideal, because it is readily held in place at all times by the first finger of the second assistant, and because it does not slip, regardless of how imperfect the patient's teeth may be.

Exploration of the trachea and bronchi. After the bronchoscopic tube-mouth has entered the trachea there will usually be encountered more or less secretion, according to the nature of the case, the anesthetic and drugs used, etc. This secretion must be removed at once, before any deeper insertion of the bronchoscope is made in order that we have the safety of sight. In foreign-body cases this is especially necessary lest the intruder be pushed down. For the same reason, sponges must be inserted only just beyond the tube-mouth, which distance can be determined by the sensation imparted to the finger and thumb when a properly fitting sponge emerges from the distal tube-mouth. Having removed the secretions by the author's "sponge pumping" process in the manner illustrated in Fig. 25, and explained under "Aspirators," the bronchoscope is carefully advanced. If the bronchoscope or the trachea become filled with secretion coughed from the lower air passages, advance of the tube must be stopped as often as necessary until the secretion is removed, lest a foreign body be overridden or a diseased area be overlooked. While it is true that the tracheo-bronchial tree is very elastic, and consequently will adapt itself in a wonderful degree to the faulty direction of the bronchoscope, yet it is essential, wherever possible, to follow the lumen as it opens up ahead of the tube mouth. As has just been said, a well-trained assistant will at the introduction of the bronchoscope have the head so held that the trachea will be in line ahead of the bronchoscope. In the further exploration of the tracheobronchial tree, the second assistant should busy himself with making sure that the head is so held that the larynx shall in the least possible degree become the fulcrum upon which the bronchoscope rests. In other words, when the position, into which the operator in pursuit of the lumen swings the bronchoscope, causes the bronchoscope to bear upon the larynx as a lever upon its fulcrum, the laryngeal fulcrum should be eased off for two very important reasons:

1. An unyielding laryngeal fulcrum limits exploration because of its distance from the upper thoracic aperture.

2. If the larynx is not eased away when fulcral pressure comes upon it, this pressure will cause subglottic edema.

Therefore a fundamental rule which must be rigidly observed by the bronchoscopist and especially by his second assistant is: *The ful-*

crum of the bronchoscopic lever is at the upper thoracic aperture; never at the larynx (Schema. Fig. 135).

To accomplish this the head and neck must gently be made to follow the direction of the proximal end of the bronchoscope.

The freedom of movement of head and neck, with synchronous undistorted status of the thoracic cage requires the Boyce position. In no other way can the same results be accomplished. The nearest approach to this position as to movability of the head and neck is the lateral recumbent position, which is very objectionable because of the varying position of the thorax, the less manageable head, and the inconvenience in the exploration of the uppermost lung or the alternative of turning the

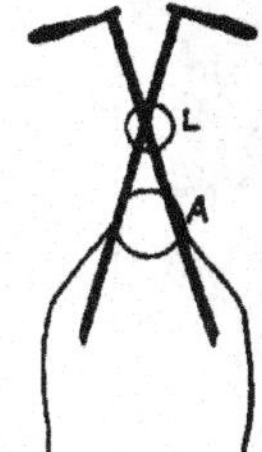

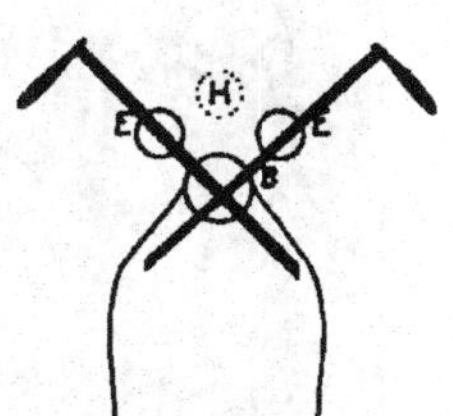

Fig. 135.—Illustrating the fallacy of supposing there is a wider range of movement possible by tracheotomic than by oral bronchoscopy. If the larynx were rigidly fixed at L, the lateral range of movement possible would be relatively slight as compared to tracheotomic bronchoscopy. But by bending the neck sharply to one side we bring the larynx from H to E, permitting the use of the entire upper thoracic aperture. This illustration also shows how the second assistant by easing away the larynx from H to E makes the upper thoracic aperture the fulcrum of the bronchoscopic lever instead of the larynx, thus preventing undue pressure on the larynx and consequent subglottic edema.

patient—a time-wasting procedure that is intolerable to anyone who has experienced the comfort, satisfaction and facility of work in the Boyce position of the patient maintained by an assistant who has worked a long time with the operator.

To accomplish the making of the upper thoracic aperture (instead of the larynx) the fulcrum of the bronchoscopic lever, the second assistant must have a good general sense of direction and must have a mental picture of the position and direction of the long axis of the part of the tube in the patient which he must gain from the uninserted portion of the tube. If the tube is deeply inserted he must mentally "line up" the position of the bronchoscope in the patient from an imaginary line drawn from the proximal tube-mouth to the bronchoscopist's right eye. This line must necessarily be a prolongation of the long axis of the bronchoscope. The axial line of the tube and the upper thoracic aperture and their relations to each other must be constantly in the mind of the second assistant.

In the descriptions before and hereafter given of various positions of the head and neck it is to be understood that these in no way inter-

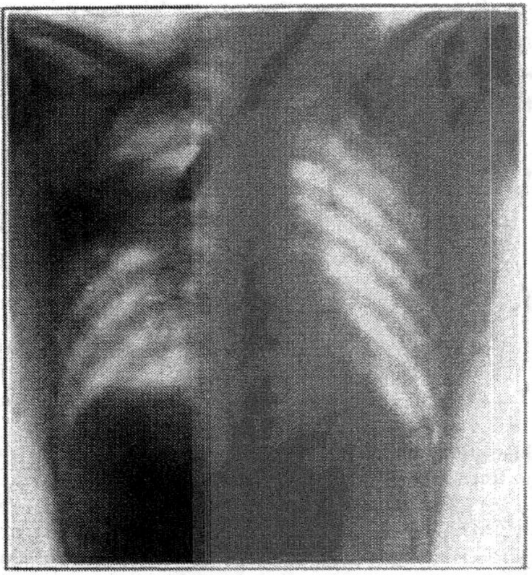

FIG. 136.—Radiograph of bronchoscope in the right upper lobe bronchus of a woman of 25 years. The bronchoscope was inserted through the mouth and the angle is shown to be as advantageous as would be possible through a tracheotomic wound. The position of the patient is easy and natural in this instance, the radiograph being made for verification of the overlay localization in a suspected case of interlobar abscess. Had demonstration been the object, the upper part of the tube could easily have been brought to the clavicle. The lesser shadow passing downward is from pus and shows the location of the middle and inferior lobe (stem) bronchi. This radiograph also shows that the limit of lateral movement is fixed by the upper thoracic aperture; not by the larynx, hence tracheotomy is of no advantage for bronchoscopy, so far as angle is concerned.

fere with the endoscopist following the lumen nor the second assistant following the operator. Yet it is necessary to know, in a general way, the positions of the patient's head and neck that will be required properly to enable a correct presentation of the desired objective point.

With all the foregoing clearly in the mind of operator and assistant we are ready to proceed down the trachea, determining as we go the proper direction by endoscopic watch of the wall of the trachea as it opens up ahead. The endoscopist should not see either wall more than the other, but with a properly directed tube should be looking directly downward into the tracheal lumen. If he sees the anterior wall, which is the usual fault, the patient's head must be elevated. If he sees one lateral wall or the other, the patient's head must be brought to the middle line. If he sees the posterior wall, which is a very rare thing, indeed, with the beginner, the head may be lowered. Of course these remarks should not be applied too strictly to cases in which a careful inspection of the tracheal wall is desired; but even in such cases it is far better to examine the general lumen of the trachea downward before making a minute inspection of the lateral wall, because it is only by keeping the lumen straight ahead that one can determine small degrees of compression or slight amounts of such diseases as perichondritis.

In passing down the trachea the following two rules must be kept in mind:

1. *Before attempting to enter either main bronchus the carina must be identified.*

2. *Before entering either main bronchus the orifices of both should be identified and inspected.*

These are time-saving and localizing expedients of the utmost importance. For quick, accurate and efficient work the bronchoscopist must at all times know exactly the particular part of the tracheo-bronchial tree that is being explored by the tube-mouth. With a natural faculty of orientation, a practical working-knowledge of the average distances, and familiarity with the endoscopic appearance of the few landmarks this is easy. These things cannot be gained from a book. It is useless to memorize arbitrary measured distances. The practical working-knowledge is best obtained from a wet anatomical preparation by draining out the fluid and then passing the bronchoscope, studying together the endoscopic and external anatomy of the dissected tree from which the lung tissue has been removed at the root of each lung.

In doing bronchoscopy on the living, after the laryngoscope is removed, the bronchoscope, which was held in the right hand for introduction, is now held between the thumb and finger of the *left* hand, the second and third fingers of which are hooked by their terminal phalanges over the upper teeth (Fig. 137). This steadies the hand and any desired depth of bronchoscopic insertion can be maintained indefinitely with ease and accuracy by the left hand alone. This serves two very important purposes: 1. The exact desired relation of the tube-mouth to a foreign body (or tumor) can be preserved exactly for the application of the forceps. 2. The right is free for the prompt use of the forceps, as soon as the desired tubal position is established. The author believes these two factors contribute largely to the success attending work with distally lighted tubes. A heavy handlamp prevents this anchoring of the tube in a fixed position by the fingers of the left hand on the teeth. Hence, the slightest movements of the patient, even the respiratory movements, may disturb the relations which are relied upon to

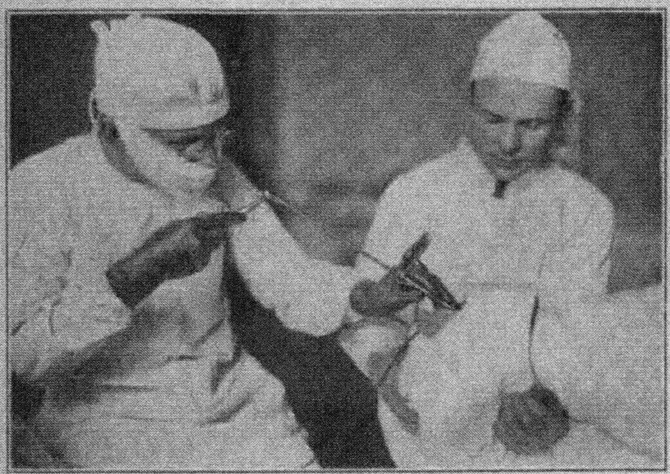

FIG. 137.—The heavy laryngoscope has been removed leaving the light bronchoscope in position. The operator is inserting forceps. Note how the left hand of the operator holds the tube lightly between the thumb and first two fingers of the left hand, while the last two fingers are hooked over the upper teeth of the patient "anchoring" the tube to prevent it moving in or out or otherwise changing the relation of the distal tube-mouth to a foreign body or a growth while forceps are being used. Thus, also, any desired location of the tube can be maintained in systematic exploration. The assistant's left hand is dropped out of the way to show the operator's method. The assistant during bronchoscopy holds the bite-block like a thimble on the index finger of the left hand, and the assistant should be on the *right* side of the patient. He is here put wrongly on the left side so as not to hide the instruments and the manner of holding them.

facilitate the accurate application of the forceps by sight. After anchoring the bronchoscope with the fingers of the left hand, the *right* is used at the collar of the proximal end (not grasping the handle) to manipulate the tube, inward, outward, downward, upward or laterally, the tube being permitted to slide between the finger and thumb of the left hand, if withdrawal or deeper insertion is needed. At any time it is instantly fixed at the desired point; for instance when a momentary view of a foreign body has been obtained, followed by disappearance due to respiratory movement, cough, a flood of secretions. It is very important under such circumstances to keep the tube there until another view is obtained. The manipulation of the tube with the right hand is important. The handle of the bronchoscope is not grasped firmly in the clenched hand as one would hold a revolver (A, Fig. 138). On the contrary it is held lightly, by the collar with the right thumb and index finger (B, Fig. 138) the other fingers either not being used at all or only to assist in rotating or balancing the instrument. The handle of the bronchoscope is needed only when it is desired to rotate the bronchoscope, and then it is used but slightly, being pushed around with the second and third fingers of the right hand while the thumb and index finger hold the collar.

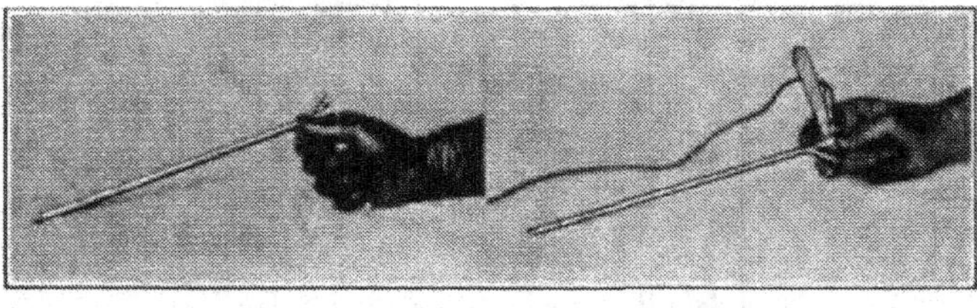

A B

Fig. 138.—A, incorrect manner of holding bronchoscope. The grasp is too rigid and the position of the hand is awkward. B, correct manner, the collar being held lightly between the finger and the thumb. The thumb must not occlude the proximal tube mouth.

Identification of the normal carina is easy when the orifices of both main bronchi are exposed. The difficulty which beginners have is due to the fact that the right bronchus is morphologically the continuation of the trachea whereas the left is, in many cases, for endoscopic purposes, a lateral branch. Hence, special care must be taken in searching for the carina to pass down the trachea with the lip of the bronchoscope toward the left (A, Fig. 139) and to make slight lateral pressure with the lip of the bronchoscope on the left tracheal wall, while the head of the patient is held slightly toward the right. This will result in exposing the left main bronchial orifice and between it and the right is the carina, which by this method should never be missed. If some detail is neglected and the left bronchial orifice is not in evidence, it is only necessary to withdraw the bronchoscope (not too far, lest it be brought altogether out of the trachea) and to start over again. Occasionally a diseased condition of the carina may cause difficulty in identification, as in ulceration, excessive deformity from the pressure of a mass of mediastinal lymph nodes, etc. In such cases the identification of the bronchial orifices can be made by careful examination. Anomalies, such as the upper lobe bronchus being given off from the trachea, might cause confusion though in the only case of this anomaly seen by the author the mistake could scarcely have been made because the orifice was found only by effort. Kahler has observed diverticula of the trachea but these pouches ought not to lead to error in identification of the carina.

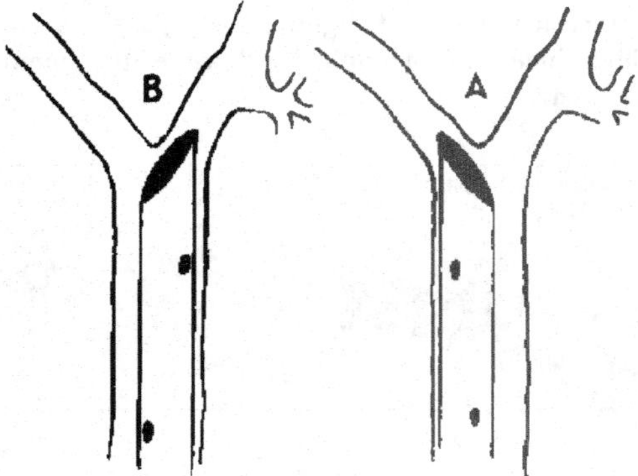

FIG. 139.—Schema demonstrating the method of entering the desired bronchus with the slanted end bronchoscope. Recumbent patient. A, entering the left bronchus. B, the beak being reversed, the bronchoscope naturally finds its way into the right bronchus. The head of the patient is to the side opposite to that of the desired bronchus, and the axis of the trachea consequently is given a position at a more obtuse angle to that of the desired bronchus than is shown in this schema, which is intended to emphasize only the use of the slanted end.

Entering the bronchoscope into the right and left main bronchi. If it is desired to enter the right bronchus, the patient's head is moved to the left and the bronchoscope is maintained in the same position as when started, namely, with the handle out horizontally to the right. If it is desired to enter the left bronchus, the patient's head is moved to the right and the handle of the bronchoscope is placed out horizontally to the left. The purpose of turning the handle in these directions is to bring the lip of the bronchoscope in proper position to facilitate the entrance of the desired bronchus, as will be understood by referring to the schema, Fig. 139.

Entering the bronchoscope into the middle lobe bronchus. For introduction, the head must be high above the table in order that the trachea shall be in line, as previously explained. When, however, it is desired to enter an anterior branching bronchus, like the middle lobe bronchus, which is usually given off more or less toward the anterior part of the right stem bronchus, below the giving off of the upper lobe bronchus, it is necessary to lower the head and to some extent the shoulders of the patient, as seen in the schema, Fig. 140. To accomplish this lowering, it is necessary to have the shoulders of the patient well out in-

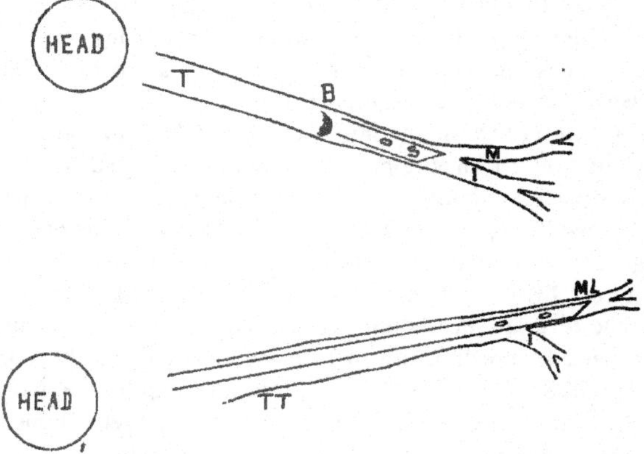

FIG. 140.—Schema illustrating the entering of the anteriorly branching middle lobe bronchus. T, trachea. B, orifice of left main bronchus at bifurcation of trachea. The bronchoscope, S, is in the right main bronchus, pointing in the direction of the right inferior lobe bronchus, I. In order to cause the lip to enter the middle lobe bronchus, M, it is necessary to drop the head so that the bronchoscope in the trachea T T, will point properly to enable the lip of the tube mouth to enter the middle lobe bronchus, as it is seen to have done at ML.

to the air toward the operator. The ridge of the patient's scapulae should be at the edge of the table. This will give the widest range of movement. In entering the middle lobe bronchus the slanted-end bronchoscope is much superior to any other shape as will be understood by looking at the schema, Fig. 141.

The method of entering the bronchoscope into the various branch bronchi is the same in principle as the entering of the middle lobe bronchus. That is, the lip of the slanted-end bronchoscope is brought to the mouth of the branch bronchus by rotation of the bronchoscope until the handle corresponds to the general direction of the branch bronchus. Then the head and neck of the patient are swung to the opposite direction more or less strongly as needed. The bronchoscope, which has been kept a little above the orifice of the branch bronchus, is now pushed downward, the lip making slight pressure on the wall as it goes, so that when the mouth of the branch bronchus is reached, the lip will slip in. If the orifice cannot be thus found, the reverse method may be used. That is the bronchoscope is inserted down the stem bronchus past where the orifice must be. On withdrawal the lip of the bronchoscope is pressed firmly against the lateral wall so that when the orifice is reached the lip will spring into the orifice, or, rather, the ridge corresponding to a carina will suddenly appear in the endoscopic image. This reverse method is especially undesirable in foreign-body cases because the foreign body may be pushed farther into the branch bronchus.

Entering the bronchoscope into the upper lobe bronchus is done by the method just described, the maneuver being facilitated by moving the tube to the corner of the mouth opposite to the side of the desired bronchus, and by displacing the head and neck far down to this opposite side, also being careful to have the lip of the bronchoscope in the proper direction (Fig. 141). If it is remembered that the fulcrum of the bronchoscopic lever is, or should be, the upper thoracic aperture (Fig. 135) there need be no difficulty in entering the stem of the upper lobe bronchus of either side (Fig. 141). A greater depth is explorable on the right than on the left side. It is not possible to get a lumen image, but the short stem can be entered as far as the giving off of the first branches, and this is the part in which foreign bodies are most likely to lodge. Even in this location they are exceedingly rare. There is no need of tracheotomy for exploration of the upper lobe bronchus because no more of it can be explored by that route nor is it more easily thus entered, as explained on a future page in discussing the relative merits of oral and tracheotomic bronchoscopy. The limitations are fixed, not by the larynx, but by the upper thoracic aperture. The orifice of the upper lobe bronchus on the left side may be looked for at about 4 cm. after passing the bifurcation. On the right side it may be 1 cm. or 2 cm. from the bifurcation, but it should be looked for at once after entering the right main bronchus. In estimating desired depths of insertion, the quickest method is to move the finger and thumb of the left hand up on the tube the required distance from the teeth. Then the tube is inserted until the thumb and finger are felt to reach the teeth. This seems simple, easy and quickly done as compared to reading numbers in a darkened room; but many operators prefer to read off the graduation marks on the outside of the tube and the endoscopist may choose for himself. The author never uses either method, preferring to gauge the depth by the endoscopic image as the tube is advanced or withdrawn.

Bronchoscopy in children. The technic of bronchoscopy in children is precisely the same as just described for the recumbent position in adults. The author of late years has not used any anesthetic, general or local, for children under six years of age. This increases the difficulties somewhat, yet it brings the risk of bronchoscopy down to nothing, eliminates complications, and it has the advantage of rapidly getting rid of secretions. The recumbent position is best, in the author's opinion, for reasons already herein given. One precaution necessary in children is to see that they do not arch up the chest. If they do, the nurse who holds the two hands, uses her right hand to press the chest

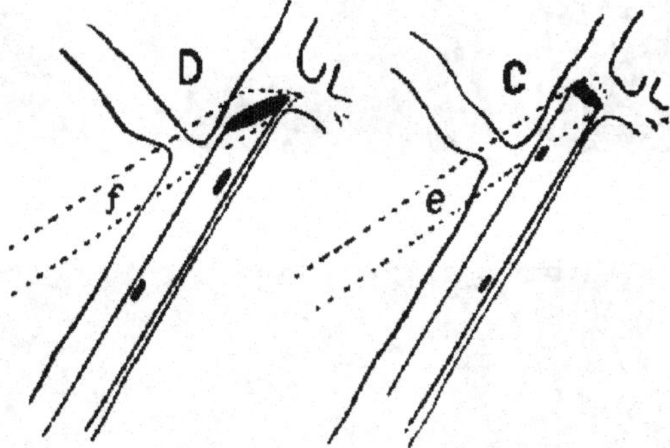

FIG 141.—Schema illustrating the advantage of the slanted-end bronchoscope for entering branch bronchi, especially the upper lobe bronchus. When the squarely cut off bronchoscope (*e*) is lowered to the most advantageous angle possible, as shown by the dotted lines, the mechanical difficulty is still great as compared to the slanted-end bronchoscope as shown by the dotted lines (*f*).

gently down on the table, without letting go the left arm of the child, carrying the child's arm with her hand. Children are particularly subject to subglottic edema, especially if too large a tube be used, or the before-mentioned precautions to avoid the fulcral pressure on the larynx are neglected. In addition, of course, all of the niceties of bronchoscopy must be practiced in the bronchoscopy of children, because of the delicacy of the tissues. The 4 mm. tube should be used as a rule for infants under about ten months. The author uses it for one year and under. The author has special forceps for the 4 mm. tube. These forceps can be seen to close; and all of the manipulations in foreign-body extraction can, and should be, done under the guidance of the eye. Brünings' state-

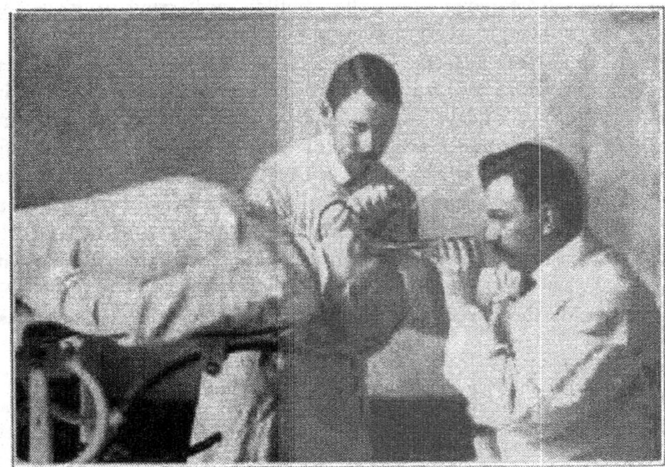

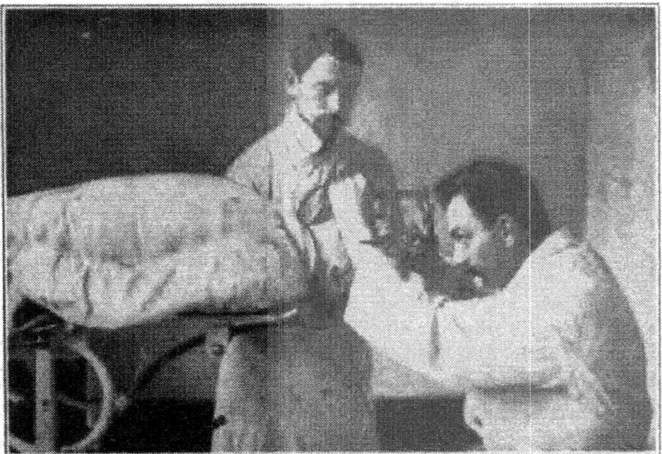

FIG. 142.—Bronchoscopy by Brünings method. The laryngoscopic tube is introduced through the glottis with the right hand. Then the inner tube is inserted with the left hand, as shown in the upper illustration. When forceps or other instruments are to be used the laryngo-bronchoscope is transferred to the left hand as shown in the lower illustration.

ment that ocular guidance "is largely an illusion" can refer only to proximally lighted tubes.

Introduction of the Brünings bronchoscope. The introduction of the Brunings bronchoscope is, in principle, precisely the same as just described up to the exposure of the glottis. At this point, the distal end of the Brünings laryngoscope, which is intentionally small for this very purpose, is itself pushed through the glottis into the trachea, then the bronchoscopic extension inner tube is inserted and pushed down the required distance and locked with the ratchet, shown in Fig. 4. In order to prevent loss of time in cleaning the mirror, Brünings advises that every time the patient is about to cough, the mirror carrier should, if possible, be swung to the operator's left side. The Brünings method differs from that of the author in the uses of the operator's hands as shown in Fig. 142. The operator protects the lips with the *left* hand, while introducing the laryngoscope grasped with the *right* hand. The epiglottis is identified. the tip of the laryngoscope is inserted beyond it, but not too far, as previously described. Then the epiglottis is lifted, (recumbent patient) and the glottis is exposed. As before explained, under no circumstances should any attempt be made to expose the glottis until the epiglottis has been identified, nor should any attempt be made to insert the instrument through the glottis until the cords are seen and identified with certainty, in at least their posterior third. Brünings considers it not absolutely necessary to wait for the complete abduction of the cords, as the beak of the instrument can be pushed through, if the instrument is exactly in the middle line. In difficult cases digital counterpressure externally on the larynx may be used to assist in exposing the cords; and in cases of incomplete anesthesia the instrument may be rotated so as to insert the wedge-shaped beak of the laryngoscope in the long axis of the glottis. Having inserted the laryngoscopic tube into the trachea with the *right* hand, the inner sliding tube is inserted with the *left* hand (Fig. 142). The laryngoscope is not removed as the bronchoscopic tube slides in at a close fit and becomes, when locked with the ratchet shown in Fig. 4, a rigid part of the laryngoscope itself. When it is desired to use forceps, swabs, aspirator or other instrument, the laryngo-bronchoscope, which up until this stage has been held in the *right* hand, is now transferred to the *left* hand so that the right is free for the use of forceps as shown in Fig. 142. Brünings states that when insurmountable obstacles to the passage of the instrument are encountered, it is usually possible to succeed by putting the patient on his left side, with the head supported. Then the instrument is passed as in the sitting position. He states that he occasionally also uses the ventral recumbent position which he finds particularly easy. The illustrations.

Fig. 142, are reproduced, by permission, from Brünings'excellent treatise, "Die direckte Laryngoskopie, Bronchoskopie und Esophagoskopie," of which an excellent English translation, by Mr. Walter G. Howarth, is published by Messrs. Bailliere, Tindall and Cox.

The introduction of the Kahler bronchoscope is precisely the same as just described for the Brünings instrument.

THE NORMAL BRONCHOSCOPIC IMAGE.

In the author's earlier publication (Bib. 269) were shown a number or normal and pathologic endoscopic illustrations which show in such a satisfactory way the living appearances that no new colored illustrations are here added.

The *color* of the mucosa as seen endoscopically varies with the degree of illumination. With a dull glowing filament the normal mucosa may seem dark red; with the bright, white light of a fully illuminated tungsten filament the same mucosa will seem pinkish white; while, with an over-illuminated filament, the mucosa may seem grayish white. The color of the normal mucosa also varies with the anesthetic. With chloroform the mucosa is paler than with ether, the difference being due not to local irritation, but to the engorgement of the vessels from the general stimulant effect of ether. Cocaine, by the ischemia it causes, if applied before the bronchoscope is deeply introduced causes the color of the mucosa to appear a paler pink. Adrenalin has an even more marked effect in whitening the endoscopic image. Neither of these act to the same extent if applied after the bronchoscopic examination has continued for some time in the examined locality. The ridges between the orifices of branching bronchi are, under all ordinary conditions, normally of a glistening whitish color with only occasionally a slight tinge of pink. Their color often leads them to be mistaken by the beginner for a thread of mucus or a foreign body, such as a bright pin.

It may be said, then, that the color of the mucosa as seen endoscopically, may, in health, vary from almost white, through yellowish pink, bluish pink, pale red to dark red, depending upon illumination and vascularity.

The *form* of the endoscopic picture depends upon the angle at which the lumen is presented, this being in turn dependent upon, (1) the position of the tube, and, (2) the position of the parts examined. As both are constantly changing, the variety of forms in the endoscopic picture is almost endless. The respiratory, bechic, pulsatory, reflex and transmitted muscular movements and compressions so modify the normal image that nothing but study of the image, as seen in the living, will educate the eye, as elsewhere mentioned. When the axes of the bronchial and the bronchoscopic lumina exactly correspond, the lumen of the bronchus seems to diminish more or less concentrically owing to perspective, and the orifices of the branch bronchi with the white shining ridge between are seen beyond (Fig. 143). These views represent complete images which are momentarily obtained. Movements of the various kinds mentioned are constantly hiding the orifices and ridges that are a centimeter or more beyond the tube-mouth. These are accurately presented images. When the axis of the bronchoscope deviates from coincidence with the luminal axis, more or less of the wall toward which

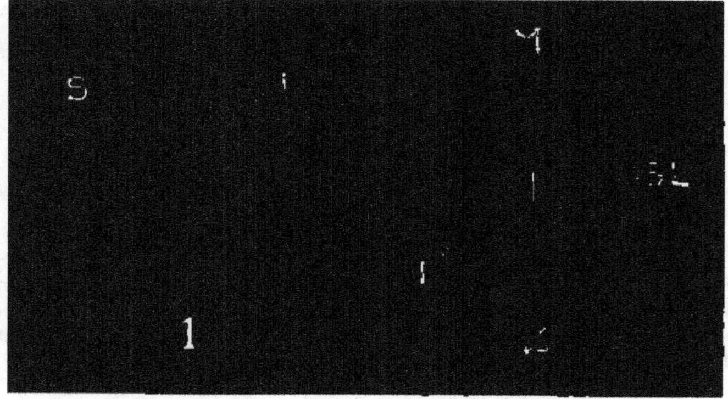

Fig. 143.—Normal endoscopic images. Semischematic. 1. Left main bronchus. S, left upper lobe bronchus. I, left inferior lobe bronchus (or "stem" bronchus), showing dorsal and ventral branches. 2. Right main bronchus. SL, superior lobe bronchus. M, middle lobe. I, lower lobe bronchus showing orifices of dorsal and ventral branches. The main bronchus (right or left) below the upper lobe bronchus is usually referred to as "stem" bronchus because there is no true bifurcation, only a giving off of lesser branches from the stem.

the tube-mouth deviates, is seen. By the form and position of the rings seen in perspective in the bronchial wall it is possible to estimate how far the luminal axis deviates from the bronchoscopic axis, and thus the direction of the particular branch bronchus may be estimated. By the same means the proper direction in which to move the tube to obtain a view directly into the long axis of the lumen is known. On the posterior tracheal wall, the "party wall," the signs of rings are absent. Elsewhere in the normal trachea the ring-like appearance is more or less marked by differences in color. The membranous inter-spaces are usually of deeper color than the prominences corresponding to the cartilage.

If the tracheal mucosa is edematous, infiltrated, or very much engorged, the rings may not be visible. The ringed appearance of the wall diminishes as we go downward until it is not noticeable in the smallest bronchi, though it is not missed because the orifices make more or less of a ringed appearance in the endoscopic image.

The posterior tracheal wall is ordinarily somewhat flattened and may even assume a convex form as it bulges forward into the trachea during cough, especially in children examined without, or with only slight, anesthesia (Fig. 144). In addition to the posterior wall, there is a flattening often visible at the aortic crossing and also at the bifurcation, these being in some instances continuous with each other. A slight flattening in the

FIG. 144.—Endoscopic view showing forward bulging of the posterior membranous tracheo-esophageal wall during cough. Patient dorsally recumbent. Not pathological. Seen mostly in children, and accentuated when the bronchoscopic tube mouth bears too much on the posterior tracheal wall.

neck at the level of the thyroid gland cannot be called pathological. All of these flattenings are usually from before backward, though the longest diameter of the tracheal cross-section is seldom exactly in the lateral plane.

The orifices of the dorsal and ventral branch bronchi are not opposite each other in the stem bronchus. The inferior lobe bronchi in some cases end in a sort of axis, where two or more branches are given off at nearly the same level, which is in contrast to the monopodic branching higher up.

CHAPTER X.

Introduction of the Esophagoscope.

Indications and contraindications for esophagoscopy will be considered under "Foreign Bodies" and under "Diseases." The remarks there made on contraindications, especially, should be read before attempting the introduction of the esophagoscope.

Anesthesia and position of the patient for esophagoscopy have already been considered in a separate chapter.

NORMAL NARROWINGS OF THE ESOPHAGUS.

He who contemplates attempting esophagoscopy for the first time should fix in his mind certain general principles, anatomical and mechanical, that are known to experienced esophagoscopists, but which have never before been put in concrete form for the preliminary study of the beginner. These may be classed under two heads: 1. The normal narrowings of the esophageal lumen as seen endoscopically. 2. The normal direction of the esophageal lumen, esophagoscopically considered.

The esophagus is not a flaccid tube through which an endoscopic tube can be rudely pushed. Nor is it a straight tube. It deviates and has certain narrowings, some of which are constant anatomic decreases of lumen. Others are due to pressure of surrounding structures that, viewed endoscopically, give one the idea that the esophagus was put through first, and then all of the surrounding structures were tamped in around it like the stones and earth around a post in a post-hole. Other narrowings, and these are the most troublesome, are the spasmodic ones, due to the contraction of periesophageal musculatures. There are, also, spasmodic contractions, less powerful, of the circular muscular fibers of the esophageal wall itself. Mehnert (Bib. 404), in a very elaborate paper on the anatomy of the esophagus, describes thirteen physiological constrictions in the esophagus. The esophagoscopist, however, will usually be able to demonstrate but five. 1. The cricopharyngeal fold. 2. The crossing of the aorta. 3. The crossing of the left bronchus. 4. The hiatus esophageus. 5. The upper thoracic aperture. Some esophagoscopists believe in a constriction at the cardia itself. In the author's opinion there is certainly no sphincter at the cardia and he cannot but think that the constriction noted by some observers is due, in some instances, to the intra-abdominal pressure; in others to mistaking for the cardia the compression produced by the narrowing of the hiatus esophageus through the action of the diaphragmatic musculature.

These narrowings are largely due to static or contractive pressure of surrounding structures. The esophagus itself is so thin-walled a structure that its narrowings, even under spasmodic contraction of its own musculature, are of less endoscopic importance than the peri-esophageal musculature, are of less endoscopic importance than the periesophageal structure. It is elsewhere stated that it is necessary to relax the esophageal musculature in order that trauma be not done during the extraction of a very large and sharp foreign body. It is true that the contractions of the esophageal musculature are sufficient to permit of its laceration by the withdrawal of a foreign body when the musculature is spasmodically contracted, yet it is the surrounding musculature acting upon the surrounding hard and soft parts adjacent to the esophagus that is in large part responsible for trauma in the withdrawal of foreign bodies as well as for the difficulties in the introduction of the esophagoscope.

The cricopharyngeal constriction. In a previous chapter it was stated that a knowledge of endoscopic anatomy cannot be learned from books; and to a certain extent it cannot be learned from the cadaver. Nowhere is this better exemplified than in the study of the cricopharyngeal constriction of the espohagus. In the cadaver this constriction is widely open; and prior to the days of esophagoscopy it was supposed to be open in life. This has been called the "mouth" of the esophagus: but, as by the "mouth" of the esophagus esophagoscopists do not refer to the crescentic crevice, (Fig 1, Plate III) visible by direct or indirect laryngoscopy back of the arytenoid eminence and aryepiglottic folds, where these meet the postero-lateral pharyngeal wall, much confusion might result and the author proposes the term "cricopharyngeal constriction." This crevice is the entrance to the hypopharynx which ends below (in the unanesthetized living subject) in a physiological narrowing. which, in life, looks as though it were being drawn together intermittently by a purse-string outside the esophageal wall. This narrowing, in the adult, is about two centimeters in extent and is noticeable both on introduction and withdrawal of the esophagoscope. As this constriction is more or less circular, though muscularly incomplete anteriorly, it might be called a sphincter; but this is objectionable because some esophagoscopists believed in a sphincter at the cardia and spoke of "upper and lower sphincter." As the author has demonstrated, the lower constriction is at the hiatal level—not at the cardia. Therefore, the author suggests as a more accurate, and hence better, nomenclature "cricopharyngeal constriction" and "hiatal constriction." If deemed justifiable, a "cardial constriction" may be added. But true sphincter there is none, in the esophagus.

The lower circular bundle of fibers of the inferior constrictor is very powerful, much more so than the orbicular fibers of the esophagus into which they merge. (See illustration in chapter on "Diverticulum of the Esophagus.") The median raphe, which receives the insertion of the oblique fibers above, is wanting below, and the contraction of these circular fibers causes the greatest difficulty in the way of introduction of the esophagoscope, and it is the one thing above all others in which continual practice is necessary in order to acquire skill and confidence. The cricopharyngeal constriction and the fact that it is caused by the inferior constrictor were recognized by Mikulicz; but it remained for Killian to demonstrate that only the circular fibers were concerned, and he also demonstrated the fact that there is a weakly supported point between the fundiform and circular fibers, at which weak point the esophageal wall is herniated to form the pulsion diverticula of Zenker, as illustrated in the Section on Esophageal Diverticulum. The author has noted in two instances of esophagoscopic perforation that inexperienced operators had pushed the esophagoscope through the wall at this same weak point. The author wishes especially to emphasize the vital importance of these two observations. (1) *If the esophagoscope is allowed to follow its natural route and is forcibly pushed downward it will certainly perforate this weak point, into which it naturally is guided by the surrounding tissues.* (2) *This tendency is to be combated, in the recumbent position, by forcing the tube mouth anteriorly (and slightly medianwards) with the left hand, as soon as the bottom of the pyriform sinus is reached, as hereinafter described.* The constriction at the mouth of the esophagus is to a great extent relaxed under profound general anesthesia; but local anesthesia has only a slight relaxing effect upon it. What little relaxation there is, is due to the slight lessening of reflex excitability. No endoscopist expects to use a general anesthetic in any but exceptional cases; and children should not have either a local or a general anesthesia because of the peculiarly grave risks they introduce into esophageal cases. Therefore, it is very desirable that the beginner in esophagoscopy should first devote especial preliminary study to the upper end of the esophagus.

The best method of studying this region, in health or disease, is with the esophageal speculum (Fig. 21) used gently. It requires considerable force to pull the cricoid forward. Killian, who tried it on a tracheotomized patient by means of a hook passed through the tracheal wound and up into the cricoid ring, described the resistance as "enormous." The hypopharynx was watched in the laryngeal mirror and could be inspected but the mouth of the esophagus could not be made to gape. The use of the esophageal speculum (Fig. 21) on the living subject and on the cadaver will, by contrast, demonstrate that the larynx is supported in position by a powerful tonic muscular activity in life. As shown by Killian, this muscular tonicity is only relaxed by central impulses such as in deglutition, emesis and singing. The hypopharynx can be studied by von Eicken's method of hypopharyngoscopy. The larynx is cocainized and a stiff steel rod bent to the "laryngeal curve" of indirect instruments and having a rounded probe point, is inserted into the larynx and used to pull the whole larynx forward, while the hypopharynx is watched in the laryngeal mirror. This in favorable cases will expose the hypopharynx down to the level of the middle of the cricoid cartilage. This cartilage usually shows whitish under the mucosa.

The apertural narrowing of the esophagus requires experience to demonstrate esophagoscopically, but is amply demonstrated by the lodgment of foreign bodies. (See Chapter XVIII.)

The aortic narrowing of the esophagus. In the living, the mouth of the esophagus will seem the narrowest part of the esophagus as seen endoscopically; but in the cadaver the aortic constriction may be the narrowest point in the esophagus. The level of this aortic constriction is determined by making slight pressure with the tube-mouth against the left anterior wall of the esophagus when the actively pulsating aorta will be readily palpated with the tube. Otherwise the aortic narrowing may not be noticed at all in the author's "high-low" method of esophagoscopy. Faulty positions, by compelling faulty tubal direction, may bring the aorta into conspicuous, even obstructive prominence. This is especially true of a low head at the start, as in the Rose position As explained later, the head should not be dropped until the tube-mouth is beyond this point. The normal aortic pulsation usually is so great that the beginner is apt to think it pathologic. The displacement of the esophageal wall by the aorta is beautifully shown in the bismuth radiographs reproduced in the Section on Spasmodic Stenosis. The aortic constriction is about 23 cm. from the upper incisor teeth in the adult.

The approximate distance in children is given in the author's esophagoscopic chart, Figs. 145 and 146.

The bronchial narrowing of the esophagus is due to the backward displacement caused by the left bronchus which crosses anterior to the esophagus at about 27 cm. from the upper teeth, in the adult. The ridge observable esophagoscopically, Fig. 6, Plate III, is quite prominent in some patients, especially those with dilatations from stenoses lower down. If the tube-mouth is made to bear firmly on the anterior wall on the way down, the ledge corresponding to the bronchial crossing can be made to come out very prominently.

The hiatal narrowing is both anatomic and spasmodic. The esophagus is narrowed markedly as compared with the suprajacent esophagus; and the peculiar arrangement of the tendinous and muscular structure of the diaphragm acts on this hiatal opening in a way to constrict it most powerfully. Besides this there is a local musculature demonstrated by Liebault (Bib. 329) that also contributes to spasmodic closure. The level of the hiatus in the adult is about 36 cm. from the upper incisors in the extended position of the head. The approximate distance in children at various ages is given in the author's esophagoscopic chart Figs. 145 and 146.

The cardia will be considered under the head of spasmodic stenoses.

The approximate distances of the esophageal narrowings from the upper teeth as given in the chart (Fig. 145) are necessarily subject to individual variation, a variation with different body-lengths in children of the same age, a variation with posture, coughing, breathing, retching, swallowing, etc. Moreover, the aorta and the left bronchus are rounded and do not cross at a right angle to the esophageal axis. For all of these reasons absolute accuracy is impossible. Therefore, the measurements were made to read in even centimeters. Notwithstanding all of these variations the distances given will be found very useful, practically, and much more accurate for the living than cadaveric tables. The chart is arranged as the operator will encounter the narrowings on the way down, with the patient in the recumbent position. The measurements were taken with the head extended

The *direction of the esophagus* is very important to the endoscopist for on a thorough knowledge of this depends the easy and safe introduction of the esophagoscope. The esophagus enters the chest in a direction decidedly backward as well as downward as shown in the schema (Fig. 64) of the direction of the trachea, which is nearly parallel, the esophagus lying behind the trachea. This backward direction of the esophagus is maintained as though the esophagus were trying to get behind the aorta, heart and left bronchus. Below the left bronchus the

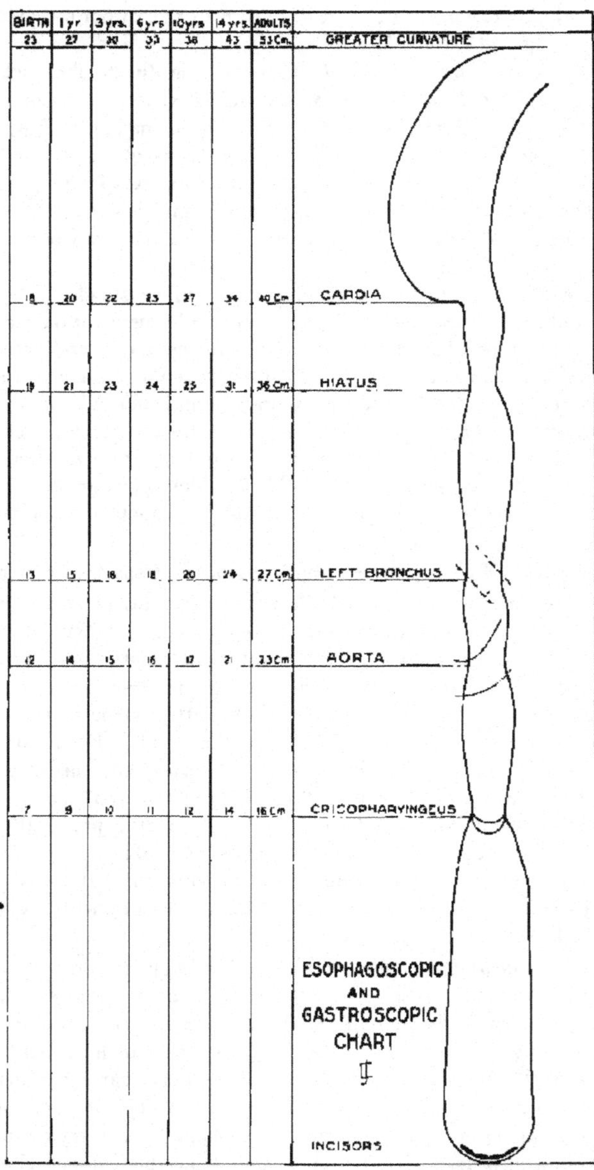

FIG. 145.—The author's esophagoscopic chart of approximate distances of the esophageal narrowings from the upper incisors prepared by the author from measurements in the living. Arranged for convenient reference during esophagoscopy in the dorsally recumbent patient.

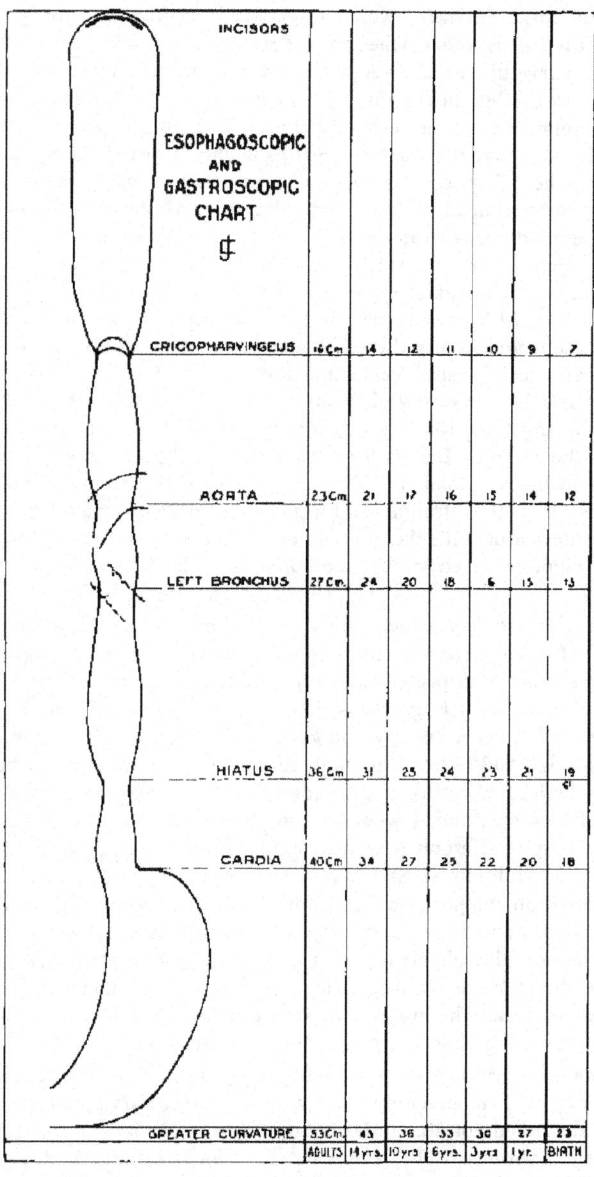

FIG. 146.—The author's esophagoscopic chart arranged for convenient reference in the sitting or laterally recumbent patient.

esophagus turns forward, which direction it maintains until it passes through the hiatus and reaches the stomach. In addition to the anteroposterior curvature of the esophagus just described, there is a lateral deviation to the left in the thorax, which partly accounts for the esophagus passing back of the *left* bronchus. The other part is accounted for by the fact that the trachea deviates slightly toward the right in approaching the bifurcation as though to get its axis more nearly in line with the right bronchus. The slight deviation of the esophagus to the left in the middle half of its thoracic portion is of less importance, endoscopically, than the very marked deviation of the lower esophagus to the left before and after passing through the hiatus. In considering the anteroposterior and lateral deviations the endoscopist must fix in his mind that the esophagus enters the chest in a backward and downward direction (anatomically) until below the level of the left bronchus, then it curves markedly forward and to the left. Mikulicz thought it necessary to put an angle of 150 degrees in his esophagoscope to get forward through the hiatus. But with the patient in the position developed for the author by Dr. John W. Boyce, the patient's anatomy is so easily controlled that the straight and rigid esophagoscope can be inserted through the hiatus with the greatest ease, by careful attention to the details hereinafter given of the author's "high-low" method of esophagoscopy.

Specular esophagoscopy. As a rule, before introducing the esophagoscope for any purpose, the hypopharynx and cricopharyngeal constriction should be inspected carefully with the speculum, Fig. 21. If this be not at hand, a fairly good inspection can be made with the laryngeal speculum. This is necessary for growths high up and for traumatism due to foreign bodies or to attempts at removal; or the foreign body itself may be located in this upper region. If so, it may be overridden by the esophagoscope, and it would be, in any event, much more easily removed through the esophageal speculum. Another very important point, especially in children, is that a retropharyngeal abscess may have burrowed down on the posterior wall until it has produced serious difficulty in swallowing; and such a condition might easily be overlooked with the esophagoscope, though plainly visible with the esophageal speculum, or with the direct laryngoscope. Of course dyspnea is much more apt to be a symptom, but the author has seen one case which was totally free from dyspnea, the child being brought for dysphagia.

Technic of specular esophagoscopy. The use of the esophageal speculum (Fig. 21) is precisely the same as direct laryngoscopy by the method described for the author's laryngoscope, in both the sitting and recumbent positions. The recumbent position is preferable for reasons previously given, and for foreign-body work is, in most instances, much more certain of successful extraction of the intruder. Secretions are less troublesome to the operator and, by not overflowing into the larynx, to the patient. Children are more easily controlled, no anesthesia being used, as elsewhere explained. Having exposed the larynx as shown in Fig. 1, Plate III, by the method shown in Figs. 78 and 92 (according to whether the patient is in the sitting or the recumbent posture) the spatular tip of the esophageal speculum is inserted into the right pyriform sinus (left in the sitting patient). From now on downward the speculum is gently insinuated as a tube, the very powerful anterior displacement necessary for direct laryngoscopy and for other methods of exposing this region is not necessary with the author's speculum because the sloping end of the speculum rides forward readily with a slight anterior pull, and exposes the cricopharyngeal constriction. This is readily identified with the speculum by the anteriorly convex, crescent-shaped fold that extends forward from the posterior hypopharyngeal wall at the level of the lower third of the cricoid cartilage (Fig. 3, Plate III). The forward projection of this fold hides the esophageal lumen below and it forms a chute which throws forward a bougie, esophagoscope or other instrument causing the instrument to override and pass the foreign body just below the lip. Strong anterior traction on the larynx does not open the lumen any wider because the posterior hypopharyngeal wall, with the cricopharyngeal folds, follows the cricoid forward, the esophagus remaining closed. In Fig. 10, Plate III, is shown the manner of drawing back this posterior fold with the alligator forceps, exposing a coin wedged in the esophagus below the fold. The speculum is long enough to be pushed on downward flattening the fold and exposing in the open trough of the speculum the posterior esophageal wall below the fold for examination or operation. A careful study of this fold and its chute-like action must be made with the speculum to be understood, because the fold, as such, is not so noticeable in the introduction of the esophagoscope, though the obstruction is felt very markedly. The weak point in the esophageal wall between the horizontal and oblique fibers of the inferior constrictor is just at the proximal base of this fold, and if the angle of introduction is bad or the force too great an esophagoscope will not be chuted forward, but will perforate and the beginner, strange as it may seem, does not discover his error. He passes his esophagoscope on downward with little resistance between the layers of tissue into the mediastinum not realizing the difference between the walls of the false passage and the esophageal wall. In one such case the author was asked to look through the esophagoscope to identify a shining gray membrane that was puzzling the surgeon by obstructing the way. The author could not identify the membrane, but on withdrawing the esophagoscope the layers of connective tissue revealed a false passage. From the depth of insertion it was probable that the membrane was the pleura though no post mortem could be obtained. There was extensive emphysema. Death apparently was due to vagitis and mediastinal emphysema. The false passage began (B, Fig. 153) just above the cricopharyngeal fold.

An excellent view of disease of the posterior wall as seen through the esophageal speculum is shown in Fig. 9, Plate III.

Technic of the introduction of the esophagoscope, patient recumbent. In his early work the author used a mandrin but he soon found that both foreign bodies and disease might be overridden; therefore, he developed the technic of passing by sight and now finds it so much easier in all cases, as well as so much safer in disease high up, and so invariably contributes to successful foreign-body removal, that he would not consent to the use of a mandrin under any circumstances. In his earlier work, it was customary with the author to apply sterile vaseline to the esophagoscope before passing. Later experience has proven this to be unnecessary, because the secretions sufficiently lubricate the instrument, and it is quite a relief not to have any greasy substance about the instrument table, or on the instruments introduced.

As in bronchoscopy (Fig. 137) the esophagoscope can be "anchored" at any desired depth by hooking the phalanges of the left fourth and fifth fingers over the patient's upper alveolus. In the author's method of passing the esophagoscope by sight five things are essential:

1. The correct "high-low" position-sequence of the patient.

2. A knowledge of the endoscopic anatomy in the living as described in this chapter.

3. A clear conception of the direction and changes of direction of the esophageal axis as herein given.

4. A good general sense of direction that enables the endoscopist to point his esophagoscope in the general direction of the esophagus.

5. A clear mental image of the esophagus and its direction in relation to the esophagoscope.

With these qualifications the endoscopist has only to follow the landmarks, to be able quickly to pass the esophagoscope on any human being whose mouth can be opened. The introduction may be divided into four stages.

1. Entering the right pyriform sinus.
2. Passing the cricopharyngeus.
3. Passing through the thoracic esophagus.
4. Passing the hiatus.

During the entire procedure the patient and second assistant are in the Boyce position (Fig. 72), the second assistant holding the bite block. During the first and second and third stages the head is held high, in the fourth stage it is dropped until the occiput is slightly below the level of the table. Hence, the author has for convenience formed the habit of calling his method the "high-low" method of esophagoscopy.

Stage 1. Entering the pyriform sinus is readily understood by looking at the schema, Fig. 147, and comparing it with Fig. 1, Plate III. The collar of the tube is held lightly between the right thumb and fingers as shown in Fig. B. 138, and the tube-mouth, guided by the left hand, is inserted posterior to the dorsum of the tongue and with the proximal end high (Fig. 148).* The operator standing, his eye at the proximal tube-mouth seeks the right pyriform sinus. (P. Fig. 147, and Fig. 2, Plate III). The landmark is the right arytenoid eminence, A, Fig. 147, which

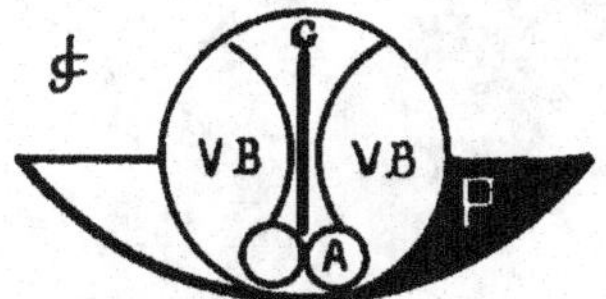

FIG. 147.—Schema for finding the pyriform sinus in the author's method of esophagoscopy. The large circle represents the cricoid cartilage. G, glottic chink, spasmodically closed. VB, ventricular band. A, right arytenoid eminence. P, right pyriform sinus, through which the tube is passed in the recumbent posture. (Compare Fig. 1, Plate III.) The pyriform sinuses are the normal food passages.

shows as a rounded mass rather larger than when seen by the indirect method. (Seen upward to the left in Fig. 2, Plate III). Great care must be taken to identify this arytenoid and to avoid hooking the tube-mouth over it or its fellow. This would prevent further insertion and if force were used the arytenoid mobility might be seriously injured. (A, Fig. 153). Having found the right pyriform sinus the tube glides in readily for 2 or 3 centimeters when it comes to a full stop and the lumen disappears. This is the spasmodically closed cricopharyngeal constriction. *During stage 1 or any of the other stages the fingers are not inserted in the mouth, except so far as necessary for the "hooking" of the phalanges.* (Fig. 137).

Stage 2. Passing the cricopharyngeus is, with the beginner, the most difficult part of esophagoscopy, especially if the patient is unanes-

*In passing the slanted-end esophagoscope (Fig. 426) in the recumbent patient, the handle of the esophagoscope must always point toward the ceiling, in order to bring the lip of the esophagoscopic tube-mouth anteriorly, so as to ride over the cricopharyngeal fold. If the lip is posteriorward, perforation is possible if violence be used.

thetized. Local anesthesia does not help much. The cricopharyngeus as seen through the esophagoscope does not resemble the image seen in the speculum (Fig. 3, Plate III). It is simply a lost lumen. Only a solid wall of mucosa is seen. Force must not be used but a steady, firm pressure is made on the esophagoscope while a strongly anterior (lifting in the recumbent position) movement is imparted to the distal end of the esophagoscope by the left hand. At the same time the lifting motion is imparted, the distal end should be guided slightly toward the middle

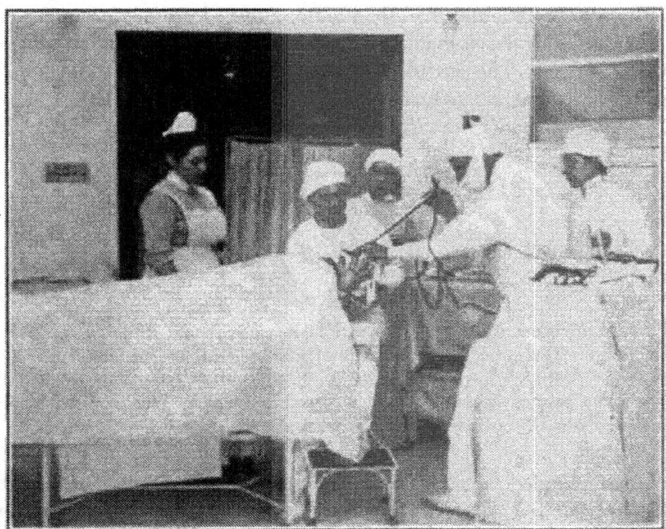

Fig. 148.—Esophagoscopy by the author's high-low method. First stage. Finding the right pyriform sinus. In this and the second stage the patient's vertex is about 15 cm. above the level of the table and in full extension.

line of the body. If the lumen is not seen, the patient should be told to take a deep breath when the lumen will usually appear. In an unanesthetized child the deep inspiration will soon be made involuntarily. A little patience here will always succeed. The author's slanted-end esophagoscope executes this second stage with particular ease, the lip being insinuated upward and forward, and the handle being held sagittally and anteriorly. The lumen is a mere slit, like Fig. 4, Plate III, though the axis of the slit may be in other directions. The folds at the sides of the slit may seem to bulge toward the operator. In many instances it is rosette-like in form with radial folds; and it varies with the instrument used.

There is usually from 1 to 3 cm. of this constricted lumen at the level of the cricopharyngeus and the subjacent orbicular esophageal fibers, after which the esophagoscope glides into the few centimeters of partially open cervical esophagus. (Fig. 5, Plate III).

Stage 3. The esophagoscope usually glides easily through the thoracic esophagus (Fig. 150). If it does not the patient's position is faulty or the esophagoscope is rubbing on the upper teeth. The levels of the aorta and left bronchus (Fig. 6, Plate III) are readily recognized by the description previously given. After passing them the lumen of the esophagus seems to have more and more of a tendency to disappear anteriorly. This is the signal for lowering the head, which has till now been kept high, for the next stage.

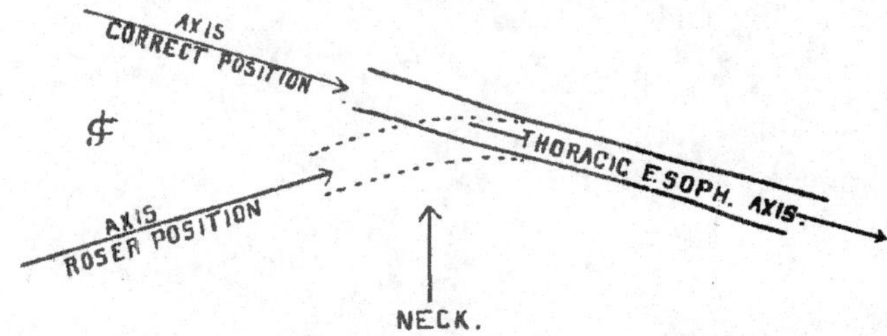

Fig. 149.—Schematic illustration of the author's "high-low" method of esophagoscopy. In the first and second stages the patient's head fully extended is held high so as to bring it in line with the thoracic esophagus, as shown above. The Rose position is shown by way of accentuation.

Stage 4. Passing the hiatus is very easy after a little practice if the directions here given are followed. It will be remembered that in the first part of this chapter the direction of the lower esophagus was given as anteriorly and to the left. To obtain this in the recumbent patient the head is dropped as shown in Figs. 151 and 152.

When the head is dropped it must at the same time be horizontally moved to the right (without rotation) in order that the axis of the esophagoscope shall correspond to the axis of the lower third of the esophagus which deviates to the left. The shoulders should also participate slightly in this movement. It is in the facility of making these movements that one of the great advantages of the Boyce position over the lateral or any other position for esophagoscopy consists; and had the author not had the advantage of "team work" with a good assistant holding the patient in the Boyce position he could not have developed this "high-low" method to its present approximate perfection. This dropping of the head was not understood by Mikulicz and in order to overcome the angle P S, Fig. 152, he put a bend in his gastroscope thinking that he had encountered the dorsal spine when his tube, which was passed blindly, encountered the resistance of the diaphragm, against which the esophagus was pushed just above the hiatus, because the direction of the tube was faulty owing to not dropping the head. Mikulicz did not use the dorsal position but doubtless he would have obtained an equivalent of

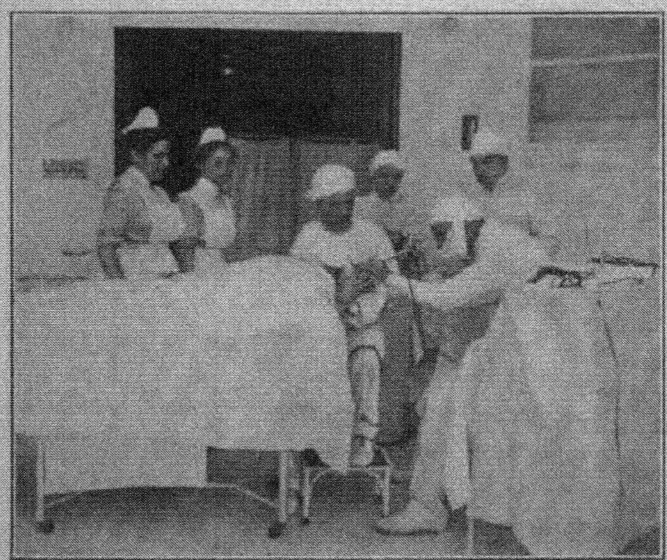

FIG. 150.—Esophagoscopy by the author's "high-low" method. Stage 3. Passing through the thoracic esophagus.

dropping the head had he been possessed of a modern open tube gastroscope passed by sight. The hiatal constriction may assume the form of a slit or more commonly a rosette (Fig. 7, Plate III), and in its rosette form has often been mistaken by esophagoscopists for the cardia, leading to the erroneous idea of a sphincter at the cardia. If the rosette or slit cannot be promptly found, as may be the case in various degrees of diffuse dilatation, the tube-mouth must be shifted farther to the left, and also anteriorly. If the tube-mouth is centered over the hiatal constriction, moderately firm pressure continued for a short time will cause it to yield. Then the tube, maintaining its same direction will, without further trouble, glide into and through the abdominal esophagus. The cardia will not be noticed as a constriction, but its appearance will be announced by the rolling in of reddish gastric, mucosal folds, Fig. 8, Plate III, and by a gush of fluid from the stomach.

The normal esophagoscopic image. The *form* of the endoscopic image has already been described, as seen at the various stages of esophagoscopy. The *color*, as in all the mucosae, is subject to wide individual variations within the limits of health, though not, perhaps, quite so wide as is seen in the pharynx. The color, of course, varies in shade

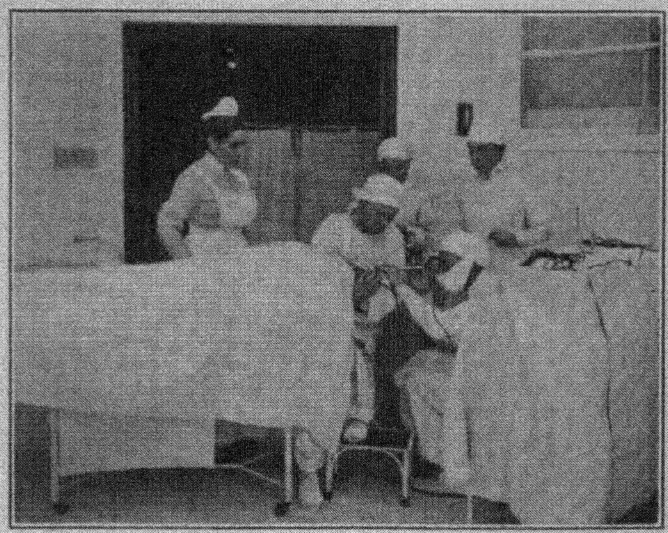

Fig. 151.—Esophagoscopy by the author's "high-low" method. Stage 4. Passing the hiatus. The patient's vertex is about 5 cm. below the top of the table.

with the intensity of the illumination, being dark crimson or brown under feeble light, nearly white under the intense light of an over-illuminated electric lamp. Under ordinary conditions with proper illumination it may be described as pink varying from yellowish to bluish pink. As the author has pointed out, a good idea of average color may be had from inspection of the inside of the particular individual's cheek under the same illumination. The esophageal mucosa glistens with surface moisture. The folds are soft and velvety, rendering infiltrations quickly noticeable. The cricoid cartilage usually shows whitish through the mucosa. As soon as the eye becomes educated to the normal appearance abnormalities of form and color are instantly noted. The gastric mucosa is pink if no food is present, but it is a darker pink than that of the esophagus. When food is in the stomach the color is crimson. These colors refer to distally illuminated images. With proximal illumination the color is said to be dark violet, probably because of the distance from the source of light.

Difficulties of esophagoscopy. Those who follow carefully the methods herein suggested should be able to esophagoscope an average patient under general anesthesia. For the first trial of esophagoscopy without anesthesia the patient should be a slender adult, with long lean neck and few upper teeth. The author urges every endoscopist to avail himself of the first esophageal case of this type, to try esophagoscopy without anesthesia. Soon he will find it needless to use either general or local

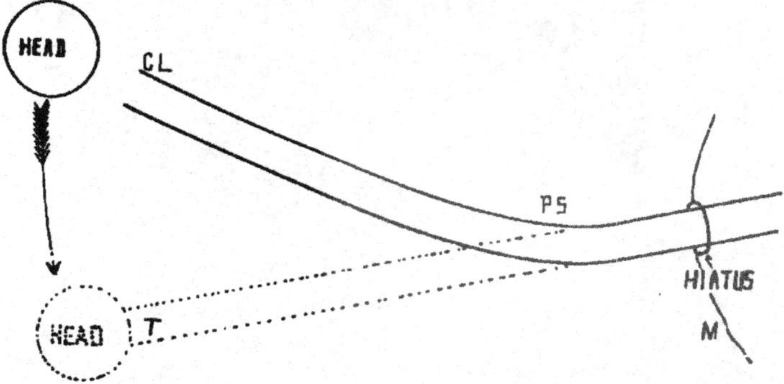

FIG. 152.—Schematic illustration of the author's "high-low" method of esophagoscopy, fourth stage. Passing the hiatus. The head is dropped from the position of the 1st and 2nd stages, CL, to the position T, and at the same time the head and and shoulders are moved to the right (without rotation) which gives the necessary direction for passing the hiatus.

anesthesia for esophagoscopy, and he will have many occasions to be glad that he has acquired the knack. Cases of esophageal malignancy quite often present the desired qualities mentioned, and many of them come for diagnosis in no condition to stand an anesthetic. The greatest difficulty arises from the faulty direction of the tube. It requires a general sense of direction and a mental picture of the direction of the esophagus within the body to get the tube started right and to find the lumen of the pyriform sinus and of the esophagus until the operator has had sufficient experience to know the landmarks and the different appearance of the folds of mucosa as he proceeds. In order to bring these into view it is necessary to remove the secretion. In the author's esophagoscope this is taken away with the aspirator without interruption, though occasionally a swab may be useful in addition. Stagnant semi-solid food in stenotic cases is best removed by the "sponge pumping" process as described for bronchoscopy. Another great difficulty arises from the spasmodic contractions of the esophageal musculature and especially of the inferior constrictor near the cricoid level, in fact, the greatest difficulty in esophagoscopy is right at this point. This and the hiatal spasm are to be overcome by patient waiting with gentle pressure on a correctly directed tube centered over the closed lumen. Forcible misdirected pressure may perforate. The beginner will often find that the esophagoscope seems to be rigidly fixed so that it cannot be either introduced or withdrawn readily. Usually this comes from contact with the upper teeth of the patient and is overcome sometimes by a little wider opening of the jaws, and sometimes by easing up on the bite block, but most often by correcting the position of the patient's head. If the beginner cannot start the tube into the right pyriform sinus, in an adult, it is a good plan to insert an adult direct laryngoscope, and after exposing the arytenoid eminences to view to insert the child size (7 mm.) esophagoscope into the pyriform sinus by sight. This is one of the best ways to learn esophagoscopy. The side-slide oval laryngoscope is the best for this purpose, leaving the slide off and keeping the speculum to the right (recumbent patient) side of the tongue so that the tongue will not crowd into the side opening. It is very rarely necessary to remove an esophagoscope once it is inserted. The author has been much surprised to learn how often some esophagoscopists remove and reinsert the esophagoscope at a seance. Once in, it should stay until the esophagoscopy is finished. If an anesthetic is used, it may be necessary to remove the esophagoscope for respiratory arrest, unless insufflation anesthesia is used. Without anesthesia no accident can occur in careful hands. Occasionally it is necessary to remove the esophagoscope to exchange it for a very small one that will go through a small stricture to get a foreign body that has lodged between two strictures. Occasionally, especially in stenotic conditions of the esophagus a large quantity of fluid will well up into the tube and it will be thought that the light has gone out because there are a number of centimeters' depth of opaque fluid over the light. As soon as this is aspirated through the drainage canal the light will be found burning as brightly as ever. If in doubt as to whether this is the case the light carrier may be withdrawn, but under no circumstances except vital dangers to the patient should the esophagoscope be withdrawn until the examination is complete. As the author uses only two sizes of the esophagoscopic tubes, one for adults and one for children.

there is no need of starting with the wrong size. Serious difficulties may arise from insufficient instrumental equipment, and unlike other departments of surgery makeshifts are usually impossible and may be dangerous. No peroral endoscopic attempt should be made without proper sized tubes for the particular case, proper forceps, sponges, batteries, etc. The operator does his patient and himself an injustice to attempt endoscopy without a complete set as to sizes of whatever form of tubes he desires to use. In his earlier writings the author stated that "If rigid economy must be practiced, much good work can be done with a 7 mm.x45 cm. esophagoscope, a 5 mm.x30 cm. bronchoscope and a 12 mm.x17 cm. laryngeal speculum." Brünings has very justly criticized this statement as "likely to beguile the surgeon" into being content with a couple of tubes selected at random; and he further states, "An insufficient equipment is often worse than none at all." In all of which the author fully concurs.

Moser has advocated the ballooning of the esophagus by the soft-rubber hand-ball of an atomizer, the air being prevented from escaping by the insertion of the window-plug (Fig. 20).

In conclusion it may be said that with the exception of inadequate equipment all of the difficulties of the introduction of the esophagoscope are overcome, as with any other purely manual procedure, by practice.

Complications following esophagoscopy for foreign bodies will be considered in a later chapter. The simple passage of an esophagoscope, if skillfully done, is rarely, if ever, followed by any complications. Slight stiffness of the neck, and irritation of the lower pharynx may be noted in sensitive subjects, especially those with short, thick necks. In diseased conditions, however, we may have complications due either to the esophagoscopy or to the condition for which it is done. Mr. Waggette (Bib. 567) reports a case of severe dysphagia following esophagoscopy in a case of extensive specific ulceration. It would seem, however, that the dysphagia might have resulted from the disease itself without the esophagoscopy. Both contingencies should be borne in mind, and a patient with disease of the esophagus should be told beforehand that his ability to swallow may grow worse either with or without an esophagoscopy. These remarks, however, do not ordinarily apply to recent foreign-body cases. Old foreign-body cases may be followed by cicatricial stenosis. If esophagoscopy is to maintain the high position of usefulness it has attained it is necessary that it shall be safe. If the rules and instructions herein given are followed, esophagoscopy is absolutely without mortality apart from the condition for which it is done. In view of this the beginner must be warned to be careful. The accidents shown in Fig. 153 can occur only through brutal disregard for the delicacy of the vanced organic disease such as hard arteries, cirrhosis of the liver, advanced tuberculosis, uncompensated heart lesions, etc., may have severe complications precipitated by esophagoscopy. A child's esophagoscope (7 mm.) skillfully passed with high head will involve the least risk in such cases.

The technic of introducing the Kahler esophagoscope is precisely the same as that of the Brünings esophagoscope.

Introduction of the Brünings esophagoscope. Brünings describes two methods of introduction, one with a mandrin and one without, the former the easier, the latter the preferable way. Brünings advises ocular introduction when mandrin introduction involves special dangers or fails to accomplish the object for which the esophagoscopy is done. He believes that ocular introduction, therefore, is indicated in the majority of cases. Brünings prefers the sitting position of the patient, though he also uses the laterally recumbent position with knees flexed. In either position the patient's head is held by an assistant. Occasionally he uses the dorsally recumbent position, but he regards this as more difficult, and in children he states that "Lying on the back must in any case be avoided." He states that a general anesthetic is always necessary in children and that they must be raised up for the introduction of the tube after they are anesthetized. In adults thorough local anesthetization with cocaine is used. The Brünings tubes should be warmed and greased with liquid petrolatum and the mirror should be warmed to prevent fogging from condensation. In introduction of the esophagoscope with the mandrin, the hand lamp, Fig. 2, is detached; the funnel-shaped proximal end of the tube is held between the thumb and finger of the right hand like a pen. The silk woven mandrin projecting beyond the distal end of the tube is passed down along the posterior pharyngeal wall into the esophagus. If the mandrin deviates into either pyriform sinus, Brünings directs the patient to swallow to centralize the tube again. When the reflex contractions at the esophageal mouth stop the advance of the mandrin and instrument, no violence is to be used. Instead, an in-and-out probing movement of the tube is used and the patient is commanded to continue regular breathing, and to swallow. If introduction fail, it is necessary to wait with the tube and mandrin in position until the spasm relaxes. This is known by the sensation of an easy advancing of the tube to slight pressure, and by the fact that the "spatula tube" of the instrument almost disappears in the mouth. Then the patient bends the head farther backward and the proximal portion of the tube is moved around to one corner of the patient's mouth, the head being slightly turned to the opposite side. If a gap between teeth is available the tube is moved into the gap. Then the mandrin is removed, the hand lamp attached and the inner tube inserted. If the latter has been in place with the mandrin inside of it, it is now pushed downward. In most instances, however, foreign bodies and disease high up are dealt with through the spatula tube alone, without using an inner tube.

In introduction by sight in the sitting patient the procedure is as described for direct laryngoscopy up to the point of exposing the larynx, the hand lamp being fitted with the tube spatula as shown in Fig. 2. This will reach to the level of the tracheal bifurcation. If it is desired to explore further, the inner tube (Fig. 4) of appropriate size and length according to the patient is inserted. After exposing the larynx, the spatular end of the tube spatula, or outer tube, is inserted in the median line and the larynx is drawn forward as the spatular end is slid down behind the larynx into the hypopharynx. Here the advance is usually opposed by spasm, bringing the posterior lip of the esophageal mouth forward and presenting an "unconquerable barrier" to further advance. While waiting for the spasm to subside the position of the patient and of the instrument are inspected to see that they are correct, with relaxed muscles, without rigid bending of the head; and the patient is told to keep on breathing quietly and regularly. Swallowing, if the patient can accomplish it, helps materially. Rotating movements of the tube are helpful in finding the lumen. Once past the constriction at the mouth of the esophagus the tube passes without further difficulty, the head being managed as before. When the full length of the spatular tube, or outer tube, has been inserted, which will bring the distal end to about the level of the tracheal bifurcation, the inner extension tube is inserted if it is desired to explore further. In the left laterally recumbent patient the manipulations are the same as in the sitting patient, because with the operator standing facing the patient, and bending the operator's head down to the right, the operator maintains the same relative position to the patient's anatomy as in the sitting position of the patient. In the dorsal position of the patient which Brünings does not advise, the operator holds the instrument with the right hand as in Fig. 142. For further details of Brünings' methods the reader is referred to Brünings' interesting and instructive book (Bib. 62) or to the excellent translation thereof by Mr. Walter G. Howarth (Bib. 208).

CHAPTER XI.

Acquiring Skill.

The purpose of this book is to tell how to do peroral endoscopy. But with all purely manual things a knowledge how to do them is merely a start. It requires prolonged practice to be able to do them well. An orchestra leader knows how the instruments should be played, yet is unable to play upon any except the one on which he has spent a lifetime of practice. Were it not for the evidence of the performance of others, a beginner's first instrumental musical attempt would lead him to think impossible many of the manual things that later are as easy to him as walking. Other and new difficulties will arise and will be overcome; there will always be difficulties worthy of continual practice in order to acquire the utmost tactile and co-ordinate dexterity. So it is with peroral endoscopy. Herbert Tilley (Bib. 545) very aptly states that, "While it would be idle affectation to suggest that neither skill nor practice is necessary for the intelligent use of the bronchoscope, yet it is very true that a little practice combined with patience and gentleness should render any surgeon competent to use the bronchoscope with reasonable assurance." While the author believes that more than a little practice is desirable, he heartily concurs in the foregoing statement because of the qualifying clause "combined with patience and gentleness." These are the great safeguards of endoscopy.

As with instrumental music certain personal qualifications will enable better endoscopic work and especially is this true in difficult foreign-body cases. Good eyesight without excessive refractive errors comes first in importance. Endless patience is an essential. A good faculty of orientation will stand the endoscopist in good stead. Mechanical ingenuity is necessary. The greatest percentage of successes will accrue to him who is so constituted as to work calmly and deliberately, yet quickly and accurately, under severe stress of prolonged work with one eye, subject to great anxieties and where a mistake or lack of promptness and accuracy may mean the death of the patient either immediately or by default ultimately. There is absolutely nothing like it in the whole realm of surgery. The operator's ordeal is well described by Ingals as follows: "The heart-breaking delays, the extreme anxiety for the patient and the knowledge that prolonged operations of this kind are dangerous, while failure may spell death for the patient, place the operator under such circumstances under an indescribable stress."

The greatest difficulty will be encountered by the surgeon who has been accustomed always to work with both hands and both eyes in an open wound. Such a one will find difficulties in working with the mirror in ordinary indirect rhino-laryngologic work, and endoscopy will present to him difficulties infinitely greater. Far be it from the author to deter any one from taking up bronchoscopy and esophagoscopy. On the contrary, it has been the author's endeavor for years to popularize these procedures with the profession and to induce every one who is willing to devote to it the necessary amount of practice, to take it up. In fact. it is because the author once said that bronchoscopy and esophagoscopy were easy, that he deems it at this late day necessary to issue a word of caution against taking up the work, especially in foreign body cases, without due appreciation of the difficulties to be met and overcome only by continual practice.

The foregoing, however, applies only to foreign body work, direct laryngeal operating, and a few other procedures like the dilatation of bronchial and esophageal strictures, exploration of the subdiverticular esophagus, and the like. It does not apply to the exposure of the larynx for diagnosis or for the introduction of intratracheal insufflation tubes, which procedures anyone can easily learn without special forehead mirror experience or special qualifications. The author believes that every laryngologist of the future will be considered incompetent if he cannot examine the larynx of any child by direct laryngoscopy, and that the rhino-laryngologist (who of necessity is trained by years of work with one eye through narrow openings) is, logically, the best man fitted for bronchoscopy and esophagoscopy, and he should be a bronchoscopist and an esophagoscopist. If. however, the laryngologist prefers not to devote the time and attention needed to do them well, he may refer cases requiring bronchoscopy and esophagoscopy to some near neighbor who is equipped; but escape direct laryngoscopy he cannot, if he desires to be called a laryngologist.* It is the author's hope and belief that perfection in direct laryngoscopy will lead every rhino-laryngologist possessed of good eyesight to be also a broncho-esophagoscopist. For foreign-body work a large instrumental outfit is necessary, but no armamentarium, however complete, will lessen the need for prolonged coordinate education of the eye and the fingers. To some extent, this might be said of surgery in general; but with endoscopy it will be very different if none of the previous training of the surgeon has been in the

*Extracted from the Author's "Rapport" at the International Medical Congress, London, 1913.

line of working with one eye while ignoring the image of the other, nor in the practice of depth perception with one eye only. Estimation of distances is under all circumstances largely a matter of personal equation, some persons being remarkably adept naturally, while others find it exceedingly difficult to make even an approximate estimate of so apparent a distance as the width of a street. Such difficulties in making estimates are, of course, enormously increased when they are to be made with one eye only and looking through a tube. Much practice, however, will enable anyone to estimate with sufficient accuracy the various depths of the tissues seen in the endoscopic image; and those with natural aptitude can develop this depth perception to an extent that seems incredible. Much as it may hurt the self-esteem of the surgeon, after his years of experience in surgery, if he wishes to do bronchoscopy for foreign bodies, he must begin at the beginning and take endless hours of practice on the dog, unless he be so heartless as to do his first tube work on human beings. Practice on human beings in the general field of surgery is very different, because the careful man, working in an open wound with both eyes and both hands, and with an experienced surgeon assisting, will do no harm. The very worst that may follow is simply a prolongation of the operation. In endoscopy, prolongation is often a very serious matter; and the errors of omission and those of commission may be fatal both by default in not removing the foreign body; in making it impossible for anybody else to remove it; or in producing fatal trauma or respiratory arrest. Master and pupil cannot see at the same time in endoscopy.

For the acquirement of skill five modes of education of the eye and fingers are available.

1. Preliminary practice with bronchoscope and forceps.
2. Practice upon the cadaver.
3. Practice upon the dog.
4. Sketching the endoscopic image.
5. Practice upon human beings.

Preliminary practice. The first step for the beginner in endoscopy should be the mastery of the mechanical details of tubes and their illumination. He should learn just the degree of illumination the lamps will stand without burning them out or shortening their "life." Carbon filament lamps will stand only an amperage that is indicated by the filament *beginning* to turn white. Tungsten filament lamps illuminate with a less amperage, but the rheostat may be run up until the filament gets quite white. If after an hour's use the glass of the lamp shows black it indicates that the lamp has been overilluminated. Some instruction by an electrician is valuable. These suggestions apply to all forms of instruments. With the Brünings and Kahler instruments the adjustment of scope should be introduced and the fully extended head gradually raised until the vertex is higher than the table. The laryngeal exposure obtained will give the key to the proper position for peroral endoscopy. Then the bronchoscopic and esophagoscopic anatomy should be studied. Particular attention should be given to appreciation of distances especially those from the glottis to the bifurcation; from the bifurcation to the upper lobe bronchi on the right and the left sides respectively; and from the right upper-lobe bronchus to the middle-lobe bronchus. The angle of branching of the larger bronchi is also important, though these angles are apt to be distorted in the cadaver. The beginner in endoscopy should make himself familiar with all parts of the tracheo-bronchial tree so that he knows instinctively how to reach any desired location. All of these things can be learned quicker and better on the cadaver than on the living and they cannot be learned at all from books.

Practice upon the dog. The next step in the endoscopist's training should be the education of the eye to the prompt comprehension of the endoscopic pictures by practice upon the dog. This will be of little use so far as the exposure of the larynx and the introduction of the bronchoscope and esophagoscope in the human being are concerned, because the dog does not present the difficulties arising in the human being from the right-angled pharyngeal turn of the air and food passages. Nevertheless, practice on the dog is of the utmost importance in training the eye and the fingers. The mentality of vision must be educated not only to comprehend the endoscopic image but it must comprehend the ever changing image promptly. The histologist must educate his eye to extreme niceties of morphologic distinctions, but he has no end of time in which to study each field. The endoscopist in making observations in the air and food passages must observe not only form but color; and most difficult of all, his object is never still a moment, never twice in precisely the same position.

It takes much practice to be sure when the forceps are at the proper depth to grasp the foreign body or particular piece of tissue. Dog work is better than cadaver work for practice in this direction, because the colors, and especially the constant respiratory, pulsatory, bechic, and, in case of the esophagus, peristaltic and antiperistaltic movements present actual working conditions. No one should think of attempting for the first time to remove a foreign body from a human being until he has at least 100 times removed a foreign body from a dog. If the operator has but little endoscopic work to do, he should practice between times on the dog in order to maintain skill. In foreign body practice on the dog, it is well to remember that this animal is peculiarly well able to rid himself of foreign bodies. He can get open safety-pins and sometimes even fish-hooks out of his bronchi. Many letters of chagrin have come to the author relating inability to find foreign bodies introduced a day or two before. If for any experimental purpose it is desired to have a foreign body remain in the canine lower air passages, it is necessary to devise a very secure anchorage. A small dog is preferable. Large dogs require longer instruments than human beings. Scopolomine 0.00065 gm. with morphine 0.0324 gm. hypodermatically is a convenient anesthetic for a small dog. It should be given an hour in advance and repeated, if necessary.

Sketching the endoscopic image. One of the best ways to educate the eye to grasp quickly the fleeting panoramic endoscopic views is to practice sketching. However crude, artistically, the effort may be, the practice of quickly observing form and color of the visible field will be of inestimable value. Practice catching the darks first and jot them down with pencil in previously scribed circles. After the habit of quickly noting the darks is formed, the noting of the lights as to their form is easily acquired, for in a measure, the lights take care of themselves because they are necessarily blocked out by the darks. The noting of the color comes next. The color of the darks is unimportant for training of the eye, though, of course, very necessary for accurate illustration. For the recognition of disease it is necessary to observe the color of the well-illuminated parts—the lights. If the sketching method of educating the eye as here outlined is practiced, it is remarkable how the eye will acquire the habit of quickly recording successive pictures of form and color. As the field of view is small the form and position of the darks and the color of the lights are taken in over different parts of the whole field simultaneously. If desired, pencil and sketch cards with scribed circles can be sterilized in alcohol for use on the instrument table, but it is scarcely justifiable to keep a patient endoscoped either with or without an anesthetic. Moreover, it is quite unnecessary, because, if the essential amount of endoscopic practice on the dog is done, the sketching can be there practiced until not only will the education of the eye be perfected, but the mental habit of recording impressions will be acquired, so that a series of a half dozen or more pictures can be sketched from memory immediately after the endoscopy is finished. Unless one has had much previous training in water or oil colors, wax crayon pencils are best, as they do not require a fixative like pastels, though their tints are not quite so accurate or so easily blended or overworked. Faber makes 60 different tints under the name of "Castex Polychrome" pencils. Numbers 31, 34, 36, 37, 49 and 52 will probably be found most useful. Blending can be done with a clean, pointed pencil-eraser. So far, no photographic method of recording endoscopic views of the air and food passages has yielded very satisfactory results, not only because of the feebleness and reddish tint of the return rays, but mainly because of the perpetual movement which prevents lengthy exposure. Until some difficult problems are overcome, pencil, crayon and brush are the only means of recording appearances.

Practice upon human beings. It is stated above that dog and cadaver practice do not help greatly in overcoming the difficulties of introduction. Dog and cadaver practice do help to some extent, because the education of the eye promptly to appreciate the endoscopic image is fundamental; but the knack of displacement for laryngeal exposure and of passing the cricopharyngeus, esophagoscopically, are yet to be learned and for these purposes only the human being will serve. Until human direct laryngoscopy is learned no attempt should be made to do bronchoscopy or esophagoscopy. Respiratory arrest during the progress of esophagoscopy, or after the withdrawal of the bronchoscope in bronchoscopy, demands that for the safety of the patient the operator shall be able promptly to expose the larynx and insert the bronchoscope for oxygen insufflation. The familiarity with the location of the pyriform sinuses and laryngopharynx under direct view is quite essential to esophagoscopy. To anyone who is skillful at exposing the larynx, the introduction of the bronchoscope is easy, and no one should attempt bronchoscopy until he has acquired sufficient skill to expose the larynx in almost any patient in 15 seconds. Seldom should it require more than 8 seconds. One ought to be able to hold the larynx in view long enough for half a dozen men to take a look. Fortunately there is, in all outpatient clinics, a goodly percentage of cases that justify direct laryngoscopy. Any patient with laryngeal paralysis of undetermined etiology or any patient with infiltration of the arytenoid region should be examined for disease of the party wall, anteriorly, and also down in the hypopharynx. Certain cases of laryngeal tuberculosis are benefited by the direct application of the galvano-cautery. Other material that can be conscientiously used will readily be found, because direct laryngoscopy in any case not dyspneic, and done under aseptic precautions is harmless. Tracheotomized cases should be regularly and carefully tracheoscoped for exuberant granulations which may occlude the tube and cause death. Erosions, necrosis of cartilage, edematous areas et cetera, due to ill-fitting cannulae are remediable. A plan for cure of the stenosis can only in this way be formulated. Such cases should be examined from above and below. Having mastered hypopharyngoscopic and direct laryngeal left-hand exposure in the human being, the student who has followed the course here laid out need have no hesitation whatever in attempting bronchoscopy or esophagoscopy in any case where these procedures are not contraindicated. The first few esophagoscopies should be emaciated adults with few teeth, and, if justifiable, should be generally anesthetized.

CHAPTER XII.

Foreign Bodies in the Air and Food Passages.

List of foreign bodies found in air and food passages. It seems to the author a sacrifice of space to list all of the foreign bodies so far found in these passages, since any substance not too large and not soluble may be encountered endoscopically; be that substance from the animal, vegetable or mineral kingdoms, or manufactured therefrom by man. Rather would it seem profitable to classify these substances by the mechanical problems of their extraction and this will be done in future chapters. It may be well here to classify the sources of foreign bodies. The following classification of Voelcker, quoted by Sir St. Clair Thomson, (Bib. 539) is comprehensive.

1. From the mouth—articles of food, bones of meat or fish, fruit stones, peas, beans, shells, seeds, ears of corn, grasses, pieces of wood or coal, coins, buttons, pencils, marbles, toys, broken pipe-stems, pins. needles, nails, tooth-plates, leeches.

2. From the stomach—vomited food or blood, or the migration of lumbrici or threadworms.

3. From the lungs—hemoptysis, hydatids.

4. From the outside—as by penetration of a pin, dart, bullet, or drainage-tube from the neck.

5. From surgical measures—detached portions of instruments, sprays, brushes, cotton-wool, gauze, sponges, antrum plugs, intubation tubes, broken-off cannulae of tracheotomy tubes, amputated tonsils, adenoids or other growths and hemorrhage.

6. Arising ***in situ***—necrosed cartilage, ulcerating sloughs, membrane, effused blood.

7. Penetration from the neighborhood—ulceration or extension of malignant disease from the pleura, thyroid gland, or esophagus, or the penetration of a tuberculous gland from the mediastinum.

To this list might be added the penetration of a foreign body from the esophagus into the trachea, of which the author has seen two instances, and the penetration of a foreign body from the tracheo-bronchial tree into the esophagus of which the author has seen one instance, that of a sharp fragment of bone the point of which was visible in the esophagus, but which was removed by bronchoscopy from the left bronchus.

Prophylaxis. Many of the foreign-body accidents are entirely preventable. If no one put into his mouth anything but food, foreign-body cases would be rare. In the author's collection only about three per cent are proper articles of food and these mostly insufficiently masticated or cooked. This does not include the foods removed from strictured esophagus. A much larger percentage are substances normally in food stuffs but not removed before eating, such as bones, shells, hulls and seeds. More care in the preparation of food and in the eating of fruits with large seeds is of first prophylactic importance. Care in the preparation of foods can easily prevent the accidental presence of pins, needles, bits of china and glass, enamelling and solder from utensils and the like. Tradesmen, such as lathers, carpetmen and upholsterers who carry tacks and nails in their mouths could just as easily have learned in the beginning some less dangerous as well as less filthy method, and apprentices should be so taught. Magazines with automatic feeding mechanisms could easily be devised that would also save time, which latter feature is the only one that would appeal strongly to the employer. Children should be taught from infancy not to put anything inedible into their mouths. A large part of the infantile education as to the physical nature of the portable substances in reach comes from testing them in the mouth; but this natural tendency can be combated as can also the infantile effort to assist dentition by biting on various substances. However, if mothers and nurses make a special effort it is remarkable how readily most children even as early as the second year can be taught by reproof. Younger children must be watched. The frequency with which pins, buttons and safety-pins are removed by endoscopists points to carelessness in leaving these things within the baby's reach. Teething rings and the toys of children should all be too large to get beyond the mouth into the air or food passages, and all toys should be regularly inspected for loose parts likely to become detached. Digital efforts at removal are frequently responsible for dislodging and forcing downward foreign bodies that could be readily removed from the pharynx with forceps. The index finger curling forward hook-like in an effort to remove an object from the laryngo-pharynx is very apt to force the object into the larynx. Parents, nurses, dentists and physicians should bear this in mind. Nurses and physicians understand fully about removing artificial dentures from the mouth preparatory to anesthesia; but they are not so often alert to the same potential dangers in case of unconsciousness from alcoholic intoxication, delirium, syncope, shock, collapse and sleep, especially the dozing or nap of the daytime.

Foreign bodies in the hysteric and the insane. We must always be on our guard against the cases which come in with the most positive assurance by the patient that there is a foreign-body present. These cases are of two classes. Those who have had a foreign body which has passed on downward and left some traumatism, the sensations of which lead the patient to believe that the foreign body is still present, and the hysteric patient who believes she, or he has a foreign body. In regard to the hysteric class, it is a great mistake to do a bronchoscopy with the hope of cure by suggestion. Such "cures" are ephemeral. The foreign-body illusion will recur with more and more persistence and amplification the more often it is removed by suggestion. As is well known, two of the most prominent characteristics of hysteria are the hunger for sympathy and the desire to mystify and astonish the physician by unusual simulations of disease. The border lines between pure hysteria and the hysteriform symptoms of paranoia on the one hand, and between the hysteriform and the suicidal symptoms of paranoia on the other hand, are too abstruse for the author. These matters concern the psychiatrist. The question that must be determined by the endoscopist is whether or not to do an endoscopy and if so whether it shall be first a bronchoscopy or an esophagoscopy in case indirect mirror examination prove negative. In case of foreign body visible radiographically, or one that has produced a visible lesion such as abscess, the question is quickly decided. In all other cases there are four safe rules to follow:

1. Consider only objective symptoms.
2. Consider only testimony of persons other than the patient as tc history.
3. In all cases of doubt make a thorough endoscopic search.
4. If endoscopy is negative do not worry about the patient's later assertion that she coughed up the foreign body that you failed to find. It is parallel with the hysteric cripples that throw away their crutches after a faith cure.

Remarkable cases of multiple foreign bodies in the stomach of the insane are not uncommon. A certain proportion of these are almost certain to be metallic, or of lead, glass or porcelain and dense to the ray. Some such bodies may be removed with the 10 mm. x 53 cm. esophagogastroscope. As a rule, however, the objects that appeal to the insane are of a kind that appears most appalling to them such as open pocketknives, sharp glass and the like. These are best removed by the abdominal surgeon by external operation. Should any object, of whatever kind, lodge in the esophagus, larynx or trachea, however, it should be removed endoscopically, and it should not be pushed down into the stomach as fatal trauma is very likely to result. In most instances it will be in the esophagus that the endoscopist will be required for foreign body work in the hysteric and the insane. The author has, however, had one case of voluntary aspiration of a foreign body into the bronchi, following a probably accidental similar aspiration.

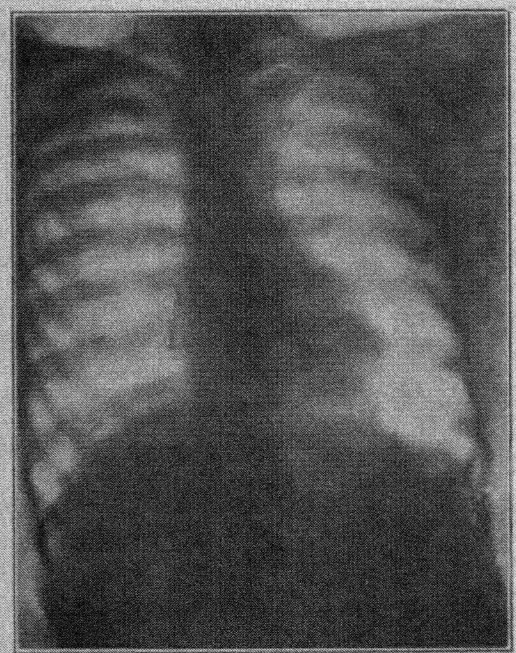

Fig. 154. Radiograph by Dr. Lewis G. Cole, showing two tacks in a posterior branch of the right inferior lobe bronchus. Tacks removed by bronchoscopy through the mouth.

A case of voluntary aspiration of a foreign body into the bronchi, removal by bronchoscopy. At the Eye and Ear Hospital, of Pittsburgh, the author removed by bronchoscopy, two tacks from a posterior branch of the right inferior lobe bronchus of a woman aged forty-one years, referred by Dr. L. G. Cole, of New York City, who made the excellent radiograph (Fig. 154). The anesthetic was ether, given by Dr. Homer

McCready. The bronchi were so full of pus that the patient nearly drowned in her own secretions. After the bronchoscopic removal of the pus the tacks (Fig. 155) were removed without difficulty, the first tack requiring one and one-half minutes and the second one two minutes, as timed by Miss Crock. At the operation the author had the kind assistance of Drs. John W. Boyce, Homer McCready, Jesse Meyer (St. Louis), Richard Lewisohn (New York). Four months after the removal of the tacks, as reported in the foregoing, the patient came to Dr. Cole's office at the suggestion of Dr. Geo. W. Bogart, stating that she had the same old symptoms, and she thought there must be more tacks there. She further said that the tacks Dr. Jackson took out were corroded, yet the last one just coughed up was bright and new. A radiograph showed one tack on each side of the thorax, Fig. 156, not so near the periphery as the previous tacks. The question then arose how could the patient get the tacks into the bronchi voluntarily, as it was clear that she was a hysteric, if not demented. Dr. John W. Boyce, in consultation

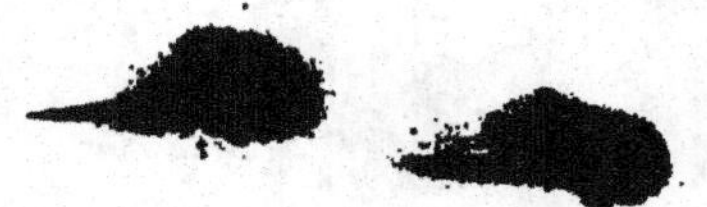

FIG. 155. Tacks removed by bronchoscopy from posterior branch of right inferior lobe bronchus of a woman aged 41 years, referred by Dr. Lewis G. Cole.

on this point, said that by throwing a number of tacks into the pharynx and taking a deep inspiration, she might get one or two down, but in so doing she would swallow many more than she could aspirate, so that, if not too late, a radiograph would show tacks in the alimentary canal in progress of passing through. An excellent radiograph by Dr. Cole showed four tacks in the abdomen (Fig. 157). The author removed the tacks (Fig. 158) from the bronchi in the French Hospital of New York City with the kind assistance of Drs. Robert C. Myles, J. H. Abraham, John McCoy, T. Taylor and Geo. W. Bogart, the head being held in the Boyce position by Dr. D. T. Sable and the anesthetic (chloroform) being skillfully administered by Dr. T. Drysdale Buchanan. There was a most intense inflammation of all the bronchial mucosa and large quantities of pus were removed. The tack in a posterior branch of the right middle lobe bronchus was readily removed, requiring about two minutes, but the second tack in the posterior branch of the left inferior lobe bronchus was exceedingly difficult safely to remove. It was imbedded in bleeding granulation tissue, and the point had perforated the opposite wall of the next larger branch. After fifteen minutes' work the author succeeded in disengaging the point and removing the tack. Two radiographs by Dr. Cole immediately after the bronchoscopy demonstrated that no tacks remained in the thorax.

Remarks. The first two tacks had, no doubt, been accidentally aspirated while putting down oilcloth as stated by the patient. The sym-

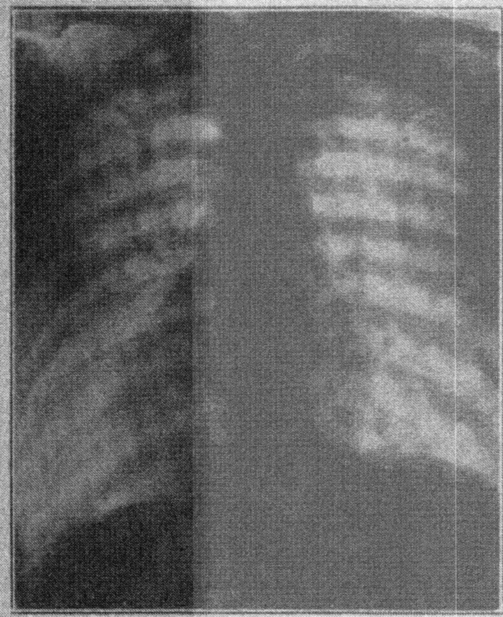

FIG. 156. Radiograph by Dr. L. G. Cole, of tacks voluntarily aspirated by the patient.

pathy, the interest, the sensational features of the case, and the anesthetic evidently appealed to the neurotic temperament of the patient, and developed the hysteria which later was most troublesomely manifest in ways unnecessary to enumerate. The case is unique in that it has never before been demonstrated that a patient could voluntarily aspirate a foreign body into the bronchi, and it teaches a valuable lesson as to how to detect the occurrence by radiography of the abdomen in cases where an accident is denied. In all hysteric and insane patients a radiograph should be made after removal of the foreign body as a matter of record.

Procedure in a case of suspected foreign body. When a patient comes complaining of a foreign body in the air or food passages the questions that must be determined are:

1. Is there a foreign body present?

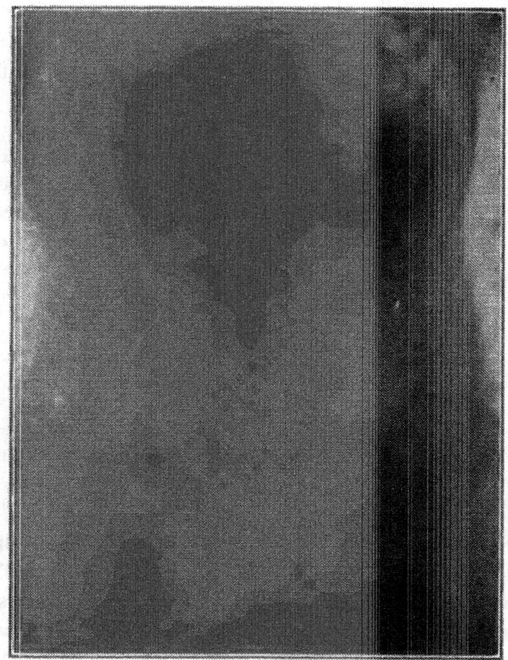

FIG. 157. Radiograph by Dr. L. G. Cole, showing tacks in the intestines in progress of passing through. Tacks were swallowed by the patient in attempt to aspirate them.

2. Where is it located?
3. Is a peroral endoscopic procedure indicated?
4. Are there any contraindications to endoscopy?
5. Shall the first endoscopic procedure be laryngoscopic, bronchoscopic or esophagoscopic?

The questions listed above are so interlaced that they must be here considered more or less collectively to avoid repetition; but to determine these questions quickly and, so far as possible, accurately requires orderly investigative procedures as applied to the individual case. The various steps as pursued in the author's clinic are detailed below, in the order given. Of course, if the foreign body is located in the earlier steps the investigation may terminate at any stage.

1. History.
2. Indirect examination of the larynx; then the naso-pharynx, then the tonsils or their neighborhood.
3. Radiography.
4. Physical examination locally in the neck and thoracically as well as generally by an internist.
5. Endoscopy.

History of the patient and deductions therefrom. Carefully taken histories are valuable statistically and for determining the question of the presence and the localization of a foreign body. To be of value statistically it is necessary that a blank should be filled out in order that a record of certain details shall not be lacking in any of the histories.

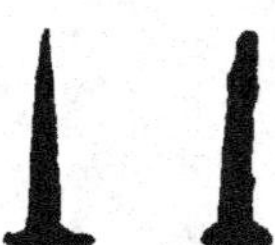

Fig. 158. Tacks voluntarily aspirated. Removed by bronchoscopy through the mouth. Covered with dried blood and secretions.

The author has used a blank of which Fig. 159 is a reduced illustration. Almost all cases come in with a history of having "swallowed" the foreign body, and we must be on our guard not to accept this as meaning that the foreign body is probably in the esophagus. As many of the cases involve the question of a foreign body not opaque to the ray, we must depend upon other things for localization. First in importance, is to find out the symptoms at the time the foreign-body accident occurred, and particularly as to whether or not there was cough or dyspnea at the time, followed with blood stained expectoration, because very often after a short period, the tolerance of the air passages manifests itself in a total absence of symptoms. It is very rare, however, that there is no coughing at the time the foreign body entered; so that a total absence of coughing, provided some one is at hand whose observation is reliable, strongly negatives the possibility of the foreign body having entered the trachea or larynx. This, of course, does not apply to patients under anesthesia, to the intoxicated, nor to any case in which a calm, reliable ob-

CASE

Name Age Date

Address Sex S. M. W.

Race Nativity Occupation

Referred by

History taken by

Diagnosis

Hospital Private case or ward case.

Admitted

Discharged

On admission

General health

Nature of foreign body

How long was the foreign body in air passage or esophagus

Immediate symptoms produced by foreign body

Symptoms following entrance of the foreign body

Attempts made to remove it before direct examination

Pulmonary symptoms

Esophageal symptoms

Other symptoms

Result of X Ray examination

Kind of method employed for direct examination

Anesthesia a. Local. b. General. c. No Anesthesia.

Operative difficulties

Instruments employed

Resulting instrumental lesion

Post-operative pulmonary and esophageal condition

Operation of particular interest

Duration of convalescence

Treatment

Result obtained

Autopsy

Bibliography

Surgeon-in-chief

Anesthetist

Assistants

Fig. 159. History sheet for foreign body cases. After the foreign body has been removed, its location is entered on the top line thus: "Case. Pin removed bronchoscopically from dorsal branch of right inferior lobe bronchus."

server was not present. The period of quiescence during which there are no symptoms, may last from a few weeks to a few months before the symptoms of chronic inflammatory conditions and irritations become manifest. The reverse of this is not, however, so generally applicable: because after some preliminary irritation in the region of the larynx exciting cough, the patient may have swallowed the foreign body, and it may have lodged in the esophagus. Then again, there may be severe dyspnea at the time either from the foreign body obstructing the larynx or from pressure on the esophagus below the cricoid where the party-wall is membranous. In one of the author's cases, a surgeon had done a tracheotomy for the removal of a foreign body supposed to be in the trachea because of great dyspnea. Not finding the foreign body in the trachea, the surgeon asked the author to pass a bronchoscope. On bronchoscopy, through the mouth, the author found nothing in the trachea or bronchi. Esophagoscopy, however, enabled us to find and remove the foreign body (a coin above which meat and other food had become impacted) in the upper third of the esophagus. The tracheotomy was perfectly justifiable and lifesaving because it was done for dyspnea, which was relieved completely; but it points a valuable lesson in regard to the dyspnea produced by esophageally lodged foreign bodies. Intermittent dyspnea or intermittent cyanosis after a history of choking on a foreign body is practically diagnostic of a foreign body in the air passages. It is most apt to occur in flat foreign bodies, which allow free passage of air when their greatest plane corresponds to the long axis of the air passages, but which are more or less obstructive when they turn sidewise. This may occur when the foreign body simply rotates in a semi-fixed position. When the foreign body is free to move and is being coughed up against the under surface of the glottis, there is, in some cases, a very decided sudden stoppage of the glottic space by the bulk of the foreign body, probably plus more or less spasm which makes a very characteristic sound that can be heard some distance from the patient. The intermittent dyspnea, in such a case, may occur not from a rocking valve-like action, but simply the intermittent occlusion of the subglottic trachea. A remarkable difference between foreign bodies in the trachea and bronchi as compared with a similar condition in the esophagus is that foreign bodies which are too small to cause dyspnea usually cause the patient no inconvenience. Even cough may be practically absent, so that the patient is almost free from symptoms. In the esophagus, on the contrary, the patient usually feels the foreign body every time he attempts to swallow, and there is usually a constant sensation of distress and annoyance. Foreign bodies which have entered the air passages usually cause coughing and a sense of suffocation at the moment that the foreign body enters the trachea; but thereafter, there is no sensation of suffocation unless the foreign body is very large, and there is usually no other sensation. When an intruder enters the esophagus, on the other hand, there is usually a sensation of something lodged in the throat and the patient is impelled to make repeated swallowing efforts in the attempt to dislodge it. Food may be regurgitated for a time and then swallowing may seem normal, leading to the error of supposing the intruder has gone down. This may be due to the relaxation of the spasm at first excited by the presence of the intruder, or it may be due to the foreign body having turned to a less obstructive position. Ingals reports a case in which small particles of corroded iron were coughed up from a nail which had been in the trachea for a number of years. While such evidence is valuable when present it must not be taken negatively. As pointed out by Iglauer (Bib. 223), the mere size of a foreign body does not preclude its presence in the trachea. Determination of the position of an esophageally lodged foreign body by the sensation of the patient is exceedingly misleading. The sensations that the patient feels may be those of the spasm excited in a relatively remote position in the esophagus, or the pains of other sensations may be reflected, but perhaps the most important factor is that the sensations of the esophagus are of a very ill-developed kind. Foreign bodies that have lodged in the larynx usually cause hoarseness in a very short time, and the cough is apt to be of a croupy character. If, however, the foreign body is of such a nature as to prop the cords apart there may be complete aphonia. and this is almost diagnostic of a laryngeally lodged foreign body. Severe dyspnea also usually points to glottic or subglottic lodgment. Foreign bodies in the larynx are usually somewhat painful as compared to those that lodge in the trachea and bronchi, which are painless. There is often a peculiar character to the cough when the foreign body prevents glottic closure by working between the cords. As is well known, the cords approximate and the cough comes with an explosive effort. This mechanism is interfered with by the propping apart of the cords and hence the cough has rather the sound of an intubated patient, though only to a slight degree. In children there is the usual tracheal cough owing to the collapse of the tracheal walls during the expulsive efforts. A very hoarse, croupy cry usually means reactionary inflammation, and to the trained ear there is a peculiar note produced in most cases by which Dr. Ellen J. Patterson and the author have been able to diagnosticate the presence of foreign bodies in a few instances. The note may be likened to a croupy cry with a metallic hiss added, though this description is inadequate to anyone who has not heard it. We do not know what produces the alteration of the ordinary croupy sound, unless it is the rush of air past the foreign body. In one such case, referred to us by Dr. C. C. Sandels, the sound amounted almost to a whistle, and was evidently due to the rush of air past the thin edge of the hollow brass cap at the "keeper-end" of a safety-pin. No radiograph had been taken and the diagnosis of foreign body in the larynx was made by us solely on the modification of the croupy cry. There was no history of foreign body and the family and their physician were astonished to see the pin. Every case with a foreign-body history should be followed up closely until the foreign body is located either in the body, in the stools, or until it is coughed up as the case may be. Under no circumstances should it be forgotten or ignored as harmless in the absence of symptoms.

Indirect examination. When a patient comes in complaining of having swallowed a pin and states he or she can feel it "here," pointing to a location in the neck or chest, the patient should be placed at once in the recumbent position and a mirror examination should be made in this position. The patient should, if possible, never be allowed to raise the head until after the mirror and Roentgen-ray examinations. When there is reason to suspect that a foreign body has entered the air passages, the patient should be kept recumbent and, preferably, face downward. Under no circumstances should the patient be allowed to sit up or to lie on either side. The reason for these precautions is to prevent gravitation. If the patient is allowed to sit erect, the foreign body, especially if of small size, will fall down into the deepest possible bronchus. If the patient is allowed to lie on the back, the foreign body will invade one of the posterior branches which are exceedingly difficult to reach. The objection to lying on the side is that this would favor the foreign body entering the upper lobe bronchus, and especially would this be the case if the foreign body should already be in one side and be dislodged and taken over into the other side. Under such circumstances, the upper lobe bronchus would be almost surely invaded if the patient were at the time lying upon the previously uninvaded side. It is probable that lying upon the face may cause the foreign body to enter the middle lobe bronchus, but in the two cases of foreign bodies in the middle lobe bronchus in the author's experience the extractions seemed easier than in other cases in which the posterior branches of the inferior lobe bronchus had been invaded. Further evidence afforded by additional cases may demonstrate that middle lobe bronchus cases are not easier. In this event dorsal recumbency would be better, but there can be no question that recumbency is advisable because of the well proven tendency of foreign bodies to work downward. Because of the branching angle of the middle lobe bronchi and of the inferior lobe bronchi, respectively, in relation to the long axis of the body, ventral recumbency does not make as steep a declivity into the middle lobe bronchus and its branches as does dorsal recumbency into the dorsal branches of the inferior lobe bronchus. The fact of there being but one middle lobe bronchus also diminishes the chances of invasion even though right sided invasion is more frequent than left as will be referred to later. Next in importance is to quiet the fears of the patient, and above all not to urge the patient to cough in the vain hope of coughing the foreign body out. Not only are the chances of success small. but the chances of a sharp foreign body, such as a pin, burying its point are great. In the event of the point becoming buried, there is very apt to be a very ratchet-like action by which the pin is forced deeper and deeper, the point preventing upward movement. In case of foreign bodies more or less cubical or globular in shape there is risk that, in coughing, the foreign body may be jammed in the subglottic space and thus asphyxia be threatened. The rule in regard to keeping the patient recumbent does not apply to foreign bodies definitely located in the esophagus, because gravity plays little or no part in the downward movement of anything in the esophagus under normal conditions. When an esophagoscope is introduced conditions are altered. Having examined the larynx first, to make sure that there is no foreign body on the brink ready to fall into the air passages below should the patient gag, the tonsils and nasopharynx and neighboring regions should be carefully examined. In all of this inspection preliminary to endoscopy, abrasions of possible foreign body origin should be looked for; and the possibility of certain kinds of foreign bodies, as needles, headless pins and the like, having entered and disappeared into the tissues should be borne in mind. In such cases discovery of the wound of entrance is of the utmost importance as facilitating removal by pursuit or by enlargement of the wound, which are justifiable in these higher regions in certain cases as hereinafter explained.

Localization of esophageally lodged foreign bodies with the bougie. Nothing can be a more useless waste of time than the blind passage of a bougie in an esophageal case, whether disease or foreign body is suspected. It usually takes less time to pass an esophagoscope and remove the foreign body or a specimen of neoplasm, or to make an accurate diagnosis of disease than it does to pass the bougie; after the passage of which one usually has accomplished nothing. The last defense of the blind bougie for diagnosis is based upon obsolete conditions. It is claimed that thus can be determined the length of esophagoscopic tube required. But there is no need of more than one tube for adults and one for children. It is also stated that high disease of the esophagus may be overridden or perforated by the mandrin of the esophagoscope unless the location is previously determined by blind bouginage. But there is no need of a mandrin in introducing the esophagoscope. The esophagoscope passed by sight is safer than the bougie. The latter is a relic of pre-esophagoscopic days.

RADIOGRAPHIC LOCALIZATION OF FOREIGN BODIES.

The author is quite unfamiliar with the technicalities of Roentgenology, and the suggestions herein given have been gleaned from experience in a large number of cases of foreign bodies (as well as of disease) the successful outcome of which has been due to marvelous work, radiographic and interpretative, of such eminent Roentgenologists as Cole, George C. Johnston, Boggs, Hickey, Grier, Foster, Gray, Bowen, Lang, Menges, Leonard, Cassabian, Pfahler, Eyman, Pancoast, Holding and others. The suggestions here given are intended for surgeons who cannot avail themselves of the work of radiographic experts. After having radiographically located a foreign body we must always remember the possibility of the foreign body having changed its position between the time the ray was taken and the bronchoscopy is done. The foreign body may have shifted to another bronchus, or it may be even in a bronchus of the opposite side.

Excellent progress has been made in the radiographic localization of foreign bodies. This is especially true in regard to the technical improvements which have rendered possible the practically instantaneous radiography, as it has quite recently been recognized (Tilley, Dundas Grant and others) that an instantaneous radiograph will often show foreign bodies not visible with longer exposures. Moreover, there is less chance for voluntary and involuntary movements of the patient, which are transmitted to the foreign body, to blur the outline of the intruder. Especially is this the case with very young children who cannot be expected to hold their breath at command. Dr. George C. Johnston has a number of times gotten a plate with beautiful definition free from respiratory movement in an extremely dyspneic child with heaving chest by snapping a number of momentary exposures at the respiratory rest periods after inspiration and before expiration. A deep inspiration held during the exposure creates an artificial emphysema which causes the foreign body to show, because it lessens the density of the thorax; though it must be borne in mind that the more horizontal position of the ribs and the displacement of the viscera, including the foreign body must be allowed for in the localization. The steady progress made by the radiographer in lateral radiography of the thorax has not only been of great aid in the general localization from bony and visceral landmarks, but also in conjunction with the caliper-guide suggested by Dr. Boyce and perfected by the author.

The author purposely omits a tabular record of the foreign bodies that might be expected to show and those that probably will not show. His reason for the omission are:

1. The casting of a radiographic shadow depends not alone upon the density of the foreign body but upon its thickness in the diameter parallel to the rays. An example of this is seen in Fig. 160 and 161.

2. A body of little density or diameter may happen to be so located that its shadow may not be overlaid by normal shadows so that it

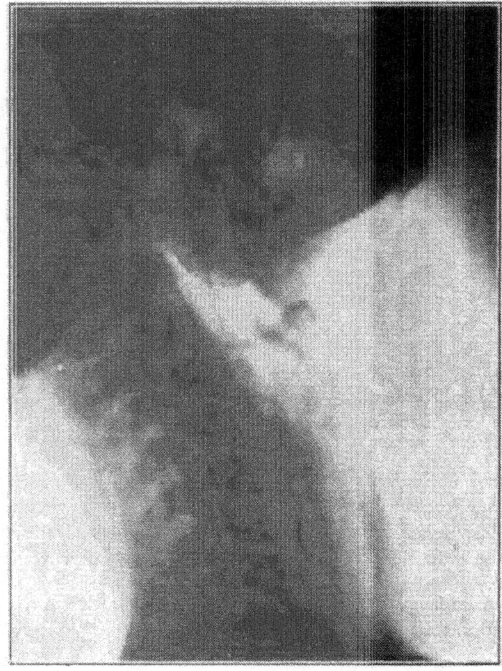

Fig. 160. Radiograph showing bone in the esophagus. Note the swelling at the esophageal walls and the clear outline of the air passages. (Author's case. See Fig. 313. Plate made by Dr. George C. Johnston.)

may show. The author has seen a large number of examples of this kind which are not here reproduced because the shadows while plainly shown on the negatives lose too much in reproduction to show.

3. Lesions secondary to the foreign body may be revealed by the radiograph and thus enable localization as in the case cited under "Pul-

monary Abscess," and under "Localization Films." In another case of the author a peanut kernel completely occluded the left upper lobe bronchus producing a shadow over the entire left upper lobe, though, of course, the peanut itself did not show. The peanut kernel was bronchoscopically removed from just within the orifice of the upper lobe bronchus, liberating a large quantity of purulent secretion.

4. The foreign body may not be the same as that of which a history is given. The most common example of this is the pin or other

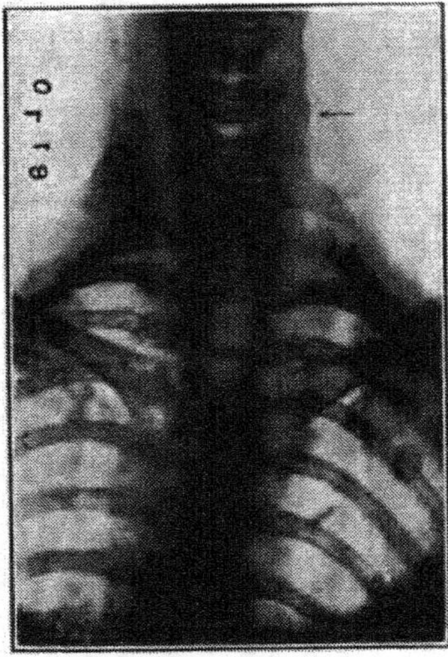

FIG. 161. Radiograph of same patient. The piece of bone, though present at the level of the dart, does not show, partly because it overlies the spine but mainly because in the lateral view the flat foreign body is seen on edge. An example of the misleading negative radiograph, and an indication for lateral as well as antero-posterior radiography.

dense object which has gotten into food and which, from the sensations and from its presence in soups, etc., the patient refers to as a "bone."

For the foregoing reasons the author, except in cases of great urgency, has a radiograph taken of every case. Unless the radiographic tube happens to be placed exactly on a line that passes through the foreign body and that is exactly vertical to the plate, there will be a misleading distortion as to the position of the foreign body relatively to anatomic shadows; because the rays passing the foreign body at a certain angle will continue to travel at that angle until they reach the plate.

Therefore, the distortion will be in direct ratio to the distance of the foreign body from the plate, and also in direct ratio to the distance of the foreign body from any landmark, anatomic or artificial. While deceptive, if misunderstood, or if the position of the tube is unknown, this distortion has been turned to good account by enabling eminent Roentgenologists (Johnston, Cole, Boggs, Grier, Pfahler, Boetjer and others) to work out plans of localization by triangulation and otherwise, by means of which the precise depth from any surface landmark desired can be determined to a nicety. In one case, in which a foreign body was buried in the inflammatory new-tissue produced during a ten years' sojourn, the author's successful extraction of the foreign body was due to Dr. L. G. Cole's accurate localization. In a similar case Dr. Menges enabled the author to find a foreign body of seven years' sojourn. In quite a number of instances Drs. Johnston, Grier, Boggs and others have similarly rendered removals possible. The limitations of this method of localizations are reached when we encounter foreign substances not opaque to the ray. Borderline cases are those in which the body is not sufficiently dense to show in more than one position of the patient, as in a case of the author (reported on a future page) in which a glass collar button could be shown only in a quartering lateral exposure, between the heart and the spine. Fortunately, a very remarkable radiograph in this position by Dr. George C. Johnston not only revealed the collar button, but, by showing the trachea and bronchi, and still more wonderful the inflammatory new tissue which blocked the bronchus above, enabled the author endoscopically to cut away the intervening inflammatory obstruction to gain access to and remove the foreign body. A radiograph, first in the anteroposterior plane and then in the lateral plane, has been very valuable in assisting in a localization of a foreign body with reference to a bronchoscope inserted to a certain definite location, which is fixed in the memory of the bronchoscopist so that he can find the same location at a subsequent bronchoscopy (Fig. 162). In doing this work, it is essential that no anesthetic ether be used, because of the inflammability of ether which might be ignited by a spark. If the foreign body is very dense to the ray the fluorescent screen may be used with results that are immediately available for work without withdrawal of the bronchoscope. Of course this method by either radiography or fluoroscopy is available only in case of foreign bodies dense to the ray. Many foreign bodies that are sufficiently opaque to show in a radiograph are insufficiently dense to show in the fluoroscope. Localization by means of a radiograph of the instrument in position at the suspected locality has been used by the author in cases of pulmonary abscess (Fig. 136). The same method may be used in esophageal cases in which the foreign body

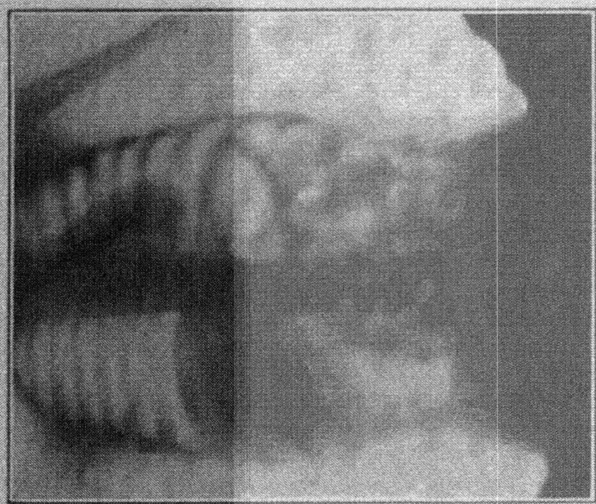

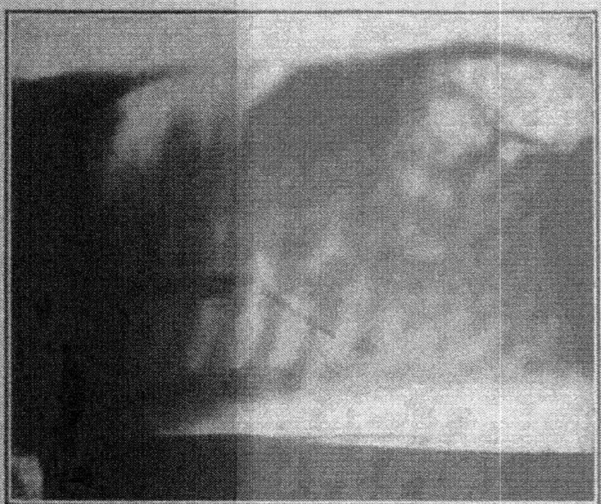

FIG. 162. Antero-posterior and lateral radiograph of recumbent patient with bronchoscope in position. Useful for localization in case of small foreign bodies so far down and far out toward the periphery that they cannot be found. The position and direction of the intruder from the tube mouth, which is at a known and subsequently findable location, locates the small branch bronchus to be searched at a subsequent bronchoscopy. With dense foreign bodies like the pin above shown, the fluorescent screen may be used, yielding immediate information.

is suspected to have wandered out of the lumen into the tissues. Care must be taken to avoid error from a foreign body being simply in a fold in the lumen. A large esophagoscope should eliminate this possibility. A subsequent radiograph with pressure of the tube-mouth against the pin will give positive evidence. A lateral as well as an antero-posterior radiograph are necessary in any case.

The statements in the earlier work (Bib. 269) in regard to unreliability of fluoroscopy as compared to radiography for foreign bodies have been borne out by further experience. A foreign body overlying the spine or behind the heart shadow may be invisible by fluoroscopy and yet show up strongly in such a location in the radiograph. In one instance, a pin behind the heart shadow showed as black as if drawn with a pen in a radiographic print, and yet was totally invisible to an experienced fluoroscopist with a proper tube. This was in an infant, and therefore a very advantageous subject in which to see a foreign body on the screen. With such results as these among the possibilities, it is useless to waste time with fluoroscopy for diagnosis as to the presence of a foreign body, because with the instantaneous exposures and rapid developing of to-day, a report may be had in 30 minutes or less from the time the radiograph is taken. Fluoroscopy, however, may be of advantage in foreign body cases in adults for another reason. An expert fluoroscopist with the recently developed apparatus can exclude aneurysm and give a report on the functional activity of the esophagus. With foreign bodies not opaque to the ray at times information can be obtained from fluoroscopic examination of the action of the diaphragm. Under average conditions there may be a slightly greater activity of one side as compared to the other, but any marked diminution of the excursion of the diaphragm on one side points to foreign body obstructing the main bronchus. This is not diagnostic but is a strong indication for bronchoscopy. Fluorescent bronchoscopy in which the bronchoscope and forceps are guided by the fluorescent shadow will be dealt with in a subsequent chapter.

In case of a foreign body, which, from its nature, would show very faintly, if at all, in the radiograph, the suggestion of Boyce to swallow a bismuth capsule, is excellent. If the foreign body is sufficiently large to be at all obstructive, the capsule will stop and remain at least for a time at the site of the foreign body. (Fig. 163). This not only shows that the foreign body is present, but it shows its position, and, furthermore, on dissolving of the capsule, the bismuth is beneficial to any traumatism or esophagitis that may exist in the neighborhood of the foreign body. In using the bismuth capsule, for the detection of a foreign body not itself opaque to the ray, it is necessary to remember that the progress downward of a bismuth capsule or any large bolus is not exceedingly rapid and may normally be seen in transit. Still more necessary is it to remember that in many cases, with a perfectly normal esophagus not containing any foreign body, the capsule may hesitate for a moment at the cricopharyngeus and also at the point where the left bronchus crosses the esophagus, and again at the hiatus. The author has noted in quite a number of cases with an apparently perfectly normal

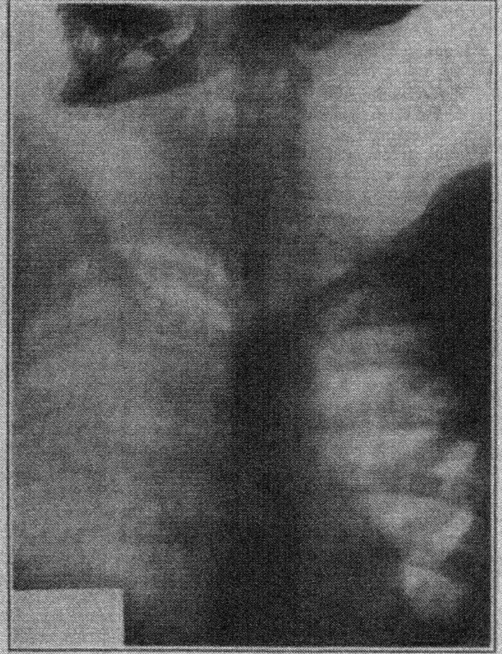

FIG. 163. Radiograph showing a method of locating a foreign body in the esophagus. The bismuth capsule was stopped in the esophagus by a foreign body that, itself, does not show.

esophagus that the ridge caused by the crossing of the left bronchus was unduly prominent, and this, in one case, was connected directly with a lodgment of the bismuth capsule for a few seconds in an esophagus which did not contain a foreign body. In view of this, it would seem to be wise in using the capsule for the diagnosis of foreign bodies not opaque to the ray to wait two or three minutes after swallowing the capsule before taking a radiograph; but, of course, the wait must not be sufficiently long to permit of the capsule dissolving. In case of small non-obstructive foreign bodies the method would not be effective, and in any case is valueless negatively. When positive it may be so from an obstruction other than a foreign body.

Interpretation of a radiograph is best done by the radiographer; a few hints to the endoscopist, however, may not be amiss. First in importance is to determine whether the foreign body is in the respiratory or in the alimentary tracts, and next in importance is to determine in what part of the respective passages the foreign body is lodged. This is extremely easy in some cases, extremely difficult in others. As a rule, it may be stated that foreign bodies more or less flat, whose plane corresponds to the lateral plane of the body, are in the esophagus and not in the air passages. This applies with a special force to the upper half of the esophagus because the esophagus is collapsed anteroposteriorly; that is, the anterior wall lies against the posterior wall. The direction of least resistance being laterally, flat foreign bodies project their longest diameter laterally. In the trachea, also, there is a slightly greater diameter laterally at the bifurcation and for some distance above it. Above the sternal notch, however, foreign bodies entering through the glottis are almost always found to have taken the anteroposterior position because of the greater axis sagittally of the laryngeal and subglottic lumina; and this position is most likely to be maintained below, because the posterior wall of the trachea is membranous and yielding. These points are well illustrated in the radiographs Figs. 164 and 165, and are especially plainly marked in lateral radiographs of foreign bodies in the esophagus as illustrated in various parts of this book. It is customary in the interpretation of a radiograph, when one lung shows dark and the other light, to consider that the dark side contains the foreign body which has occluded the main bronchus with perhaps compensatory emphysema on the opposite side. Iglauer (Bib. 222) reports a very interesting case where this reading was erroneous because the foreign body had, by a valve-like action, imprisoned more air in the obstructed side, so that there was a very marked emphysema shown by the radiograph on the obstructed side.

Calcified glands are exceedingly common and may, in some instances, lead to error. As pointed out by Dr. George C. Johnston, in connection with one of the author's cases, that of a molar tooth in the bronchus of a boy, calcified glands are always rounded in form, so that in case of any body not of rounded form, there is little likelihood of error; but it must be remembered that the foreign body must be considered from every point of view, as irregular-shaped bodies may throw a rounded shadow in certain positions. Furthermore, calcified glands are rarely single, so that any suspicious shadow is apt to be duplicated, if due to a calcified gland. Von Eicken, in a very interesting paper (Bib. 563), reports a case in which a shadow was thought by the Roentgenologist to be due to a calcified gland, and so it proved to be. There was, nevertheless, in

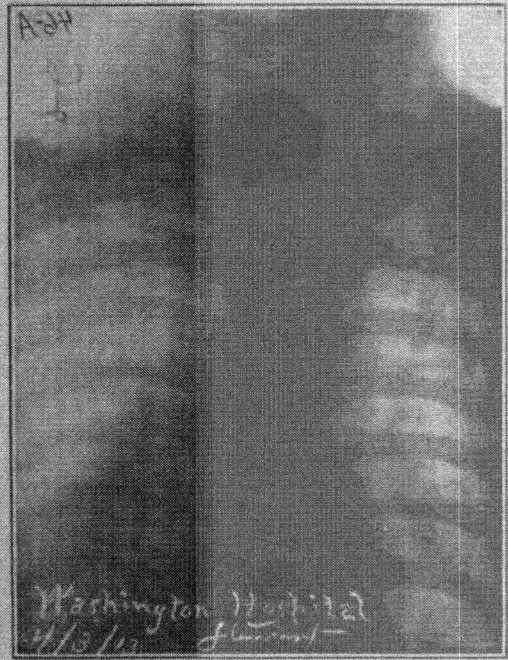

Fig. 164. Radiograph of a coin (half-dollar) in the esophagus of a child of 14 years. This illustrates the method of localization of foreign bodies in the esophagus. It is utterly impossible for a flat body of this size to be tracheally lodged thus in the lateral plane of the trachea.

the case a foreign body (bone) which did not show in the radiograph, but which was discovered and removed by bronchoscopy.

Positive films of the tracheo-bronchial tree as an aid to localization. A large foreign body in a large bronchus needs accurate localization, not but that it could be found bronchoscopically in every case; but accurate localization enables the bronchoscopist to go at once to the known location and thus greatly shorten the period of endoscopic search which

may be a vital point. There is another class of cases, however, in which the intruder may never be found if there has been no accurate localization. Small foreign bodies, or those small in one diameter, following the general rule of foreign bodies in the air passages, keep on going downward until they get into the smallest possible bronchus. Thus needles and small headed pins get very far down and very far out toward the periphery of the lung and into a very small branch bronchus of which

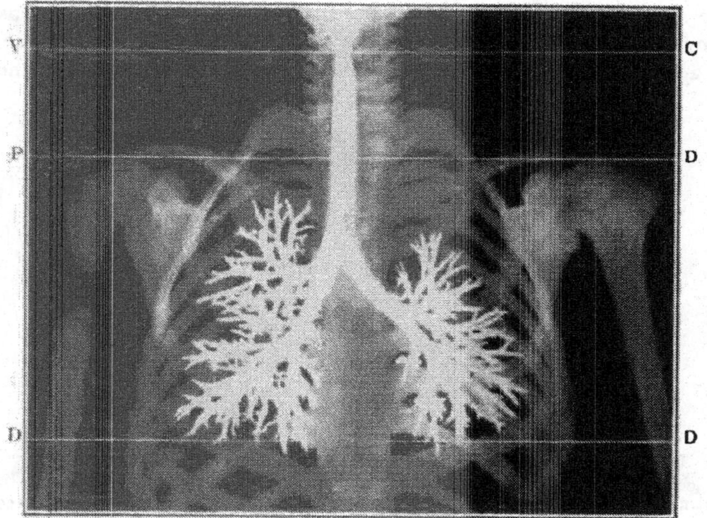

Fig. 166. Illustration of a positive film used for overlaying to assist in localization of foreign bodies or lesions in the thorax. The lower white line (D, D) corresponds to the diaphragm, the middle line (P D) to the dome of the pleura. These lines assist in placing the overlay. The upper line (V C), corresponding to the vocal cords, is occasionally useful. Twelve photographic enlargements are on hand so that a film of the size (rather than the age) is available for any sized patient. The few minute branches that go below the line, D, are those posterior to the apex of the dome.

there are many. To search all of these with a probe or minute tube consumes a large amount of time. The author has devised for help in these cases a positive transparent film of the tracheo-bronchial tree (Fig. 166). The film being a "positive" the tree is transparent. The film is laid over the negative of the patient showing the foreign body, when the foreign body will show through the transparent tracheo-bronchial tree of the overlying positive film. In placing the film, bony landmarks are not reliable because of the wide variation due to the phylogenetic recency of the upright posture. Visceral landmarks are necessary. The two important visceral landmarks are the dome of the pleura and the dome of the diaphragm. It is needless to say the tracheo-bronchial tree necessarily lies in the body of the lung between these two landmarks, and lines corresponding to these are placed on the film. Twelve photographic enlargements and reductions are on hand so that a film of the size (rather than age) is available for any sized patient, the size being chosen by matching the size between the dome of the pleura and that of the diaphragm as shown on the radiograph of the patient. All this work is done, of course, in a darkened room, with a strongly illuminated shadow-box; and in the

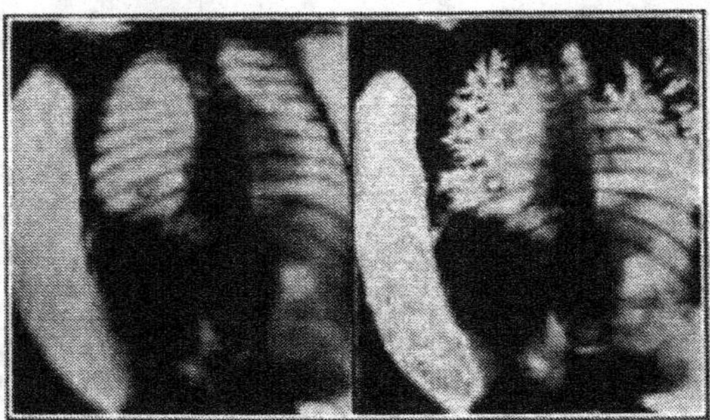

FIG. 167. Illustrating on the left, abscess (retouched). On the right the abscess is localized in the right inferior lobe bronchus by the method of overlaying. The localization coincided with the endoscopic findings when the abscess was evacuated bronchoscopically.

event of the foreign body showing very faintly on the radiograph of the patient, it is strengthened by an ink-mark on the uncoated side of the negative, which can be readily erased afterwards if desired.

Corroboration of the usefulness of these films has been forthcoming from a number of sources. (See article by R. C. Lynch in New Orleans Med. and Surg. Journal, Dec., 1913).

To prevent error in the use of these films, as with any method of interpretation of a radiograph, it is necessary to be on guard against false localization due to displacement of the lung by atelectasis, and especially by the compensatory emphysema on the other side. Another source of error, of course, is that the positives of the tracheo-bronchial tree are made from the tracheo-bronchial tree of a cadaver, whereas bronchoscopic study of the tree shows that it is not quite in the same position in the living. The injection preparations of Brünings come nearer those of the living tree than any other that the author has been able to find, and therefore he has used them in making the positive films.

Caliper-guide method of localization. This method, suggested by Dr. John W. Boyce and perfected by the author is intended primarily for bringing the tube mouth in close relation with a small foreign body that cannot be found because it is in a minute bronchus of which there are too many for each to be searched. In conjunction with the lateral radiograph the caliper-guide will bring the point of the bronchoscope, afterward at bronchoscopy, in close relation with the foreign body, thereby greatly diminishing the number of small bronchial tubes to be searched; this method being used, of course, only in case of small foreign bodies

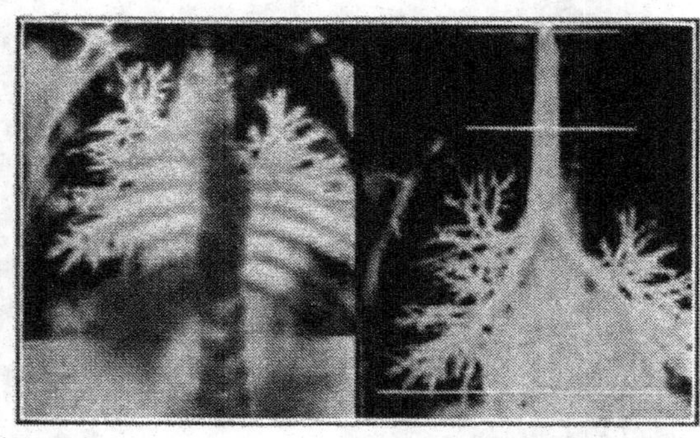

FIG. 168. Illustrating a positive radiographic film of the tracheo-bronchial tree used for overlaying to assist in localization of a foreign body. The left hand illustration shows the film laid over a negative of a patient in whose left main bronchus was a pin. Localization verified by bronchoscopy. The shadow of the pin is strengthened with ink.

which have fallen into a very small bronchus far down or far out near the periphery of the lungs. The lateral placement of the point of the bronchoscope depends upon a mark placed on the skin by the radiographer who determines the point by an anterior-posterior radiograph (Fig. 169).

Value of negative radiography. The negative report from the radiographer remains to-day as it always has been, unreliable, because many bodies are not opaque to the ray, and, moreover, the foreign body may not be the same as that of which we get a history. In addition to this, even metallic bodies at times do not show. For instance, in one of the author's cases, that of an enormous woman of 53 years, expert radiographers, for a period of two years, made quite a number of exposures that failed to demonstrate a tack which they finally demonstrated to be present (Fig. 170) and which the author removed bronchoscopically. Such occurrences will doubtless be less and less frequent because of the steady advance in the technical perfection of radiography. A number of

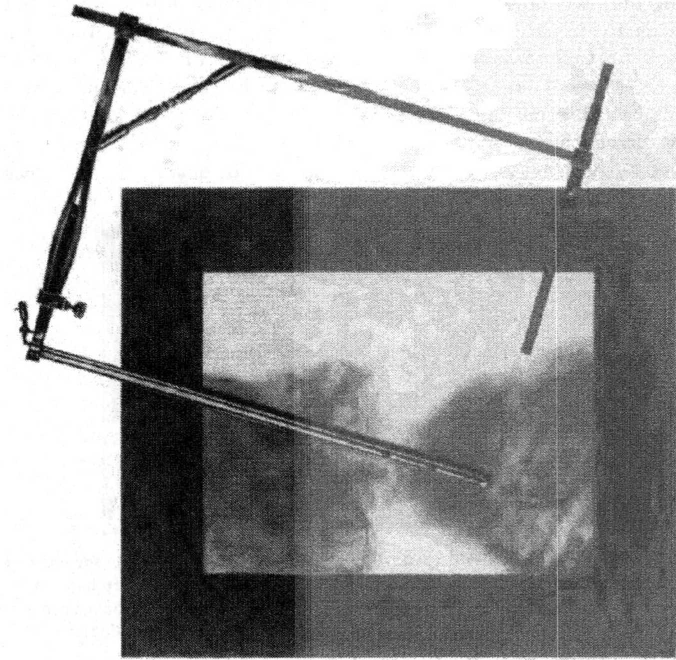

FIG. 169. Illustrating the position of the caliper-guide in getting the adjustments by which the point of the bronchoscope can be brought, later at bronchoscopy, in close proximity to a foreign body. For use in case of small foreign bodies in minute bronchi. Suggested by Dr. John W. Boyce and perfected by the author. Inadvertently, in making the illustration, a radiograph of an esophageally lodged foreign body (safety-pin) was used, but the principle is illustrated just as well.

recent cases have made it quite clear that it is necessary to do a bronchoscopy if there is any reason to suspect from the history that there is a foreign body located somewhere in the air-passages or in the esophagus, notwithstanding a negative ray finding and a total absence of symptoms, for it is remarkable how tolerant the trachea, bronchi and the esophagus become to the presence of foreign bodies after the initial symptoms immediately following the accident have subsided. A negative X-ray may be very misleading, because, as shown by Frank C. Todd (Bib. 541) a radiograph may not include the region in which a foreign body is located. Notwithstanding the fact that there was no clear history of a foreign body having been seen in the child's possession, and despite the negative radiograph, Dr. Todd bronchoscoped the child without a general anesthetic and skilfully removed the tack. J. W. Murphy (Bib. 397) reports

FIG. 170. Radiograph showing tack in bronchus of a woman of 53 years. This tack failed to show in radiographs taken by expert radiographers at intervals for a period of two years before getting the tack to show. Tack removed bronchoscopically by the author.

experiments demonstrating the fact that the composition of which most buttons are made did not show in the radiograph, and that with physical signs, sensations of the patient, and the radiograph all negative, the foreign body, nevertheless, was present. In one of the author's cases (illustrated on a subsequent page) the metal part of a shoe button showed but the composition part did not. As before mentioned it is needless here to consider in detail the different kinds of foreign body as to their density to the ray, because a radiograph should be taken in every case; and if negative an endoscopy should be done anyway if there is reason to suspect a foreign body. Those who are interested in the relative densities are referred to the interesting article of von Eicken (Bib. 563).

Physical examination of the chest. Should the foreign body be located by radiograph, physical examination of the chest is, nevertheless, necessary for two reasons. 1. The data to be obtained will be, when sufficient has been accumulated, invaluable for other cases in which the foreign body is not dense to the ray. 2. The condition of all the viscera in the thorax and elsewhere should be known before endoscopy. The notes on the physical signs of foreign body, by Dr. J. W. Boyce (Bib. 269, p. 90), have stood the test of further experience. In case of complete occlusion of one bronchus, there may be a very marked diminution of the respiratory excursion of the thorax on the affected side, as observed by Dr. John R. Simpson in one of the author's cases. The same signs have since been observed in a number of other cases. The author is utterly incompetent to make a physical examination of the chest by auscultation and percussion. But comparing the findings of very competent physical diagnosticians with the author's endoscopic findings, he is strongly impressed with the fact that foreign-body cases are nearly always associated with a large amount of secretion because of the difficulty in expectoration, and especially is this the case in children. In some instances, physical signs of solidification have completely cleared up after the author has bronchoscopically removed a large quantity of secretion. This accumulation of secretion is especially liable to occur in the lower lobe, and (H. T. Price) it may be limited to one lower lobe even when the foreign body is in the trachea. In some instances the intruder was known to have been in the trachea for a number of weeks. This prolonged sojourn negatives the hypothesis that the foreign body might have been in a lobe of one lung at a previous time, resulting in the excessive secretion. It seems certain that the secretion had drained downward and accumulated because of the difficult expectoration, and that some peculiarity either in form or position of the right or the left bronchus, or some difference in ciliary action has favored the greater accumulation on one side as compared with the other. A number of interesting facts bearing on the physical signs produced by the lesions following prolonged sojourn of a foreign body in the lung will be given along with the case reports in the section devoted to this class of cases. The similarity to the physical signs of pulmonary tuberculosis is remarkable. Bronchiectasis may be present with its physical signs.*

*A unique case in which Dr. George L. Richards diagnosticated a foreign body on physical and laboratory findings, in the absence of a history, is recorded in the Transactions of the American Laryngological, Rhinological and Otological Society, 1915.

ERRORS TO AVOID IN SUSPECTED FOREIGN-BODY CASES.

1. Do not reach for the foreign body with the finger, lest the foreign body be thereby pushed into the larynx, or the larynx be thus traumatized.

2. Do not make any attempt at removal with the patient in any position other than recumbent with the head and shoulders lower than the body (Fig. 73a).

3. Do not hold up the patient by the heels, lest the foreign body be dislodged and asphyxiate the patient by becoming jammed in the glottis.

4. Do not fail to have a radiograph made, if possible, whether the foreign body in question is of a kind dense to the ray or not.

5. Do not fail endoscopically to search for a foreign body in all cases of doubt.

6. Do not pass an esophageal bougie, probang or other instrument blindly.

7. Do not tell the patient he has no foreign body until after radiography, physical examination, indirect examination, and endoscopy all have proven negative.

CHAPTER XIII.

Foreign Bodies in the Larynx and Tracheobronchial Tree.

Etiology. In the air passages, which are not intended for solids, foreign bodies that get in through natural passages can only do so by passing the normal safeguards which are mainly reflexes. Hence anything which interferes with these reflexes is the chief etiologic factor. Sleep, anesthesia, intoxication, syncope, delirium, mechanical interference of masses of disease as in malignancy, tuberculosis, etc. The reflexes may interfere with each other; as, for instance, the sudden inhalation which precedes or follows coughing, laughing, sobbing, and unusual exertion. The protective reflexes act chiefly in two groups. The laryngeal closing reflex and the bechic reflex. Laryngeal closure for normal swallowing is chiefly in the tilting and closure of the upper laryngeal orifice. The ventricular bands help but slightly and the epiglottis and the vocal cords not at all. Foreign bodies going in with the inspiratory blast, must run the gauntlet of the following guards:

GAUNTLET TO BE RUN BY FOREIGN BODIES ENTERING THE LOWER AIR PASSAGES.

1. Epiglottis.
2. Upper laryngeal orifice.
3. Ventricular bands.
4. Vocal cords.
5. Bechic blast.

The epiglottis makes somewhat of a fender, efficient in proportion as it hangs backward toward the posterior pharyngeal wall. The upper laryngeal orifice, composed of a pair of movable ridges of tissue has almost a sphincteric action, besides its tilting movement. The ventricular bands can approximate under powerful stimuli. The vocal bands act similarly. The one defect in the efficiency of both sets of bands in barring out intruders is the tendency to take an inspiration preparatory to the cough excited by the contact of a foreign body. This inspiration is not invariably taken, however. A slight explosive cough can be taken without inspiration, especially if it start near the end of an inspiration, but following this or any other coughing effort is a deep inspiration which is probably the most efficient factor in the entrance of foreign bodies into the lower air passages.

Gottstein collected statistics which showed that 66 per cent of the cases of foreign bodies in the air passages occurred in children. This may be in part due to a less degree of automatic protection to the entrance of foreign bodies in the air passages; but doubtless is, to a greater extent, due to the fact that children are prone to play, run, laugh and attempt to speak with various foreign bodies in the mouth. It does not seem probable that children put foreign bodies in their mouths more frequently than adults when it is considered how many women are in the habit of putting pins in their mouths especially when dressing, and how many workmen place small foreign bodies, such as tacks and nails and the like in the mouth. Of course in infants there is a well known tendency to put everything into the mouth, as this seems to be one of the means by which the infant mind acquires knowledge of material things. Soluble material, such as candy, or foods which very quickly disintegrate, such as bread, toast, and the like, need cause no uneasiness, as they are very soon coughed up and expectorated. Meat, if composed purely of muscular fiber or fat, is practically always expectorated. If, however, it is firmly attached to periostium or bone or cartilage, it may constitute a foreign body for which bronchoscopy should be done. It is quite remarkable that all strictly food substances are rather rare in the bronchi, while the portions of food which should be and usually are rejected, are not at all uncommon, such as the seeds of fruits, the shell of nuts, bone and the like. Of course it is not meant to refer here to the various food substances such as dried maize, beans, peas and the like, which are put into the mouth by children in play and not strictly for food. It is well known that any light particles of dust usually are largely removed by the cilia, while heavier particles of dust become encysted as in anthracosis. Just where the border line exists between the foreign body of such small size that it may become encysted, and the larger bodies which will form an abscess, has never been determined, and it is very difficult to determine because the smaller bodies which form an abscess usually become disintegrated, or are lost in pus and are never discovered. It seems quite certain that a large proportion of the non-tuberculous pulmonary abscesses are due to this cause. In the author's collection, pins are the most frequent of foreign bodies in the bronchi. Next comes various forms of hardware, and then various vegetable substances, bones and coins. Peanut kernels are among the most fatal of foreign bodies, and this does not seem to be due to comminution and multiple abscesses, so much as to the peculiar irritating effect of the peanut kernel upon the tracheo-bronchial mucosa. A metallic body will be tolerated for a long time with little reaction, whereas a peanut kernel will set up violent local reaction in a few days as shown by the author's cases to be cited later.* Dr. E. W. Carpenter (Bib. 73) reports the case of an infant of sixteen months that was asphyxiated by the pus liberated from an abscessed lung following the aspirat' n of a peanut. J. A. Stucky (Bib. 511) and many others report fatal cases. Metallic bodies if of such shape as completely to occlude a bronchus, usually cause rapidly developing fatal abscess by the stagnation of secretions which cannot be coughed out. On the other hand foreign bodies that do not occlude the lumen may produce little reaction for a long time, provided the lumen is not occluded by the reactionary swelling of the mucosa. Sooner or later this occlusion occurs, however, and the patient usually succumbs. Considering the millions of people who are carrying about with them loose teeth or loose artificial dental attachments it is a very remarkable thing that relatively so few foreign bodies to be classed as dental find their way into the air passages. Large artificial dentures are by no means uncommon in the esophagus and of course by reason of their size they could not well get into the air passages. In the author's opinion it is a great tribute to the skill of dentists that so few foreign bodies are to be classed as dental. Teeth may be knocked loose in a fall and be aspirated as in one of the author's cases. In another case he treated laryngeal stenosis that followed an abscess caused by impaction of a tooth in the subglottic region. The rootless deciduous tooth had shot out of the dental forceps in the hands of a skilful dentist. Dried vegetable substances such as beans, peas and maize soon occlude the lumen and are rapidly fatal. Those interested in the further pursuit of this interesting phase of the foreign body question are referred to the excellent article of D. Bryson Delavan (Bib. 107) which also gives a number of references. An excellent article on the experimental pathology of foreign bodies in the lungs was written by George B. Wood. (Bib. 585.)

Why do foreign bodies lodge at certain localities in the air passages? Lodgment at some of the most frequent sites is accounted for by seemingly adequate reasons. The factors may be classed in two main divisions:

1. (a) The size and shape of the foreign body; whether long, broad, pointed, angular, disk-like, etc. (b) Its surface, whether rough

*So uniformly is this observed that the term "peanut bronchitis" has come into common use in the author's clinic.

or smooth. (2) Its physical properties, resiliency, plasticity absorptivity, etc.

2. The anatomic peculiarities of the various localities. (a) Angles, arcs. (b) Fixed and motile narrowings.

The size, shape and surface of the foreign body has less to do with the particular site at which it is most likely to lodge than have the anatomical regional peculiarities. A pointed body may catch at any location if the point be downward as it often is in the esophagus. In the air passages, however, pins are almost invariably head downward, and by a ratchet-like action, the point preventing return, work tow: :d the lowest point. In the air passages the narrowness, quiescent and spasmodic of the larynx halts many foreign bodies which may be retained because of peculiarities of their shape, or by a projection; or by entering a ventricle. As in one of the author's cases, that of a safety-pin, one part may drop through the glottis while another part not passing through, the intruder is prevented from going either way. Having passed the cords a foreign body may be wedged in the subglottic space, either on its way down or when it is shot back upward by the bechic blast. Below the subglottic space the next point of frequent lodgement is the bifurcation. Lodgement here is due rather to the shape of cross-section, elongated laterally with two openings laterally below, causing the intruder to be caught crosswise. More often it is the effort of the intruder to enter either the right or the left bronchus, both of which are smaller than the trachea. The bronchi do not diminish between branches. That is, the diminution is at the points of subdivision (monopodic branching, not true bifurcations), and between these the bronchus is cylindroid, not tapered. Therefore a foreign body usually halts with its largest diameter at or immediately below a point where a lateral branch is given off.

Greater frequency of right-bronchial invasion. The right bronchus is invaded by foreign bodies more frequently than the left. Statistics collected by Gottstein show that 75.4 per cent of foreign bodies entering the bronchi were in the right bronchus. Von Eicken found 70.2 per cent· Preobraschensky, 69 per cent. Morrell Mackenzie, 62.5. The reasons for this are anatomical and physiological.

1. The greater diameter of the right bronchus.
2. Less angle of deviation of the right bronchus.
3. Situation of the carina to the left of the long axis of the trachea.
4. The action of the trachealis muscle.
5. The greater volume of air going into the right bronchus on inspiration.

The first three of these factors are shown in the schema Fig. 171, The right bronchus is in size and direction the continuation of the trachea; the left bronchus in many cases simulating a lateral branch of the trachea rather than a bifurcational half. The situation of the carina to the left of the long axis of the trachea is important. Heller and V. Schrötter found the carina to the left in 57 per cent, in the middle line in 42 per cent and to the right in 1 per cent. Sir Felix Semon and Morrell Mackenzie's joint results were: left, 59 per cent, middle line, 35 per cent, right, 6 per cent. These statistics are all based on the cadaveric anatomy. The author feels certain that the living anatomy shows a much more marked preponderance of left-sided situation of the carina.

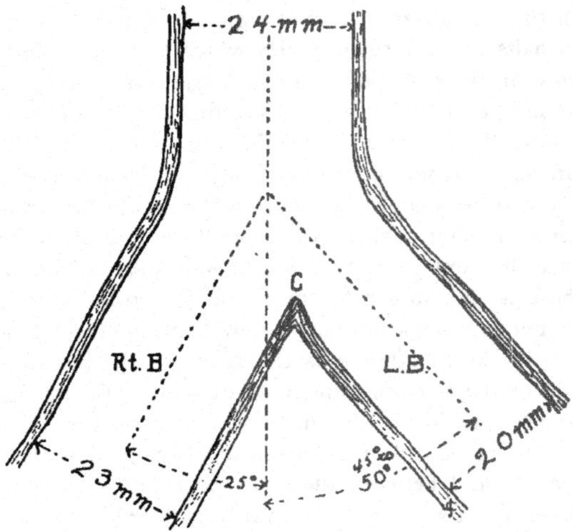

FIG. 171. Schema showing three anatomical reasons for the greater frequency of right-sided lodgement of foreign bodies in the bronchi. The right bronchus (Rt. B.) is almost as wide (23 mm.) as the trachea (24 mm.) and it deviates much less than the left from the long axis of the trachea. The carina, C, is to the left of this axis. (After Sir St. Clair Thomson.)

He regrets that he did not keep a record of this point in all of his bronchoscopic cases. But in 40 cases where he kept a record the carina seemed more or less to the left in all but one and in that case the carina seemed central. These cases were without known pathology that could alter the position of the carina. The observation is submitted with acknowledgment of the possibility of error, because of the alteration of position of all the thoracic viscera due to position of the patient, the bronchoscopic tube and the pulsatory and respiratory movements. Furthermore, the observations were incidental and no time was taken to insure accuracy. From general observation and the instinctive habits of work, the author has come always to move the head to the right to get into the left bronchus while the head is not moved to the left simply to cause the bronchoscope to enter the right bronchus. It always goes there naturally with the head in the middle line, though, of course, the author's custom of turning the lip of the bronchoscope to the right for entering the right bronchus assists. The action of the musculature at the carina in drawing the carina to the left and thus reducing the size of the left bronchial orifice is thought by Snow to be one of the chief factors in the preponderance of foreign bodies in the right bronchus. The fifth factor mentioned above does not seem to have received the attention it deserves. In one of the author's cases, that of an extremely dyspneic child, there was demonstrated by physical examination by Dr. H. T. Price very little air going into the right side and none at all into the left. The foreign body was in the subglottic space. This case seems to prove what theoretically would seem probable from the greater size of the right lung, that there is a greater volume of air rushing through the right bronchus at each inspiration.

Why is the middle lobe bronchus relatively so rarely invaded by foreign bodies? The middle lobe bronchus is rarely invaded. The author has seen but two such instances, in over two hundred cases of foreign body in the bronchi. The relative rarity of invasion possibly is due to the fact that the middle lobe bronchus is given off anteriorly, consequently gravity tends to lead the foreign body into posterior branches because the patient does not lie on his face but on his back. This theory of the author has never been positively proven because foreign bodies are rarely radiographed soon enough after the accident, i. e., before the patient has lain down. Excluding the effect of gravity, the angle of the giving off the middle lobe bronchus does not seem less favorable for the invasion by a foreign body than do some of the dorsal branches of the inferior lobe bronchus which are so frequently invaded. True, in looking down the lumen of the right stem bronchus the orifice of the middle lobe bronchus is not seen, which would lead one to think that it is out of the direct route of the invader. To some extent, however, this is also true of the dorsal branches of the inferior lobe bronchus. The inspiratory air blast entering the middle lobe bronchus possibly is not quite so great. It is hoped that future observation will clear up this point. William Bruce Smith reports an interesting case of middle-lobe bronchus invasion.

Spontaneous expulsion of foreign bodies from the trachea and bronchi. Fortunately for the patient, but unfortunately for other patients, foreign bodies are occasionally coughed up. Still more unfortunate is the fact that no distinction ordinarily is made between a foreign body coughed out of the larynx and the much rarer event of one coughed up from the bronchi. It is for the latter reason that statistics are almost valueless. There have been too few cases of spontaneous expulsion where the location of the intruder was precisely known. Manifestly the expulsion of a large, light foreign body in the larynx or subglottic trachea is no basis for deduction as to a specifically heavy foreign body in a minute bronchial branch at the periphery of the lung. In these days of safe and easy bronchoscopy with an enormous percentage of successes, no one, who is well informed, for one moment considers the advisability of waiting for a foreign body to be coughed up; but in the event of bronchoscopy failing to remove the intruder, the very high mortality of thoracotomy for foreign body, together with a certain percentage of failures to find the intruder by external operation; and, furthermore, as there may be present at consultation someone who will recite a case where the foreign body was coughed up—for these reasons, it is wise to consider the possibilities. The chance of the bechic expulsion of a foreign body depends largely on its nature. Sharp foreign bodies, such as pins lying point upward, have never been known to be coughed up, for the reason that the pin will stick at the very first angle encountered. On the other hand, smooth, rounded bodies have a tendency to be tightly fixed in the bronchus, and the absorption of air below causes a negative pressure which pulls the foreign body tighter and tighter into the bronchus with less and less air below, and consequently less and less chance for expulsion. The patient cannot draw in air enough beneath the foreign body for the expulsive efforts. In the third class might be considered the foreign bodies that are quite heavy, such as bodies of iron, pewter, lead, and the like. These are very rarely ever coughed out because of the little surface they present relatively to their weight. The expiratory blast has not sufficient force, relatively to the surface against which the force is applied, to expel the intruder. We come then to the class of foreign bodies which are not heavy nor sharp-pointed nor so smooth as to lodge tightly, thus preventing air from being drawn below them, and we find such bodies are the most likely to be expelled. The chances are better before than after such a body has reached the smallest bronchus it can enter. It is not so tightly impacted at first unless its size is so large as to nearly occlude the trachea or bronchi. In that case it is drawn in by the inspiratory blast and accumulates energy on the way according to the well known law of physics. This accumulation is less, directly as the actual weight, and also as the specific weight, except in cases of foreign bodies which fit quite closely to the tracheal or bronchial lumen. This accumulated energy in travel cannot occur in expulsion until after impaction is released, because it does not begin until the body has begun to move. Hence there is a great disadvantage in expulsion as compared to inhalation of a foreign body. This is not sufficient to overcome the relative advantage which should accrue from the fact that an expulsive effort in coughing is very much greater in power than any inspiratory effort can be, the difference being probably twice as much in a coughing expiratory pressure. Then we have the absorption of air drawing the foreign body downward in the case of round foreign bodies which fit the bronchial lumen, either at first or after swelling has taken place. This accounts for the fact that corks and similar substances, though of low specific weight, are rarely coughed up. Pins almost invariably enter the air passages point upward and the point constitutes a ratchet-like mechanism which resists any other movement than downward; and moreover, the pin offers but little surface upon which the expiratory blast in coughing may act. Furthermore, to get out at all, it must proceed with its long axis more or less in the axis of the passage through which it must go. Anyone who will attempt to throw any sort of a pin point first, will find that the head of the pin, being heavier, very promptly begins to turn round in advance of the point. With practically all pins this would be impossible in expulsion through the air passages for want of space, and the turning would cause the point to stick even if the passage were straight. On the contrary, a number of bends and turns have to be accomplished. For these reasons, a pin that has gotten down to the bifurcation or below, practically never is coughed up, and if it is in the trachea it is almost certain to reach the deeper air passages in a very short time by the combined action of gravity and the ratchet-like action of the point. Another factor against the coughing up of a foreign body is that of gravity. This led in the prebronchoscopic days to the holding up of the patient by the heels in order to let the foreign body fall out. This was occasionally successful within a few days of the accident, though it sometimes caused a spasm of the glottis and demanded immediate tracheotomy. Of course such a procedure is not to be considered in these days of bronchoscopy; but the fact that it sometimes succeeded indicates the effect that gravity has in interfering with the coughing out of foreign bodies. As elsewhere mentioned, the dog has a vastly more effective mechanism for ridding his bronchi of foreign bodies than is possessed by human beings. To what extent the more nearly horizontal trachea and bronchi of the dog is concerned, has not yet been determined. It seems probable, however, that the erect posture of human beings, which is, phylogenetically, very late, is in a measure responsible for the very inefficient efforts of nature to cough out foreign bodies. Another factor which favors the inhalation of a foreign body and retards its expulsion is the well known physiological action of the glottis. During inspiration the glottic chink is widened to the maximum, while on expiration it is only partially open and it does not open to the maximum even during the expulsive efforts of the cough. Moreover, the foreign body itself, being driven up against the under side of the vocal cords, or even against the tracheal wall, has a strong influence in exciting reflex contraction which closes the glottis. Still another impediment to the expulsive efforts of the cough is the fact that the bronchi contract very greatly during cough and the trachea also contracts to a certain extent. This contraction has been witnessed by every bronchoscopist, as it is one of the difficulties with which he has to contend in bronchoscopy. Perhaps one of the most important factors in the defeat of the bechic expulsion of foreign bodies is the fact that after each coughing effort there is a deep inspiration, during which the bronchi are dilated and the inspiratory blast has the effect of carrying the foreign body deeper and deeper, aided by the negative pressure below.

In deciding the chance of spontaneous expectoration of a foreign body in the bronchi it is necessary to remember the very inefficient coughing and expectorating mechanism of children.

Summarizing, we divide for prognostic purposes all foreign bodies into three classes:

1. Those of high specific gravity.
2. Those of low specific gravity, (including hollow bodies with relatively large surface).
3. Those of intermediate specific gravity.

In the first class we may tell our patient that there is almost no hope of the intruder ever being coughed up in case of adults and absolutely none in infants and very small children. In the second class there is a chance of expectoration in older children and adults, almost none in children, none at all in infants. In the third class of substances the chances of expectoration of the foreign body in either adults or children are remote. Long, thin, pointed and relatively heavy bodies like pins and needles are never coughed up from below the glottis. In any case, the author's later experience confirms his earlier statement (Bib. 269); namely, "We do full justice to our patients when we tell them that while the foreign body may be coughed up, it is very dangerous to wait; and, further, that the difficulty of removal increases with each hour the body is allowed to remain."

Magnetic extraction of foreign bodies. Many of the mechanical problems, and also the problem in certain cases of finding the foreign body, would be solved if magnetic extraction were feasible. It has yielded such wonderful results in ophthalmology that its use in bronchoscopy at least seemed worthy of development. Ten years ago the author experimented quite thoroughly and the results of the experiments were published in *The Laryngoscope* (Bib. 233). Only four of the conclusions need be mentioned here, namely:

1. The foreign body must be of iron or steel, partly or wholly.
2. The body must be free to move.
3. The attraction of the magnet for the foreign body is no greater than that of the foreign body for the magnet, hence:
4. The probabilities of magnetic removal are directly as the size of the foreign body, within the limits of size permitting mobility.

It will be seen by the foregoing that the magnet is only useful in precisely those cases which are most favorable for bronchoscopic methods. Unfortunately magnetic extraction does not assist in those cases beyond the limits of bronchoscopy. R. C. Lynch (Bib. 350) reports a successful case of magnetic extraction, as does also Iglauer (Bib. 221).

Mortality and results of bronchoscopy for foreign bodies: In considering the mortality of bronchoscopy, two facts stand out prominently. The first is that we should distinguish between the mortality of the method on the one hand, and the mortality from the lack of promptness and precision in performing it. For instance, the reports of four of the fatal cases show that the patients died upon the table of asphyxia for want of a prompt bronchoscopy.

Ingals, who is a pioneer bronchoscopist of large experience, writes: "Owing to numerous cases that come to my knowledge where inexperienced men have performed bronchoscopy with fatal results, and owing also to my recollection of the difficulties I experienced in the beginning of this work, I think it is highly desirable that some statement be made which would deter the inexperienced from undertaking these operations needlessly. I believe the fatalities with inexperienced people would run between 10 and 20 per cent if all cases could be collected."

Von Eicken collected 300 cases of bronchoscopy for foreign bodies up to and including the year 1908. The total mortality from all causes is given as 13.1 per cent. His statistics show for the pre-bronchoscopic period, 52 per cent. This brought into strong contrast the wonderful results of bronchoscopy even in the hands of beginners, as many of the cases were, and is a tribute to Killian, the father of bronchoscopy. The statistics of 1909 and 1910 were collected by Kahler, consisting of 291 cases with a mortality of 27, making 9.6 per cent. Of this mortality, not a single case could be attributed directly to bronchoscopy, but rather to the results of the foreign body itself or of blind methods of removal attempted prior to the bronchoscopy. The statistics of these two years, as compared with those collected by Kahler of the time prior to 1909, show clearly the improvement in technic and instruments, as well as in the personal skill of the various operators. As Brünings points out, if it is desired to get at the exact mortality of bronchoscopy *per se*, it will be necessary to include in statistics only the cases in which the foreign body has not been long present, because of the secondary changes that take place after a more or less prolonged sojourn of the foreign body. In preparing a "Rapport" for the International Medical Congress (Bib. 270), the author collected 171 cases of bronchoscopy for foreign bodies done in the United States (European statistics being in charge of the co-rapporteur, Prof. Killian) by various operators. In the 171 cases there were nine deaths (5.3 per cent). This does not include four deaths due to asphyxia for want of promptness in performing bronchoscopy. Of these, 156 were removed, 140 by peroral bronchoscopy, 22 by tracheotomic bronchoscopy. Of the fifteen unsuccessful cases, twelve were failures to find the foreign body known to be present, and only three were failures to remove it when found. In the twelve cases mentioned as failures to find the foreign body are included four in which the foreign body had been seen when higher up. After escaping into the deeper, minute bronchi it could not be re-located bronchoscopically, though still showing in the radiograph. The statistics of the author's own clinic and of his cases elsewhere, which are not included in the foregoing, are as follows: Of the last 182 consecutive cases of bronchoscopy for foreign body there was a total of three deaths (1.7 per cent) from any cause whatever within one month, though a few of the cases could not be followed this long. Of the 182 cases all were peroral bronchoscopies. Of the 182 cases, the foreign body was removed in 177. Of the five failures to remove foreign bodies known to be present, all were failures to find a small foreign body that was in a small branch bronchus close to the periphery of the lung. Two of these cases were recent. The percentage of the author's failures will doubtless increase in the future, since he now gets the cases upon which others have been unsuccesful and doubtless he will be equally so; though he has hopes that the elsewhere mentioned recently perfected means of locating small bodies in small bronchi near the periphery will diminish for every one the number of cases in which the intruder cannot be found.

Indications for bronchoscopy in suspected foreign body cases. It would be a mistake to elaborate many fine points of distinction as to the indications for bronchoscopy in suspected foreign body cases for three reasons: (a) A foreign body may be present without any demonstrable signs or symptoms. (b) In all cases of doubt a bronchoscopy should be done anyway. (c) Disease may be found to account for foreign body symptoms. The first two reasons are so abundantly proven as to need no citation of cases. The third reason (c) may be supported by two cases selected from among a number because the bronchoscopic diagnosis was of fundamental therapeutic importance. A man of forty years was referred to the author for removal of a wooden toothpick which was thought by the patient to be the cause of a cough of sudden onset following "choking on a toothpick." No foreign body was found but an indurated ulcer at the carina lead to a diagnosis of lues which was verified later. Mr. H. J. Davis reports an interesting case in which a fourteen-year-old child insisted that she could feel a pin in her chest. The radiograph was negative but on passing the bronchoscope he found a diphtheritic membrane in the trachea though none was present higher up.

Acute disease, such as the bronchopneumonia of children and unexplained "edema of the lungs," may in a few cases suspected of foreign body origin be indications for bronchoscopy.

The simulation of tuberculosis, chronic pleurisy with effusion, bronchitis, asthma, bronchiectasis and other chronic lung affections by prolonged sojourn of a foreign body renders bronchoscopy indicated in certain cases of these diseases. Instances have been reported by the author and others where these diseases have actually arisen secondarily to the presence of a foreign body. Of course it is not meant to urge bronchoscopy for foreign bodies in all cases of the diseases mentioned except bronchiectasis; but bronchoscopy is indicated in any case where there is a possibility of foreign body origin and in certain cases it is indicated for assistance in diagnosis and treatment of the diseases independently of a foreign body element. A radiograph may confirm or negative the indication. This matter is more fully considered in connection with the problems presented by bronchial foreign body cases of prolonged sojourn. The various indications for bronchoscopy in suspected foreign body cases may be summed up as follows, though this is by no means a complete category:

1. The appearance, in the radiograph, of a foreign body or of any suspicious shadow.

2. In any case in which there is a clear history of the patient having choked on a foreign body, and in which the foreign body was not afterwards found.

In this connection, it must be borne in mind that foreign bodies may be multiple, as in one case of the author, in which a bronchoscopy was not done because after the accident a gourd seed was found in the stools. Three months later he removed a gourd seed from the bronchus. The child had been playing with a whole mouthful of gourd seeds.

3. In any case in which there are signs of stenosis of the trachea or of a bronchus.

4. Any case suspected of bronchiectasis.

5. In the absence of any foreign body history, the patient giving symptoms of pulmonary tuberculosis, in which the bacilli cannot be found in the sputum and especially if the physical signs are at the base, particularly the right base, and above all, if there are also physical signs of pleural effusion.

6. In case of doubt, bronchoscopy should be done anyway.

Contra-indications to bronchoscopy for foreign bodies. The author has had no cause to modify his views previously expressed (Bib. 269), namely, that there is no absolute contra-indication to bronchoscopy. In some cases of extreme exhaustion, for instance when a patient who has already had too many bronchoscopies, it may be advisable to delay until the patient recuperates. Pneumonia of any form is certainly no contra-indication. It has been the author's custom to remove the foreign body even at the height of pneumonia, and invariably the influence of the removal of the foreign body has been good, rather than otherwise. Pulmonary abscess and other local lesions due to the presence of the foreign body itself, far from being contra-indications, are indications of the strongest kind for immediate bronchoscopic removal of the intruder. Gangrene of the lung is not a contra-indication to bronchoscopic removal of a foreign body unless the patient is moribund. Guisez has successfully treated gangrene of the lung bronchoscopically. It goes without saying that if the patient is dying from obstruction due to the foreign body, an immediate bronchoscopy is indicated; but if the patient is moribund from other causes, bronchoscopy is contra-indicated until the patient has rallied. Serious organic disease, such as aneurysm, does not constitute an absolute contra-indication, for unless the patient's immediate condition is serious from the aneurysm, he will live longer with the foreign body out than in. The author has had three foreign body cases in each of which a diagnosis of the vague syndrome called "status lymphaticus" had been made by a competent internist, and yet nothing unusual was noticed at the bronchoscopy, nor afterward. In a number of other foreign body cases a slight degree of thymic compression was noted incidentally at bronchoscopy. No anesthetic was used in any of these cases. The author quite agrees with Clark that "status lymphaticus" is no contra-indication. When a patient is in bad general condition, but not dyspneic, the question arises whether it is wise to wait for the patient to recuperate before doing the bronchoscopy for removal.

The situation is best illustrated by the following case: Three days after having aspirated a pin, an infant was sent from a distant city where it had been subjected to an oral bronchoscopy of one hour's duration, followed by a tracheotomy and a tracheotomic bronchoscopy of two hours' duration on the day after having aspirated the pin, involving an ether anesthesia of one hour's duration the first day and of two hours' duration the second day. Then it was subjected to a day's travel. When the child arrived it was quite exhausted from the various ordeals and the interference with regular nutrition. The question arose whether under these circumstances it were better to do the bronchoscopy at once or to wait for recuperation. The only objection to waiting was that the difficulty of removal usually increases steadily with each day that elapses after the inspiration of a very minute foreign body into a very small bronchus. For this reason, immediate bronchoscopy was decided upon and successfully executed through the mouth. There was no increase in the exhaustion and the child rallied well and was sent home a few days later. Had the foreign body been of larger size, instead of in a small bronchus which could have easily swollen shut by a few days longer wait, the author and his medical advisors would have decided on waiting for the child to rally before subjecting it to any further ordeal. Fortunately, we were able to do the work without anesthesia. Had a general anesthetic been required, it doubtless would have involved very great risk in the exhausted condition of the child. Had dyspnea been present, of course immediate bronchoscopy would have been obligatory and no question of delay could have been considered for one moment. In view of such experiences as these, the author feels that the question should be decided on the following basis: In cases without dyspnea, where a large foreign body is present in a child very much exhausted from any cause, it is better to wait, under careful watching, for recuperation; and if general anesthesia is to be used, it is quite imperative to wait. If, on the other hand, the foreign body is of the nature of a small pin or needle that has invaded a very small bronchus far out toward the periphery of the lung, it is better to proceed at once without any anesthesia, general or local. If there is dyspnea present, immediate bronchoscopy is absolutely imperative, and it must be done. without any anesthesia, general or local. We are, of course, speaking of children only; in adults there would be little or no danger in the use of a local anesthetic. In passing, it may be mentioned that in cases such as the one cited above, the inefficiency of the infantile cough in the removal of secretions must be borne in mind as mentioned under "Drowning of the patient in his own secretions."

Choice of time to do bronchoscopy for a foreign body. The choice of time to operate is as soon as possible after the accident. The difficulties of removal increase steadily from that time onward. The bronchi will swell shut and the orifices will be entirely obliterated temporarily by edema, later by the organization of granulation tissue, or the granulation tissue will, by its bleeding, render much more difficult the bronchoscopic removal, or the secondary changes, such as strictures, will enormously increase the difficulties. The patient's health will deteriorate, making him a less favorable subject for bronchoscopy, and occasionally the foreign body may escape from the bronchus into the tissues, though this is a rare accident. In case of bodies liable to expand or become friable by absorption of moisture, as dried beans, peas, maize and the like, every moment lost decreases the patient's chances. This does not justify hasty or ill-planned efforts without equipment; but, as Emil Mayer says, "Such a patient should be looked upon as constituting an emergency case to be operated upon at once." Solid bodies that by their shape are apt to occlude a bronchus, even though they do not swell, are to be operated upon at once, also, because of the serious effect of atelectasis and stagnation of secretion below the intruder, and, most important of all, because of the drawing downward of the foreign body by negative pressure which, with the swelling of the mucosa above as shown in Fig. 182, makes removal more and more difficult the longer the delay.

The duration of a bronchoscopy. Endoscopists are now agreed that prolonged bronchoscopy in children is inadvisable and that a number of shorter sittings is safer. This has no reference to the question of subglottic edema which will be separately considered. The author has frequently prolonged bronchoscopy to one hour's duration in children; but as a rule, a half hour from the time the bronchoscope passes through the larynx, should be the limit except in exceptional instances, in a child under two years of age. Over two years of age, a bronchoscopy of an hour, without anesthesia, general or local, is practically without risk. Drug shock, especially the paralyzing effect morphine and chloroform have on the respiratory center, renders a bronchoscopy of over fifteen minutes' duration hazardous. In an adult, the author has, in one instance, prolonged the bronchoscopy to three and a half hours, using a very little bit of cocaine solution a number of times, applied only to the neighborhood of a foreign body in the bronchus.

This matter of duration is so important, and is so greatly influenced by various factors, that it is quite necessary for bronchoscopists to record the duration of their endoscopies in order to get data for a working basis. The author has such a record for most of his cases.

The endoscopic appearances of foreign bodies in the air passages. Those who have never tried it may not realize that the endoscopic detection of a foreign body is, even when presented, not always easy to the inexperienced. Prolonged training will enable the experienced endoscopist instantly to recognize any departure from the normal, even though the exact nature of the condition may not be at once realized. This is a valuable time-saving acquisition to be striven for. It must be remembered that, as is well known to all artists, color depends largely on the intensity, quality and direction of the illumination. Moreover, it is often not the true color of the foreign body itself that presents, but the foreign body as seen through a filmy coating of secretions which may be tinted with pus, blood or dissolved material from the foreign body itself. Therefore, the tube must be advanced slowly and carefully, all secretions being sponged away ahead of the tube-mouth so that the *wall* as well as the lumen can be carefully studied, not for the foreign body alone, but for evidences of traumatism or inflammatory lesions due to its presence. As stated above, the color of a foreign body as seen endoscopically, varies with the degree of illumination. As a rule, however, iron and steel bodies look black even after a few days' sojourn, no matter how highly polished they may have been when they entered. Nickel-plated objects, as a rule, do not tarnish so readily. Silver objects turn black very quickly, just as steel and iron bodies do. Brass substances corrode quickly and soon look dark brown or black. The glint even of nickel-plated bodies is soon dulled by secretions, so that taking it all in all, the endoscopist will usually find all sorts of foreign bodies to be grey, or, more often, almost black in color, with the exception of very recently aspirated brass, gold and bright copper substances, which may show for a few days in nearly their natural colors. As a rule, however, the bronchoscopist who is looking for a brightly shining, whitish glint will be deceived by the refraction of air bubbles and the spurs at the giving off of the different branch bronchi. As pointed out by Waggette (Bib. 567), it is necessary urgently to warn the beginner not to mistake the sharp, white, cartilaginous division between two branches for a foreign body. With a corroded steel or iron body, showing black, this is not likely to occur; but if the operator has in mind the bright silvery whiteness of the ordinary pin, for instance, he is very apt to make such a mistake as Mr. Waggette warns against. As shown by D. R. Patterson (Bib. 439), the natural color of a foreign body mav be such as to render its contrast with the surrounding mucosa so slight as to make prompt recognition difficult. This is an important point to keep in mind.

Bronchoscopic finding of a foreign body in the tracheo-bronchial tree. Finding a large foreign body recently aspirated presents no especial difficulties. One of long sojourn may be hidden by secondary processes; and the problem then presented will be separately considered. Small foreign bodies are in some cases very difficult to find. Not because of any difficulty in seeing a minute object when such objects can be brought in line with the observer's eye, but because small foreign bodies may be located "around the corner" in a small branch bronchus, into which we do not directly look. When a small foreign body, such as a needle or a pin, has penetrated a small bronchus, there may be secretions emerging from the little bronchial branch that will betray the presence of the pin, but quite as often there is nothing in the way of local appearances to guide. Under such circumstances, the methods of localization referred to in a previous chapter should be used to limit the number of bronchi to be searched to a very few. In the absence of such means, it certainly is not justifiable to search every bronchus in the entire lobe, and still less is it justifiable to go with the forceps or probe into every bronchus. Having narrowed down the number of small bronchi to be searched to a few, each of the few orifices must be looked into in the manner shown in the schema Fig. 172. The bronchoscope, B, is introduced as far as possible into the inferior lobe bronchus and the endoscopist sees ahead the orifices of two or more branches, (D.) none of which, however, shows any evidence of invasion of the pin, which is below the level of the visual axis, and is hidden by the intervening tissue, C. When we have reason to suspect such a condition of affairs from the radiographic localization, either by the radiograph with film overlay, or by radiograph with the bronchoscope in position, the tissue, C, must be pushed backward out of the way by the lip of the bronchoscope. In doing this, it is necessary to raise the head of the patient and in certain instances it will be necessary to raise the head and shoulders, the head being flexed forward on the thorax. In this position, the bronchoscope, as shown at M, will afford a view of the point of the pin (E.). The large amount of resiliency of the bronchial tissues permits of such manipulation without injury, provided the manipulations are gentle. It is very easy to rupture a bronchus by pushing the tube with too much pressure into a bronchus not sufficiently large to admit the tube. Blind probing for exploration of bronchi suspected to contain the intruder is dangerous unless done with extreme caution. If any orifice seems at all suspicious the conical-ended bronchoscope (Fig. 18) may be used, or a closed, plain, straight forceps (Fig. 28) may be introduced carefully as a probe. If the intruder is felt the forceps jaws may be expanded and the foreign body seized, but great care must be used. Under no circumstances should strong traction be made. In minute bronchi a foreign body is rarely firmly fixed because its distal part is necessarily small or it could not have entered. If a spur between two bronchial openings is grasped, slight traction will give an elastic sensation that can readily be recognized as quite different from the yielding of a foreign body that is free to move. Of course, a pin whose point is upward, as practically all are, may stick into the bronchial wall, preventing withdrawal. This would give the same sensation of elasticity, which is due to the elastic mobility of the lung. This blind

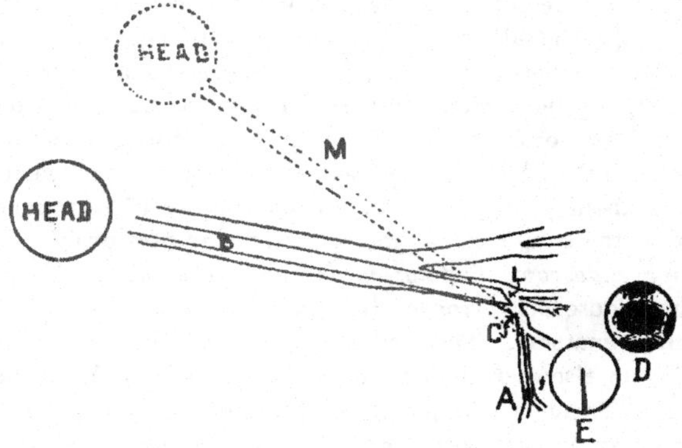

FIG. 172. Schema illustrating the author's method of bringing into view a pin (A) located "around the corner," and hidden by the tissue (C) from the observer, who, in looking through the bronchoscope, B, sees only empty orifices (D). By raising the patient's head very high, the lip, L, of the bronchoscope displaces the tissue, C, permitting the observer to see the point of the pin as at E. The schema was drawn by the author after thus finding a pin in a small dorsal branch of the inferior lobe bronchus. He has used the principle many times since in branches diverging at various angles and twice in the upper-lobe bronchus.

groping is dangerous. Particular care must be used not to mistake the grating sensation of the probing forceps sliding over the inner wall of the bronchoscope for the contact of a foreign body. Under no circumstances is it justifiable to use toothed forceps for probing.

When a pin is located so as to have its long axis corresponding to the long axis of the bronchoscope, the point of the pin presenting toward the operator, the pin may be difficult to see, though as a rule there is movement enough to the whole tree to throw the pin at various angles so that it is only for a moment that the pin's axis exactly coincides with the visual axis. Usually also, the color of the pin is black from corrosion. A very recently aspirated bright pin may, however, be mistaken for a string of mucus or a division spur. Much more often, however, the reverse mistake is made; the white line of a spur, or a thread of mucus is thought to be the foreign body, until the eye has become educated to these illusions.

It is a mistake to be constantly withdrawing and inserting the bronchoscope. The author in 208 cases of foreign body in the bronchus did not remove the bronchoscope in a single instance until entirely through with the bronchoscopy. This is not mentioned boastfully but to correct the prevalent misunderstanding of the subject. The author cannot bring to mind any reason why, starting with a properly selected tube, the bronchoscope should be removed. It is a time-wasting procedure even if it does take but a few moments. If there should be any trouble with the light, the light carrier can be withdrawn; but this should not be necessary more often than once in thirty or forty cases; and not oftener than once an hour in any case. Properly illuminated, the life of a lamp is about 40 hours. The sponging away of secretions from the field keeps the lamp clean at the same time, as previously explained.

Negative endoscopic findings in foreign body cases. Many cases come to the endoscopist erroneously believing that a foreign body has lodged in their anatomy. These cases may or may not need endoscopic search as herein elsewhere indicated; but if searched it should be thoroughly done. There is another class of negative cases, in which the foreign body has probably been present at some time or other. These require very careful work. In the trachea and bronchi, evidence, in the form of local reaction, justifies the most careful and persistent search, because the chances are all in favor of the foreign body still being present, possibly hidden in swollen mucosa or in a closed-off bronchus, either of the same side or even on the other side. In other words, traumatism or reaction found in a bronchus indicates that the foreign body is present, but it does not necessarily localize it to the side on which the traumatism is seen, because of the well known tendency of foreign bodies that are free to knock in the air passages to be aspirated into the opposite side. In all cases of doubt as to the localization of the foreign body we must do a bronchoscopy as well as an esophogoscopy, doing first the one indicated by the preponderance of evidence. Furthermore, in any case where all the data point almost conclusively to the foreign body being in the esophagus or in the air passages, as the case may be, and failing to find it in the search of the one, we must then search the other before giving a positive opinion that a foreign body is not present, because none of our diagnostic means are absolutely reliable negatively. In the esophagus both pyriform sinuses and the sub-cricopharyngeal space must be searched with a large tube or speculum. The possibility of sharp-pointed bodies having wandered out through the esophageal wall must be borne in mind. Such bodies usually are metallic and hence radiographically discoverable; but occasionally a rib bone of a fish will thus wander and will not show. The author had one such case, also a case of a toothbrush bristle. In none of these was an esophagoscopy done. Mr. E. D. Davis reports the case of a boy with a pin that could not be found esophagoscopically, but which seemed, radiographically, to be in the retropharyngeal space. In conclusion we may say that no case can be considered to have been endoscopically explored unless the trachea, right and left, main, inferior and upper bronchi and the middle lobe bronchus (present on the right side only) shall have been examined, to the greatest depth reachable. Nor are we ready to give a negative opinion then. The hypopharynx and esophagus must be explored from the arytenoids to the stomach. This, however, must not be misconstrued into advising that thorough exploration must be completed at one seance.

Inasmuch as we know that certain foreign bodies, such as small pins, may be present in the bronchi, as shown by the radiograph, and yet not be discoverable by bronchoscopy, how shall we be certain, in case of a foreign body not opaque to the ray, that it is not present on the strength of not being able to find it bronchoscopically. If the foreign body is of such small size that it can enter a small bronchus far out at the periphery, it is impossible to be certain. If, on the other hand, the history mentions a nonfriable foreign body of such size that it cannot enter a bronchus too small for a bronchoscope to follow it, we may be certain, after a careful search, that it is not present if not found. If the body is liable to be comminuted by maceration this does not hold absolutely true. One other point which will aid sometimes in deciding the question is that we may be able to state from the appearances of reaction around a small bronchus, that it probably contains a foreign body. This is only available, however, when there has been no previous bronchoscopy which could have caused irritation by probing that bronchus, and of course the error must be avoided of mistaking traumatism of a foreign body which had been coughed up for the traumatism of the reaction of a foreign body which is still present.

*Oral or tracheotomic bronchoscopy. Which?** Unfortunately the statement has crept into the literature that in infants or small children it is preferable to do a tracheotomic bronchoscopy. In the opinion of the author this is due to two things: 1. The ignoring of the precautions mentioned under subglottic edema. 2. The fact that when this statement

*Abstracted from the author's Rapport at the International Medical Congress, London, 1913.

was originally made, illumination was not in the relatively perfect condition that is seen on the instruments of to-day. In making this statement, the author hopes he will not be misunderstood as referring to any difference between distal and proximal illumination. He means simply that the light on all forms of instruments to-day is far superior to what it was in the early days. At that time it made a great difference whether the tube was a long or a short one. To-day, it is questionable whether anyone can tell by looking through the lumen whether the tube is 30 cm. or 50 cm. The author has often tested this and found the observer unable to tell with a pair of concealed tubes which was the longer and which was the shorter, even though one was an 80 cm. gastroscope. Therefore, a short tube has no advantage so far as illumination is concerned. In regard to the manipulation of forceps, etc., an additional length of 10 to 14 cm. is of no advantage whatever. It is true that a somewhat larger tube can be used through a tracheotomic wound than through the glottis with safety to the subglottic structure, but Dr. Ellen J. Patterson and the author have found that a tube of 4 mm. internal diameter is amply large for delicate manipulations under the guidance of the eye, such as the placing of a hook through the eye of a shoe-button in the bronchus of a child six months of age. If one is not accustomed to work through small tubes, doubtless it is better to do a tracheotomic bronchoscopy than to force a large tube through the larynx. In upper lobe bronchoscopy, almost as favorable an angle can be obtained by shifting the tube to the opposite corner of the mouth, as could be obtained by a tracheotomic bronchoscopy, provided the assistant holding the head, and the operator have worked years together so that they co-operate and the head of the patient is carried along with the tube to the extreme opposite position from the lobe to be explored. All of these things are readily demonstrated on the patient, but unfortunately the statements in the early literature have led men into hasty tracheotomy rather than to develop the necessary technic to work with exceedingly small tubes and to avoid damage to the subglottic area Out of 706 bronchoscopies for all purposes, no one in the author's clinic has ever done a tracheotomy for the purpose of bronchoscopy. One tracheotomic bronchoscopy done by the author for a foreign body was in a case where the general surgeon had already done a tracheotomy for the compressive stenosis due to a goitre. In that case the author failed to find the foreign body, a small pin. In one other case, also in his early work, he did a treacheotomic bronchoscopy in a foreign body case tracheotomized for dyspnea. Both cases failed to convince the author that there is any advantage in the tracheotomic route. With these two exceptions, it has always been our custom to insert the bronchoscope through the mouth, even in the cases already tracheotomized for dyspnea. Very often patients come in with such severe dyspnea that it is unwise to leave them over night without a tracheotomy. In such cases, the absolute rule in tracheal surgery to do a tracheotomy always early, never late, is followed; but in the first management of the case we have always found that a bronchoscope introduced through the mouth is much better for the temporary relief of dyspnea, insufflation of oxygen, etc. In foreign body cases previously tracheotomized the bronchoscope introduced through the mouth we have found much more freely manipulated and much more satisfactory to work with because the patient's head is very much less in the way, and all of the movements and manipulations are the usual ones in peroral endoscopy. The author hopes the foregoing will not be regarded as boasting. He feels sure that other endoscopists just simply have not tried oral bronchoscopy in infants, but have been misled by early statements based upon different conditions, and especially different instruments. The production of subglottic edema by oral bronchoscopy in children was due to faulty position, too large tubes and other preventable factors that will be considered in a later section. The preference of some operators for tracheotomic bronchoscopy has been due to the erroneous position of the head used in oral bronchoscopy. As elsewhere mentioned, the direction of the trachea is backward as well as downward. It follows that a tube introduced through the anterior part of the neck will necessarily be of a great advantage compared tc a tube which is introduced through the mouth if the head of the patient is very low. If, on the other hand, the head (recumbent) is very high, there is absolutely no advantage in direction in the tracheotomic route. The head has usually been held too low in oral bronchoscopy. Figure 162 illustrates the needlessness of tracheotomy so far as reaching a foreign body is concerned (it was necessary in this case for other reasons). The bronchoscope shown in the radiograph is passed through the mouth and shows the bronchoscope at a farther angle toward the periphery than was necessary to reach the pin. A tracheotomy had been done by the previous operator in the hope that a tracheotomic bronchoscopy might succeed when he failed at an oral bronchoscopy. The author worked through the mouth only, and while he was equally unsuccessful in finding the pin, the point here made is that so far as reaching a foreign body is concerned there is absolutely no advantage in angle by the tracheotomic route. The radiograph was not made for the purpose of demonstration but as an aid to the working out of the problems in that particular case. Had demonstration been the object, the distal end of the bronchoscope could easily have been moved out to the patient's left beyond the heart shadow, there being absolutely nothing in the oral route to prevent such an angle. So far as any advantage in lateral movement is concerned, the error has been made of not realizing the wide range rendered available by the Boyce position. The range is shown schematically in Fig. 135 and actually in the living patient in Figures 136 and 162. Sharp foreign bodies, especially those with hooked extremities, or such as may require a complicated procedure for removal, do not demand a tracheotomy, but simply more careful work. In the hands, however, of the endoscopically inexperienced, it is perfectly justifiable in such cases to do a tracheotomy; and it should by all means be done in preference to rough and violent removal after an indiscriminate forceps seizure of the foreign body at any point that may present. Extremely large foreign bodies do not necessarily demand tracheotomic bronchoscopy. Any intruder that has gone down through the glottis can be brought up the same way, if turned to the position of least resistance. Thymic tracheostenosis, thyroid anomaly, acute or chronic laryngeal stenosis and many other conditions may demand tracheotomy and the author would be the last one in the world to argue against its prompt and early performance. But in this chapter are presented reasons why it is needless for the passage of a bronchoscope. In conclusion the author would strongly urge the bronchoscopist not to resort to tracheotomic bronchoscopy at the second trial. If the first bronchoscopy is not successful after fifteen or twenty minutes in a child it is better to desist, wait a few days and repeat the oral bronchoscopy at least twice before resorting to the tracheotomic route. The author feels sure that a large number of the reported cases where the first bronchoscopy was oral and the second, tracheotomic, the second bronchoscopy would have been just as successful if it also had been oral. On the other hand, the author regards tracheotomy as perfectly justifiable in any case in which the surgeon in charge deems tracheotomy for any reason whatsoever indicated for the best interests of the patient. In stating his personal views he recognizes the advisability of everyone deciding such questions for himself, apropos of the particular case.

COMPLICATIONS AND AFTER-EFFECTS OF BRONCHOSCOPY.

After-care in endoscopic foreign-body cases. All foreign-body cases should have a special nurse night and day so that a careful watch may be maintained at all times. The possibility of the patient drowning in his own secretions, or of respiratory arrest, should be borne in mind and under no circumstances whatever should the patient be permitted to leave the hospital before all danger of complications is over. In the majority of cases the patient could go home the same evening without injury but occasionally complications may occur and it is better to be on the safe side.

General reaction. There is in the majority of instances no general reaction following a bronchoscopy in a patient whose temperature, pulse and respiration are normal at the beginning. Occasionally there is a reaction to 100° F. The chart in such a case is reproduced in Fig. 173. If, however, bronchopneumonia, septic pneumonia and other

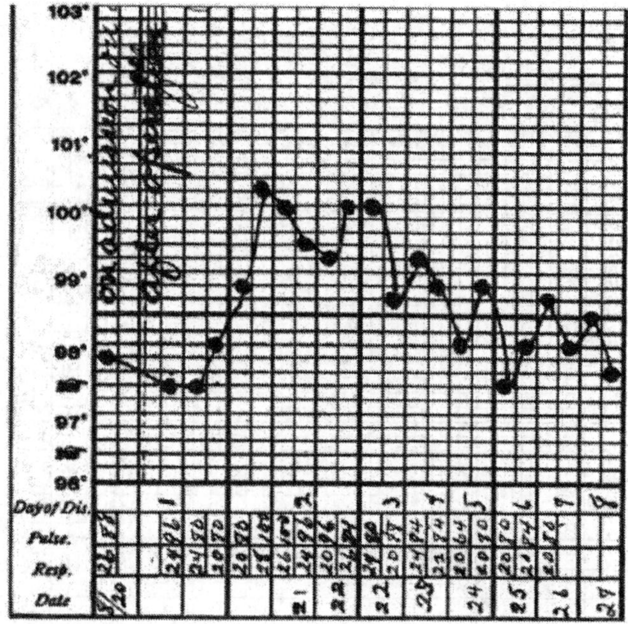

Fig. 173. Chart of a maximum reaction seen after bronchoscopic foreign body removal. Patient normal as to temperature, pulse and respiration before operation.

acute conditions are present, we may have a severe reaction, though it is very rarely fatal. Lesser degrees of virulence of infective inflammation present prior to bronchoscopy may produce only moderate reaction as shown in Fig. 174, which is quite typical. Out of 31 cases of children in which the larynx and trachea seemed to be perfectly normal, but in which a foreign body was found in the bronchi, there was no reaction in any instance. The temperature did not rise to 100 in any but one case and the children seemed normal in every way as to breathing, appetite, and general condition. In one instance there

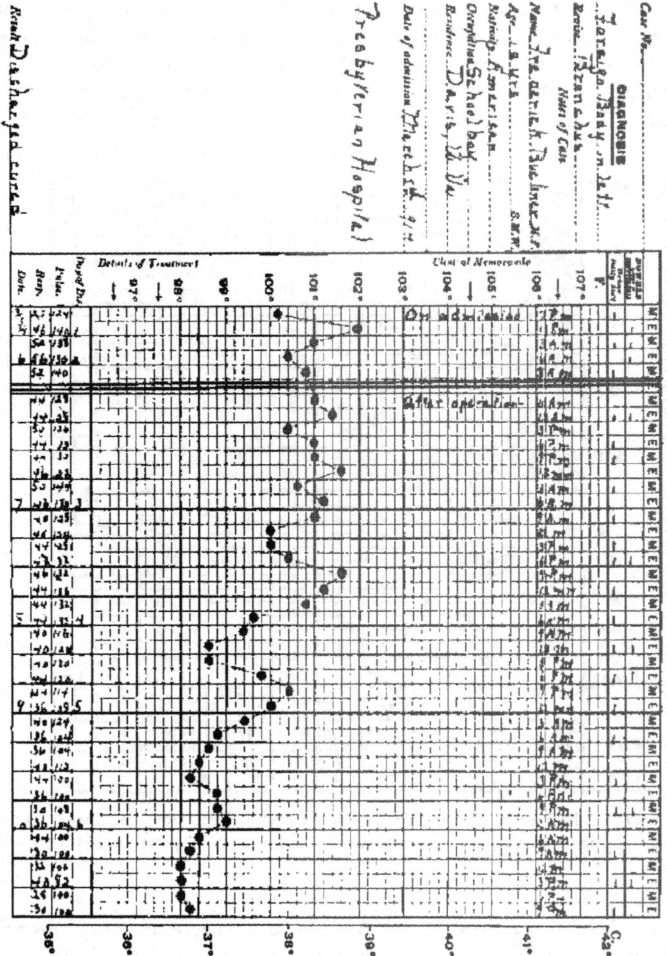

FIG. 174. Chart after bronchoscopic foreign body removal in a case in which there existed previously a moderately virulent infective tracheobronchitis.

was a rise in temperature to 103. As there was in this instance no cough, no hoarsenes, marked respiratory rise nor other sign pointing to the air passages, but on the other hand gastro-intestinal disturbances, which were promptly relieved, followed by prompt subsidence of the temperature elevation, Dr. Price concluded that the condition was one of gastro-enteric trouble and not a reaction from bronchoscopy. On the other hand, in another group of 26 cases, which, on first examination, were seen to have an intense laryngitis or tracheo-bronchitis, either from previous attempts at removal or from the foreign body being thrown about the interior of the air passages, there was a prompt reaction following the bronchoscopy with a rise of from one to two degrees in the already elevated temperature. This rise and the reaction was most severe in the cases associated with copious pus formation. In three of these cases a peanut kernel was the offending substance, and this particular foreign body seems to have a peculiarly irritating effect upon the mucosa of the lower air passages. From the foregoing statistics, as well as from the general recollections of clinical observations, the author feels justified in the following conclusions:

1. Bronchoscopy carefully done in children, without an anesthetic, general or local, is unassociated with any reaction worthy of consideration, provided the child beforehand is normal as to temperature, pulse, respiration and nearly so as to the local conditions in the larynx, trachea and bronchi, and provided the technic is strictly aseptic.

2. General systemic reaction including temperature elevation, advance in pulse rate and respiratory frequency may be anticipated in any case where the temperature is already above 100, and especially in such cases as have a severe local inflammatory condition in the larynx, trachea or bronchi.

3. The most severe reactions are due to absorption through abrasions of the epithelium. These abrasions, when occurring from the foreign body, cannot, of course, be avoided, but abrasions in bronchoscopy, except in exceedingly complicated removals, need not occur if great care be taken, not only in the performance of bronchoscopy, but also beforehand, to see that all of the instruments are free from roughness and sharp corners or angles. Von Schrötter (Bib. 565) reports a rise of pulse to 140 with rapid, irregular heart action but without dyspnea, due to the patient having swallowed a considerable amount of air during bronchoscopy, causing a dilatation of the stomach. The symptoms all subsided after a rest in bed.

Shock. To the writer's knowledge no accurate experimental work has been done in regard to the degree of shock, if any, in bronchoscopy and esophagoscopy. Taking Crile's definition of surgical shock as a "low blood pressure," the author has never seen a single instance in any way approaching surgical shock, in a case where there had been no operative measures other than the endoscopy. A number of cases have had severe fatigue; especially noted in children after a prolonged bronchoscopy. When the author first noted the interesting observations of Yandell Henderson on the acapneal hypothesis of shock, the author was surprised that nothing of the kind had ever been noted after bronchoscopy without anesthesia. Careful observation, however, revealed the fact that respiration far from being excessive is so much interfered with by spasm, cough, and holding the breath that it seems certain that there is a hypopnea instead of a hyperpnea. This observation is not intended as applying in one way or the other to the theories as to the nature of surgical shock. They merely go to show that unless unduly prolonged there is nothing approaching surgical shock from a carefully done bronchoscopy or esophagoscopy when no trauma is inflicted. There may be, and doubtless is in many cases, a drug shock. Sargnon reports a case where a tuberculous pulmonary hemorrhage supervened preventing the bronchoscopic extraction of a pea, the patient dying twelve hours later. Pulmonary tuberculosis cannot be regarded as a contraindication to the removal of a foreign body and it was perfectly right and proper in this case to make the attempt. Undoubtedly the hemorrhage would have supervened anyway in a very short time so that such a case can hardly be regarded as strictly a death from bronchoscopy. Mosher reports central hemiplegia during bronchoscopy under ether.

Local reaction. Ordinarily the only local reaction noted is a slight laryngeal congestion producing slight hoarseness which disappears in a few days. If dyspnea, without pneumonia, supervene it is usually due to one of three things:

1. Drowning of the patient in his own secretions.
2. Laryngeal edema.
3. Subglottic edema.

Impending drowning of the patient in his own secretions is a complication seen by the author in a number of cases. The subject has so many important bearings that it is separately considered under "Diseases of the Trachea and Bronchi." Suffice it here to say that it is the first thing to be thought of in dyspneic cases and is quickly relievable by the "sponge pumping" process. In a number of instances, the child has become dyspneic within 24 or 36 hours after the bronchoscopy, but on passing the bronchoscope, a large quantity of secretion was removed with complete re-establishment of quiet respiration and the disappearance of the dyspnea. It is especially to be anticipated in cases of peanut kernels and other secretion-producing foreign bodies.

Edema of the supraglottic larynx sufficient to become obstructive is quite rare. The only case of the kind that required tracheotomy, in the author's experience, was in an elderly patient with advanced nephritis

Subglottic edema. The causes of this complication in the author's opinion are:

1. The use of over-sized tubes.
2. Undue violence in insertion of the bronchoscope.
3. Faulty position of the patient, the long axis of the trachea not being in line with the bronchoscope as the latter enters the trachea.
4. Faulty position of the patient after the bronchoscope is introduced resulting in undue pressure by making the larynx the fulcrum of the bronchoscopic lever instead of the upper thoracic aperture.
5. Trauma by extraction of the foreign body wrongly placed with reference to the long diameter of the glottis.
6. Trauma in the application of local anesthetics through the glottis before the bronchoscope is introduced.
7. The anatomic and physiologic nature of the subglottic tissue is a contributing cause.
8. Infective trauma by the foreign body itself prior to the bronchoscopy is undoubtedly a contributing factor.

Von Eicken has reported a number of cases in which a subglottic edema present before bronchoscopy increased after bronchoscopy so as to require tracheotomy. Logan Turner has scientifically determined that the development of inflammatory edema of the larynx is dependent upon three factors. 1. The intensity of the inflammatory process producing it. 2. The site of the infection. 3. The anatomic arrangement of the loose submucous cellular tissue of the larynx. The bearings of these observations upon subglottic edema after the sojourn of a foreign body in the subglottic region, or in the trachea where it is intermittently coughed upward toward the glottic chink and aspirated backward again, is self evident, but it is hoped that still further study by this eminent authority will throw further light upon the occurrence of subglottic edema without general laryngeal edema, after bronchoscopy, as reported by a number of authors.

The author may be biased but he believes that the production of subglottic edema is lessened by distal illumination by permitting the use of very small tubes and by doing away with the heavy handle, thus permitting of the utmost delicacy, and, most important, the thick strong heavy laryngoscopic tube is not introduced through the larynx. The thinnest Brünings bronchoscope at the laryngeal part of the tube during bronchoscopy is 7 mm. and this Brünings states "Cannot be used until the child is from 4 to 5 months old." Consequently in very young infants tracheotomy has to be resorted to because as Brünings states: "No reliance can be placed on the employment of tubes narrower than 7 millimetres." This can only apply to proximally lighted tubes which require not only a relatively large lumen for illuminating purposes but require a relatively thick and heavy laryngoscopic tube outside the bronchoscopic tube, because by this system the laryngoscopic tube itself is pushed through the glottis. By the author's method the bronchoscopic tube is too thin and light to be used to produce the displacement necessary to expose the glottis, and with distal illumination, a 4 mm. tube is quite practical for anyone who will practice with it a while. The author has done a number of peroral bronchoscopies for diagnosis in suspected thymic pressure cases in new-born infants without any ill effects from the use of the 4 mm. distally illuminated tube. In the author's clinic, both Dr. Ellen J. Patterson and the author use tubes of 4 mm. and 5 mm. internal diameter, for children under 6 years of age, the 4 mm. tube being for infants under one year. Our youngest patient from whom a foreign body was removed was an infant of 2½ months. This was a common pin removed from the right bronchus with a tube 4 mm. internal diameter. Since 1911, not one case of subglottic edema has occurred in the practice of either Dr. Ellen J. Patterson or the author in 36 successful removals of foreign bodies in the trachea and bronchi of infants under one year. Every case was done by oral bronchoscopy. This freedom from subglottic edema, we believe, is due to the use of small tubes, close attention to the details of introduction and manipulation herein given; and, especially to the aid of good assistants—in other words to "team work." Stanton A. Friedberg in a recent case reports the use of a distally illuminated 5 mm. tube in an infant of 3 months, for the peroral bronchoscopic removal of a safety-pin from the right bronchus. Considering the nature of the foreign body this is one of the most remarkable cases recorded, and is the youngest patient from whom a safety-pin has been removed. Dr. Friedberg states, "What pleases me most is the facility with which an upper bronchoscopy was performed on such a young child." Killian, himself, recently has recognized the disadvantage in children of adding the bulk of the heavy laryngoscopic tube to the bronchoscopic tube in the larynx and has devised an excellent set of very small single tubes for children, (Fig. 175), to obviate the bulk of the double tube. These tubes Killian inserts with a mandrin and illuminates with a Kirstein headlight; though the tubes are also arranged to fit the Brünings or Kahler hand-lamp. Faulty direction of the tube on introducing may easily cause trauma by gouging into the subglottic wall, if the axis of the bronchoscope and that of the trachea do not coincide at the moment the tube passes the glottis. In ten different publications within the last two years, the operators stated they placed the patient in the Rose position. If the patient actually was in the Rose position, he was just exactly rightly placed for the bronchoscope to gouge into the subglottic wall and to risk a production of subglottic edema, especially if the head of the patient was a little more to one side than the other. Mention is made in the chapter on introduction of the bronchoscope, of the necessity for, and method of, avoiding the use of the larynx as a fulcrum and the bronchoscope as a lever, because not only is the bronchoscopic freedom of movement thus hampered but the incidental trauma is a fruitful source of subglottic edema. The operator, who expects by means of heavy handles, and special leverage to get along with an illy trained assistant by dragging his patient around with his instrument until he can find the lumen he seeks, will have frequent subglottic edemas; and if he cannot improve the technic he had better do a tracheotomic bronchoscopy in order to leave the larynx out of harm's way. Bronchoscopy should be a gentle art.

Treatment. When subglottic edema is present, the patient should be closely watched and secretions should be promptly removed, though if it is certain that the trouble is due solely to the subglottic swelling, it would

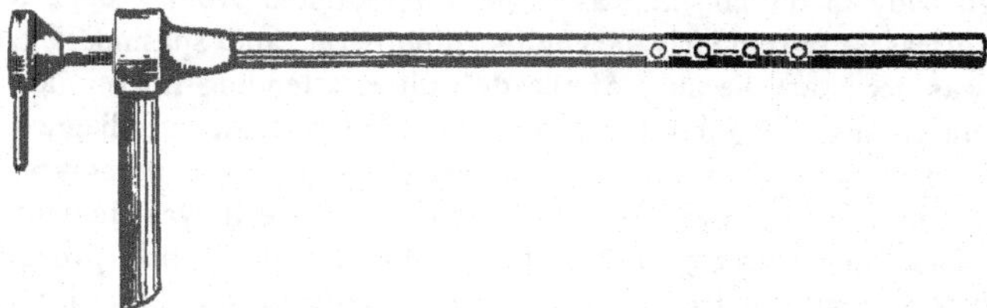

FIG. 175. Killian's new tubes for children. What resembles an inner tube is really a mandrin for insertion, to obviate the use of the bulky double tube. They will fit the Brünings or Kahler handlamp; but Killian uses the Kirstein headlight. Six sizes are required.

4.5 mm.	for children	54 to 57 cm. body length.
5. mm.	" "	58 to 64 cm. " "
5.5 mm.	" "	65 to 70 cm. " "
6. mm.	" "	71 to 85 cm. " "
6.5 mm.	" "	86 to 100 cm. " "
7. mm.	" "	101 to 120 cm. " "

perhaps be better not to pass the bronchoscope for the removal of secretions, but to proceed to a tracheotomy. Intubation should never be used, as it is not safe in these cases and is very likely to lead to an after stenosis. The same may be said of a very high tracheotomy in which the reaction around the cannula may result in a stenosis from perichondritis or cicatricial contraction which will require a long period of treatment for cure. When done for subglottic edema, the tracheotomy should be below the second ring of the trachea.

The patient should be decannulated in a few days. Should the edema become chronic and prevent decannulation, direct galvano-cauterization as elsewhere herein explained, should be done. The treatment of other complications are within the province of the internist and pediatrist.

CHAPTER XIV.

Removal of Foreign Bodies from the Larynx.

Symptoms and diagnosis. The older laryngologic works contain lengthy descriptions of signs and symptoms by which the presence of a foreign body in the larynx was to be differentiated from neoplasm and other diseases, particularly laryngitis, diphtheria, and spasmodic croup. This was necessary because of the difficulties attending mirror laryngoscopy in children. To-day the promptness and certainty of diagnosis by the direct method of examination has rendered all this unnecessary. In the earlier days the usefulness was limited because it was thought that anesthesia was necessary: but as the author has abundantly proven, no anesthetic, general or local, is necessary for a diagnostic direct laryngoscopy in any infant or older child. The prompt, safe and successful removal of foreign bodies from the larynx is one of the greatest achievements of direct laryngoscopy. Not only is it exceedingly difficult to see the larynx of a child, but even if seen, removal by the indirect method is of such extreme difficulty that tracheotomy has usually been done in days past in preference to attempting indirect removal without general anesthesia, and of course general anesthesia is absolutely contraindicated because of the laryngeal obstruction. On the other hand by the direct method foreign bodies can be removed from the larynx of children without any anesthetic, general or local and without tracheotomy. Another great advantage of the direct method is that in case of impacted foreign bodies which have to be rotated for safe removal, the rotation is easily accomplished by means of the straight instruments. This was impossible with the angular instruments required by the indirect method. Such a case is shown schematically in Fig. 176, which illustrates the difficulties presented by the firm lodgement of a safety-pin in the edematous larynx of an infant of 8 months. Notwithstanding the achievements of the direct method it is still quite common to have children with foreign bodies in the larynx given antitoxin on an erroneous diagnosis of laryngeal diphtheria. Of course, if for any reason a direct laryngoscopy is not to be had promptly because of lack of instruments or of familiarity with their use, it is perfectly right to give antitoxin rather than delay 24 hours for a diagnosis, but when the day shall have arrived that every laryngologist and every pediatrist will be able to examine the larynx of any child without any anesthetic, general or local, the necessity for "a shot in the dark" will cease to exist. Harmon Smith (Bib. 509) reports a very interesting case of a closed safety-pin. The patient had not only been given antitoxin for diphtheria, but had been intubated. The intubation tube was coughed out, leaving the pin *in situ*. Harmon Smith discovered and removed the pin by direct laryngoscopy, and very justly urges that, in all cases in which cultures are negative and no membrane is in evidence, the larynx and the trachea should be examined by the direct method "if for no other reason than to exclude the presence of a foreign body." Almost every endoscopist has had a similar experience. When we add to such occurrences the great number of papilloma cases the neglect of direct laryngoscopy begins to assume the aspect of serious lack of efficiency. In one case reported repeated operations for papilloma had been previously done, the fungations having been mistaken for neoplasms.

Many cases of foreign body in the larynx are immediately fatal as the columns of the newspapers show. Many others are extremely dyspneic when they come to the laryngologist. No physician or surgeon should hesitate to do an immediate tracheotomy in such cases. In lesser degrees of dyspnea the child must be carefully watched until preparations for direct laryngoscopy can be made, because of the risk of a sudden increase of dyspnea from a shift of the foreign body, drowning of the patient in his own secretions, spasm, edema, etc. Preparations for a tracheotomy should also be made, not that the direct laryngoscopy, if carefully done, would ordinarily provoke stenosis, but the foreign body might be shifted. It is well to remember that these cases often come in exhausted because for days and nights they have been too busy fighting for air to either eat or sleep. It requires but little to cause them to give up the fight because of exhaustion. For this reason also it is never wise to prolong the examination. They cannot stand for long the spasmodic reflex closure of the glottis.

Preliminary examination. As previously stated, in every case of foreign body, regardless of whether it is expected to be in the larynx, trachea, bronchi or esophagus, indirect mirror examinations should be made, if the patient be old enough. The patient should be recumbent. In a number of cases where a foreign body was suspected by the patient, a local lesion has been found; in three instances tuberculosis had produced no symptoms until the patient strangled on some article of food which was thought to have entered the larynx. On the other hand, especially if granulations are present, the endoscopist must be on his guard against making a diagnosis of disease from the appearances of inflammatory changes which may be secondary to the presence of a foreign body. Quite a number of such cases have been reported and the author

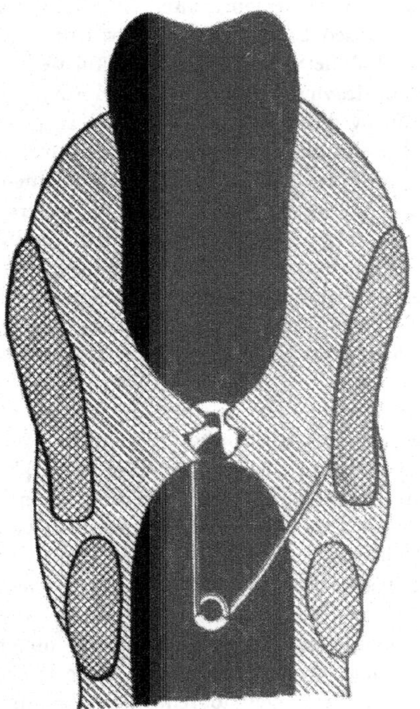

FIG. 176. Schema showing lodgement of a safety-pin in the larynx of a male infant eight months of age. The pin was pushed downward, rotated and removed with its greater plane sagittally. Rotation would have been impossible with the angular instruments necessary in direct methods.

has seen two cases of foreign body in the larynx that simulated tuberculous perichondritis. If, however, a foreign body is discovered by the indirect method, the removal should not be attempted by the indirect method unless the operator be one of those experts who by long practice with indirect operating have developed an unusual degree of skill. If an indirect attempt is made the patient must be recumbent in the author's position, (Fig. 73a). Quite a large proportion of foreign bodies in the lower air passages have been dislodged and lost downward.

Technic of direct laryngoscopic removal of foreign bodies. Differing from foreign bodies elsewhere the first step is not to study out the mechanical problem. Because of the risk of loss downward, it is best to seize the foreign body as soon as seen and to proceed to study how best to disimpact the intruder. If the larynx contain suspicious granulation tissue it is as well to remove it, as removal will cause no more bleeding than sponging, and in the event of no foreign body being found the examination of the tissue may contribute to the diagnosis. The mechanical problems of disimpaction are similar to those in the trachea and bronchi and need not be extensively considered here. Because of the chink-like lumen of the glottis and the frequency with which part of a foreign body gets hooked below the lateral glottic borders, rotation is more frequently required for disimpaction. Rotation will also be required for foreign bodies engaged in one ventricle or transfixed with one end in each ventricle. Rotation is best accomplished with the rotation forceps. (Fig. 210). The problem of the foreign body hooked below the glottis is well illustrated in the schema, Fig. 176. In this case trauma would have resulted from its being brought up through the glottis, so it was rotated so as to bring its greater plane sagitally, permitting easy and harmless withdrawal. Not infrequently a child will come in completely aphonic from a foreign body wedged in the subglottic space and projecting upward between the cords which, in consequence, cannot approximate. Usually such a position of the foreign body results from coughing the intruder up from below. Careful work with the alligator forceps. the patient being recumbent, will usually succeed, especially if no anesthesia is used. The application of a local anesthetic may mechanically dislodge the intruder, and the relaxation of a general anesthetic may release it. In some cases it will be found that a tracheally lodged foreign body can be easily seen through the glottis and can be removed by inserting the alligator forceps during inspiration. This should only be done, however, where there is no great dyspnea, and where the foreign body is small in one diameter and large in the other, allowing plenty of air to pass on each side, and also allowing a ready grip with the forceps inserted so that the jaws will open at right angles to the longest presented diameter. The intruder must be turned so that its longest diameter comes sagitally through the glottis. For this, Mosher's forceps are excellent.

CHAPTER XV.

Mechanical Problems of Bronchoscopic Foreign Body Extraction.

The greatest triumph of bronchoscopy over thoracotomy is in the low mortality of bronchoscopy. Esophagoscopy presents a similar triumph. The problem is not simply to remove the foreign body. A strong forceps and main strength would do that. The problem is the removal without endangering the patient's life. A careful study of the mechanical problems presented will always discover a safe method of removal. In view of this, the temptation to remove the body at all hazards once it is grasped, must be resisted. The endoscopic extraction of a foreign body is a mechanical problem pure and simple. A bad mechanic will either fail to remove the foreign body or will kill the patient or, alas, will do both, as has already happened a number of times, to the undeserved discredit of bronchoscopy and esophagoscopy. Being a mechanical problem it can be best illustrated by reference to every day experience in mechanics. For instance, a cap-screw is broken off flush with the surface of the cylinder of an automobile engine. The repairman who is not a mechanic will pound away with a punch in an effort to turn the screw out. He breaks the entire engine casting by hasty, ill-planned or rather unplanned efforts at removal. The good, careful mechanic will carefully cut a slot in the broken screw. This slot will enable him to use a screw-driver, by means of which he will remove the screw without damage to the engine, in less time than it took the unmechanical repairman to ruin the entire engine. Unfortunately, endoscopic work has been done on the basis that, left *in situ*, the foreign body would probably be fatal; consequently, any violence in removal was justifiable. The basis is indisputable, but the inference is erroneous. In the solution of the mechanical problems involved, as well as in their execution, the utmost pa-

*Lecture given by the author before the New York State Medical Society, Section on Laryngology, New York City, April 30, 1914. Revised and supplemented.

tience is necessary. The hasty, brilliant man may remove the foreign body, but the removal may be fatal to the patient.

As Brünings has well said, "The description of operative technic, which affords such an unlimited scope to the person of skill, ingenuity and talent for mechanical adaptability, encounters quite special difficulties."

Only general rules can be laid down; and the author wishes particularly to warn any one from taking any of the following suggestions as absolute for application to a case which may present itself. Every case must be dealt with upon its own merits, and variations from any rules will naturally suggest themselves to the mechanically inclined. The author can say this, however, that every statement made herein as to mechanical problems, unless otherwise stated, is a note made at the time when the particular plan had resulted in a successful issue. Past experience becomes a guide for future procedures, but it is a guide that must not be followed implicitly without reasoning as to whether or not it is applicable to the particular case in question. It must be remembered, also, that there is more than one way of doing things mechanical, though, as applied to foreign body extractions, it will usually be found that one plan is better than another, because of the personal equation of the operator. For instance, nearly every endoscopist has his own pin closer. The chapter of case reports will contain notes of how the mechanical problems were dealt with.

The lip of the bronchoscope and esophagoscope is one of the most important factors in the solution of the mechanical problems of foreign body extraction. Under the manipulation of the well-trained left hand, co-ordinating with the forceps, hook or snare in the right hand, the endoscopist has a *bimanual*, eye-guided control that can accomplish what seems wonders to anyone whose work has been limited to square-ended tubes and unaided right-handed forceps manipulations. The bimanual control is possible only because of the lip of the slanted tube-mouth. This lip is of the greatest aid in making a space at the side of a foreign body where the intruder impinges on the bronchial wall, for the insertion of the forceps jaw. It forms a shield or protector that can be slipped under the point of a pin or other sharp foreign body and can make counter-pressure on the tissue while the forceps are disembedding the point of the foreign body. In many other ways it can be used to assist once the habit of working with a knowledge of its direction in relation to the handle is mastered by practice. The lip cannot be seen as such in looking through the tube. One of the most important points in foreign body extraction is to introduce the tube until the distal end arrives at the proper distance above the foreign body. What constitutes the proper distance varies in the different cases. So far as merely seeing the object is concerned, the tube need, ordinarily, not be very close to the foreign body. But the mechanical problem of removal is closely concerned with the distance of this rigid tube-mouth, and the tube must be "anchored" in the chosen place by the left third and fourth fingers hooked over the upper alveolus (Fig. 137), while the right thumb and first two fingers make lateral pressure to swing the bronchoscope, if needed, to displace swollen mucosa, open the lip of a bronchial orifice or the like. Never go into any foreign body case hastily or unprepared with the idea of taking a preliminary observation. Often the first sight of a foreign body is the best you will ever get. If not immediately removed it may become more difficult later, through being hidden by mucosal swelling, dropping into a smaller bronchus, passing down the esophagus, etc.

The use of hooks will be mentioned in connection with various mechanical problems. The Lister hook is very useful. Small probe pointed hooks are excellent but a right angle is sufficient for most purposes. Hooks with a curve greater than a right angle are very apt to become engaged in small orifices and to be very difficult in removal.

The use of forceps in endoscopic foreign body extraction. The author uses two different strengths of forceps. The regular forceps is so strong and firm that the full amount of strength of an ordinary man's fingers can be applied without bending or breaking the forceps. These are necessary in foreign bodies which present a hard, smooth conical end towards the operator, the strength of instrument being necessary not for traction but to prevent the forceps slipping off such bodies. These forceps, however, are not so well suited to extremely delicate manipulations because they are larger in size. The more delicate forceps are just one-half the dimensions of the larger ones and they will suffice for ordinary extractions, but they must be used with consideration and care, or they may get bent or broken. Or, indeed, the delicate or friable foreign bodies may get bent or broken. As in all other mechanical problems, and practically all of the problems in foreign body extraction are mechanical, the operator must use judgment and adjust the means to the end. It is absolutely essential, for accurate work, that the forceps be seen to close upon the foreign body. This is one of the chief reasons why the author prefers distal illumination. The illumination of the field is just as good after the forceps are introduced as it was before, and all the operator has to do is to look past the near part of the forceps. The practiced eye will, in every case, see the jaws close under the guidance of the eye, even in the 4 mm. tube, of whose lumen the forceps occupies nearly one-half of the entire diameter. The crevice remaining is sufficient because the illumination is uninterfered with. However reliable the sense of touch, there are many things in foreign body extraction in which the sense of touch alone will not be a sufficiently accurate guide to safety and success. Most important is development of the ability to gauge depth with one eye alone. Those who have never tried it think that this is easy, those who have tried it only once, think it is impossible. Those who have the natural aptitude to begin with and who devote a sufficient length of time to it, can develop this sense to an extent that seems incredible. When one sees a foreign body for which one has been searching there is naturally great eagerness to seize it and remove it. This impulse must be resisted and a careful study of the size, shape and position of the foreign body and its relation to surrounding structures must be clearly determined before any attempt at extraction is made. To seize it and tear it out regardless of the harm that may be done is to court disaster, for however successful it may be in a possibly considerable number of cases, the endoscopist is bound to encounter other cases in which such a procedure will be fatal, and needlessly fatal. In approaching a foreign body with the forceps, to grasp it, careful watch should be kept by the eye to see that the forceps do not touch the foreign body before the jaws are expanded, as this may have the effect of driving the foreign body more deeply. The forceps are inserted through the bronchoscope closed and are allowed to expand when they are within a few millimeters of the intruder. In using forceps, the tube mouth must not be so close to the foreign body as to hinder the expansion of the forceps jaws, unless the intruder be small, such as a pin or a needle, in which case ample expansion can be had within the tube. This is the better way to work in case of pins or needles, because the points can be more or less fixed by the pressure of the tube while the forceps are being placed. The first trial of forceps extraction is always the best opportunity for removal, because of secretions, possibly blood stained, set free as soon as the foreign body is disturbed. Therefore, the proper placing of the forceps on the proper part of the foreign body to insure its extraction, should be planned before the forceps are inserted. As explained under esophagoscopy, the point at which the foreign body is seen makes a great difference with certain foreign bodies which should be allowed to turn in order to present their least diameter to the cross section of the bronchus; and also, in certain cases, to turn where a point or rough place on the foreign body will do no harm. For permitting rotation, it is necessary to use forceps such as the author's "rotation" forceps, Fig. 33, in order that the foreign body may be free to turn. For use with the laryngoscope or esophageal speculum the author's alligator rotation forceps are used. (Fig. 210.)

When the forceps have slipped off a foreign body during attempted extraction, the bronchoscope has usually been slightly withdrawn. At this point extreme caution is necessary. The first thing to remember is never to push the bronchoscope immediately downward again. On the contrary, it should be withdrawn a centimeter or two. Then the secretions and blood, if any, should be carefully sponged away and a good clear view of the tracheal or bronchial lumen obtained. Then, being sure the foreign body is not being overridden, the bronchoscope is slowly advanced and each step of the way is searched until the old location is reached. If the bronchoscopist were hastily to push the bronchoscope down to the place where the foreign body was previously seized, the foreign body might easily be overridden, its point, if any, caused to puncture or to enter a lateral branch, or it might be lost in the secretions requiring prolonged search. Precipitate grabbing with the forceps never accomplishes anything and may do serious and even fatal damage. It is well to see that the thumb nut of the forceps is in place, and to look carefully to the angle of closure of the forceps, to make sure that they grip properly. The proper closure is illustrated in Fig. 31.

Lateral movements of the forceps by the author's method. In making lateral movements of forceps, the tube mouth, either the lip or the short side, is used, as required. The bronchoscope is swung in the required direction as a lever on its fulcrum (Fig. 135) carrying the distal end of the forceps strongly sidewise. This maneuver, devised by the author, has been exceedingly successful, and has led him to wonder at the statements made that lateral movements of forceps are impossible. In combination with the side curved forceps (Fig. 29) some otherwise difficult maneuvers become easy.

Bringing the foreign body through the glottis. Stripping of the foreign body from the forceps at the glottis in cases where tube, foreign body and forceps are withdrawn together, is so frequently reported that it deserves special consideration. This accident is due to one of four causes:

1. The foreign body was not being brought out with its largest diameter in the sagittal plane of the glottic chink.
2. The forceps were not most advantageously applied.
3. The forceps were mechanically imperfect.
4. The foreign body was not kept close up to the tube mouth, thus allowing the glottic tissues to close tightly on the forceps between the tube mouth and the intruder.

The remedies are obvious in each class of case, except in class 2. To make sure of proper grasp accurate closure of the forceps under ocular control is the greatest safeguard. In addition, however, it is well to test the firmness of grasp of the forceps against the end of the tube before starting to withdraw forceps, tube and foreign body all together, because if the grasp is insufficient, it is better to know it before withdrawal is attempted than to have the intruder become wedged in the glottis, or to lose it back in the trachea. In the case of small objects, if scraped off by the glottis, they may drop back into a new location where removal and finding may be still more difficult. For these reasons, it is best to assure one's self that the grasp is firm before the foreign body is removed from the locality in which it is found. As a rule, it is unsafe to attempt to test the grip of very soft friable bodies by withdrawing them against the end of the tube, except with the utmost gentleness, because of the likelihood of crushing. When a foreign body is stripped off the forceps on withdrawal it may become jammed in the glottis in such a way as to occlude breathing completely. It is therefore wise to have always at hand the alligator jawed forceps which can be used promptly through the direct laryngoscope. In the event of the foreign body not being of such shape as to occlude the glottis this method of removal will be the most convenient anyway and as pointed out by D. R. Paterson, the circumstance may be even fortunate in preventing the loss of the foreign body downward. Nevertheless, it will require prompt action in some cases to avert disaster. The accident of stripping off the foreign body at the glottis often makes the situation much more complicated by the large quantity of pus and secretions that are liberated by the loosening of the foreign body, which had been occluding the bronchus. In such case, a careful removal of the secretion by "sponge pumping" as mentioned under "Aspirators" is necessary. Then careful search is resumed. Usually the foreign body will be found not to have gone so deeply. If large, it may stop at the bifurcation, even though it had previously been much lower. Most foreign bodies require time to work their way downward. Care must be used not to override the intruder as explained in connection with "Use of the forceps." The accident of dropping from the grasp of the forceps during process of bronchoscopic removal seems from the literature to have been quite a frequent accident and in some instances it has proven fatal. Often the foreign body will be found to have dropped into the opposite bronchus from that in which it was first lodged, the reason being probably, that the negative pressure is very much less in the bronchus of the first invaded lung because secretions have accumulated and in cases of long standing there may be obliteration of a large amount of lung tissue, whereas the negative pressure is increased by the compensatory activity of the sound side. To prevent this dropping into the main bronchus of the opposite side, Brünings has suggested the use of a "bronchus protector" which is like a bottle brush. It is inserted into the sound bronchus before attempting the removal of the foreign body from the invaded bronchus. Its brush-like form permits of respiration but will prevent the entrance of a foreign body of any appreciable size. Hinsberg reports an interesting case in which a plum stone in process of removal from the right bronchus slipped from the forceps and dropped into the left bronchus from which he could not remove it. The patient died within a few hours. It was found at autopsy that the right lung was atrophied, the patient having existed almost solely on the left lung, the use of which was suddenly lost when it was occluded by the falling backward of the foreign body. Ingals (Bib. 225) reports two cases in which the foreign body in process of bronchoscopic removal slipped from the forceps and prolonged search in the trachea and bronchi failed to find it. The search was given up and the bronchoscope withdrawn. In one of the cases after withdrawal the foreign body was found in the patient's mouth and in the other case it fell out on the floor. This points a very valuable lesson that should always be borne in mind. After a foreign body has slipped from the forceps seemingly at the glottis, on withdrawal of the bronchoscope, forceps and foreign body all together, it must be remembered that there is a possibility that it really came through the glottis and may be in the pharynx or perhaps swallowed. This, however, must not prevent us from prompt reinsertion of the bronchoscope especially with foreign bodies which may cause dyspnea, but if a preliminary search fails to find the foreign body in the trachea or bronchi very careful search of the pharynx should be made with the finger and if the bronchoscopy has already lasted a considerable time it is better to desist and have another radiograph taken because the foreign body may have been swallowed.

Extraction of pins, needles and similar long pointed objects. In case of such bodies as pins, tacks, nails and the like, whose points are presenting and thus the mechanical problem clearly apparent, we may proceed at once to raise the point with the lip of the bronchoscope so as to get the point into the lumen. It is usually better that the forceps be not used to seize the point until the point is in the lumen, as otherwise the intruder will almost certainly get crosswise of the tube mouth. For the same reason a pin, needle or similar object must be first studied from a distance lest the tube mouth override the proximal end of the pin. In other words the nearest end must be searched for first, and the rule should be to look, not for a pin, but for the *point* of a pin. One pull with the forceps on the middle portion of a pin has caused the point to perforate, enormously increasing the difficulties of removal and in some instances resulting fatally. (Fig. 177.) Even if grasped near the point, if the grasp is exactly "on end" there is a strong tendency for the point of a pin to hook over the outside of the tube mouth. In such a case, as soon as the forceps grasp the pin, the pin should be pushed downward, if necessary to free its point, or if this is unnecessary, the tube can be slightly withdrawn so that the point will not become hooked over the edge of the tube in withdrawal. To still further prevent this hooking over the edge, it is often necessary to move the lip of the tube mouth rather strongly in the direction of the point. The author usually prefers the pushing downward of the pin with the forceps to disengage it, when safely possible; but it may be disengaged by putting a hook below the place where the point disappears into the mucosa and by withdrawal upward the point can be forced out. (Fig. 178.) This, of course, is not

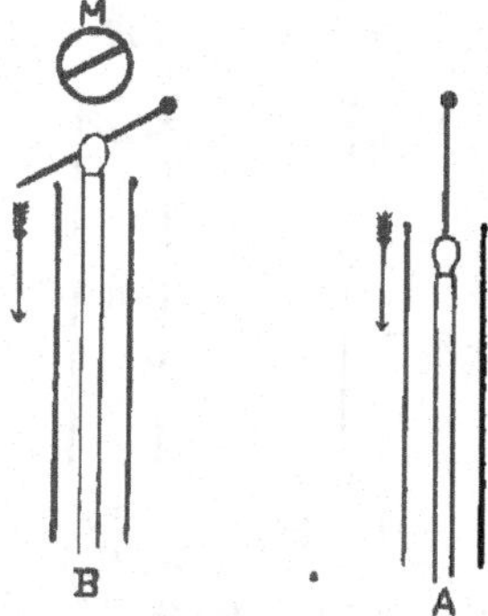

FIG. 177. Schema illustrating one phase of the error of grasping a long foreign body in the middle, upon first seeing it across the tube mouth as at M. It gets crosswise of the tube mouth, like a "toggle and ring," and the point cannot be drawn into tube mouth for protection.

permissible if the point is deeply embedded. For the grasping and withdrawal of pins the side-curved forceps (Fig. 29) are admirably adapted. The side curve enabling a grasp sidewise when the pin is lying in contact with one bronchial wall as it usually is. They can also be used closed as a hook. Pins, especially the glass-headed steel pins in common use, are very prone to drop down into the smaller bronchi and to disappear completely from the ordinary field of endoscopic exploration. Pins with slightly larger heads not dropping so deeply, and yet going into the branches of the stem bronchus, are very prone to appear and disappear during endoscopy, in a way that makes them, at times, quite difficult to find and remove. Cough will throw the point into view, but the point will immediately recede before it can be grasped by the forceps. This ap-

...chi. the up and ... greatest degree ... the insertion of ... pressure with the ... ugh. The axis of ... are inserted in such ... grasping. In one ... the ribs raised

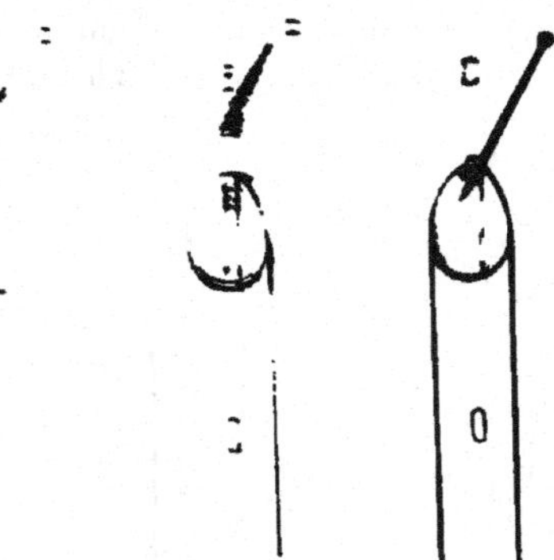

...em of the pin, needle (P), tack or ... the forceps, H, is pulled up- ... und, and the point, M, of the ... the difficulties of removal or ... the forceps, H, they are *pushed* ...aged, and the lip of the broncho- ... if the pin is prevented by its ... extracted by traction with a ... may be used instead of the ...traction is then done with the

...gh to cause the point of a ... In two cases the rise of ...pulsion forced the lung up- ... to cause the pin point to ...maintained with the broncho- ...duced and the next emer- ...stantly seized and the pin ...cases. In one instance, the ...n became transfixed across the lumen of the bronchoscope through the breathing apertures and into the opposite wall, requiring breaking of the pin by pushing on the forceps. The relative position of the apertures has since been changed to prevent such a possibility. Ingals has devised a very ingenious corkscrew-like instrument which will bring a pin into the corner of the lumen in cases where a point is deeply buried.

In the bronchi, it may not be possible to push the foreign body sufficiently far down to disengage the point. Under such circumstances, if the point cannot be liberated by the methods already mentioned, the pin must be cut or broken. Casselberry has devised a very ingenious forceps

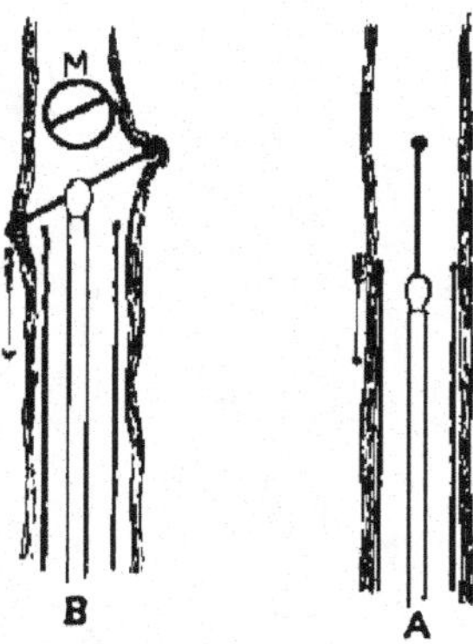

FIG. 179. Schema illustrating a serious phase of the error of hastily seizing a transfixed pin near its middle, when first seen as at M. Traction with the forceps in the direction of the dart in schema B will rip open the esophagus or bronchus inflicting fatal trauma, and probably the pin will be stripped off at the glottic or the cricopharyngeal level, respectively. The point of the pin must be disembedded and gotten into the tube mouth as at A, to make forceps traction safe.

for the purpose of cutting pins, and at the same time retaining the point. Before using, these forceps should be tested upon a pin to make sure that, after cutting the point can be held in the forceps and not get lost. In use the forceps must be held closed after closing in order not to drop the pin in three pieces. Yankauer has devised a method of dealing with the crosswise fixed pin by pulling it into the tube of a combination tube and hook forceps, which seems a promising though as yet untested method. It is intended for untempered pins which will bend without breaking. He has successfully used an instrument shaped like a tack-drawer for extracting the embedded point of a tack; and this should be equally useful for an embedded pin point.

angle projecting at the branch bronchus. This is especially true of bodies like the upholsterer's tack, of which every bronchoscopist of experience has had one or more cases. These tacks hold like a "mushroom anchor," and great care must be taken that traction is being made in the proper direction. The direction of traction can be modified by the position in which the forceps are placed, as previously described; and it can also be modified by the movement of the head of the patient and the bronchoscope in the proper direction. The lip of the bronchoscope can also be used for the moving out of the way of the obstructing tissues, as elsewhere described, and as illustrated in Fig. 172. The shortness of a tack may permit it to turn more or less sideways in the bronchus, the point entering

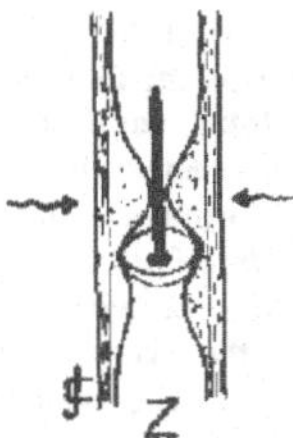

FIG. 179b. "Mushroom anchor" problem of the upholstery tack. If the tack has not been *in situ* more than a few weeks the stenosis at the level of the darts is simply edematous mucosa and the tack can be pulled through with no more than slight mucosal trauma, *provided* axis-traction only be used. If the tack has been *in situ* a year or more the fibrous stricture may need dilatation with the divulsor (Fig. 46). Otherwise traction may rupture the bronchial wall. The stenotic tissue in cases of a few months' sojourn may be composed of granulations, in which case axis-traction will safely withdraw it.

the mucosa or a lateral branch. This permits the head in some instances to present its edge toward the observer. Great caution is required in such instances. If the head is seized as at A, Fig. 180, serious trauma may result in withdrawal, by the ripping effect of the point, and the chances of its getting dragged out of the grip of the forceps are great. If it is grasped by the stem we have the "toggle and ring" action against the tube mouth (Fig. 177), and unless the tack is very short the point will cause trauma. The best method in the author's experience with such cases is to push the presenting edge of the head downward and laterally so as to bring up the point as far as possible. Then a hook (or the closed side curved forceps) is inserted under the shank as close to the point as possible and thus the point can be brought up in the clear so that it can be seized with the forceps and withdrawn into the tube mouth. If the head is too large to enter, the point is thus protected while forceps and bronchoscope are withdrawn together.

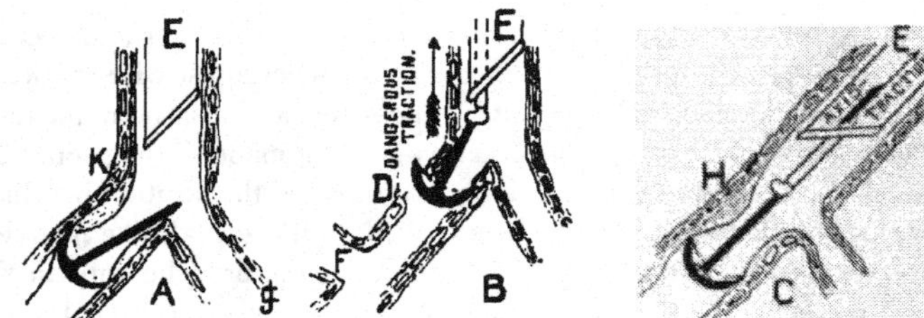

Fig. 179c. Schema illustrating the "mushroom anchor" problem of the brass-headed upholstery tack. At A the tack is shown with the head bedded in swollen mucosa. The bronchoscopist, looking through the bronchoscope, E, considering himself lucky to have found the *point* of the tack, seizes it and starts to withdraw it, making traction as shown by the dart in drawing B. The head of the tack catches below a chondrial ring and rips in, tearing its way through the bronchial wall (D) causing death by mediastinal emphysema. This accident is still more likely to occur if, as often happens, the tack-head is lodged in the orifice of the upper lobe bronchus, F. But if the bronchoscopist swings the patient's head far to the opposite side and makes *axis-traction*, as shown at C, the head of the tack can be drawn through the swollen mucosa without anchoring itself in a cartilage. If necessary, in addition, the lip of the bronchoscope can be used to repress the angle, K, and the swollen mucosa, H. If the swollen mucosa, H, has been replaced by fibrous tissue from many months' sojourn of the tack, the stenosis may require dilatation with the divulsor, Fig. 46.

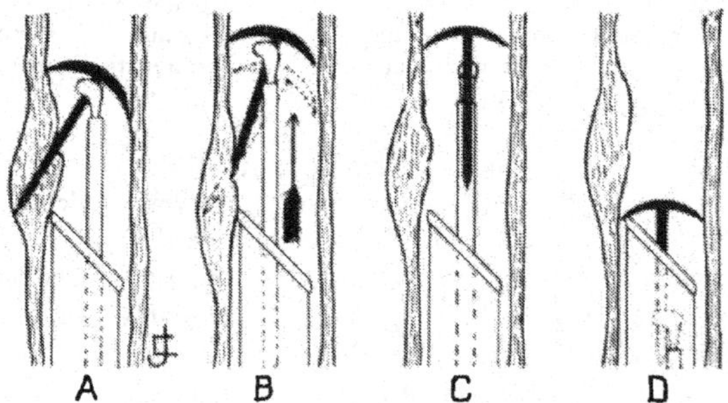

Fig. 179d. Problem of the upholstery tack with buried point. If pulled upon, the imminent perforation of the mediastinum, as shown at A, will be completed, the bronchus will be torn and death will follow even if the tack be removed, which is of doubtful possibility. The proper method is gently to close the side curved forceps on the shank of the tack near the head, push downward as shown by the dart, in B, until the point emerges. Then the forceps are *rotated* to bring the point of the tack away from the bronchial wall. It is usually better at this stage to release the tack and grasp it firmly near the point for withdrawal, D. During stages A, B and C the tack is grasped very gently.

In making the lateral movements referred to, the tube mouth is used to push the forceps sidewise, the bronchoscopic lever being swung on its fulcrum (Fig. 135). Articles of jewelry, such as stick pins, usually require the same care that pertains to pins, in regard to getting the point safely into the tube mouth. In withdrawal the head is apt to catch as mentioned in regard to tacks, and the direction of traction must be modified accordingly. Nails of any except the smallest sizes are easily found and usually present the same problems of extraction as mentioned

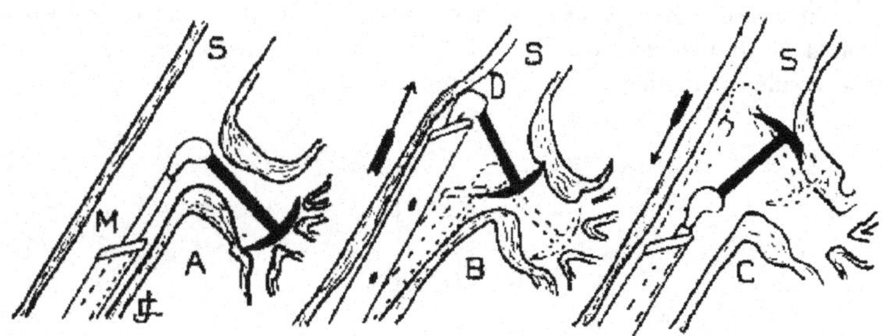

Fig. 179e. Schema illustrating the "upper-lobe-bronchus problem," combined with the "mushroom-anchor" problem and the author's twice-successful method for their solution. The patient being recumbent, the bronchoscopist looking down the right main bronchus, M, sees the point of the tack projecting from the right upper-lobe-bronchus, A. He seizes the point with the side-curved forceps; then slides down the bronchoscope to the position shown dotted at B. Next he pushes the bronchoscopic tube-mouth downward and medianward, simultaneously moving the patient's head to the right, thus swinging the bronchoscopic lever (Fig. 135) on its fulcrum, and dragging the tack downward and inward out of its bed, to the position, D. Traction, as shown at C, will then safely and easily withdraw the tack A very small bronchoscope is essential. The *lip* of the bronchoscopic tube-mouth must be used to pry the forceps down and over, and the lip must be brought close to the tack just before the prying-pushing movement. S, right stem-bronchus.

for pins. Their points are usually not sharp but their shape renders it necessary to get the point into the tube mouth to prevent "toggle and ring" action. The side curved forceps (Fig. 29) usually get a better hold than straight jaws, and they can be used to better advantage in lateral movements and in grasping pins, nails and tacks. Nails lodged head uppermost may present the problem of annular edema (Fig. 182).

Jervey (Bib. 274), by a very ingenious method, extracted a very large nail by carefully disengaging the point and getting the nail into the bronchoscope for half the nail's length and then pressing the nail tightly to the wall of the tube by means of a hook firmly rotated.

Hollow metallic bodies. For foreign bodies presenting an opening toward the observer, no instrument has proven more efficient than the excellent one of Killian (Bib. 269, p. 26). Different endoscopists will prefer different handles, but the grooved expansile holder shown, fitted to a suitable handle, cannot be excelled for firmly grasping and holding such foreign bodies. An additional merit is that most of such bodies, when so held, are in the best position for removal, whereas if grasped by their edge there is more or less traumatism apt to be inflicted by other portions of their edge, if thin. If a large cylindrical hollow metallic body does not present its opening toward the operator, it may present the problem of annular edema, Fig. 182. It may be turned if not too long, but as a rule the method, Fig. 182, is preferable.

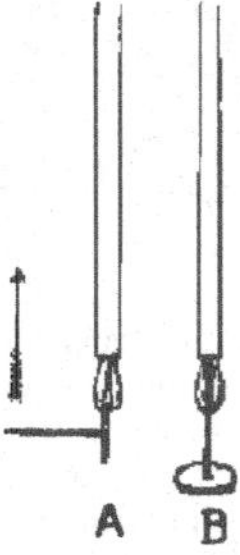

FIG. 180. Schema of the mechanical problem of tack extraction from the bronchi. If the edge of the head presents, the point being in a branch bronchus or imbedded in the wall, traction upon the head in the direction of the dart will produce trauma and will probably be unsuccessful. After turning, the point is seized as at B, and traction is safe and successful.

Removal of open safety pins from the trachea and bronchi. The removal of a closed safety pin presents only the ordinary mechanical problem of the long foreign body that must be grasped on end to prevent the "toggle and ring" difficulty. When the safety pin is open, but with point down the problem is quite easy of solution. The near or spring end of the pin is grasped and pulled into the bronchoscope which closes the pin. If the pin cannot be withdrawn completely into the tube it must at least be drawn in until the "keeper" end of the pin is close up against the tube mouth, not only to prevent the loss of the pin at the glottis, but to prevent trauma by the usually sharp and hook-like "keeper." When we have to deal with an open safety pin lodged point up we have a difficult problem, the proper execution of which is one of the most interesting in bronchoscopy. If the pin is grasped and pulled out without closing the pin, the point will inflict severe and probably fatal trauma. If the pin is in the cervical trachea the patient will be subjected to less risk in a removal by tracheotomy than by a ruthless endoscopic extraction. If an experienced and careful bronchoscopist is available, tracheotomy is a great injustice to the patient. If the intruder is in the thoracic trachea, tracheotomy is absolutely contraindicated, and, moreover, quite unnecessary. The pin must be closed and removed or the point must be protected by the lip of the bronchoscope, as shown at C in Fig. 178 in dealing with the point of straight pins. Then the point of the safety pin is grasped with the side curved forceps, Fig. 29, and pulled into the bronchoscope. This leaves the "keeper" end out, but as the hook-like end is down no trauma will be inflicted in withdrawal. But the pin will almost certainly be lost at the glottis if care is not taken to be sure that the greater plane of the keeper corresponds to the sagittal plane of the glottis. If the safety pin is a small one it may be entirely pulled into the bronchoscope by the forceps applied to the point. Large pins are too stiff for this and rupture of the bronchus might result from the attempt. Closure of an open safety pin lodged point upward is not a difficult procedure for those who will preliminarily practice it. The author's method is shown schematically in Fig. 181. The most essential precaution is to select from the set of three a closer that has a ring of the proper size for the particular pin in question. The ring should be large enough to admit the spring end of the pin, but should be no larger than necessary. This is best determined by trial with a similar pin, if one is brought by the patient, or by trial with a pin of similar size and shape as determined with the aid of a radiograph. Due allowance must be made for radiographic magnification, if any. The ring of the author's pin closer is oval which is of fundamental importance. Many clumsy imperfect models are sold under the author's name. In case of an infant too small to admit a bronchoscope large enough to admit the closer through the lumen, the closer may be passed into the trachea first and allowed to lie on the posterior tracheal wall and interarytenoid space while the bronchoscope is passed through the glottis anterior to the stem of the closer. The fork is removed after the pin is closed and the removal is accomplished with forceps. Should the endoscopist, from insufficient practice or constructive imperfection of the particular instrument at hand, be unable to close the pin completely, he can at least bring the point away from the wall and then the point can be guarded by pushing the bronchoscope down over it. The point can then be seized with forceps if necessary, though it will usually be found that the pin is tightly held by keeping the bronchoscope and pin closer in exact relation to each other after the fork is re-

[illegible]

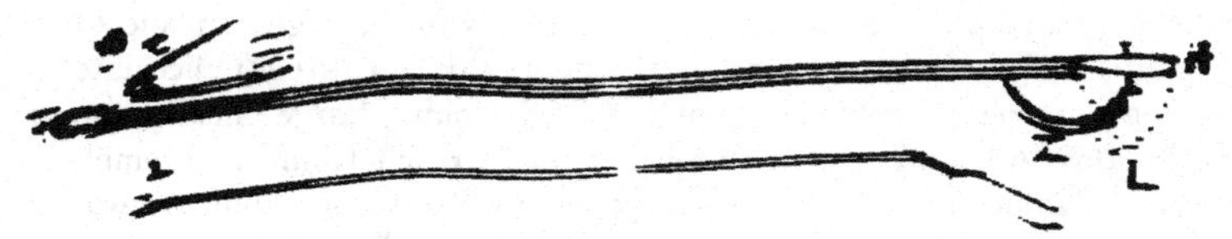

[illegible] until the [illegible] slotted [illegible] there with the [illegible] spring loop. [illegible] of the pin [illegible] the center.

[illegible] the esophagus, in which [illegible]

[illegible] in the trachea.

[illegible] though they must be [illegible] If lodged point up [illegible] manner. The slightest pull [illegible] sinking the points into the wall. The author [illegible] hook to deal with, but he has worked out a number of methods which will be mentioned in connection with esophageal foreign body problems. The author's experience with the double pointed tack and staple has led him to favor turning this kind of intruder end for end by means of the rotation forceps, Fig. 33, or the full curved hook shown at C in Fig. 158, applied to the far (curved) end of the tack or staple. This is only feasible with a relatively short intruder or a large [illegible] With a long staple in the infant trachea the best method is to "coax" the intruder along gently under ocular guidance, never making traction enough to bury the point deeply, and lifting the point with the hook whenever it shows any inclination to enter the wall. This is not difficult to do in the trachea, but extreme dexterity is needed thus to get the intruder through the glottis. Should the endoscopist fail in this, or have doubts as to his ability to accomplish it, he is justified in doing a tracheotomy for removal *after*, not before, he has brought the intruder up to the subglottic region. The child must be kept in the Trendelenberg position in order to prevent the intruder dropping again into the thoracic trachea and a bronchoscope must be left in the glottis during the tracheotomy to forestall spasmodic stenosis. Under no circumstances should the intruder be violently pulled through the glottis point first. Mortality will almost certainly follow. Tracheotomy for the insertion of a bronchoscope for the removal of inverted double pointed tacks from the thoracic trachea or from the bronchi is a mistake. Better work can be done through the mouth up to the point of getting the tack into the subglottic region. In certain locations turning is facilitated by diverting the points into branch bronchi as in the case illustrated by Figs. 181a, 181b and 181c.

The extraction of tightly fitting foreign bodies from the bronchi. Annular edema. Bodies such as corks, pebbles, marbles, Job's tears, beads and the like are propelled into the lower air passages with considerable force by the inspiratory blast, especially by the deep inspiration following cough. This impaction prevents further ingress of air, and the absorption of air below adds a negative pressure which increases the impaction and the tightness of the fit aids in quickly producing an annular mucosal swelling (A, Fig. 182) which covers the presenting part of the intruder so that all that is seen is a small surface in the center of an acute edematous stenosis. If application of the forceps (F, Fig. 182) is attempted they will not expand sufficiently to take in the intruder because of the annular edema A. The author in such cases uses a forceps (K) having very stiff expansive spring jaws so that when protruded from the forceps cannula they will expand with sufficient force to press out of the way (in the plane of their own expansion only, not annularly), the swollen mucosa so as to permit of seizure of the foreign body, as shown at B. The jaws of these forceps are narrow, because it is easier to press outward a narrow portion of the swollen mucosa than a wide one. Of course the jaws must not be so narrow as to cut, and in using the forceps it is necessary to use great care to prevent damage. All use of such instruments must be under the guidance of the eye. Another very effectual way (Fig. 183) is to repress the swollen mucosa at one point with the lip of the bronchoscope so that a hook may be passed

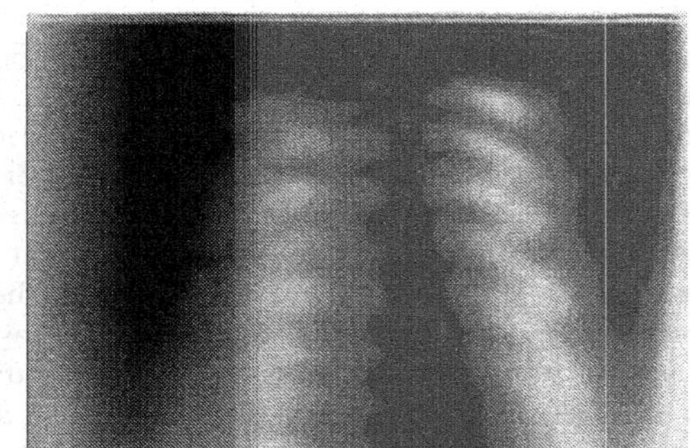

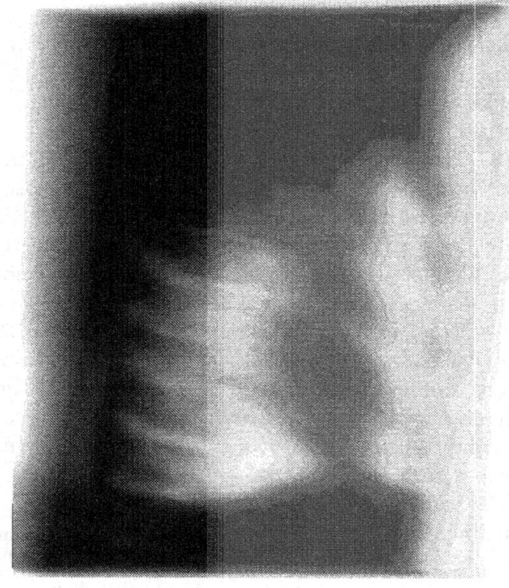

below the intruder which is drawn upward to a wider place where the forceps can be applied, or in some instances it can be imprisoned against the tube mouth. One of the most difficult mechanical problems is where a foreign body that completely occludes a bronchus into which it is tightly drawn by the absorption of air below, and that in addition has a conoidal

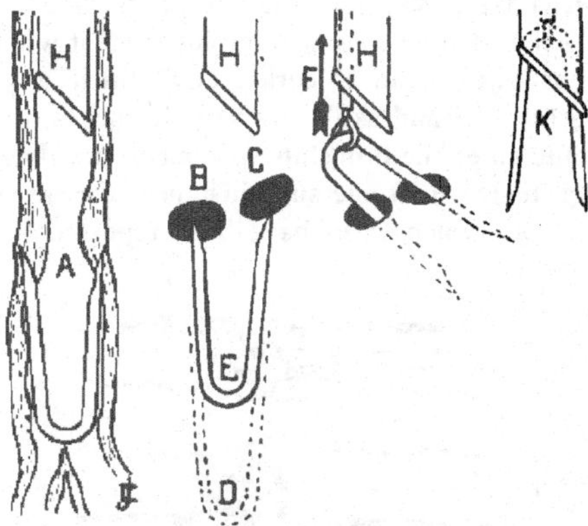

FIG. 181b. Schema illustrating a new method of removal of bronchially-lodged staples or double-pointed tacks. H, bronchoscope. A, swollen mucosa covering points of staple. At E the staple has been manipulated upward with bronchoscopic lip and hooks until the points are opposite the branch bronchial orifices, B, C. Traction being made in the direction of the dart (F), by means of the rotation forceps, and counterpressure being made with the bronchoscopic lip on the points of the staple, the points enter the branch bronchi and permit the staple to be turned over and removed with points trailing harmlessly behind (K).

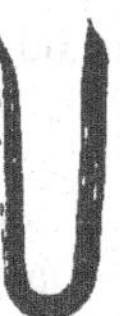

FIG. 181c. Staple (actual size) removed from the right lung (see Fig. 181a), bloodlessly through the mouth, by bronchoscopy, after version as shown in Fig. 181b.

form toward the operator. The problem is difficult, especially if the intruder is hard and smooth because the forceps cannot get a large surface of contact and hence slip. Patience, however, will succeed. Eventually a sufficiently tight hold will be maintained to withdraw the foreign body, notwithstanding the negative pressure which has pulled it down and which is still resisting its withdrawal. The author's heavier forceps are used for this because tactile sensibility is not so essential as in friable bodies. Strong forceps are needed, not for traction but for firm holding on a hard smooth surface of a presenting cone. An illustrative case of the author is the lump of coal removed from the bronchus of a Marathon racer (see Chapter XXI). In the case of a rubber pencil eraser Richardson (Bib. 448) used a screw-pointed instrument which he screwed into the rubber as one would a corkscrew. Such a procedure, of course, requires great care and skill. In some instances, the largest possible tube that would enter the bronchus without injury, has been used to liberate the foreign body. In some such instances the intruder has been coughed into the tube. Such cases have been reported by Tilley (Bib.

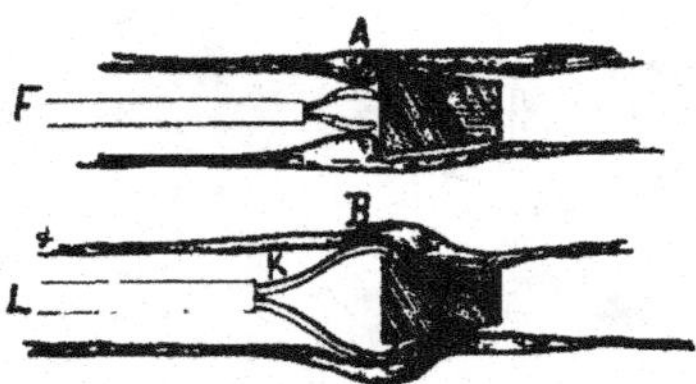

Fig. 182. Schema illustrating the problem of a tightly impacted foreign body (C), above which an annular edema (A) prevents sufficient expansion of the forceps, F. Pushing on the forceps may force the foreign body into the mediastinum or pleura. A special forceps (L) with very narrow and stiff-springed expansile jaws (K) is used to displace the edematous mucosa (in the plane of their expansion only) as at B, so that they can be pushed down over the foreign body sufficiently for a good grip on the foreign body (D).

546), Geo. L. Richards, Beck and others. As pointed out by Ingals (Bib. 226) oversized tubes must be used with caution, and this may be said of every endoscopic procedure. A very interesting and quite unique case of the aid of gravity in bronchoscopic foreign body extraction is that of Goldstein (Bib. 185) in which by placing the child in the Trendelenberg position a marble after disimpaction was skillfully dragged down hill with a bent bronchoscopic probe.

Extraction of soft friable bodies from the tracheo-bronchial tree. Bodies that are soft, either by nature or from maceration in the secretions of the tracheobronchial tree, besides the difficulty of disimpaction present the difficulty of removal without crushing and permitting the fragments to scatter. The essentials for successfully dealing with this problem are extremely delicate forceps unopposed by springs and a well developed sense of touch on the part of the operator. As elsewhere mentioned, heavy spring opposed forceps prevent all delicacy of touch and manipulation. The form of jaws used in Killian's "bean" forceps Fig. 32 is very useful in the removal of friable bodies and the author uses jaws modeled after these adapted to his forceps. In the removal of friable foreign bodies, if they are by accident broken up by too firm a grasp of the forceps, the question will arise how long the search should be continued for every minute fragment. As a rule, fragments smaller than 2 mm. in diameter have a very good chance of being coughed up with the secretions which surround them. In some instances, however, foreign bodies of this size and smaller will cause multiple abscesses, so that, as a rule, the bronchoscopist should persist in his search until he

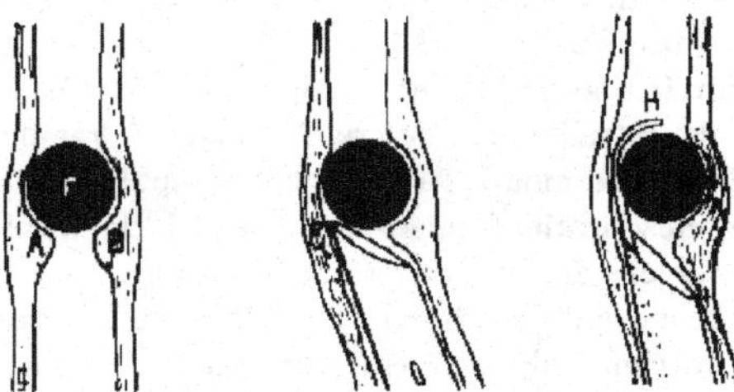

FIG. 183. Schema illustrating the use of the lip of the bronchoscope in disimpaction of foreign bodies. A and B show an annular edema above the foreign body, F. At C the edematous mucosa is being repressed by the lip of the tube-mouth, permitting insinuation of the hook, H, past one side of the foreign body, which is then withdrawn to a convenient place for application of the forceps. This repression by the lip is often used for purposes other than the insertion of hooks. The lip of the esophagoscope can be used in the same way.

has removed every fragment that he can find. Doubtless quite a large quantity of small particles of friable foreign bodies, such as peanuts, will be removed along with secretion by the author's "sponge pumping" method elsewhere described for the removal of secretions without an aspirator. The sponges and secretions should be saved and washed to find the particles after bronchoscopy. Neither the occasional success of this nor the chance of a foreign body being coughed up should, however, make one feel warranted in deliberately breaking a friable foreign body, which cannot be considered as otherwise than a disaster. Claw forceps are particularly undesirable and beans should always be seized with the plain foreign body forceps or "bean forceps" of delicate construction. By delicate pressure with these, crushing can be avoided, whereas with claw forceps the perforation of the claws is almost certain to cause the breaking up of the intruder. In dealing with soft friable bodies of round shape of which the swollen mucosa overlaps the presenting end the stiff-springed forceps above described cannot be used with sufficient delicacy and the points would comminute the intruder. The tube mouth must be placed in gentle contact with the foreign body and then moved laterally so that the lip of the bronchoscope will draw aside a little crevice between the intruder and the bronchial wall, in order that a hook may be inserted at one side of the foreign body, which is, by means of the hook, withdrawn to a wider place in the bronchial lumen where the delicate forceps jaws (Fig. 183) can be, when fully expanded, closed over the foreign body. The mechanical spoon (Fig. 40) is substituted for a hook, if the intruder is in the main bronchus of an adult. Unless the swelling of the bronchial mucosa, and also of the bean or similar absorbent foreign body is very great, the author has usually found it possible to use forceps in the extraction of the foreign body; but the manipulation must be extremely delicate, otherwise the intruder will be crushed and its fragments scattered. The distance of the tube mouth during such manipulations is necessarily, at the beginning, close to the foreign body. When the mechanical spoon, the hook or the forceps are properly placed, the tube must be withdrawn ahead of the foreign body as the latter is brought upward, unless it is desired that the foreign body shall enter the tube. Holding of large soft intruders tightly against the tube mouth cannot be done in case of very friable foreign bodies without risk of crushing them. It is feasible in the less friable bodies. Herbert Tilley reports (Bib. 546) the bronchoscopic removal of a green pea from the right bronchus of a man aged 63 under local anesthesia, by a very ingenious method. The bronchoscope was passed down to the pea against which it was firmly pressed. A closely fitting plug of cotton wool soaked in liquid paraffin (petrolatum) was passed down the bronchoscope until it reached the foreign body. Then by a sudden but sharp movement of withdrawal of the piston-plug the pea was sucked into the lower end of the bronchoscope and removed together with the tube. Winslow (Bib. 575) reports the recovery of a desperate case after the bronchoscopic removal of the pulp of an almond from the left bronchus of a child two years of age. Friable bodies such as egg shells and thin glass, of each of which the author has had cases, require an extremely delicate touch, for which the extremely delicate forceps are necessary.

Removal of small animal objects from the tracheo-bronchial tree. The author has never had occasion to remove an insect. Flies and small beetles are occasionally inhaled; but are usually promptly coughed out. Leeches seem to be of not rare endoscopic occurrence in Europe. Sargnon, Guisez and others have reported cases. Masterman, quoted by Sir St. Clair Thomson (Bib. 539) states that a ten or twenty per cent solution of cocaine will cause a leech to loosen its hold from paralysis. Doubtless ascarides and other living parasites would be equally susceptible. In grasping any form of animal tissue the plain foreign body forceps (Fig. 28) or the side curved forceps (Fig. 29) are best. The broad surface will hold without comminuting the intruder.

Extraction of foreign bodies from the upper-lobe bronchus presents interesting problems because of the impossibility of obtaining a lumen presentation. Fortunately, it is exceedingly rare for foreign bodies to disappear wholly into the upper-lobe bronchus. Of the author's six cases all but one had been pushed there by previous operators. If a portion of the foreign body projects the intruder can be removed by the method shown in Fig. 179e. A foreign body that has disappeared completely within the upper-lobe bronchus can be removed by the author's upper-lobe-

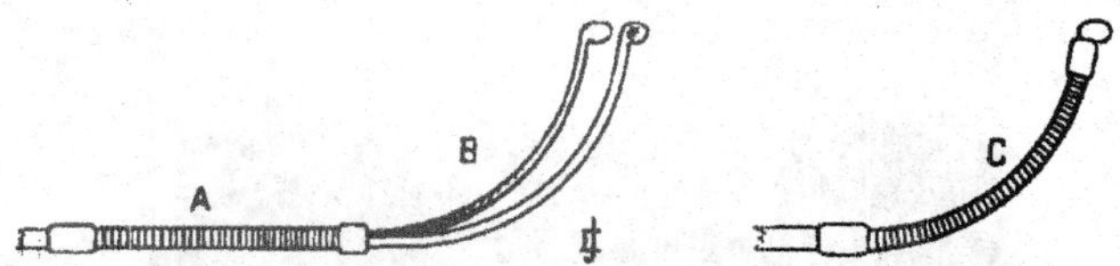

FIG. 183a. The author's upper-lobe bronchus forceps for reaching "around the corner" in the bronchoscopic extraction of foreign bodies. The jaws, B, can be straightened out in passing them through the bronchoscope but will spring back into their original shape on emerging at the distal bronchoscopic tube mouth. The end of the forceps cannula, A, is a spiral tube so as to pass over the curved jaws as shown at C.

bronchus forceps (Figs. 183a, 183b, 183c) guided by the collaboration with a fluoroscopist looking through the double-plane fluoroscope devised for the author by Dr. George W. Grier.

RULES FOR ENDOSCOPIC FOREIGN BODY EXTRACTION.

1. Never endoscope a foreign body case unprepared, with the idea of taking a preliminary look.

2. Approach carefully the suspected location of a foreign body, so as not to override any portion of it.

3. Avoid grasping a foreign body hastily as soon as seen.

4. The shape, size and position of a foreign body and its relations to surrounding structures should be studied before attempting to apply the forceps. (Exception cited in Rule 10.)

5. Preliminary study of a foreign body should be from a distance.

6. The first grasp of the forceps being the best, it should be well planned beforehand so as to seize the proper part of the intruder.

7. With all long foreign bodies the motto should be "Search, not for the foreign body, but for its nearer end." With pins, needles and

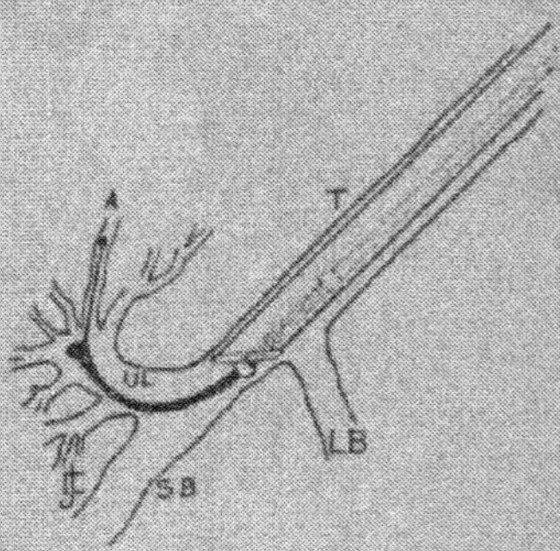

FIG. 183b. Schematic illustration of the author's upper-lobe-bronchus forceps in position grasping a pin in an anteriorly ascending branch of the upper-lobe bronchus. T, trachea; UL, upper-lobe bronchus; LB, left bronchus; SB, stem bronchus.

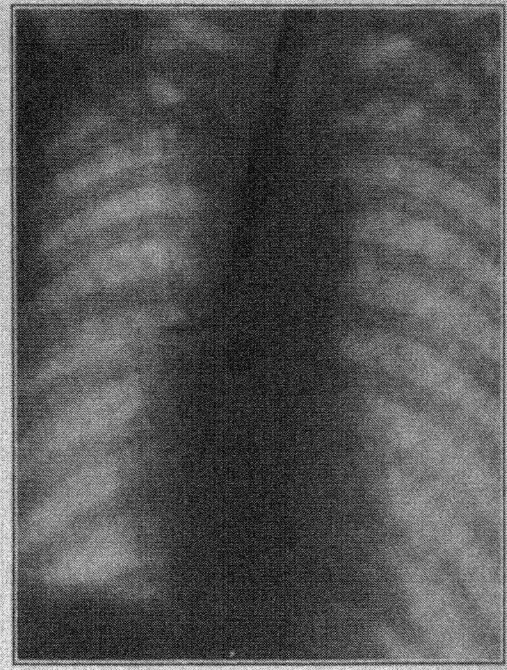

FIG. 183c. Upper-lobe-bronchus forceps in position in the living patient. Radiograph originally made for localization, but incidentally showing curve resumed on forceps after emerging from the bronchoscope.

search always for the point. Try to see it

foreign body grasped near the middle
a "toggle and ring."

mortality to follow failure to remove a for-
probably fatal violence in removal.

foreign bodies, because of the likelihood
may be seized by any part first presented, and
mined afterward.

laryngeal cases should be dealt with only
(Fig. 73a).

may be needed in a bronchoscopic case, or
esophageal case. Both kinds of tubes should be
case before starting. It is the unexpected that
endoscopy.

on a foreign body unless it is properly grasped to
without trauma. Then do not pull hard.

if you cannot remove the foreign body.

choscopy. In cases of foreign bodies which can-
oscopically, and yet which show clearly in the ray.
be passed to the suspected region and a probe may
bronchus too small for the bronchoscope to enter. If
density as to show in the fluoroscopic screen, the
a prompt answer as to the localization, and this
valuable if both a horizontal and a vertical screen can
combination of screens would be valuable for fluoro-
guiding of forceps for the removal of foreign bodies
small peripheral bronchi that the intruder could not be
cally. Personally, however, the author questions the ad-
losing forceps by any other means than by the endoscopic
the eye. It happens only rarely that the foreign body is
fluoroscopic screen. When not visible fluoroscopically, a
should be taken with the probe in situ. Having limited by
previously mentioned, the number of bronchi to be searched,
pist can usually memorize two or three bronchi for separate
find by remembering the place it is possible to tell which one
nchi is invaded. The best probe for this purpose, in the au-
perience, is the very small forceps which are only half the size
gular forceps. They are used closed which gives a very safe

George W. Grier has devised for the author a double-plane fluoroscope
to be very useful in cases of foreign bodies that are in such minute
that they cannot be found, and in cases of upper-lobe bronchus invasion
intruder is dense to the ray. General anesthesia should not be used
he inflammability of ether and because the patient should hold his
mmand.

probe pointed instrument, and if the intruder is found it can at once be seized. If not found the forceps will show in a radiograph. The author has had two cases in which extraction of bronchially lodged foreign bodies was previously tried by other endoscopists. Both were foreign bodies of moderate size lodged in the right stem bronchus and not difficult of removal. In one case fluoroscopic bronchoscopy had been unsuccessfully tried for over an hour under ether anesthesia. In the other case two unsuccessful attempts under ether had been made, one of an hour and the other of an hour and a half. It only required a few minutes in the author's clinic in each instance to remove the foreign bodies without anesthesia, general or local, under ocular guidance by oral bronchoscopy in the regular way. Tracheotomy had been done for the previous unsuccessful fluoroscopic bronchoscopies. For obvious reasons, the author does not care to publish further details. Sufficient is here given to emphasize the practical point that the author wishes to make. Namely that fluoroscopic bronchoscopy is so deceptively easy from a superficial theoretical point of view that it has been used unsuccessfully in cases easily handled in the regular endoscopic way. The author has been able to collect 12 cases of fluoroscopic bronchoscopy for foreign bodies of which the following is an analysis:

Statistics of fluoroscopic bronchoscopy for foreign bodies by various operators:

Foreign body removed in	8	(66.7 per cent).
Foreign bodies not removed	4	(33.3 per cent).
Number of cases fatal within a week	5	(41.6 per cent).
Of fatal cases foreign body removed in	3	(60 per cent).
Of fatal cases foreign body not removed	2	(40 per cent).

From the foregoing it is clear that fluoroscopic bronchoscopy because of its high mortality and its low percentage of successes, has nothing to justify its use in any bronchially lodged foreign body case until after regular Killian, ocularly guided, endoscopic bronchoscopy has failed. Personally the author would not use it until after another endoscopist besides himself had failed. Its use is, of course, only possible in case of bodies very dense to the ray and such as can, by posture, be seen clear of the heart and spinal shadows. Practically all of the cases reported have required tracheotomy. Fluoroscopic bronchoscopy is an improvement on the old method of using forceps blindly through the tracheotomic wound; but it is a step backward as compared to Killian bronchoscopy, and, because of its high mortality and lack of success, it is justifiable only when Killian bronchoscopy has failed.

Brünings has devised a lead-ended probe for radiographic localization.

CHAPTER XVI.

Foreign Bodies in the Bronchi for Prolonged Periods.

Cases of foreign bodies of prolonged sojourn, say a year or more, in the bronchi require special consideration. Just what length of sojourn is to be regarded as "long," is, of course, difficult to say. The secondary changes which make the difference requiring special consideration set in after a few weeks, in some cases and a few months in others, but bronchiarctia, bronchiectasis and abscess, in the author's experience, have been encountered only after a period of a year or more.

Etiology. The causes leading to the prolonged sojourn of a foreign body may be classified under three heads:

1. Ignorance of its presence.
2. Inability to make a diagnosis when suspected.
3. High mortality attending efforts at removal in the pre-bronchoscopic days.

The cases hereinafter reported as well as common experience show that, strange as it may seem, practitioners are heedless of, and even scoff at. the patient's suspicions that a long previously aspirated foreign body is the cause of present symptoms. This is largely due to failure to recognize and to teach in colleges the fact that there is a prolonged symptomless quiescent period after the aspiration of a foreign body into the lungs. When a patient states that he has neither felt anything nor coughed for months after the suspected accident, theoretically the presence of a foreign body in a bronchus seems impossible; yet, practically, we know that is just the usual course of such cases. The difficulty of diagnosis prior to the days of radiography, and still existing in cases of intruders not dense to the ray, has been an important factor in the etiology of the cases we now see. Another important factor is that prior to the days of bronchoscopy the then state of intrathoracic surgery rendered intervention inadvisable until after abscess formation. For surgical safety, as well as because the abscess often could not be located prior to the development of radiography, waiting for invasion of the pleura was usually advised.

*Pathology.** Doubtless very minute bodies become encysted or invade the interlobular connective tissue, as in anthracosis, but aspirated foreign bodies of larger size apparently rarely, if ever, become encysted, though, as in one of the author's cases, the foreign body may migrate and become somewhat "pocketed." It is evident from bronchoscopic findings that a foreign body too large for anthracosis, by gravity, as well as by aspiration, reaches the smallest bronchus it can enter, where it stops. Later negative pressure draws it still further downward. By mechanical irritation alone, or, more likely, from this combined with pyogenic organisms carried down with the foreign body, there results a productive inflammation which first completely occludes the involved bronchus with swollen mucosa (plus the bulk of the foreign body itself) ending in abscess of the lung below the foreign body. Later, sloughing or ulceration follows in the tissues surrounding the foreign body, permitting the slow escape of discharges, which because of the lessened expulsive cough effort from below consequent on the obstruction, tend to accumulate, producing the condition of bronchiectasis above the obstruction. In time, the obstruction owing to the productive inflammation becomes a cicatricial stricture. Below the stricture, the abscess cavity becomes, in a sense, a bronchiectatic cavity, also. The loss of the cilia and even of the epithelium itself follows, and increases the stagnation of the secretions. The bronchial wall may be destroyed by ulceration and chondrial necrosis, and the foreign body may wander. The law of gravity would lead one to expect to find the foreign body at the bottom of the cavity in the formation of which it has been the chief etiologic factor. In two of the author's cases it was at the top, close under the stricture. The following seems a plausible explanation: The abscess, of course, forms below the obstruction, but by the time the substrictural bronchiectatic cavity has been produced, the foreign body has become sufficiently fixed, by organization of a part of the surrounding granulation tissue, to hold the body in its place at the top of the cavity which it has caused. The development of a stricture above the foreign body is plausibly explained by the ulceration which is more or less annular. Such ulceration in any channel or tube in the body always results in more or less constriction of the lumen when the scar tissue contracts. That it does not occur to the same extent immediately below the foreign body is probably due to the conditions which cause the substrictural bronchiectasis. The reader interested in the etiology and pathogenesis of

*Abstracted (with revision and additions) from a paper read by the author at the meeting of the Laryngological Section of the American Medical Association, June, 1912.

bronchiectasis is referred to the excellent article of C. P. Howard (Bib. 214). In some cases communication with the subjacent bronchi is permanently closed by inflammatory sequelae, and the abscess may become walled off and so remain for years. Sooner or later, however, if the patient survive, the abscess, probably, will burst into the same bronchus or a branch, or it will burst into the pleura. There seems to be a strong tendency for foreign bodies to work toward the periphery as shown by the consecutive radiographs in one of the author's unsuccessful cases. This seems to be the tendency whether the abscess is closed off from bronchial drainage or not, but the history of nearly all cases seems to show that drainage is usually interrupted for a greater or lesser time, so that all cases are closed abscesses for part of the time. Atelectasis of the occluded lung area is usual with foreign bodies that occlude a bronchus, and, if prolonged, eventual functional destruction by the secondary processes is the usual result. Emphysema and not atelectasis may in rare instances follow the presence of a foreign body as shown by Iglauer (Bib. 223). Cases of foreign bodies, such as pins, that because of their small diameter are not obstructive, usually are not quickly followed by secondary changes, as noted by James W. MacFarlane at thoracotomy. Eventually, however, secondary inflammatory sequelae will cause occlusion of the invaded branch bronchus and all the sequelae of a pent up infected focus may be looked for. Gangrenous bronchitis and pneumonitis have been recorded as following the aspiration of a foreign body, but they are very rare sequelae.

A distinction should be made between an area of "drowned lung" (natural passages full of pus) and a true abscess cavity.

Prognosis. If unremoved the foreign body will almost certainly prove fatal. If removed most cases will recover without further local treatment. A few will require bronchoscopic attention to drainage. All cases will need a general antituberculous regime, and if this can be followed the prognosis is good. In a small percentage of cases extensive secondary changes as in one of the author's cases (Edward M.) an infective embolus from the lung or endocardial focus, before complete resolution has ensued, may lodge in a vital spot and end fatally, just as sometimes happens without bronchoscopic or other removal.

Indications for bronchoscopy for foreign body of prolonged sojourn. Bronchoscopy for removal is urgently indicated in every case in which there is any expectoration. In cases with a history of intermittent expectoration of foul pus, it is better to do the bronchoscopy during the discharging period, rather than in the dry interval, so that following the pus to its source will lead the bronchoscopist to the foreign body. Feebleness, even approaching a moribund condition, is no contraindication, as shown by the author's case (Mrs. K.), provided no anesthetic, general or local, is used. In cases in which there is a long period of cessation of discharge even though the patient is in good health, an exploratory bronchoscopy is indicated. If in such a "dry" case, a thick barrier is found bronchoscopically with no fistulous opening, and the radiograph shows an abscess close to the external wall of the chest, external operation by the general surgeon may be indicated. Of course, it is not known how frequently foreign bodies may be the cause of bronchiectasis, but the similarity of the symptoms in bronchiectasis and in foreign bodies in the bronchi, would certainly render exploratory bronchoscopy advisable even in a case with a radiograph negative as to foreign body. The same may be said of circumscribed pulmonary abscess, especially if tuberculosis can be excluded, though it is not impossible that a tuberculous process may exist primary or secondary to foreign body lodgment.

In all cases of doubt bronchoscopy is a harmless procedure that should be done anyway.

Symptomatology and diagnosis. After the aspiration of a foreign body into the trachea and bronchi, there is a longer or shorter period of perfect health in which the patient has no symptoms whatever. It is often difficult to convince the family, and even the family medical advisor, that a foreign body can be present and not produce any cough, bloody expectoration, dyspnea, rise of temperature, or any other symptom. Nevertheless, nearly all small foreign bodies that reach the bronchi do not produce any such symptoms for a variable period of weeks or sometimes months. Then begins a gradual turn to failing health, the exact cause of which is often unsuspected. There may be slight cough with scanty expectoration, slight temperature elevation, some malaise, with slight loss of weight, and altogether a picture of incipient tuberculosis, which, indeed, has been, undoubtedly, the diagnosis in many cases. The close parallel between the symptoms noted in these cases and in pulmonary tuberculosis even to the clubbing of the fingers (see case of Edward M.) would seem to render it advisable to suspect the presence of a foreign body in every case of seeming tuberculosis, in which no bacilli are found in a purulent sputum, and especially if the symptoms are confined to the lower lobe, particularly the right lower lobe. This would still leave out the cases of foreign body in which a tuberculous infection has preceded, or, more often, followed the aspiration of a foreign body. Two of the author's cases (Brooks G. and Mary N.) had such marked signs of pleurisy that they had been previously tapped without getting fluid. Ingals reports a similar case. The erroneous diagnosis of pleural disease in these and other cases of foreign body in the lungs has been ably pointed out by Boyce (Bib. 14).

The use of the radiograph as a routine procedure would certainly seem indicated in the diagnosis of thoracic disease.*

Treatment. Pus, granulomata, blood and stricture are the obstacles to be overcome in dealing with foreign bodies of long duration. As large a quantity of pus as possible should be removed by posture and voluntary cough before bronchoscopy. As a rule the morning is the worst time to operate because of the accumulation over night. By afternoon much pus can have been expectorated. Children can be held up by the ankles during coughing paroxysms. Adults may be placed on the sound side, pillowless, on a bed elevated high at the foot. Antibechics, bad at any time, should be especially forbidden during the forty-eight hours preceding bronchoscopy. What pus remains should be removed at the first stage of bronchoscopy by the author's "sponge pumping" process previously herein described. For this, work without anesthetic is a great help. If anesthesia is used, as the author did in some of the adult cases, the cough reflex should not be altogether abolished. It is very essential in the preliminary examination to use the sponges very gently in getting out the pus, so as to avoid, if possible, traumatism to the granulations, which may cause quite a good deal of bleeding and thus obscure the field. Of course, after the first survey of the field, it is often necessary to remove the granulations with forceps. During this, the sponging can be fairly vigorous, but removal of the granulations should not be begun until after the preliminary survey. It will require, in some instances, as much as three-quarters of an hour to get the field entirely clear of granulation tissue, pus and secretion, and to get the blood wiped away and the bleeding stopped. This is usually time well spent, because it enables more prompt work when the foreign body finally comes into view. The difficulties of contending with abundant granulation tissue, is well described by Ingals, as follows: "The moment this tissue was disturbed, bleeding occurred which obscured the field of vision and caused great delay from the necessity of swabbing away the blood. This is one of the greatest difficulties when granulomas are encountered in these cases, and one which occupies at least nine-tenths of the operators time. When bleeding has been checked and the field of vision once more cleared, the next portion of granulation tissue that is removed causes a repetition of the whole procedure; and this is likely to occur repeatedly before the foreign body can be seen." This statement has absolutely nothing to do with the form of distal illumination which Ingals uses.

*Just as these pages go to press, Dr. George L. Richards made a diagnosis of a foreign body in the lung upon an unexplained leucocytosis, cough, negative sputum examination and physical signs of bronchial obstruction. Diagnosis verified by radiographic finding and bronchoscopic removal of a tack of the aspiration of which the patient had no recollection.

There is no form of illumination which will permit the observer to see through a pool of blood.

The probability of location of the foreign body at the top, instead of at the bottom of the abscess cavity in strictured cases, is a point of greatest importance, as without the advice of Dr. Boyce on this point, the search in two of the author's subsequently mentioned cases would have been prolonged, and might have been futile; because the foreign body was not in either instance free in the cavity. On the contrary, it was fixed and bedded in granulation and fibrous tissue, external to the bronchial wall, through which it had eroded its way. The location of the intruder outward under the overhang of the cicatricial stricture rendered the finding of the foreign body difficult, if not impossible, without dilatation of the superjacent stricture. No useful forceps could have been inserted through the strictures, in the two cases referred to; the foreign body could not have been found and certainly could not have been withdrawn. If withdrawal were possible, trauma would have been extensive, and probably fatal. The dilatation of the purely cicatricial tissue of the stricture was harmless. Further, and very important, the dilatation improved the drainage, so that Nature could care for the lesions resulting from the long sojourn of the intruder.

The method of dilatation by divulsion used in these cases possesses the following advantages:

1. It is safe because it is under the guidance of the eye and the trained touch, by which both the direction and the extent of the dilatation are accurately limited at will.

2. It does not require tracheotomy in any case.

3. There is no danger of pushing the foreign body downward as is possible in certain cases, if anything in the shape of a bougie were to be used. Pushing a foreign body downward not only makes removal more difficult but involves serious risk of rupturing the bronchus.

4. It is, obviously, better adapted than tent dilatation to foreign body cases, and is, in any case, much safer and simpler.

The method is simple. The divulsor, Fig. 45, is inserted, under guidance of the eye, into the stricture which is stretched to the maximum expansion of the instrument. Then the larger divulsor, Fig. 46, is used to its maximum. This will permit the entrance of the closed side curved forceps, Fig. 29, with which the cavity can be probed. When the intruder is felt the forceps can be expanded and the intruder grasped; and if it does not come readily through the stricture the forceps can be rotated, if the foreign body be not such as to cause dangerous trauma. A tack or pin wrongly grasped cannot be pulled through a firm cicatricial stricture. It is necessary to release the hold at the top (near end in the recumbent patient) of the cavity, and examine the position and shape of the foreign body and get a fresh hold planned according to the mechanical problem presented. In some instances the cavity can be explored by gently forcing the conical ended tube (Fig. 18), into the already partially dilated stricture. In case of tacks lodged point upward the point may project upward through the stricture. If traction demonstrates a firm strictural obstruction, the dilator, Fig. 46, which is hollow may be pushed down outside the stem of the tack, and the stricture dilated without risk of pushing the tack downward. The conical ended tube may be used, the point of tack seized and then the stricture dilated by forcing the bronchoscope, forceps and tack all down together, before withdrawal.

In one case of prolonged sojourn the stricture was so firm and unyielding that prolonged intubation with metallic tubes was required. A tracheotomy was done and the tube inserted, removed at intervals of a few days and reinserted under local anesthesia. For further details see Brünings' book (Bib. 62) or Mr. Howarth's excellent translation (Bib. 208).

In one of the author's cases (Mrs. K.) recited below, instead of a stricture there was a mass of cicatricial tissue with small fistulae filled with buds of granulation tissue. This plug of cicatricial tissue, as shown by the radiograph, was about two centimeters in depth and beyond lay the foreign body. Fortunately the accurate advice of the radiographer, Dr. George C. Johnston, enabled the author to excise this intervening tissue and thus to reach and extract the foreign body. Without the guidance of an extraordinarily good radiograph showing the bronchus for a sufficient distance above the tissue barrier, thus giving a line of direction, such removal is exceedingly hazardous as to both life and successful foreign body removal. Fluoroscopic guidance is unsafe unless the fluoroscopy is done by two independent fluoroscopists, one for the vertical and one for the horizontal screen, while the bronchoscopist follows the dictates of the endoscopic image and of this general sense of direction. Even under these circumstances the procedure is hazardous.

Particular care must be taken not to lose the foreign body from the grasp of the forceps. The risk involved is especially great if the intruder be large enough to be obstructive because if it should enter and occlude the sound bronchus, the diseased side may be so atrophied as to be useless and the patient may die before the intruder can be again grasped and removed. This accident happened to Hinsberg.

After-care. Local treatment has not been necessary in the author's cases, of 2, 7, 10 and 26 years respectively. If, however, there seems to be a serious degree of bronchiectatic pus retention, or the patient fails to improve, after a few months, a radiograph should be made and compared with one made immediately after the foreign body removal. All of the author's cases were thus examined and all were making such excellent progress that nothing further was done. In case, however, of serious lack of drainage repeated dilatations and intubations of the strictural obstruction to drainage is indicated. This was done by Killian and Brünings in the case referred to and will be necessary in a certain proportion of cases.

General treatment after the removal of a foreign body of prolonged sojourn is quite essential. Milk, eggs, rest in bed out doors are indicated. In fact the entire anti-tuberculous regime is highly efficient.

AUTHOR'S BRONCHOSCOPIC CASES OF FOREIGN BODY OF PROLONGED SOJOURN.

Brass fastener removed by oral bronchoscopy from right bronchus after seven years' sojourn. Mary N., aged 23, was seen in consultation with Drs. J. Solis Cohen, D. Braden Kyle and Tello d'Apery. The patient gave a history of continual cough and foul, yellowish expectoration for about a year and a half, during which time she had an irregular temperature elevation and had lost weight. For seven years she had been subject to severe cough with expectoration during the winter, these symptoms disappearing in summer. The diagnosis of pulmonary tuberculosis had been made by a number of physicians. The foregoing is in brief the history she gave on admission to Jefferson College Hospital.

Radiographic examination. Dr. Solis Cohen in consultation with Dr. d'Apery found both apices free from disease. The only abnormal physical signs were slight impairment of resonance at the right base, with diminished voice and breath sounds. As these, in his opinion, did not sufficiently account for the symptoms, he referred the case to Dr. Willis F. Manges for radiographic study. Dr. Manges in a beautiful stereoscopic radiograph (Fig. 184) showed a stricture of the right bronchus, with a metallic body resembling an upholsterer's tack, point upward, below the stricture and behind the bronchus. The patient remembered having "swallowed" a price tag fastener seven years before, but as she was told that it would pass harmlessly, she had forgotten the occurrence. She had had no symptoms whatever until the winter following the accident. Symptoms recurred each winter.

Bronchoscopy. At Jefferson College Hospital before the members of the American Laryngological Association, the author passed a bronchoscope through the mouth. The trachea was full of foul, purulent secretion which was removed by "sponge pumping," the patient being kept only partially under ether to gain the aid of the cough reflex.* The last of the secretion removed from the right bronchus was mixed with blood. The right main bronchus, just below the orifice of the middle lobe bronchus, was occluded by a firm stricture, the lumen of which was a mere slit, extending about 3 mm. laterally, and with no appreciable antero-posterior diameter, the anterior and posterior edges being in contact. At each coughing effort, bloody secretion was forced through the slit. The stricture was dilated with the author's divulsors, in the direction of the narrowest diameter. Then the source of the bleeding and the blood-stained secretion was found to be a mass of granulations located below the stricture and posteriorly. Below this was a large cavity from which a quantity of very thick pus was removed. This pus was not foul like the tracheal pus. (Possibly the author's olfactory sense was by this time obtunded.) On exploration, with bronchoscopic lateral displacement, the mass of granulation tissue at the top of the cavity posteriorly was found to protrude from an accessory cavity, extending posteriorly and medianward, outside of the bronchus. On removal of the granulation tissue, the foreign body was found and removed. It proved to be a price tag fastener (Fig. 185).

Pathologist's report. The granulation tissue removed was examined by Dr. Ernest W. Willetts, who reported as follows: Specimen consisted of several very small pieces of tissue. Microscopic examination shows a covering of stratified squamous epithelium which has normal appearance but is thickened considerably at some points. Beneath the epithelium there was a mass of connective tissue showing many mast-cells, fibroblasts, new blood-vessels and some older, more fibrous areas. There is also considerable round-cell infiltration. The process appears to be a chronic inflammatory one, the exact nature of which is not evident from microscopic examination."

Subsequent history. The patient made an entire and complete recovery, and one year afterward, Dr. d'Apery reported that she was working at her occupation in the stocking factory, in possession of perfect health, the cough and expectoration having been totally absent for the past winter, the first out of seven winters. The patient was exhibited the following year at the meeting of the American Medical Association and now, three years later, is still in perfect health.

Lead-alloy collar button in right bronchus ten years. Removal by oral bronchoscopy. Brooks G., aged eighteen years, small, frail and undeveloped for his age, gave a history of pneumonia eight years before (1903), followed by pleurisy and empyema, which one year later (1904)

*This and the two following cases occurred a number of years ago. In later cases the author has found it advantageous to work with local anesthesia in adults, without any anesthesia in children.

was tapped and drained. Only a very small amount of pus was obtained and drainage during three months was very unsatisfactory. Temporary improvements were followed by relapses. Chills were attributed to a supposed malarial infection while living in Virginia. An eminent internist diagnosticated pulmonary tuberculosis, since which time treatment had been chiefly climatic, by residence in Arizona. The boy never re-

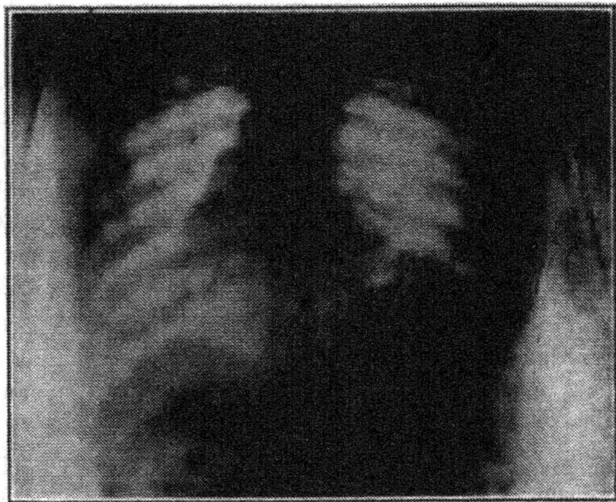

FIG. 184.—Radiograph by Dr. Willis F. Manges, (Philadelphia) showing price-tag fastener which had been seven years in the right bronchus of a girl of 23 years. (Mary N.). Fastener removed by oral bronchoscopy after bronchoscopic dilatation of the bronchial stricture (Author's case).

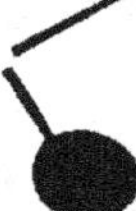

FIG. 185.—Price-tag fastener lodged for seven years in the lung of a girl aged 23 years. Removed bronchoscopically through the mouth after dilatation of the overlying bronchial stricture. Only one branch wire shows in the radiograph, because the two were in line (Author's case).

gained his health sufficiently to dispense with a nurse. He was frail and suffered continually from cough, usually with purulent sputum, frequently pink-stained, and occasionally of foul odor. He had low, irregular temperature elevation very suggestive of tuberculosis, but sputum examination was always negative. Dr. J. C. Roper, of the New York Hospital, after careful sputum examinations, found no tubercle bacilli and no elastic tissue.

Report of physical examination (Dr. James L. Edgerton and Dr. John W. Boyce). Patient is frail, underweight, pigeon-breasted, and has marked dextrocardia; apices free from disease. Physical signs are confined to base of right lung. Low down posteriorly, and extending to edges of lung, both breath and voice sounds were increased with a suggestion of amphoric breathing and whispered pectoriloquy. No change in percussion note. We are unable to demonstrate either tympany, cracked-pot note or Wintrich's change of tone when mouth is open.

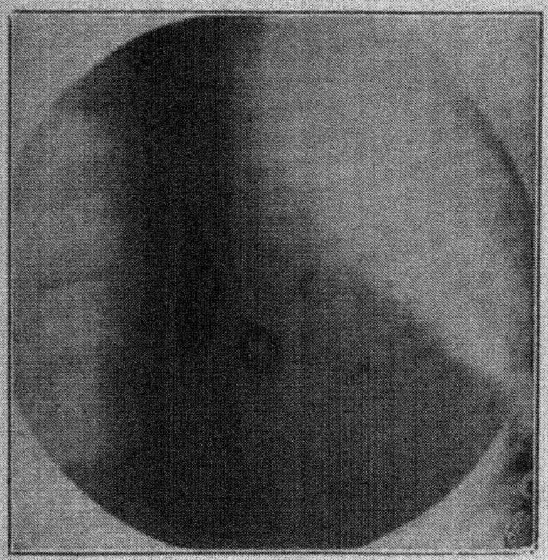

Fig. 186.—Radiograph by Dr. Lewis Gregory Cole (New York) showing lead collar button (minus head) in right lung of a boy of eighteen years. Removed bronchoscopically through the mouth, after divulsion of the overlying stricture (Author's case).

Such was the history and the condition of the patient when taken to Dr. James L. Edgerton, of New York City. Unlike his predecessors, Dr. Edgerton did not conclude that all the physical signs were attributable to the secondary changes, following the supposed empyema of eight years before, and sought the aid of Dr. Lewis Gregory Cole, of New York City, who located with wonderful accuracy by radiographic triangulation, a portion of a lead collar button, midway between the angle of the scapula and the spine, 6.4 cm. from the posterior wall of the chest. The collar button consisted only of a base and post, without a top, giving the appearance of a rivet as seen in the radiograph (Fig.

186). The parents remembered that the child had "choked ten years (symptoms eight years) previously on the collar button; and they had reiterated to numerous medical attendants their suspicion that the collar button might be the cause of all the symptoms, and in recent years they had even requested that a radiograph be taken." But the scoffing at lay opinions had silenced them. Dr. Edgerton brought the boy to the author.

Bronchoscopy. On passing the bronchoscope through the larynx, a large quantity of very foul, blood-stained pus was continually being coughed up from below. This coughing could, of course, have been stopped by deep general anesthesia, but the cough reflex was preserved under slight ether anesthesia, as an invaluable aid in ridding the lower air passages of the foul secretion, which obscured everything. After the fluid was removed from the trachea by "sponge pumping," it was easy to see that the pus was coming from the right bronchus. This bronchus was pumped out and then it could be seen that almost all the right bronchus was a bronchiectatic cavity with a cicatricial bottom, at the right edge of which was a small strictural opening, about 2 mm. in

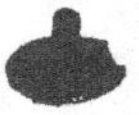

Fig. 187.—Portion of lead collar button (kind used by laundries) removed by oral bronchoscopy, from the lung of a boy (Brooks, G.) aged eighteen years (Author's case).

diameter. A cicatricial web occluded about two-thirds of the bronchial lumen just above the stricture and this web at its right end curved downward forming part of the edge of the stricture. The apertures of the upper and middle lobe bronchi seemed more than usually oval in outline, though of this it was difficult to be certain, and the time could not be spared for careful examination, since it was practically certain that the collar button was below the stricture, which therefore must be dilated. The divulsor (Fig. 45) was passed and readily entered the lumen of the stricture. The divulsion to the full extent of the instrument (1 cm.) did not require great force. After the withdrawal of the small dilator, the large dilator (Fig. 46) was introduced and expanded and allowed to remain *in situ* for a few minutes. Next, the cavity below the stricture was wiped out with small bronchoscopic swabs. Basing his judgment on the fact that the physical signs as above given were below the point at which Dr. Cole located the foreign body, Dr. Boyce advised the author that the collar button would be found at the top and not the bottom of the abscess cavity. Acting on this advice, a small patch of granulation tissue was found immediately under the overhanging left edge of the dilated strictural openings. During exploration of this granulation tissue with the jaws of the forceps (Fig. 29) the collar button was felt and removed. At the first attempt, the tip of the post of the button came away, permitting the removal of the balance of the button (Fig. 187) edgewise. The boy returned to his home a few days later, and four months afterwards, entered college in fairly good health. One year after the operation he was reported by Dr. H. W. Fenner, of Tucson, Arizona, to be free from cough and expectoration and otherwise healthy and normal in every way. Two years later he won the tennis championship of Colorado after a long and arduous training and tournament. Now, three years after the removal, he is in good health and averages up to normal development for his age except in height. Radiographic study by Dr. Cole at various stages of convalescence gave accurate graphic data on local progress, and the skillful care of Drs. Edgerton and Fenner contributed largely to recovery.

Brass-headed tack in right bronchus two years. Removed by oral bronchoscopy.

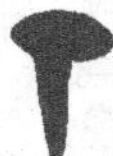

FIG. 188.—Brass-headed tack that remained for two years in the bronchus of a woman of 52 years. Removed by oral bronchoscopy (Author's case).

Mrs. J., aged 52 years, referred by Dr. J. J. Richardson. Two years previously patient had choked on a tack. For a time there were no symptoms, then chronic bronchitis supervened, followed ever since by irregular fever and chilliness. Occasional expectoration of blood. Repeated radiography failed to reveal the tack, until a week before admission, when the radiograph (Fig. 170) was made. Dr. N. H. Clark reported: "Breathing diminished throughout right chest, marked at base in front, almost absent at base in back. Marked auscultatory signs of bronchitis on right, moderate on left." At the Presbyterian Hospital the author at oral bronchoscopy under ether anesthesia found the right inferior lobe bronchus below the orifice of the middle lobe bronchus occluded with a fungating bleeding mass of granulation tissue. Quite free bleeding followed excision of this. After about seventy minutes of work all of the granulation tissue was removed and a dry field was obtained. Careful search over this field revealed on the posterior wall a small spot where a granulation bud had been nipped off at the orifice of a dorsal branch bronchus. In the center of the red spot was a black spot which proved to be the point of the tack. The side-curved forceps were insinuated into the bronchial orifice and the intruder withdrawn by a firm grip of the point of the tack (Fig. 188). There was expectoration of blood for a week. The temperature continued to rise occasionally but in about a month came permanently to normal, the cough and expectoration ceased in about three months and now, after almost two years, the patient is reported by Dr. Richardson to be in perfect health.

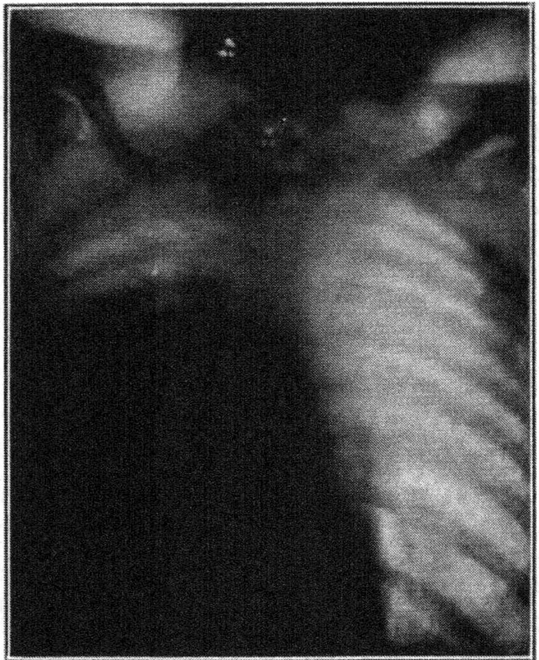

Fig. 189.—Radiograph of Mrs. K., showing left pyopneumothorax which was due to the bursting into the pleura of a foreign body abscess of the lung in a woman of 48 years. Collar button was in the lung but did not show through pus shadow (Author's case).

Glass collar button in left bronchus for twenty-six years. Removed by oral bronchoscopy without anesthesia, general or local. Mrs. K., aged 48 years, was admitted to the Presbyterian Hospital with a history of having "swallowed" a pearl collar button twenty-six years previously. There was some cough and bloody expectoration at the time of the accident and for about a year subsequently. This was before the discoveries of bronchoscopy and roentgenoscopy. No further pulmonary symptoms were noted for twenty-four years. During the twenty-fifth year there was an attack of "pneumonia" in treating which the attending physician (a very competent man) ridiculed the patient's idea that the button could still be in the lungs. In the early part of the twenty-sixth year, under the care of a third physician, a second attack of pneumonia occurred,

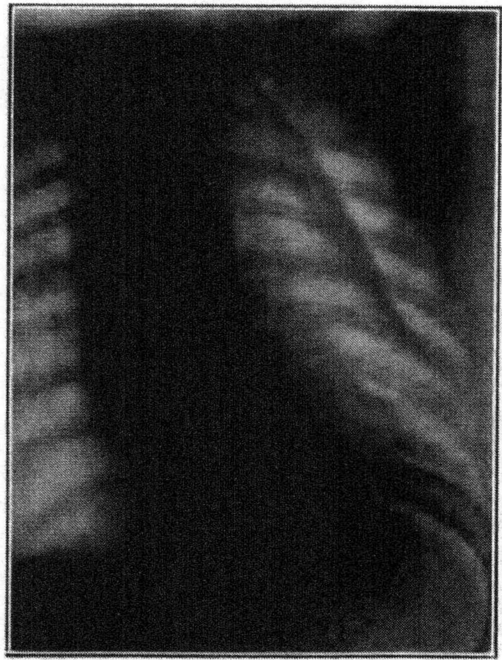

Fig. 190.—Radiograph of Mrs. K., after external drainage of the abscess by Dr. J. Hartley Anderson. Foreign body (collar button) present did not show. The dark line from the first rib downward and outward toward the drainage tube is the thickened visceral pleura seen on edge. The lung is collapsed as far as the pleural adhesions will permit.

followed by pain in the left side, bloody, foul expectoration, fever and emaciation. Again the patient's story of the collar button was ridiculed. Extremely feeble and emaciated, she fell into the hands of Drs. Thomas L. Ray and S. B. Pierce who, on the physical signs, made a diagnosis of lung abscess and pyopneumothorax. Suspecting foreign body origin, they referred the case to the author.

On admission to the Presbyterian Hospital, the woman's temperature was 102°, pulse 140, respirations 40. Sputum was profuse, thick, foul and of dark gray color. A radiograph (Fig. 189) by Drs. Johnston and Grier showed a dense shadow over the left lung, which they believed to be pus. Dr. John W. Boyce corroborated Dr. Pierce's findings and urged immediate drainage of the pleura by rib resection and a wide open-

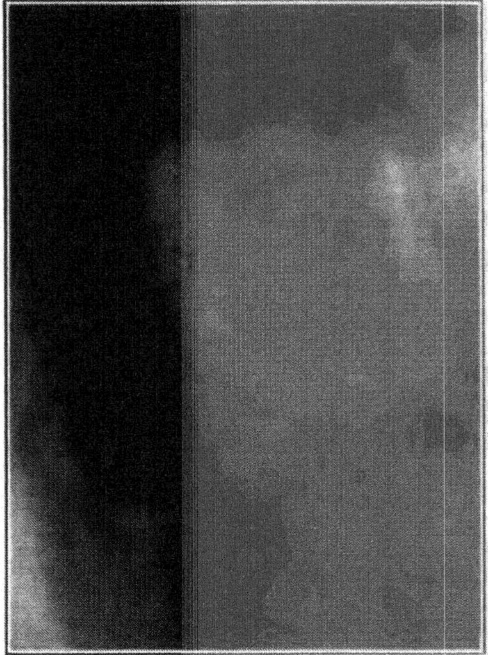

FIG. 191.—Quartering lateral radiograph by Dr. George C. Johnston showing collar button in the lung between the heart and the spine. (Same patient as Fig. 190).

ing. This was done by Dr. J. Hartley Anderson, evacuating over a quart of putrid pus. Drs. Johnston and Grier then made another antero-posterior radiograph (Fig. 190) which showed that the pus was well drained, but did not show a foreign body. In further search they made a diagonal radiograph (Fig. 191) which showed a collar button between the heart and the spine, in direct line with the stem bronchus of the left side. Dr. Johnston stated that there was tissue overlying the foreign body and that in order to reach the foreign body it would be necessary to remove this tissue in a direct line with the axis of the stem bronchus. With the assistance of Drs. Patterson, McCready and McKee, without anesthesia, general or local, I passed a bronchoscope through the mouth and found the inferior lobe bronchus occluded just below the orifice of the upper lobe bronchus by a cicatricial mass containing three apertures through which reddish granulations, that bled when wiped, were protruding. Clearly, dilatation, as practiced in previous cases, was useless and, with the accurate localization and advice of Dr. Johnston as a guide, the author excised tissue endoscopically with biting forceps until a rather large cavity full of granulations was reached. Excising the granulations and wiping away blood, foul pus and secretions, the collar button (Fig. 192) came into view bedded in granulation tissue, from which it was readily removed through the mouth along with the bronchoscope and forceps. The foul odor disappeared in about four weeks, cough and expectoration lessened, and both have now disappeared. The lung has completely filled

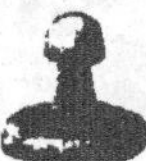

FIG. 192.—Glass collar button removed from the lung of Mrs. K. by oral bronchoscopy without any anesthesia, general or local. It had been in the lung for twenty-six years.

with air as shown radiographically. The external pleural fistula persisted for a number of months, but healed completely and now, one and one-half years later, Dr. Pierce reports the patient to be in perfect health and weighing 175 pounds.

The points of special interest are:—

1. The extremely long sojourn of the foreign body in the lung; the longest, to the author's knowledge, yet recorded.

2. The freedom from symptoms after the first year, for so long a period, twenty-four years. This is exceptional.

3. The bursting of a foreign body abscess into the pleura, while doubtless not of the greatest rarity of occurrence, has been recorded in only a few instances.

4. The foreign body did not follow the discharging abscess into the pleural cavity.

5. The necessity of the most expert ray work. It was only the quartering lateral radiograph that could show this foreign body, and all ordinary work would have been negative. Good lateral radiographs are exceedingly difficult to make of adult subjects.

6. The necessity in such cases of draining pus collections in order to get a radiograph of a foreign body, which would not show through the purulent shadow.

7. The feasibility of endoscopically removing a tissue barrier in order to reach an abscess cavity in the lung, when guided by both an accurate radiographic localization and ocular evidence through the tube that the tissue to be removed is pathologic.

8. The advantage of working without an anesthetic. This patient was *in extremis* and an anesthetic was not to be thought of. Moreover, the peroral bronchoscopy was no more painful than the filling of a sensitive tooth cavity, for which no one requires an anesthetic. The air passages were full of pus mixed with blood from the granulations. The

Fig. 193.—Enlarged view of fingers from a photograph of hands of Edward M., showing "clubbing" of the finger ends. (Author's case). Photographed by Dr. H. H. Fischer.

coughing of the unanesthetized patient greatly assisted in removing this by the "sponge pumping" method.

Nail in left bronchus four years. Removed by oral bronchoscopy without anesthesia, general or local. Edward M., aged ten years, referred by Dr. Robert L. Morehead, of New York City. Four years previously the child, then six years old, aspirated a nail, followed by paroxysms of coughing and gradually failing health. Sputum examination negative as to tubercle bacilli. Mixed pus cocci and saprophytes were present. Dr. H. T. Price reported the results of his physical examination as follows:

Child fairly well developed, rather languid, color good, head large, fingers markedly clubbed (Fig. 193), toes not so large, slight cough at intervals of half to two minutes. Breath very offensive after coughing, especially if a paroxysm occurs. Pigeon breast, rather emaciated chest, indrawn on left side (Fig. 194). Apex beat tumultuous in sixth interspace and about one inch to left of nipple line. Heart much enlarged to left barely compensating with a mitral regurgitation transmitted to left and all over left side and back. Jugular pulsation. Child cannot lie with comfort on account of posture causing coughing spells,

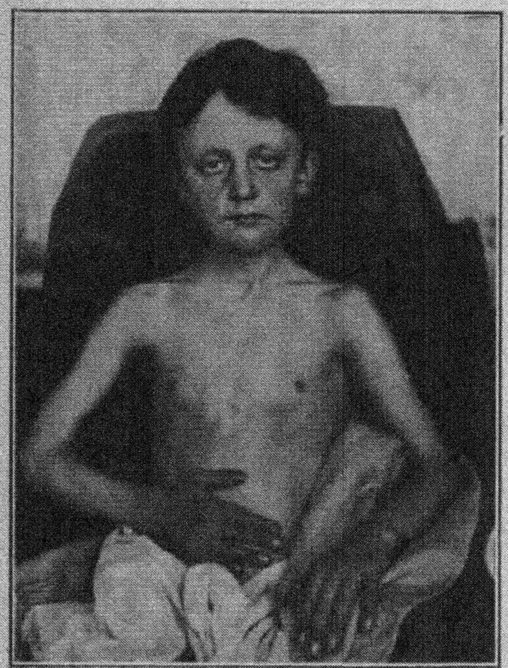

Fig. 194.—Photograph of Edward M., aged ten years, who for four years had a nail in a dorsal branch of the posterior lobe bronchus. Note emaciation, "pigeon breast," indrawn on left side, clubbed fingers. (Author's case. Photographed by Dr. H. H. Fischer.)

nor can he lean forward without distress. Right lung negative as to dullness, normal breathing, but few rales on deep respiration. Left chest dull all over. Very little air entering upper lobes. A few rales on deep inspiration. Lower lobe, breathing of bronchial type with large moist rales, suggesting cavity, about ninth rib and two inches from spine. Abdomen negative.

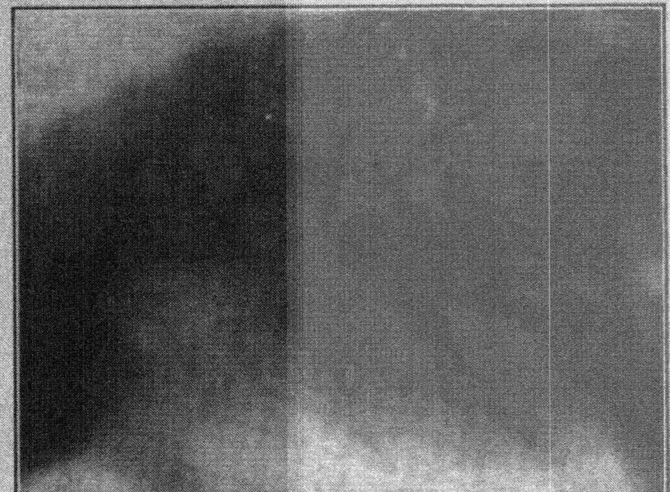

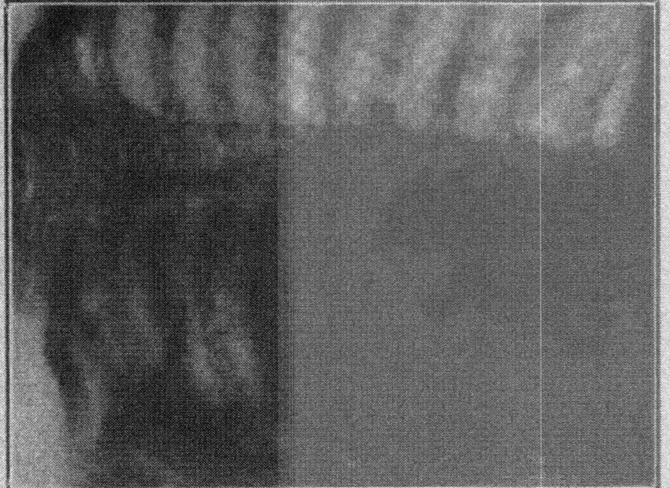

Radiographs taken in Brooklyn showed the nail in the center of a large shadow that included nearly all of the left lung (Fig. 195). At the Presbyterian Hospital the author passed a bronchoscope and encountered a large quantity of very foul pus. After removal of this and the excision of granulations the nail was found in a large cavity. There was no stricture and the removal presented no particular difficulty. The child returned to New York the next evening. Dr. Moorehead reported later that the child did well for three weeks, his condition was improved, and his cough and expectoration very greatly diminished. Suddenly, about a month after the nail was removed, he had a convulsion and on the following day, two more. Complete paralysis of the left arm, left leg and left side of the face developed and he died five days after the initial

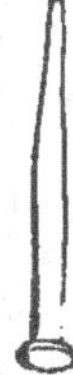

Fig. 196.—Drawing of nail removed from lung of Edward M. by oral bronchoscopy without anesthesia, general or local.

convulsion. A consultant neurologist stated that it was undoubtedly a case of embolism of the middle cerebral artery. No autopsy was permitted.

Remarks. This case shows clearly that removal of the foreign body cannot be expected always to be followed by recovery in a case with an extensive virulent pus focus in the lung. The emaciated wretched condition of the child shows the havoc that can be wrought by a foreign body in the lung. The close simulation of tuberculosis might be very misleading in case of a foreign body not radiographically visible. The source of the embolus might have been the lung or the heart. Occurring over three weeks after bronchoscopy it could have had no relation thereto.

CHAPTER XVII.

Unsuccessful Cases of Bronchoscopy for Foreign Bodies.*

After a monotonously long series of successful cases, the bronchoscopist is apt to think there are no limits to bronchoscopic foreign body removals. Sooner or later, however, he will discover that there are very decided limitations. These limitations so far as present experience shows, are all the failure to find a small body that has entered a minute bronchus far down and far out toward the periphery. In such cases, the localization methods of the author's films, Boyce calipers, fluoroscopy, etc., having failed, the question arises whether it is advisable to incur the risk of endoscopic excision, with the aid of two fluoroscopes, one for the lateral and another for the vertical plane. Naturally the risk of such a procedure will depend upon the nature of the tissue intervening between the foreign body and the end of the bronchoscope, and this, in turn, will depend upon the location of the intruder. With foreign bodies in the larger bronchi near the root of the lung, it is not to be thought of, but here endoscopy is rarely, if ever, unsuccessful. At the extreme periphery of the lung the danger is less, and is largely concerned with the contingency of opening a vessel that will permit blood to be retained to break down later, as well as the immediate risk of hemorrhage. The author has planned such an operation but has not yet encountered an endoscopically unsuccessful case of foreign body so located that the endoscopic operation seemed to involve less hazard than thoracotomy.

Theoretically, it might be supposed that the shortening of the bronchi that takes place in pneumothorax might be sufficient to cause the point of a pin to emerge from the invaded bronchus into the larger one of which it is a branch. In one of the author's cases (Miss J.), this did not occur. (Compare Figs. 199 and 200.) The question arises, what shall be done if the bronchoscopist fails to find the foreign body after having used all the methods of localization mentioned? The writer

*Revised from author's paper read before the American Laryngological Association, May, 1914.

feels that duty to a fellow creature demands that at least one other skillful bronchoscopist should try before deciding upon either leaving the foreign body alone to nature, or sending the patient to the general surgeon for thoracotomy. Up to the present writing, the author has had five failures and he congratulates himself upon his not having advised either of these alternatives without the patient having the benefit of the efforts of another bronchoscopist. In his first failure, Prof. Killian had previously failed, and the author had with him at the time of his own attempt, Algernon Coolidge, Jr., who made a careful search at the author's request after the author's failure to find the foreign body. In the second case, Cornelius Coakley had previously attempted to find the foreign body. In the third case, Samuel Iglauer and J. W. Murphy had both attempted to find the foreign body, and in the fourth case, Dr. P. M. Hickey had attempted to find the foreign body. In the additional case the patient was taken away from the hospital by the father, who positively refused to leave it until another bronchoscopist could be called. In the four cases enumerated, after the efforts of the expert bronchoscopists mentioned had failed to find the foreign body, the author felt that, with his own efforts failing also, the patient had been given the benefit of everything that bronchoscopy had to offer, and it remained to consider the next step.

In deciding this question, it is first necessary to consider what will happen if the foreign body is allowed to remain. This has been gone over analytically by Delavan, Roe, Wood and others in the pre-bronchoscopic days and by Clayton, Clark and Marine more recently, as elsewhere mentioned. Because of its brilliant achievements, bronchoscopy has been universally accepted, and for that reason, but very few foreign bodies have remained in the bronchi when their presence was known. The cases where bronchoscopy has failed have been limited to cases in which the foreign body could not be found, and these have invariably been very small bodies far down and far out at the periphery. In this location, the most probable result is that an abscess will form and that it will burst through into the pleural cavity. It then becomes a question whether thoracotomy shall be done at once upon the failure of bronchoscopy or whether the abscess formation with invasion of the pleura shall be awaited. The chief arguments against waiting are that the patient may not survive sufficiently long for the development of the abscess and the reaching of the pleura. Furthermore, the foreign body may not follow the abscess into the pleural cavity as seen in the case of Mrs. K., reported in a previous chapter. In that instance the foreign body was easily removed through the mouth because it was large and consequently easy to find. Because of its large size, also, it had not reached the point near the periphery after the original accident, and it took twenty-six years for the abscess to reach the pleura. During the wait for an abscess to reach the pleural cavity, there is, of course, the possibility that the foreign body may slough loose and be coughed out. Such a possibility is remote in any case and in case of some bodies, as pins, it is impossible. Furthermore, (Delavan, Bib. 107) lesions may be established which will result in the death of the patient even after the foreign body has been gotten rid of. (See case of Edward M., in Chapter XVI). Nature can cure appendicitis and can amputate a limb, but no one knowingly takes the risk of waiting. Apropos of this, a very interesting collection of thirty-two cases is reported by Clarke and Marine, in which gangrene of the lung followed the aspiration of a foreign body. Their analysis is as follows: "Of thirty-one cases, the foreign body was a tooth twice, a pin once, a piece of wood once, a button twice, a head of grain or grass seven times, a bit of evergreen twice, a fruit stone twice, a bone ten times; not mentioned, four times; that it occurred with equal frequency in adults and children; that it remained in the bronchus before gangrene set in from four days to five months, usually under three weeks. Gangrenous process lasted from three days to four years, most frequently from two to four weeks; the outcome was death in twenty-one cases, recovery after thoracotomy in two, and spontaneous recovery in four cases. The foreign body was coughed up in five cases, four of which subsequently died and only one recovered." To these statistics is to be added the case that Clarke and Marine themselves observed, in which a man died of pulmonary gangrene seventeen days after aspirating a fragment of bone, death occurring two days after the first appearance of putrid expectoration. Viewing the question impartially from all sides, the author believes, first, that large foreign bodies, which necessarily stop in the trachea or larger bronchi, can always be removed by bronchoscopy, therefore, thoracotomy is absolutely out of consideration. In case of small foreign bodies far down and far out at the periphery, after two expert bronchoscopists have failed to find the foreign body, the intruder should be removed by external operation, and the sooner after the bronchoscopic failure, the better, because of the usually early development of septic processes around an aspirated foreign body. Modern developments and especially the intratracheal insufflation anesthesia, originated by Meltzer and Auer, and developed by Elsberg, Janeway and others, have placed thoracotomy on a plane never before obtained, and while the pleural shock remains, the mortality is very much decreased and the operation has reached the stage where it is justly entitled to consideration in cases where two expert bronchoscopists have failed. It is certainly preferable to taking the chances of leaving the foreign body alone. Formerly, there was great difficulty in finding the foreign body after the lung was open, but in the modern operation with the very large flap and ample opening, where the entire lung can be handled, the chances of not being able to find the foreign body are very small. In the event of a foreign body reaching the pleura either with or without pus, it should be immediately removed by pleuroscopy (q.v.) or by thoracotomy, without waiting for adhesive pleuritis.

As to the details of thoracotomy, the author has never done the operation and never will. He begs, however, to make four suggestions. 1. In these days of insufflation intratracheal anesthesia, the bronchoscopist is of no use in the operation. Any aid in localization he may be able to afford is better given verbally by naming the approximate location of the invaded bronchus. 2. The best method of visceral localization is by the author's transparent films, because after collapse of the lung, the relation of the visceral to the bony anatomy is entirely changed. To know the bronchus invaded simplifies the search. 3. The best method of location of the osteoplastic flap is by the method of Lewis Gregory Cole and other expert radiographers. 4. As the infective risk is slight, and the operative risk is greater than the square of the duration of the operation, the thoracotomy, especially in children, should be done without gloves. However trained the gloved touch, no one can argue that a pin cannot be found quicker in the lung without gloves than with them, especially in the case of infants and children where the largest possible opening will not permit the use of the whole hand. Extraordinary care in preparation of the hands will make the hands reasonably safe from infective risk in this, the only operation in surgery where gloves may kill the patient.

THE AUTHOR'S UNSUCCESSFUL CASES.

Of the author's five unsuccessful cases, one was before the development of bronchoscopy to a reasonable degree of efficiency, and four cases have occurred since. All were failures to find a small foreign body in a minute bronchus far down and far out toward the periphery. The author hopes that his elsewhere mentioned, recently perfected means of localization will in the future be of assistance in lessening the number of unfindable foreign bodies, though these methods were used in the last case of the four and failed to enable success. In each of these four cases removal had been previously attempted by skillful bronchoscopists of large experience. Had the author alone failed on these four cases he would feel that they were personal failures. On the contrary they should be considered as failures of bronchoscopy and should be analyzed as such in order that bronchoscopy, like any other department of medical science, shall profit by its failures.

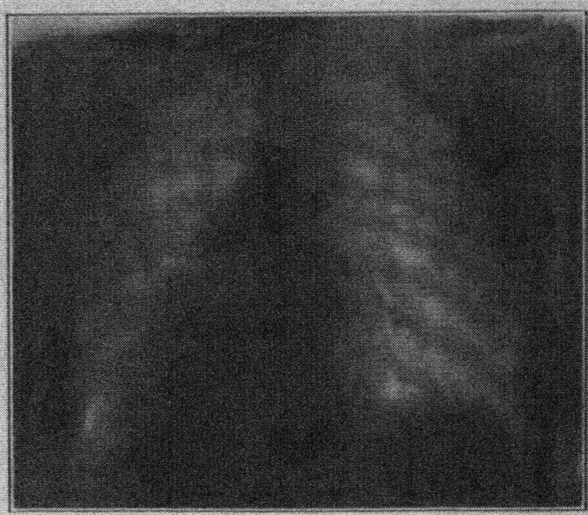

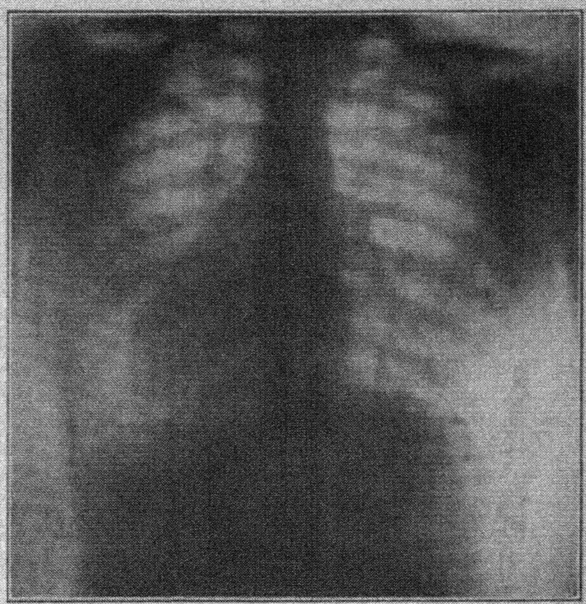

FIG. 197.—Radiograph of pin in right lung of a girl, aged eighteen years. The pin could not be found at bronchoscopy. (Miss C). Lower radiograph shows how the pin had migrated towards the pleura at the end of two years.

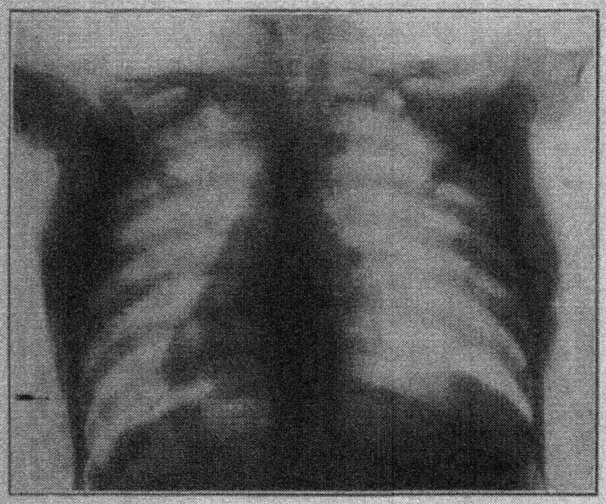

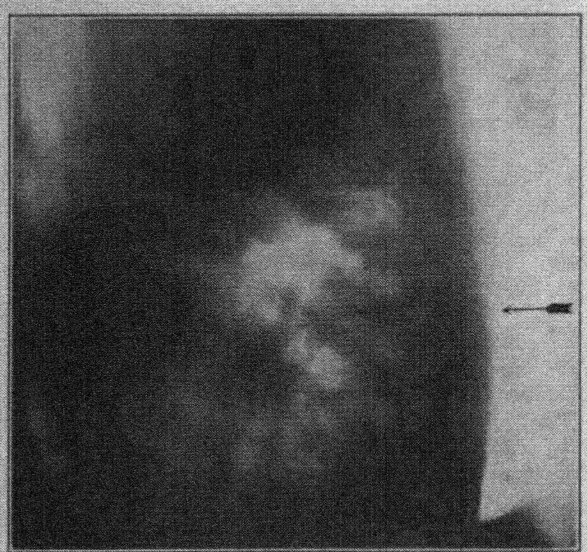

Fig. 199.—Radiographs, anteroposterior and lateral (by Dr. Lange of Cincinnati) showing pin in posterior branch of left inferior lobe bronchus of Miss J. The pin is retouched for clearness.

Miss C., aged eighteen years, referred by Dr. Edward S. Bacon. Patient had aspirated a pin four weeks previously. No cough, expectoration or other symptoms. Dr. Bacon saw the pin endoscopically in the right bronchus immediately after the accident, but was unable to disimpact it with all the traction he deemed safe. A few weeks later the pin was, radiographically, found to have gradually worked its way toward the periphery of the lung. Prof. Killian, who was the guest of the American Laryngological Association at the time, made an unsuccessful bronchoscopic attempt at removal. A few weeks later the author passed a bronchoscope. Ether was used at the start, but was discontinued after about fifteen minutes. The author was honored by the presence of

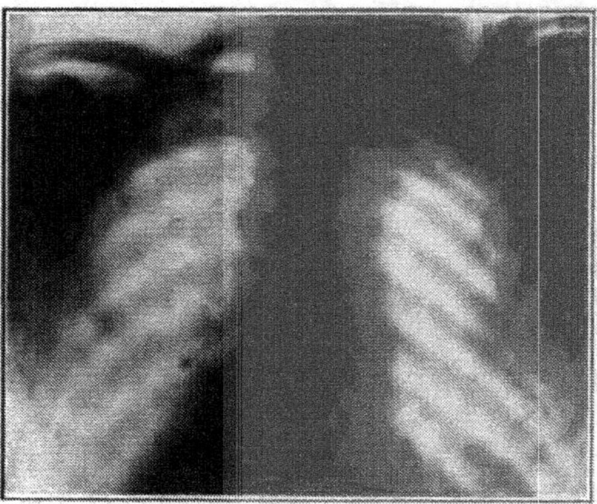

FIG. 198.—Radiograph of Mrs. S. showing pin in posterior branch of inferior lobe bronchus. Pin could not be found at bronchoscopy. (Retouched for clearness).

Algernon Coolidge, Jr., one of the pioneer bronchoscopists. Neither of us could find the pin which was plainly evident in the radiograph (Fig. 197). We found the bronchi of the left lung all normal in appearance. The mucosa of all the right bronchi was congested and swollen. The orifices of the branch bronchi were diminished to about half the normal size, as estimated by comparison with the opposite side. As Dr. Coolidge pointed out, there were no localizing signs, such as emerging pus, to lead one to suspect one bronchus more than another. A few were carefully explored by the author with negative results. The search occupied about an hour and a half. There was no reaction and the patient left the hospital. Her health was fair at the end of a year. Occasional "jagging" pains were felt and there was some cough. At the last report the pin was gradually working toward the pleura.

Mrs. S., aged forty-three years. Seen in consultation with Dr. Cornelius Coakley, at St. Luke's Hospital, New York City. Patient had a strumic stenosis for which a tracheotomy had been done by Dr. Farquar Curtis. A pin had been aspirated into the bronchus two months before admission, and the excellent radiographic work of the

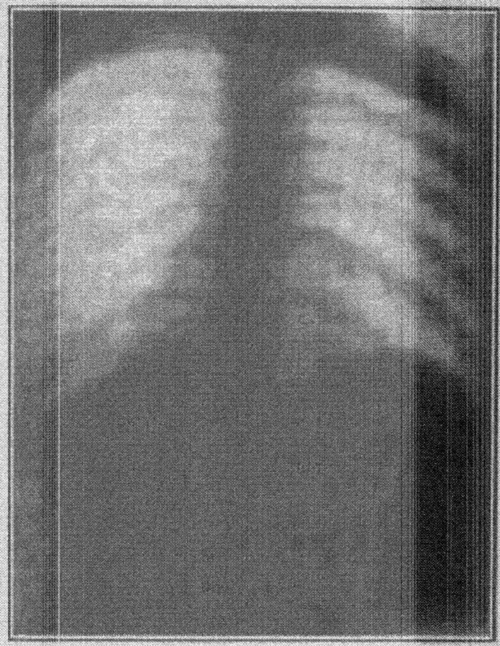

FIG 200.—Radiograph showing displacement of pin after pneumothorax. (Case of Miss J). Retouched for clearness. (Author's case).

hospital radiographer had located the pin posteriorly very low in the left lung (Fig. 198). Dr. Coakley had made a careful and skillful search without finding the pin. The author was equally unsuccessful. There were no localizing signs. In one of the bronchi the author thought he felt contact of the pin but it could not be sufficiently confirmed to justify using the forceps. The patient died one and one-half years later, after refusing external operation for pulmonary abscess.

After the foregoing was written and while this book is in press the author has had another unsuccessful case. Drs. Henry Janeway, Harmon Smith and Sidney Yankauer had failed to find a metallic foreign body which showed plainly in excellent lateral and anteroposterior radiographs (by Dr. A. S. Holding) and they honored the author by calling him to the case. Bronchoscopy by the author at the New York General Memorial Hospital was equally unsuccessful in seeing the foreign body. Dr. A. S. Holding fluoroscopically saw the intruder upward and outward and forward from the bronchoscopic tube-mouth when the latter was in the left upper-lobe bronchus, thus definitely locating the foreign body in an anteriorly ascending branch of the left upper-lobe bronchus. A subsequent thoracotomy confirmed the localization; but the patient succumbed.

From this case it is fair to conclude that a foreign body may get so far toward the periphery in the upper lobe-bronchus as to be beyond the limitations of bronchoscopy. Out of six upper lobe-bronchus cases, in the author's experience, this is the only one that invaded so far as to be beyond reach.

CHAPTER XVIII.

Foreign Bodies in the Esophagus.

Part of this subject was considered in a previous chapter (XII) on the general subject of foreign bodies in the air and food passages. A number of important points require additional consideration.

Etiology. In the esophagus the lodgment of foreign bodies is influenced by five factors.

1. The shape of the foreign body (pointed, rough, etc.).
2. Resiliency of the foreign body (safety pins, etc.).
3. The size of the foreign body (a large meat bolus).
4. Narrowing of the esophagus, spasmodic or organic, normal or pathologic.
5. Paralysis of the normal esophageal propulsory mechanism.

The modes of action of the foregoing list of causes are self-evident. but numbers three and five require further consideration. As a rule, when ordinary food lodges in the esophagus, there is a strong suspicion that there is some organic trouble present, such as compression by an aneurysm, or a malignant, or a cicatricial or a spasmodic narrowing. In one of the author's cases a deckhand, eating a very hurried meal, had an enormous bolus of meat lodge in the esophagus at the crossing of the left bronchus, completely occluding the gullet. The pyriform sinuses were full of secretions and a large quantity of secretions was brought through the aspirator before the esophagoscope reached the bolus at the crossing of the left bronchus. After the esophagoscopic removal of the meat, the esophagus seemed normal and free from compression or stricture. The man had never had any trouble in swallowing before, and has had none since, although three years have elapsed. It seems quite evident that it was only the enormous size of the bolus which caused it to lodge, and it is probable that it passed the cervical narrowing in more or less elongated form but broadened out as it reached the thoracic esophagus, during the negative pressure of an inspiration, and in this more expanded form, it completely occluded the narrowing at the crossing of the bronchus. Paralysis of the esophagus, at first thought, might be thought not to interfere with the downward passage of any substance and yet even liquids will not go down a paralyzed esophagus as mentioned under diseases of the esophagus.*

Why do foreign bodies in the esophagus lodge most frequently at certain localities? As in the air passages, the greater frequency of lodgment of foreign bodies in certain localities is governed by factors which may be classed in three main divisions:

1. (a) The size and shape of the foreign body, whether long, broad,

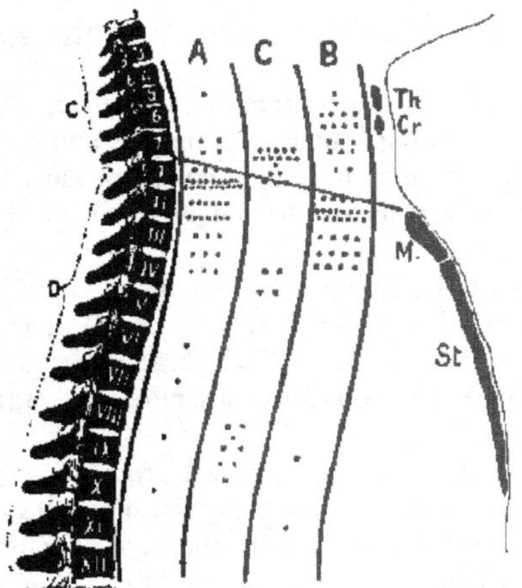

FIG. 202.—Schematic illustration of the site of lodgment in 135 cases of foreign body in the esophagus, from statistics collected from literature by H. Burger. Th., thyroid cartilage. Cr., cricoid cartilage. M., manubrium. Column A shows the location in those cases where relation to the spine was mentioned. Column B shows the position of the intruder when this was given in relation to the thyroid, cricoid, manubrium or sternum. In column C are indicated the cases where the localization was given in more general terms. (After Sir St. Clair Thomson).

pointed, angular, disk-like, etc. (b) Its surface, whether rough or smooth. (c) Its physical properties, resiliency, plasticity, absorbtivity, etc.

2. The anatomic peculiarities of the various localities. (a) Angles, arcs. (b) Fixed and motile narrowings.

3. Paralysis of the esophageal propulsory mechanism.

An interesting tabulation of reported cases of esophageally lodged foreign bodies is shown schematically in Fig. 202, which is reproduced

*Age as an etiologic factor is shown by the fact that of the author's 43 cases of bones in the esophagus all but 2 were in adults; whereas, of 38 cases of esophageally lodged coins, in the author's experience, all were in children.

from Sir St. Clair Thomson's excellent book. Of course, a considerable latitude for inaccuracy must be allowed, because of the necessarily inaccurate localization in perhaps the majority of published reports. Nevertheless the grouping of almost all of the cases in the upper third of the esophagus is very striking and coincides with the experience of all esophagoscopists. Most of the very few cases of lower lodgment encountered have been pushed down by blind methods. Various reasons have been assigned for the lodgment of almost all foreign bodies in the upper third; but none of them appeal to the author as being satisfactory. His own opinion is that it is a physiological narrowing due partly to spasm. but mainly to the fact that the cervical esophagus is normally collapsed and is not subject to the negative pressure that expands the intrathoracic portion of the esophagus. Not only is the musculature of the cervical esophagus more powerful in its contractions, but it is a collapsed tube. The mediastinal esophagus, on the contrary, is being pulled open and thus the foreign bodies, unless of very large size, are relieved and readily find their way downward. Against the theory that it is simply the quiescent narrowness of the cervical esophagus that holds the foreign body, is the fact that there is plenty of room for quite a large esophagoscope to override the foreign body and pass it without the inexperienced operator being able to see the foreign body at all. If the esophagus were narrow at the point and retaining the foreign body only by the smallness of its lumen, one would suppose this overriding could not occur. One point that indicates that there is a large element of spasm in the lodgment of foreign bodies in the esophagus, is the fact that operators who use general anesthesia have a much larger proportion of foreign bodies escape downward than those who do not. Since abandoning anesthesia for the removal of esophageally lodged foreign bodies (except in the case of very large bodies) the author has not had a single case of escape of the intruder downwards during esophagoscopy. From esophagoscopic observation in other than foreign body cases one would suppose that foreign bodies would lodge in the clutch of the cricopharyngeus but, in the author's experience, this is not nearly so frequent a locality as the upper thoracic aperture. We may conclude, then, that it is the physiological narrowing at the upper thoracic aperture. This narrowing disappears under anesthesia in the recumbent position and is not demonstrable by cadaveric anatomy; hence, probably is partly muscular and partly the crowding of the adjacent viscera into the fixed and narrow upper thoracic aperture. It is probable that the anatomic changes associated with the phylogenetically late upright posture of man is associated with the physiological narrowing which causes foreign bodies to lodge at the upper thoracic aperture.

Symptoms of foreign body in the esophagus, and indications for esophagoscopy. It would be a waste of valuable space extensively to consider here the symptoms of esophageally lodged foreign bodies. They form no basis for the determination as to whether an esophagoscopy should be done or not, for symptoms may be entirely absent, even in cases of rather large intruders. If the patient has swallowed a foreign body, that body must be found in the anatomy or in the stools. A very small foreign body may cause regurgitation and complete inability to swallow even water. This occlusion may be due to spasm, swelling of the

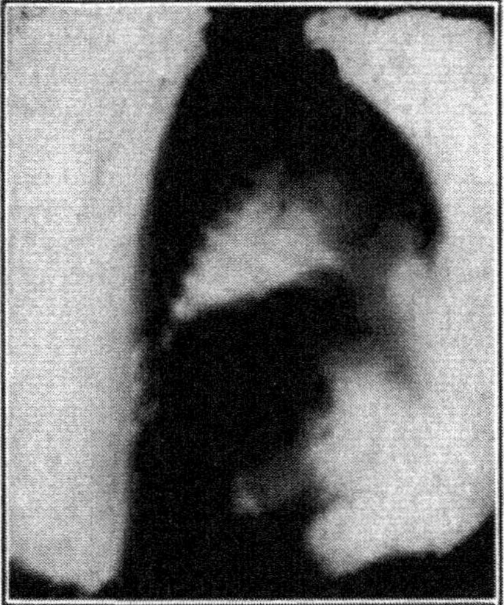

FIG. 203.—Lateral radiograph showing lodgment of a collar button in the esophagus at the usual location, at the upper thoracic aperture—not at the crico-pharyngeal narrowing. Location corroborated at esophagoscopy. (Author's case).

esophageal walls, or to augmentation of the size of the intruder by expansion with absorbed moisture, or by accumulation of food about the intruder. Coins may cause intermittent occlusion by change of position. They usually permit food to pass and they often show a bright streak down the center third of one or both sides where the passing food has kept the surface bright, while at the lateral thirds, which are more or less buried in the folds of the mucosa, corrosion or oxidation darkens the coin. This is most noticeable in silver coins, in which the lateral thirds are darkened by the formation of silver sulphide on the surface. (See illustrations of coins in case reports in a subsequent chapter.)

This shows that foods pass flat objects like coins quite readily as a rule. Occasionally, however, occlusion is complete from the outset. Carpenter (Bib 73) reports one such case in which nothing could be swallowed in the three days between lodgment and esophagoscopic removal. On the other hand a foreign body which has remained long *in situ* may give rise to no symptoms whatever and if the lodgment has been in childhood, growth and development may possibly permit the child to swallow sufficiently well that no difficulty is noticeable, as in a case reported by W. G. Porter, in which a half-penny had remained in the esophagus of a child for eight years, who then was brought for indefinite gastric symptoms, not for dysphagia. Dyspnea may be a symptom of an esophageally lodged foreign body. In one of the author's cases a large foreign body produced so much compression of the trachea that the trachea was explored first and found to be very much stenosed because of the forward pressure on the membranous party wall by the intruder. Cough is one of the symptoms of foreign body in the esophagus that must not be forgotten. It may be due to reflex irritation, to secretions overflowing into the larynx from the occluded esophagus, or to perforation, traumatic or, later, ulcerative, of the party wall causing leakage of food or secretions into the trachea. In one of the author's cases, elsewhere herein reported, the mother said the child "coughed until it vomited." What really happened was the leakage of the nursling's food through the ulcerative foreign body fistula from the esophagus into the trachea resulting in the coughing up of the milk. In foreign body cases in which there is complete obstruction the author's symptom of esophageal occlusion may be present. It consists in the pyriform sinuses, one or both, being filled with secretion as noted on indirect mirror examination in the erect posture. This is, of course, a symptom only of occlusion, not necessarily by a foreign body. It is due to retention of fluids which otherwise are constantly draining down through the esophagus.

The localization of the foreign body as to whether it is in the esophagus or in the air passages is considered under the head of bronchoscopy for foreign bodies.

Prognosis. A foreign body lodged in the esophagus may prove quickly or slowly fatal or may remain for many years if its size, shape and position permit food to pass. E. A. Peters reports the case of a man dying two hours after a tracheotomy done for edema of the glottis, secondary to hemorrhage down along the spine, from the puncture of the jugular vein by a pin swallowed with food. Adelman cites nine cases and Chiari twenty-one cases of perforation of the aorta by foreign bodies in the esophagus. The perforation may be shortly after the lodgment, in the case of sharp bodies, such as pins, needles and sharp bones; or more slowly by erosion and ulceration. Many cases of foreign bodies in the esophagus have been quickly fatal through perforation and septic mediastinitis. Many others have caused death through suppuration extending to the trachea with consequent edema and asphyxia. In cases of prolonged sojourn of the foreign body in the esophagus thickening

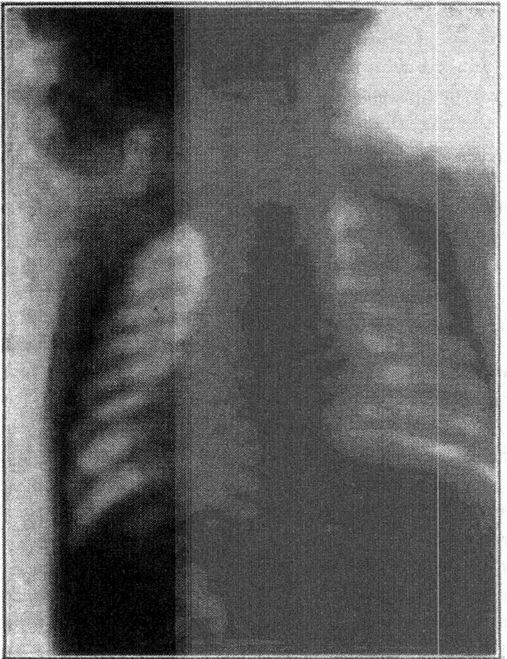

Fig. 205.—Radiograph of foreign body (cuff link) part of which had ulcerated through from the esophagus into the trachea of a three months old infant. Removed partly by oral bronchoscopy and partly by oral esophagoscopy without anesthesia, general or local. (Author's case).

and hyperplasia of the esophageal wall result from nature's effort to protect the surrounding tissues. Sooner or later, however, if not removed, the foreign body causes death. Every large museum has specimens of this kind, and the most frequently seen foreign body is the artificial denture. The foregoing remarks, however, apply chiefly to the pre-esophagoscopic days. To-day, with the radiograph and the esophagoscope, foreign bodies are discovered and promptly removed. Dr. D. Braden Kyle reports a very remarkable case in which he very skillfully removed an artificial denture that had been in the esophagus for seventeen years (Fig. 215). The patient's condition was very serious, and but for the timely work of Dr. Kyle, the patient would have succumbed. Perforation of the upper esophagus may result in cervical cellutitis of varying degrees of intensity. Abscess may result in any of the surrounding tissues, either from direct infection or from secondary necrosis of the tracheal or laryngeal cartilages from infective perichondritis. One such case was referred to the author by Dr. Greenfield Sluder for an opinion. A tooth brush bristle and a bit of necrotic cartilage were discharged from an abscess at the mouth of the esophagus of a physician of about forty years of age, after a number of years of ill health. The fistula is still unhealed. Joseph White (Bib. 573) reports a similar case followed by laryngeal stenosis. Many cases are fatal within a short time from perforation and mediastinal abscess. The author has had two cases in which a foreign body ulcerated through from the esophagus into the trachea. One of these has been reported (Bib. 269). The other one is as follows:

Cuff link that ulcerated from the esophagus into the trachea. Infant C., aged three months. Referred by Dr. J. A. Sullivan. Parents said child "coughed until it vomited." Dr. Sullivan was about to prescribe for the bronchopneumonia present when the parents said they had missed a cuff link for six weeks before and notwithstanding this indefinite statement and the age of the child (only six months at the time), the doctor sent the patient to Dr. George C. Johnston who found the cuff link radiographically (Fig. 205) and referred the case to the author. As the symptoms seemed altogether tracheo-bronchial, the author passed a bronchoscope first and found the smaller part of the button in the trachea with the stem passing backward towards the esophagus. Withdrawing the bronchoscope the author passed an esophagoscope and found the larger part of the button in the esophagus with the stem passing forward toward the trachea. On re-examination with the bronchoscope it was found that the smaller end of the button was loose on the stem. With forceps it was soon twisted off and withdrawn through the glottis with the forceps and bronchoscope. The esophagoscope was introduced into the esophagus and the larger portion of the button with the stem was removed without difficulty (Fig. 206). The temperature which had ranged about 103° before the broncho-esophagoscopy remained about the same for about a week and then slowly and gradually subsided. One year later the child was reported perfectly healthy.

Remarks. The symptom "coughing until it vomited" was quite evidently due to the leakage of the milk from the esophagus into the trachea, where the cough thus excited expelled the milk from the mouth, while the portion aspirated produced the broncho-pneumonia. Considering the vague history of missing a cuff link, and the age of the child (then only six weeks) the practitioner is to be complimented.

The prognosis as to esophageal function after cases of prolonged sojourn of foreign bodies is closely related to the length of sojourn. The longer the intruder has been *in situ* the greater the likelihood of stenosis. In D. Braden Kyle's unique case of seventeen years' duration, Fig. 215, the stenosis required after-treatment which Dr. Kyle carried out so skillfully as to get an excellent ultimate result. Prognosis may be made very grave from ill-advised interference, especially blind bouginage and external esophagotomy, as will be cited under treatment. The prognosis after esophagoscopy is excellent as shown by the statistics given in this chapter.

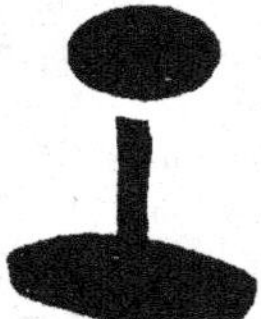

Fig. 206.—Cuff link shown in Fig. 205.

Even if the foreign body becomes dislodged and moves downward the patient is not safe. It may cause intestinal perforation (Fig. 207). So long as the intruder remains in the body the prognosis must be guarded.

Treatment. If for any reason immediate removal is contraindicated, bismuth subnitrate should be given dry on the tongue in small doses frequently repeated. It will adhere to denuded surfaces. Calomel may be advantageously added to the first few doses. Removal is the only treatment to be seriously considered. With the relatively high mortality from external esophagotomy, it certainly seems as though the operation is rarely if ever justifiable in foreign body cases. Compared to other operations in the neck, it has a very high mortality. Furthermore, it has happened more than once that an external esophagotomy done on the strength of a radiograph, has failed to find the foreign body because the latter has passed on downward into the thoracic esophagus, where it cannot be reached otherwise than esophagoscopically, and one such case has been recorded in which the patient died from an external esophagotomy at which the foreign body was not found. In view of these things, those who have had most experience in dealing with the esophagus regard esophagotomy as unjustifiable until after esophagoscopy has failed, and the author's personal opinion is that any and every foreign body that has gone down through the mouth into the esophagus can be brought back the same way, unless it has already perforated the

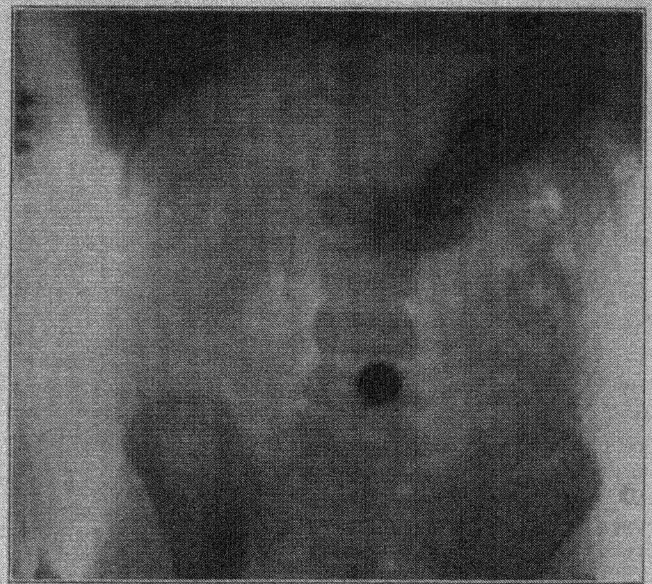

FIG. 207.—Needle in the intestine. Death resulted from septic peritonitis following perforation. Esophagoscopy was opposed by the family physician when the needle was in the esophagus. The position of the stomach is shown by the bismuth shadow. Laparotomy advised when needle remained in one place in intestine for 6 days.

esophageal wall, in which event it is no longer a case of a foreign body in the esophagus. Furthermore, external esophagotomy requires a general anesthetic, which, because of its relaxation may permit the foreign body to move downward. In contrast to esophagotomy, esophagoscopy does not, as a rule, require general anesthesia, and while it may be occasionally found that the foreign body which shows so plainly in the radiograph has moved on downward to a lower position, or even into the stomach itself, no harm has been done. In case of its simply having moved to a lower position, it is just as readily removed with the esophagoscope as if it were at the higher point where originally seen in the radiograph. The most favorable statistics give a 20 per cent mortality for external esophagotomy in adults. The mortality is still higher in children, in some statistics as high as 42 per cent. Comparing such mortality with the two or three per cent mortality in esophagoscopy, the operation of external esophagotomy for foreign bodies has been rightly recommended only after failure of esophagoscopic extraction. Doubtless blind attempts at removal have increased the mortality of both procedures but as it has probably increased them both in the same ratio the relative percentages still hold good. It must be borne in mind, also, as pointed out by John C. DaCosta (Bib. 101) the esophagoscope in the hands of the inexperienced may be more dangerous than external esophagotomy. A recent book on surgery has advised the passage of a bougie to determine whether the foreign body is present, and if present to push it down. It should be unnecessary at this late day to warn against blind bouginage in foreign body cases. Citation of a few cases will suffice. One death from perforation with the bougie which did not push down a foreign body is reported by Arrowsmith. The patient was moribund on admission and told of the efforts of a physician to push the foreign body down. Mr. Waggette (Bib. 567) refers to a case in which a sharp piece of bone was overriden by the bougie passed by competent surgeons. If the bougie will thus override the foreign body in the hands of competent surgeons, and in certain hands may cause death, its use cannot be too often condemned as both inefficient and dangerous. Emerson (Bib. 134) reports the fatal case of perforation of the esophagus and aorta by a chicken bone after blind bouginage in a general hospital. The author can cite two cases. In one case, seen in consultation, a child of two years was dying from acute esophagitis. A penny had lodged in the esophagus five days before. Forceps had been passed blindly, without an esophagoscope. Two days after this utterly unjustifiable procedure, the temperature was 104°, pulse 150. When the author saw the patient, five days after operation, the temperature was subnormal, pulse fluttering and uncountable, sloughs were being vomited, and the child was sinking away in the profound shock of a traumatic esophagitis. The author concurred in wording the death certificate: "Death from acute esophagitis following the swallowing of a penny." It was really due to the absolute ignorance of the family physician who had never heard of esophagoscopy, and its safety in trained hands. In another case a child of six years was admitted to the Presbyterian Hospital with the history that five days before she had choked and vomited at dinner. It was supposed that a piece of bone had lodged in her throat. Two physicians had worked for two hours with instruments on the anesthetized patient, but had failed to remove any foreign body. The child's temperature was 101° F., pulse 128, and respiration 28. Appearance septic, breath foul, and swallowing difficult and very painful. Inspection of the pharynx showed a putrid gangrenous mass of mutilated tissues, too severely lacerated to justify examination. Discoloration and swelling externally simulated a "Ludwig's angina." Septic symptoms steadily increased and the child died five days after admission. Post mortem showed an abscess in left hypopharynx, gangrenous esophagitis, and bodies of three vertebrae partially denuded, the lowest damaged being the sixth. Macroscopically and microscopically, it was clear that the condition was due to recent trauma, and not to tuberculosis or other disease. No foreign body was found. This case gave a typical example of acute esophagitis from blind efforts at removal of a foreign body. Whether a foreign body had been present or not is not the point. It is one of the sad duties of the esophagoscopist to see little children brought in dying or seriously ill from rough, unjustifiable, brutal attempts to remove a foreign body by such relics of obsolete surgery as the Graefe basket, the coin catcher, Bond's forceps, bristle probangs, etc. It may be thought that the bristle probang should not be included here. Possibly its use may not be very dangerous in the adult, but in infants it has been fatal. The author has in his collection of esophagoscopically removed foreign bodies a number of bristles left behind from predecessor's probangs. Sir Felix Semon, with his acute observation and analytical mind, pointed out, years before the development of esophagoscopy, the danger of attempting to push down a foreign body that was lodged in the esophagus. He reported cases in which the foreign body had escaped such efforts and others in which the foreign body had been forced to perforate. He also pointed out that no foreign body, the presence of which has been actually detected, ought to be allowed to remain impacted, even if at the time it does not produce any serious symptoms. These two principles remain to-day fundamental in dealing with foreign bodies impacted in the air and food passages. Yet it is astonishing how, even to-day, practitioners will tell patients "to go home and forget about it" in some instances, while in others they will produce fatal traumatism by usually unsuccessful blind groping efforts. Emetics are inefficient and dangerous.

There is but one method of removal worthy of serious consideration and that is by esophagoscopy. It should always be used first. If it fail, which will be very rarely, then external operation is to be considered in cervically lodged foreign bodies.

CHAPTER XIX.

Esophagoscopy for Foreign Bodies.

*Mortality and results of esophagoscopy for foreign bodies.** Of 193 cases of esophagoscopy for foreign body by various operators, the intruder was removed in 155. Of the 38 not removed, 26 went down. There were 12 deaths (7.8 per cent). It is interesting to note that of the twelve deaths from esophagoscopy for foreign bodies, eight were for bodies in the upper third, four of the patients dying during operation, and in all four the foreign body was not removed until after death. All had been given chloroform, though this was probably only indirectly the cause of death. In seven of the eight, the esophagoscopy was done by operators whose total number of cases was less than three. In the large clinics (from previously published statistics) out of 210 cases of foreign bodies in this location, all were removed but twelve, and these went down. The mortality in the large clinics was 3 per cent. It is also interesting to note that in the present series of cases there were two deaths from laceration of the esophagus from violent removal of large foreign bodies, an artificial denture in one case, a large and rough bone in the other. In both instances the operators stated, in effect, that they believed they could have succeeded in devising methods of safe removal, had they realized the danger of esophageal trauma. Of the 206 cases of esophagoscopy for foreign bodies in the hospitals of Pittsburgh and in the author's work in other cities the foreign body was removed in 198, and escaped downward in eight. There were four deaths, one in a woman of 56 with advanced nephritis; the other three deaths were in patients admitted with severe laceration of the esophagus, from previous attempts at esophagoscopy. Four other cases seen *in extremis* are not included because owing to profound shock no esophagoscopy was done. There is not, and there never will be, an absolutely safe esophagoscope that can be used otherwise than with care and caution, for even the soft stomach tube has

*Abstracted, with additions, from the author's Rapport to the International Medical Congress, London, 1913.

caused perforation and death. But all endoscopists are now agreed that skillfully done under the guidance of the eye, esophagoscopy is practically without mortality, if considered apart from the trauma incident to foreign bodies and their extraction.

Indications for esophagoscopy in suspected foreign body cases. Esophagoscopy is indicated in every case in which a foreign body is known to be or suspected of being in the esophagus.

Contraindications to esophagoscopy in foreign body cases. There is no absolute contraindication to esophagoscopy for the removal of foreign bodies unless the patient is moribund from esophageal trauma from ill-advised blind efforts at removal; a state which, while less common than formerly, is still not unknown. If the patient is in bad condition from this cause, it is better to give stimulants, elevate the foot of the bed, keep the patient warm with blankets and hot water bottles and use all other means to counteract the shock of acute traumatic esophagitis before removing the foreign body. Bismuth taken dry on the tongue is the best local treatment in these cases. If there is a serious state o water hunger from occlusion of the esophagus by a foreign body tl esophagoscopy should be postponed until some water can be gotten ir the circulation. Water-starved patients make bad subjects for any p cedure and as the state is not fully understood the following case ma cited in the words of the pediatrist, H. T. Price. who was associated the author in the case of cherry stone occluding the previously stric esophagus of a girl of five years. No food or water had been swa for five days.

Report by Dr. Price. "Condition was alarming. Child una up when placed in a chair, eyes sunken and staring, color (yellowish). skin dry and harsh, lips very pale, child spoke wi seemed bewildered. Pulse almost imperceptible, no further made. Ordered normal saline solution by hypodermocly nine sulphate hypodermically. Seen about an hour later what better. pulse had better volume but was rapid. saline given by high enema, all retained and child re room. During examination child's condition contin no water expelled in spite of straining. Immedia cherry stone. while on the table child swallowed wa ily into stomach and condition steadily improve danger' from water hunger abo hours a ular

Aneurysm, serio re
sure, history of a
cautious esoph
esophagoscopy

if there is surgical emphysema, irritability, increasing fever, increasing rapidity of respiration, severe pain in the chest, aching in character, the foreign body has probably perforated and esophagoscopy is of questionable advisability, though in one such case the foreign body had not yet escaped and was caught and removed by the author. The above mentioned symptoms may be due to pleural perforation, in which case pneumothorax can be diagnosticated by physical signs and by radiography.

Endoscopic appearances of foreign bodies in the esophagus are the same as those previously mentioned in connection with foreign bodies in the air passages except that the color and form of esophageally lodged foreign bodies may be modified by accumulation of food debris or by bismuth given for radiographic or therapeutic purposes. Quite frequently the first view of a foreign substance will be a whitish or grayish mass of food debris mixed with secretions. The reader is referred to the comments on the difficulties due to the color of a foreign body in the bronchus which apply with equal force to intruders in the esophagus. Kahler reports a case in which a nodulation due to the calcification impressions of the thyroid gland were mistaken for a foreign body in the esophagus.

ESOPHAGOSCOPIC EXTRACTION OF FOREIGN BODIES.

Anesthesia, preparation of the patient, position of the patient, technic of introduction of the esophagoscope and of the esophageal speculum have all been considered in prior chapters. The "Rules" mentioned under bronchoscopy for foreign bodies are applicable to esophagoscopy for the same class of cases. As there mentioned it is unwise to go into any foreign body case insufficiently equipped with the idea of taking a preliminary look. Everything likely to be needed for the extraction of the intruder in question should be sterile and ready for immediate use. A second trial may find the problem incomparably more difficult. There should also be ready, in every esophageal case, a direct laryngoscope and a bronchoscope, for adult or child as the case may be. The foreign body may be in the air passages, either primarily or by erosion as in the case previously cited; or, more important still, respiratory arrest may result from overriding or displacement of the intruder by the esophagoscope or by efforts at disimpaction, faulty position of the patient, etc. In such cases prompt insertion of a bronchoscope and bronchoscopic oxygen insufflation may save life without a tracheotomy. Tracheotomy instruments should always be upon the sterile instrument table as a matter of routine. Those who are prompt and skillful in bronchoscopy will not need them and, indeed, it is exceedingly rarely that respiratory arrest occurs in esophagoscopy, especially if no anesthesia is used; yet it is a good general rule in all tracheo-esophageal cases to have tracheotomy instruments always prepared as a routine procedure for the rare cases of urgent necessity.

The author has among his personal armamentarium, two lengths of esophagoscopes, one for children and one for adults. It is impossible, in looking through the tube to tell whether a short or the long tube is being used, and so far as instrumentation is concerned, there is no advantage in short instruments, provided the long ones are properly constructed. The little light is close to the foreign body and perfectly illuminates the field, no matter how many instruments are introduced in the tube. All that is necessary is to look past the instruments. The instrument does not lessen the illumination. In using the long tube, if the foreign body is not found at the level where it shows in the radiograph, the entire esophagus is at once explored clear through to the stomach, and even the cardial end of the stomach can be searched. So far as introduction is concerned, a long tube is easier of manipulation than a short tube. A tube of large diameter is always preferable, because with it one is much less likely to override the foreign body; but on the other hand, a tube of large diameter is much less easy of introduction. For complicated removals, such as the closing of safety pins, the cutting of fishhooks and the like, of course the manipulations are much easier through a tube of large diameter. These considerations, however, must not lead us to endanger our patient by the use of too large a tube. The author uses a tube of 7 mm. internal diameter in children and 10 mm. diameter in adults. In no case is it wise to use a mandrin in exploring the esophagus for foreign bodies. A mandrin makes introduction somewhat easier for the beginner, but it is very likely to cause the overriding of a foreign body in the cervical esophagus, and there is always risk of a diseased esophageal wall whether a foreign body be present or not.

Sponging with the long sponge holder should be done very carefully, lest the foreign body be hidden in the secretions and be dislodged by the sponging. It is usually unnecessary to sponge at this stage because the aspirator in the wall of the esophagoscope is draining away the secretions. If small food masses are seen, it is almost certain that the foreign body lies just below, and these food masses should not be wiped away but should be picked out with the forceps lest the foreign body be disturbed. When the tube mouth reaches the proximity of the foreign body, it will be noticed if the foreign body is of sufficient size to distend the esophagus, that the esophagus seems to roll in over the foreign body which only shows in the center of the rather small lumen of the esophagus. As the tube mouth approaches more closely, this folding in of the mucosa will be distended and the foreign body comes more largely into view. If the foreign body is a coin or something of that nature, not involving any special problem on removal, it is best not to approach too closely with the tube mouth; but to insert the forceps just as soon as the foreign body comes into view. The forceps jaws should always open in the up and down direction, regardless of the plane in which the foreign body is to be seen. With all flat objects, this will bring the forceps in the correct position. In case of foreign bodies situated in other planes, or to be seized in other planes, it is better not to rotate the stilette of the forceps to make the jaws open in any other plane; but rather to place the handle in the position required for the jaws to open in the proper direction. The advantage of this is that the jaws always open in the same way, making it very much easier to follow their movements by sight. Special problems of removal will be considered later.

Difficulties. The difficulties of introduction of the esophagoscope have been previously considered. The difficulties of removal will be considered as mechanical problems. But a few words must be said of difficulties in finding a foreign body known to be present.

"Overriding," or failure to find a foreign body known to be present. One of the most difficult things for the beginner in esophagoscopy to understand is how a foreign body, especially one not of minute size, can "get lost" in the esophagus. The author is often asked how it is possible for an esophagoscope to be passed many times into the esophagus, and not reveal a penny, for instance, which a radiograph shows to be present. The explanation is found in the anatomy of the esophagus. If the esophagus were a tube of equal size throughout with rigid walls standing patulous without folds, or if an esophagoscope large enough entirely to fill the lumen were passed, the foreign body would promptly present itself at the tube mouth. But, as shown in Fig. 145, the esophagus is constricted at certain points which prevents the passage of an esophagoscope large enough to fill out its collapsed walls at the larger portions in which small foreign bodies such as needles, pins, and fish ribs may be hidden. But this is not often the explanation of failure to find coins. More often coins and similar objects are just below the plica cricopharyngeus which latter makes a veritable chute in throwing the end of the esophagoscope forward to override the foreign body and to interpose a layer of tissue between the tube and the coin so that contact at the side of the tube after the tube mouth is passed is not felt. Another hiding place for foreign bodies, especially those of small size, is the pyriform sinuses. Food naturally passes through both pyriform sinuses and there is so little room directly back of the cricoid that the esophagoscope is usually passed through one of the two sinuses, generally the right. Therefore if a foreign body is not found on the passage

downward, the distal end of the tube should be kept pressing to the left on withdrawal so as to explore the left sinus on the way out. Of course if the radiograph should show the intruder to be in the left pyriform sinus the esophagoscope may be passed that way though the retrograde search has the advantage of not risking the pushing of the intruder downward. A better method, however, in all cases of high foreign bodies is to use the esophageal speculum, Fig. 21. This instrument has enabled the author to remove, in three instances, the particularly elusive rib bones of fish after skilful esophagoscopists had failed. In one instance two good tube workers had each tried for two hours under general anesthesia to remove a fish rib which was promptly revealed, not by superior skill on the author's part, but by the advantage yielded by the use of the esophageal speculum. The bone was sticking deeply in the esophageal wall just below the plica cricopharyngeus. Coins that have been in the esophagus a few weeks show a polished streak up and down the middle third of their anterior (rarely posterior) surface evidently corresponding to the usual course of food in swallowing, the esophagus not being fully dilated, and the lateral edges of the coin being clamped in the lateral folds of the esophageal wall. In some instances the esophagoscope overriding the tube, probably follows the same route (anterior to the coin intruder). When a silver coin has been in the hypopharynx the central third is darkened by sulphides, while the lateral thirds, corresponding to the pyriform sinuses are bright from passage of the food at the sides of the upper part of the hypopharynx. The intruder may be overridden because it is hidden by secretions, or by being buried under the mucosa or under inflammatory tissue. These are unusual and in most instances the trouble will be found to be the chute-like effect of the cricopharyngeus or the lurking of the foreign body in the other pyriform sinus or in the undilated folds of the esophagus, to all of which the use of an esophagoscope of relatively small diameter contributes. Summarizing, the chief factors in overriding of an esophageally lodged foreign body are:

1. The chute-like effect of the plica cricopharyngeus.
2. The lurking of the foreign body in the unexplored pyriform sinus.
3. The use of an esophagoscope of small diameter.
4. The obscuration of the intruder by secretion or food debris.
5. The obscuration of the intruder by its penetration of the esophageal wall.
6. The obscuration of the intruder by inflammatory sequelae.

Extraction of foreign bodies with the esophageal speculum. Almost all of the esophageally lodged foreign bodies are to be found at or above the sternal notch. Of these, fully one-half can be removed with the esophageal speculum. It must be remembered, however, that, in a radiograph, a foreign body may look much higher than it really is. Doubtless this is the reason why so many deplorable, even fatal, attempts at blind removal with forceps are made. It *seems* an easy task to reach it with almost any kind of forceps—even a hemostat. When an esophagoscope is passed, the reverse mistake is usually made. The foreign body is reached, possibly overridden without being seen, before the operator realizes that he is down to the level indicated in the radiograph. A correct estimate is made more difficult by the distortion dependent upon the position of the radiographic tube. If the tube be placed exactly over the foreign body, that is, if the intruder and the center of the radiographic tube are on the same vertical line, there will be no distortion. But as this cannot be done without knowing beforehand the location of the intruder it would require a repetition of the radiography. For practical purposes it may be said that any foreign body that is not more than one centimeter below the lower border of the cricoid cartilage in a child, or more than two in an adult, is more easily dealt with by the esophageal speculum than by the esophagoscope provided the esophagoscopist has mastered the use of the speculum. But all cases can be dealt with by the long esophagoscopic tube, and thorough mastery of it will be more successful than partial mastery of each. In infants the child's size laryngoscope may be used as an esophageal speculum.

The introduction of the esophageal speculum is described in a previous chapter. Certain points should, however, be emphasized. The author prefers recumbency of the patient. The head of the patient must be elevated above the level of the table and should be extended fully but not violently. The speculum is held in the operator's left hand as shown for the laryngeal speculum in Figs. 89 and 90. The tip of the instrument, which should be very smooth, is slid into the right pyriform sinus along the posterior hypopharyngeal wall with only enough anterior lifting with the tip to open up the lumen ahead. No amount of lifting can pull the cricoid cartilage away from the spine, and all the displacement required is to lift the walls of the right pyriform sinus. This at times requires what to some may seem a considerable degree of power, but it is in no case as much as required for a good exposure of the larynx by direct laryngoscopy by the dorsolingual route. When the bottom of the pyriform sinus is reached, it will be known by the obstruction due to the cricopharyngeal fold coming forward from the posterior (lower in the recumbent patient) wall and seeming to cause the lumen entirely to disappear. At this stage the tip of the speculum should be guided slightly toward the median line and lifted. Too powerful lifting here again is to be avoided because the cricopharyngeal fold will follow all the more. It is better to push the speculum, not too forcibly, with the thumb and finger of the right hand while the left hand exerts sufficient lifting motion to find the lumen. Just at this point, it is especially necessary to proceed cautiously as the foreign body very often lies immediately below the spasmodically contracted plica cricopharyngeus. If this spasm suddenly relaxes, the foreign body may be pushed downward by a sudden advance of the speculum. The head of the patient at this stage must be noted to see that it is high. If not, it must be raised for the reasons explained in the schema, Fig. 149. As soon as the tip of the speculum passes the plica cricopharyngeus this fold will obscure the view of half the lumen. The plica should be pushed posteriorly with the closed alligator forceps (of Mosher or Paterson) used simply as a repressor, as the tube advances (Plate III, Fig. 3). As soon as the foreign body is seen, if it be a coin, smooth button, or the like, it may be at once seized with the alligator forceps. If it be a sharp, rough, irregular or transfixed body it must be seized according to the mechanical problem presented. In case of such bodies, instead of the plain alligator forceps the author's alligator rotation forceps (Fig. 210) should be used (closed) for the retraction of the plica cricopharyngeus so as to be ready to seize the foreign body in such a way as to permit of the rotation of the intruder as explained under "Mechanical Problems."

Mechanical problems of esophagoscopic removal of foreign bodies. If any argument were needed against the blind attempts at removal, it is the consideration of the various admirable solutions of mechanical problems that have been devised for endoscopic use. To any one who will review this subject, the use of blind methods is preposterous, almost criminal. The esophagus is, surgically, the most intolerant organ in the body. It must be dealt with in the most careful, gentle way, always under the guidance of the eye. The greatest triumph of esophagoscopy over every other method of dealing with foreign bodies in the esophagus is in the low mortality of esophagoscopic methods. The thought that if left, the body probably will be fatal anyway, does not justify violence. A careful study of the mechanical problems presented will always discover a safe method of removal. In view of this, the great temptation to remove the body at all hazards once it is grasped, must be resisted. Most of the mechanical problems and their solution as considered in connection with bronchoscopy for foreign bodies, are equally applicable to esophagoscopy.

As in bronchoscopy side movements of the forceps are accomplished by the leverage of the endoscopic tube, the mouth of which can be used to force the distal end of the forceps in any direction angular to the long axis of the esophagus.

Extraction of foreign bodies fixed crosswise in the esophagus. Bodies fixed crosswise in the esophagus present much the same problem and are removable upon the same principle as those fixed crosswise in the bronchi, to which section the reader is referred. There are, however, some problems of crosswise fixation that are peculiar to esophagoscopy. For instance, in the esophagus there is no limit to distance to which a long foreign body may be pushed downward to disengage the point. In the bronchi, however, a long foreign body may already have one end down as far as it can go, so that disengaging the buried upward-projecting point by pushing the foreign body downward becomes a difficult matter. One of the most important things in the

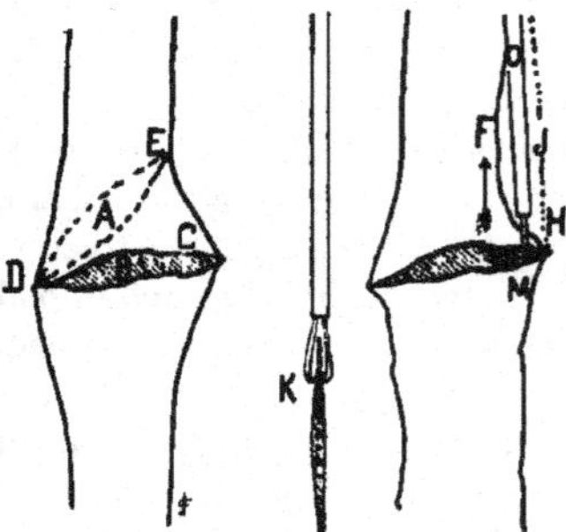

Fig. 208.—The problem of the horizontally transfixed foreign body in the esophagus. The point, D, had caught as the bone, A, was being swallowed. The end, E, was forced down to C, by food or by blind attempts at pushing the bone downward. The wall, F, should be pushed laterally out to J, permitting the forceps to grasp the end, M, of the bone. Traction in the direction of the dart will disimpact the bone and permit it to rotate. The author's rotation forceps are used as at K.

removal of a foreign body from either the esophagus or the tracheobronchial tree is to determine at what point the foreign body should be seized in order that it shall come out without injury to the tissues. Therefore, in all cases except those of smooth disk-like bodies, it would be a serious error not to get a good view of the foreign body before attempting to seize it with the forceps. In case of thin, sharp foreign bodies, such as bones, needles, double pointed tacks, pins, dentures, safety pins, and the like, found, as they often are, crosswise in the esophagus, very careful work is necessary (Fig. 208). Foreign bodies reach this position probably by one point, for instance, D, sticking in the esophageal wall. The foreign body is then in the position shown at

A, by the dotted line. The force of the subsequently swallowed food continually pushes the upper point, E, downward until it reaches the maximum stretch of the esophagus, as shown at B. To remove such a body, it is necessary to catch one of the ends, either D or C, never by the middle, B, as traumatism would be almost certain to follow the latter procedure. If either end of the intruder is higher, this is the end to seize. When the intruder is first seen it is usually the central part, B, that is in front of the tube mouth. In order to apply the forceps at the end, M, it is necessary to move the esophageal wall, F, out to the position shown by the dotted line, J, by swinging the esophagoscope as a lever, the proximal end of which moves in a direction oppo-

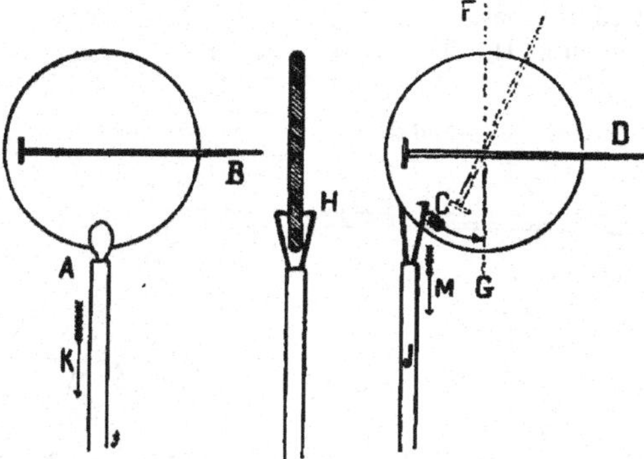

FIG. 209.—Solution of the mechanical problem of the button or other disk-like object with a sharp point. If withdrawn with a plain forceps applied as at A, the point, B, will rip open the esophageal wall. If grasped at C, the point, D, will rotate in the direction of F and will trail harmlessly behind. To permit rotation, the author's rotation forceps are used as at H.

site to that desired for the lower end. Pins lodged in the esophagus, are, in the author's experience, almost invariably found point downward, exactly opposite to their position in the trachea and bronchi. The probable reason for this is that in the air passages gravity acting strongest in the head of the pin causes it to fall head lowermost. In the esophagus, which is a collapsed canal, there is less chance for gravity to act effectively, and, more important, pins going head first probably do not lodge, hence, pass on through; whereas, if they start point first, the point will stick into the lateral wall. It is the lodged cases that come to the esophagoscopist. The importance of this as a mechanical problem lies in the necessity for caution in the esophagoscopy lest the head of the pin, impinging on the esophagoscope, may cause the point to perforate, either by the direct push of the esophagoscope against the pin or the counterpush of the heaving upward of the esophagus in reflex movements of vomiturition or vomiting.

Extraction of broad foreign bodies having a sharp point. As illustrated in Fig. 209, if the forceps were used to grasp the foreign body flatly by the portion which presented, as shown schematically at A, Fig. 209, the point, B, would rip the esophagus open. If, on the other hand, the button were caught with forceps which touched only at the points and these points were applied to one side, as shown at C, as soon as the traction was made, the point, D, would rotate to the position shown by the dotted line, F G, and would be withdrawn harmlessly. Free rotation is permitted by the forceps which touch the foreign body only at the point, as shown at H. The forceps used for this purpose are the au-

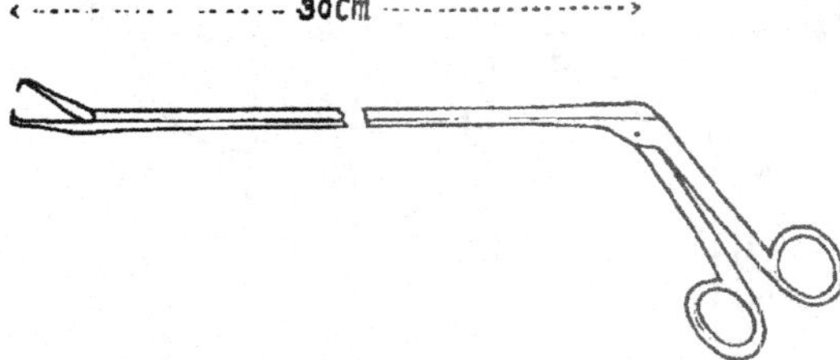

FIG. 210.—Author's rotation forceps (short form) for permitting foreign bodies to rotate to the position of least harm and least resistance. For use through the esophageal speculum.

thor's rotation forceps shown in Fig. 33. For use with the esophageal speculum, the author's alligator form of rotation forceps, Fig. 210, are more convenient. These forceps are dangerous to use otherwise than by sight, because of the possibility of trauma.

Extraction of open safety pins from the esophagus. If lodged point downward it is necessary only to pull the pin into the esophagoscope to close it, but in so doing the hook-like protector end of the pin may cause trauma. It is better to hold the near end of the pin with the forceps while the esophagoscope is pushed down over the pin. An open safety pin lodged point upward in the esophagus presents certain peculiar elements of danger, and peculiar difficulties of removal. When the esophagoscopist sees the pin in the esophagoscope, the temptation to seize it and remove it is great. To do so is almost certain death. Besides the risk of septic mediastinitis and pleuritis, there is the immediate surgical risk. Two such cases have come to the writer's knowledge by communications. In one instance, death was from hemorrhage into the mediastinum. What vessel was perforated was not known. From the location of the pin, it was probably the aorta. In the other instance, shock from esophageal trauma was the cause. In adults or older children, the pin can be closed before removal as described in connection

FIG. 211.—Radiograph by Dr. George C. Johnston, showing open safety pin, point up, in the esophagus of an infant, aged eleven months. Pin was passed into stomach, turned and removed esophagoscopically. Pin retouched for clearness. (Author's case).

with safety pins in the bronchi. The author has had a number of such cases. In infants, the esophagus is already in such a state of tension by the stretching spread of the spring (E, Fig. 212), that perforation is certain if the dilatation of the insertion of an instrument be added. The solution of the mechanical problem of safe removal when the first undernoted case presented itself, led the author to devise a new method which is practicable for anyone who has practiced gastroscopy. Republication here of a report (Bib. 256) of the first two cases will suffice to illustrate the method.

Elizabeth G., aged eleven months, referred by Dr. August Soffel and Dr. C. C. Sandels. Admitted to the Eye and Ear Hospital August 13, 1909, with a history of having swallowed a safety pin. A radiograph (Fig. 211), by Dr. George C. Johnston, showed the pin to be of large size and spread so widely open that it seemed certain, considering

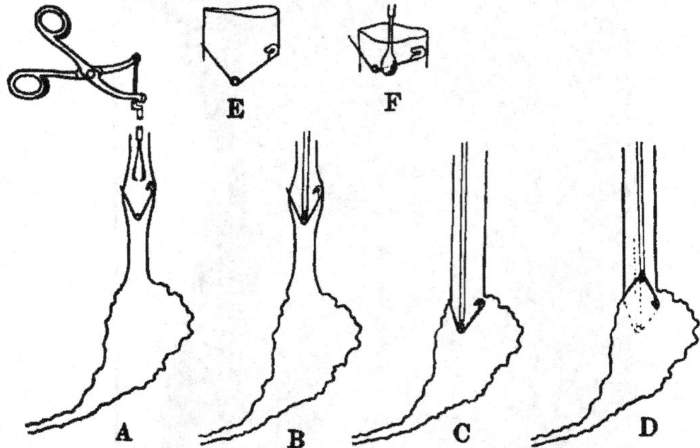

Fig. 212.—Schema showing the author's method of removal of upward pointed esophageally lodged open safety pins by passing them into stomach, where they are turned and removed. The first illustration (A) shows the rotation forceps before seizing pin by the ring of the spring end. (Forceps jaws are shown opening in the wrong diameter). At B is shown the pin seized in the ring by the points of the forceps. At C is shown the pin carried into the stomach and about to be rotated by withdrawal. D, the withdrawal of the pin into the esophagoscope which will thereby close it. If withdrawn by flat-jawed forceps as at F, the esophageal wall would be fatally lacerated.

the age of the patient, that the esophagus was perforated. The temperature 102.4, the respiration 40, the pulse 140, weak and irritable, all plainly indicated acute esophagitis. To use the safety pin closer, which, because of the small esophagus, would have to be passed external to the tube, before the insertion of the tube, was not to be thought of for the reason previously given. The author had made the forceps shown in Fig. 33. Passing the esophagoscope under ether anesthesia, the pin was quickly located, surrounded by an area of acute esophagitis. The point was buried the full extent of the taper. Under ocular guidance, the author seized the pin by the ring, as shown at B in Fig. 212. Following with the esophagoscope, the pin was pushed downward, thus withdrawing the point of the pin from its bed in the esophageal wall and gently carrying the pin, securely held, but free to move, down into the stomach as shown at C, Fig. 212. Withdrawal of the forceps turned the pin by the keeper and the point striking the wall of the stomach; and the pin was pulled into the esophagoscope sufficiently far to close it, though it was too large to be removed through the tube. The esophagoscope, forceps and pin were all withdrawn together. Dr. Homer McCready, who manipulated the aspirator, reported no stain of blood in the secretions. The entire procedure required but seven minutes. The fever subsided in a few days and the child went home well.

Remarks. The action of the forceps will be understood from Fig. 212. If the ring were seized with the ordinary flat-jawed forceps (as at F), the pin could not be turned without risk of losing it and causing delay. The special rotation forceps hold the pin securely at the ring but allow it to turn freely without letting go. The pin cannot turn the full 180 degrees, but it can turn far enough to allow it to be drawn into the tube where it is safely housed for removal. If a small pin, it can be withdrawn through the tube as in the second case. The question may be asked. Why is it safer to turn the pin in the stomach than in the esophagus? There is more room, so that there is no pressure on the point of the pin, the pin being free to turn; and, most important, the stomach wall is thick and strong as compared to that of the esophagus, though we must not be tempted into roughness by this. Gastroscopic manipulations must be gentle.

Margaret K., aged fourteen months, referred by Dr. F. L. Ives. A radiograph (Fig. 214) by Dr. L. Gregory Cole, of New York City, showed the pin to be lodged point upward in the esophagus. At the Eye and Ear Hospital, two days after the swallowing of the pin the author removed it by the same method as in the previous case, but, being smaller in size, the pin could be withdrawn through the tube. The child returned home well on the second day. Illustrations of the pins are shown in Chapter XXI.

So far the author has not lost the pin from the grip of the forceps while at work on a case. Twice, however, in demonstration work defective forceps allowed the pin to escape. It was thus discovered that the forceps must be made exactly as shown in Fig. 33.

D. R. Paterson has devised a very ingenious method of passing a small tube over the point of the safety pin and then catching the safety pin by the other limb and thus removing it safely, the little tube, forceps, pin and esophagoscope all being brought out together. Mosher, Hubbard and others have devised very ingenious pin closers.

Extraction of double pointed tacks and staples lodged point upward in the esophagus. If very short these objects could be turned by grasping them by the lower or curved end. A safer method and one that must be adopted in case of longer tacks or staples is to carry the in-

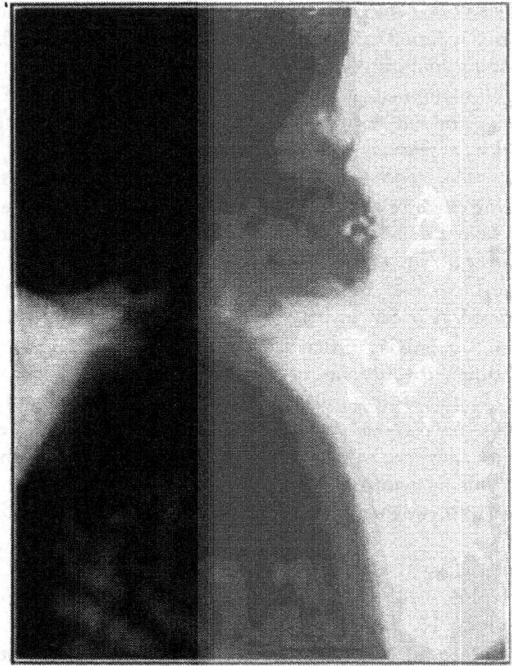

FIG. 213.—Lateral radiograph (by Dr. George C. Johnston) of a safety pin in a child of 11 months, demonstrating the esophageal location of the pin in this case and the great value of the lateral radiograph of foreign body cases. (Author's case. See Figs. 272 and 212.)

truder down into the stomach there to be turned as described for safety pins. The safety pin or rotation forceps (Fig. 33) must be used. Under no circumstances should such an intruder be pulled upon with the ordinary forceps.

Extraction of fish hooks from the esophagus. The author has never yet had to deal endoscopically with a fish hook, but there are four methods by which the mechanical problem can probably be solved. The first of these is that by which D. R. Paterson removed a fish hook from the level of the body of the fifth dorsal vertebra of a boy aged thirteen years. The hook had the usual gut leader about nine inches in length projecting from the patient's mouth. Dr. Paterson passed the esophagoscope over the gut leader and then threaded a bronchoscopic aspirating tube over the leader so that when passed down to the level of the hook the bulbous extremity of the aspirating tube fitted into the curve of the

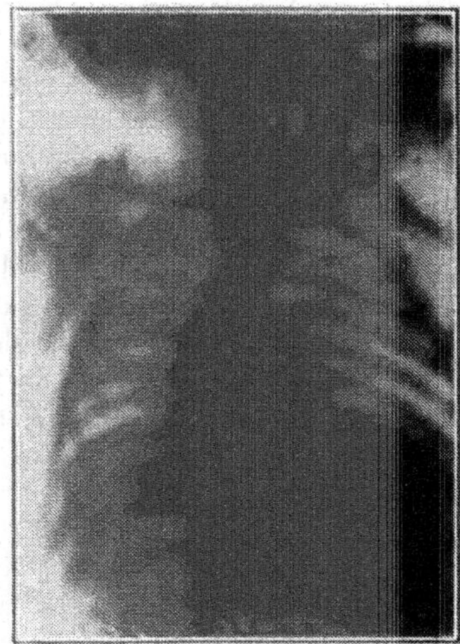

FIG. 214.—Radiograph by Dr. L. Gregory Cole, (New York), showing safety pin in the esophagus of an infant aged fourteen months. Passed into the stomach, turned and removed under esophagoscopic guidance. (Author's case).

hook which was thus safeguarded and withdrawn. In the event of encountering a hook that has an eye instead of the gut leader, forceps could be used to thread a braided silk through the eye and then the distal end being brought up we would have a double thread coming out the mouth. Over this double thread the aspirating tube could be passed as was done by Dr. Paterson in his case. In the event of the eye being too large to pass through the aspirating tube, a similar tube could be readily constructed for the purpose with a larger lumen, or a flattened lumen, if necessary. A second method would be to use the pin cutting forceps, Fig. 34. These, however, would probably not extract the fragment, if the barb was buried in the esophageal wall, though if properly constructed they should hold the fragment if the barb was not buried. The loss of the point with the barb would certainly be a risky procedure because of the certainty of the barb working its way through distant tissues. While the patient might possibly escape serious injury from this cause, the author believes that the third method will be found the easiest and the most practical as well as the most certain. This consists in passing the fish hook down into the stomach, turning it and bringing it out with the curve end first, the point trailing behind, if too large to pull the entire curved part of the fish hook into the distal end of the esophagoscope. This procedure would be precisely the same as mentioned in regard to safety pins and fence staples. This has been so readily accomplished by the author in dealing with safety pins and staples that he feels quite certain that it could be even more readily done in the case of the fish hook. Pressure downward with the forceps after grasping would certainly extract the barb. A fourth method would be by catching the point and barb in the tissue forceps, Fig. 35, after pushing the hook downward sufficiently to disembed the barbed end. Thus protected with the box-like covering of the tissue forceps the intruder could probably be withdrawn harmlessly. As before stated the author has had no opportunity to deal with the fish hook problem in the human being but he has practiced these procedures until he believes that each of them can be done upon the human being by very careful work. For such manipulations he would deem a general anesthetic advisable unless absolutely contraindicated.

Extraction of foreign bodies of large size from the esophagus. The removal of very large, rough and sharp bodies, such as bones and artificial dentures, from the esophagus deserves special consideration. Many cases have been needlessly (and occasionally unsuccessfully) operated externally. The esophagus is a highly spasmodic tube. One of the functions of nausea is to relax the esophagus and prevent spasm in order to facilitate vomiting though, of course, vomiting can occur without nausea. When the attempt is made to withdraw a foreign body spasm is excited and constriction occurs. This has been frequently demonstrated to others by the author. When a body is large, sharp and rough the spasm excited is much greater and even if it were not, constriction means more with such a body than with a small, smooth, round one. It ought not to require much argument to convince anyone of the necessity of the relaxation of deep general anesthesia for all cases of esophagoscopic removal of large, sharp or rough foreign bodies. With such relaxation any intruder, no matter how large or sharp, that has gone down through natural passages can come up the same way; provided that, in the withdrawal, as occurred naturally in the intrusion, the intruder is turned to the most favorable position. It is necessary to relax not only the esophageal musculature itself but also the musculature which acts upon the surrounding hard and soft anatomic structures, such as the action of the constrictors on the cricoid cartilage and even the diaphragmatic musculature in the rare cases of withdrawal of a foreign body from below the hiatal level. In case of small foreign bodies, the relaxation of deep anesthesia may lose the intruder downward. In large impacted bodies there is no likelihood of this, but procedure must be careful to avoid respiratory arrest as before mentioned.

Millspaugh (Bib. 383) in a very interesting paper, reports the removal of a large vulcanite plate on which were two teeth, demonstrating clearly what careful manipulations can do in the removal endoscopically of these large foreign bodies which heretofore have been considered as demanding external operation. The interesting case of esophagoscopic removal, by Dr. D. Braden Kyle, of a vulcanite tooth plate is reported in a subsequent paragraph.

In exceptional cases it may be necessary to comminute a large foreign body, as was done by Killian with rare skill in case of a vulcanite tooth plate.

Extraction of meat and other foods from the esophagus. Meat in the esophagus, after it has become macerated, can sometimes be removed very readily with forceps. In many cases, however, the mechanical spoon, Fig. 40, will be found very much better, inasmuch as it can be placed below the meat, the spoon turned up and the meat pulled *en masse* into the mouth of the esophagoscope.

Extraction of foreign bodies from the strictured esophagus. At first thought, it might seem unusual to have the combination in the same case of a stricture of the esophagus and a foreign body. Yet such a combination is by no means infrequent. Foreign bodies of relatively small size will lodge in a strictured esophagus, but would pass through a normal gullet. Children, especially, will fail to masticate food thoroughly, or will allow the foreign body, such as chewing gum, grape pulp, including the seeds, orange seeds, watermelon seeds, and the like, to slip down. The author had one case where he removed, at different times, four different foreign bodies from the esophagus of one child undergoing treatment for stricture. The situation becomes still more complicated when the patient has an upper stricture relatively larger than the lower one, and the foreign body passing the first one lodges at the second, and still more difficult is the case if the second stricture is considerably below the first and not concentric. Under these circumstances, it is best to divulse the upper stricture mechanically with the divulsor shown in Fig. 52, when a small tube can be inserted past the first stricture, thus at the same time simplifying the removal and accomplishing one stage of the treatment for the stenosis. In some of these stricture cases bismuth may completely occlude the lumen of the stricture when given in the large quantities sometimes required for a radiograph. This is much less apt to follow a mixture of bismuth with milk than with bread or porridge. In either case it is not difficult to remove the bismuth esophagoscopically, using the sponges in the sponge holder, and, if necessary, the mechanical spoon until the lumen of the stricture is reached, when the opening may be found with a small probe, and afterwards small olives can be passed. The surplus bismuth should be removed upward so as not to occlude the canal again. Usually such patients can regurgitate a large part of the contents of the esophagus, and it remains only for the esophagoscopist to clean out the remainder by the means mentioned.

Extraction of foreign bodies after prolonged sojourn in the esophagus. The leading case is that of D. Braden Kyle (Bib. 319). A tooth plate had remained in the esophagus for eighteen years. A physician called shortly after the accident assured the patient that the teeth were not in the esophagus on the strength of a negative result with bougies and probangs. The tooth plate was located radiographically (Fig. 215). With the esophagoscope, Dr. Kyle found the foreign body eighteen centimeters from the upper teeth. The upper edge was covered with fibrous tissue. At four sittings, Dr. Kyle in his careful, skillful way disimpacted and removed the tooth plate from its bed. The patient had slight difficulty in swallowing for a time, but in three months could readily swallow semisolid food.

In these cases of prolonged sojourn of the foreign body in the esophagus, the inflammatory exudate will contract after the foreign body is removed and stricture of greater or less extent is almost certain to follow, so that in all such cases, it is wise to keep a close watch on the patient, and if stricture follow, it should be treated by the same methods as other cicatricial stenoses, to be considered later.

Foreign bodies buried in pharyngeal and esophageal tissues. In cases of needles, headless pins and the like having entered and disappeared in the tissues of the pharynx, they should be followed through the wound of entrance if this can be found. Otherwise, they should be searched for by finger palpation aided by accurate localization with both an anteroposterior and a lateral radiograph. When thus located an incision should be made crosswise to the long axis of the pin. This is imperative, because if the incision is parallel the chances of striking the pin are remote. Two cases of this kind were seen in the author's service at the Eye and Ear Hospital. In one of these, previously reported (Bib.

269, page 127), a double pointed pin had wandered from the wound of entrance and was removed from the posterior wall of the laryngopharynx. In the second case, that of a needle in the tissues back of the hypopharynx of a woman of forty years, the needle was accurately located by anteroposterior and lateral radiographs by Dr. Russell H. Boggs. It could not be palpated because of its depth; but by an endoscopic estimate of the radiographically determined distance of the center of the long axis of the needle upward from the cricoid cartilage, a crosswise incision with the long laryngeal knife (Fig. 85) passed through the esophageal speculum (Fig. 21), the author was so fortunate as to strike the

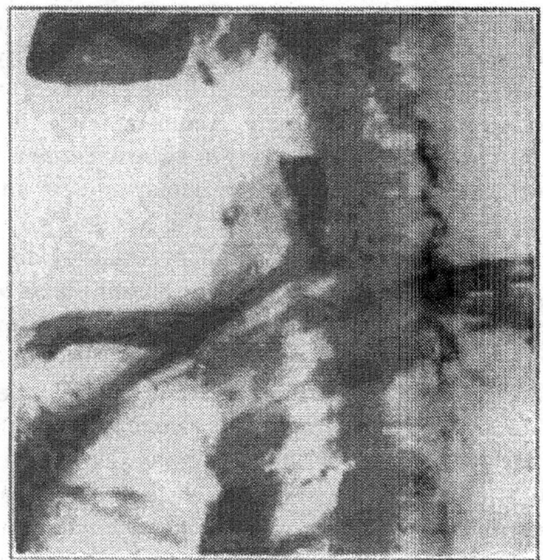

FIG. 215.—Radiograph showing tooth plate in the esophagus where it had been for 18 years. (Removed by Dr. D. Braden Kyle).

needle at the first incision. The wound was covered with bismuth subnitrate by insufflation. Bismuth was ordered in five grain doses dry on the tongue every hour. Healing was complete in about a week, without any rise of temperature or complication except slight subcutaneous emphysema which subsided in a few days. When foreign bodies have invaded the intrathoracic periesophageal tissues, it is unwise to make an incision to reach them, and even through the wound of entrance it is unwise to pursue them far. It is, however, justifiable in cases in which there is local or radiographic evidence of a buried foreign body, carefully to explore the wound by instrumental palpation. The best exploring instrument for this purpose is the forceps, Fig. 28, which are inserted closed. Should the exploration transmit the sensation of a foreign body the forceps are expanded and the foreign body is seized. This exploration refers only to recent cases with a visible wound of entrance or those in which the wound channel is marked by granulation tissue. Where the foreign body has perforated the anterior esophageal wall at any point above the tracheal bifurcation, the foreign body may be found in the trachea of which an instance is elsewhere herein reported. If there is no wound visible, fluoroscopic aid for localization may be sought as elsewhere mentioned, but great care must be used.

As pointed out by Ingals (Bib. 226)—"An operator must not too readily conclude that something which to him appears unnatural is the wound through which a coin or button that cannot be found has made its way into the esophageal wall, for in the great majority of cases it would be very much more likely that such a foreign body was hidden by a fold of edematous tissues." Under no circumstances is it justifiable to explore except in the most gentle way an apparent wound in the esophageal wall and even careful exploration should not be attempted until the entire esophagus has been explored for the foreign body and a radiograph has been taken to determine whether or not the foreign body has emerged through the esophageal wall. The author has seen five cases of abscess of the esophagus from foreign body traumatism and in two of the cases the foreign body was lodged inside the abscess. In one such case of the author, referred by Dr. Clarence M. Harris, the patient was unable to swallow. Upon passage of the esophagoscope the esophagus was found occluded at the level of the lower border of the cricoid by a smooth rounded swelling on the apex of which was a small crater-like opening. The pressure of the tube caused pus to exude and the abscess was thus completely evacuated. The patient had no further difficulty in swallowing though there was slight odynphagia for a few days during which bismuth subnitrate and calomel were given. Complete recovery resulted in one week. No foreign body was found in the pus and it was quite clear that the abscess resulted simply from the infective inflammation of the puncture of the foreign body, a bone.

Fluroscopic esophagoscopy seems to the author an unjustifiable procedure. In case of foreign bodies that have entered bronchi too small for an endoscopic tube to enter, the foreign body cannot be found except by relatively blind endoscopic methods and therefore fluoroscopic bronchoscopy may have a legitimate, though limited, field of usefulness. But in the esophagus where every square millimeter of surface is explorable by sight, fluoroscopic esophagoscopy is a step backward that is unjustifiable. A possible use for the fluoroscope in this connection would be in a case of a foreign body having wandered out through the esophageal wall, in which case it is no longer a foreign body in the esophagus. To pursue it under fluoroscopic guidance would be more dangerous than external operation. If the latter is not advisable at once the wanderings of the invader can be watched radiographically and operation deferred until the foreign body reaches a favorable location. In case a foreign body shows clearly in a radiograph, after the esophagoscopic search has proven negative and no wound of entrance is discoverable, it is advisable to use the fluoroscope to obtain accurate localization of the position of the foreign body simply to explore the wound endoscopically under ocular guidance to the limited extent such exploration may be deemed advisable. Unfortunately this can be done only in very recent cases and even in these the intruder may have traveled far, so that it may be nowhere near its wound of entrance. It is usually pins, needles and similar slender, sharp pointed bodies that escape through the esophageal wall. The author had one case, that of a common pin that had escaped—all but the head. He was fortunately able in this particular instance to find the head endoscopically and remove the pin; but he can easily see how information from the fluoroscopist working jointly with the endoscopist could, in such a case, give assistance of the utmost value, especially with the double-plane fluoroscope devised for the author by Dr. Grier.

In cases of bodies of irregular shape the fluorescent screen affords no evidence whatever that the foreign body is being so seized that it will not lacerate the esophagus during withdrawal.

As mentioned by D. R. Paterson injury has been done by fluoroscopic esophagoscopy. While successful in some cases with smooth foreign bodies the fluorescent screen does not enable the operator to make sure that he is not seizing any mucosa along with the foreign body. As stated by D. R. Paterson and concurred in by all other esophagoscopists of experience "It is surely more in accordance with surgical principles to see a foreign body *in situ*, and so define its relations to the surrounding esophagus."

Complications and dangers of esophagoscopy for foreign bodies. Asphyxia from pressure of the esophagoscope, plus the bulk of the foreign body, or, in some instances, by the foreign body alone without any esophagoscopy, is a possibility. The danger of the esophagoscope causing asphyxia is enormously increased by general anesthesia. The author's schematic representation of this (Bib. 269, p. 147), has been abundantly born out by frequent reports of deaths on the table during esophagoscopy, and especially esophagoscopy under general anesthesia. Such a possibility is very much greater with chloroform than with ether, because of the stimulant effect of ether on the respiratory center, and the paralytic effect of chloroform. Cocaine poisoning, due to the use of an anesthetic solution, or of too strong a solution, has been reported. The uselessness of local anesthesia for esophagoscopy has been elsewhere mentioned. If local anesthesia is ever needed for esophagoscopy, it certainly can be needed only in the one pyriform sinus, through which the esophagoscope is to be passed. In making the application to the pyriform sinus, there will be enough of the solution applied to the pharynx inevitably by the spread of the secretions, so that no special application is needed, except in the pyriform sinus. Such a limited application can involve no special risk in adults. Children are very susceptible. Septic mediastinitis with cellulitis of the neck has been seen three times in consultation by the author. He advised, in each case, and upon request, performed in one of the cases, a drainage of the region back of the esophagus by a long incision along the sternal mastoid muscle, with dry dissection deep down along the esophagus until the perforation was found. In two of the cases, perforation had been caused by the foreign body; in one instance spontaneously, and the other in removal. The third case was caused by perforation by the blind passage of a bougie. In both of the cases emphysema, with intense dyspnea, followed immediately after the accident, requiring tracheotomy in two of the cases. The cellulitis developed within forty-eight hours. All of the cases recovered after drainage. Perforation of the esophagus by either the foreign body or by the esophagoscope, may occur. The foreign body, especially sharp pointed pins and bones, may erode its own way through the esophagus either by ulceration or even by direct puncture, but much more frequently, the introduction of instruments blindly, or even occasionally the introduction of the esophagoscope may force the foreign body through the wall. Very careful work will prevent any assistance to perforation during esophagoscopy, but the possibility should be borne in mind. In regard to perforation of the wall with the esophagoscope, such a thing is exceedingly rare in skillful hands and with a sound esophageal wall. It must be borne in mind, however, that the esophageal wall may be weakened by ulceration, or by malignant disease, or aneurysm so that the tube will meet with practically no resistance in making a false passage. As elsewhere mentioned, the greatest danger exists in the neighborhood of the cricoid level from the contraction of the annular fibers of the cricopharyngeus. The most serious accident that can occur is a gangrenous esophagitis which is almost invariably fatal. Such a complication can occur only from the most gross and brutal attempts by one who is not only totally ignorant of the procedure, but is not ordinarily careful in his manipulations and who is not careful of his aseptic technic. The worst case of gangrenous esophagitis that the author ever saw was due to blind attempts to remove a foreign body which probably was not present. Forceps had been used blindly on what the surgeon told the relatives was a bone that he could feel. At autopsy, the bone proved to be the cervical vertebrae, the bodies of three of which were denuded. The surgeon, who had never previously handled an esophagoscope attempted esophagoscopy, and failing in that, resorted to the blind use of powerful forceps. The symptoms are, profound shock, high temperature early in the case and a subnormal temperature later, a weak rapid pulse, great restlessness, low moaning or muttering delirium, and quite characteristic is the putrid odor of the breath.

Treatment. The treatment of acute esophagitis consists in rest, sterile liquid food, and the administration of small doses of bismuth and calomel frequently repeated. The calomel may be discontinued when it acts too freely on the bowels, and the bismuth continued alone. Local applications of cold, such as with an ice bag, can be used where the trouble is in the cervical esophagus. Rest of the esophagus is best accomplished by gastrostomy for the giving of food and liquid, but in the class of case now under consideration, gastrostomy would be rarely advisable. The teeth and mouth should be kept in as clean condition as possible, and alcohol, 25 per cent, should be used to rinse the mouth at least once an hour. This, with sterile food, will limit the activity of the mixed infections, which are the most dangerous complications after esophageal trauma. Emphysema does not usually require any special treatment for the leak soon becomes obliterated and if no infective conditions follow, the emphysema will usually subside itself. An occasional case, however, may be encountered where it is necessary to puncture the skin in many places in order to liberate the air, though the author has never yet seen such a case. In the event of the pleura being perforated, immediate signs of shock and pleuritis are apt to develop and pneumothorax will show its characteristic signs within twelve hours. If tapped immediately, there may be, in this short time, the characteristic fecal odor from bacterial activity. If the mediastinum has not also been infected, a prompt opening of the pleura may save the patient.

CHAPTER XX.

Pleuroscopy.

Pleuroscopy for foreign bodies. The author has, in one instance, removed a foreign body, a primer from a shotgun cartridge. Figs. 216 and 217, from the pleural cavity through a small opening made in the chest by Dr. J. Hartley Anderson. This was done immediately after the accident and there was no odor or pus at any time. General anesthesia was given, and the child, after the chest opening was made, was placed in the sitting position in order that the foreign body would fall to the diaphragm. Healing was prompt and the air began to enter the lung on the fifth day. The child made a prompt recovery, and now, about three years after the operation, is in perfect health. In this class of cases, pleuroscopy promises excellent results if done immediately, before infection or inflammation has set in. Only a small opening is necessary, and this does not involve anything like the shock consequent upon the large osteoplastic flap. The only shock is the pleural shock, which is slight, and which in the author's case was present anyway because there was already a pneumothorax before the chest was opened. The instrument used by the author was the adult esophageal speculum (Fig. 21) with handle detached. This instrument gave a large view, and the spatular end was very convenient for moving the lung out of the way, as the greatest difficulty encountered was in the manipulation of the lung, which was flopping about like a live fish dangling at the end of a fishing line. A small drain was put in as a precaution. The absence of pus or any considerable quantity of secretion raises the question as to whether or not it would have been better to have closed the wound tightly and aspirated the pleural air. It would seem that the possibility of a valve-like action of either the parietal or the visceral pleura permitting leakage and compression of the mediastinum and other lung, seriously impairing the negative pressure needed to make the other lung serviceable, would involve grave risk.

Whether done by pleuroscopy or not, immediate removal of a foreign body as soon as it is discovered in the lung is advisable.

Pleuroscopy offers no hope of finding foreign bodies still in the lung.

Pleuroscopy for disease. Pleuroscopy for exploration and treatment of pleural diseases is quite feasible through a relatively small opening without rib resection. It is, of course, to be thought of only when

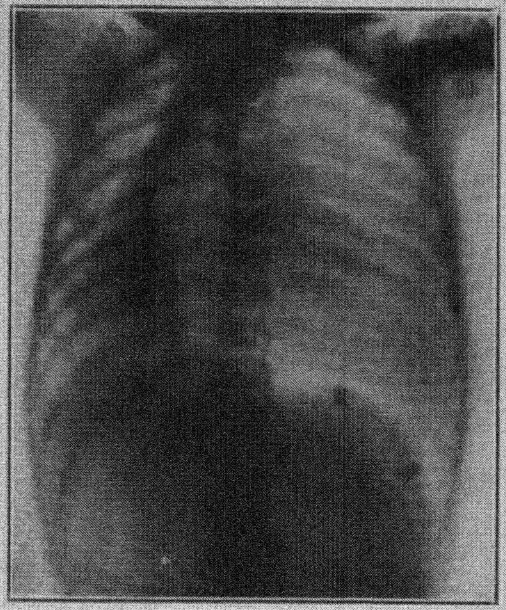

FIG. 216.—Radiograph showing foreign body (primer) at the bottom of the pleural cavity of a child of four years. Foreign body (Fig. 217) removed by pleuroscopy. (Author's case.)

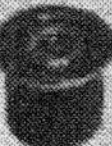

FIG. 217.—Primer removed from the pleura of a boy of four years by pleuroscopy.

for some reason, a large opening is not desired. Most pleural diseases, however, require a large external opening for drainage and these permit inspection without endoscopy, though even in case of large openings the esophageal speculum by its light and its spatular use in the moving aside the lung is a great aid to exploration in the otherwise dark pleural cavity.

HARDWARE.

Illustration.	Age.	Foreign body.	Location.	Anesthetic.	Tube.	Problem.	Forceps.	Point of Seizure.	Result.	Time.	Route.	Remarks.
Fig. 218.	12 Yrs.	Tack.	Left inferior lobe bronchus four days.	Cocaine.	7 mm.	Imbedded point.	Side curved.	At point.	Extraction. Cure.	40 min.	Oral.	
Fig. 219.	41 Yrs.	Two tacks.	Posterior branch inferior lobe bronchus (Points up) Few weeks.	Ether.	7 mm.	Imbedded in edema	Straight.	At point.	Extraction. Cure.	3½ min.	Oral.	Pus copious.
Fig. 220.	41 Yrs.	Two tacks.	Middle lobe bronchus. Post. branch inferior lobe bronchus. Few days. (Points up).	Ether.	7 mm.	Both Imbedded in edema. Point of one imbedded.	Side curved.	At point.	Extraction. Cure.	17 min.	Oral.	
Fig. 221.	52 Yrs.	Brass headed tack.	Post. branch inferior lobe bronchus. 2 yrs. (Points up).	Ether.	9 mm.	Imbedded in granulation tissue, free bleeding.	Side curved.	At point.	Extraction. Cure.	70 min.	Oral.	No stricture though in situ two years.

HARDWARE—Continued.

Illustration	Age	Foreign body.	Location.	Anesthetic.	Tube.	Problem.	Forceps.	Point of Seizure.	Result.	Time.	Route.	Remarks.
Fig. 222.	8 Yrs.	Tack (Brass headed).	Left stem bronchus (Point up).	None.	7 mm.	"Mushroom anchor." Caught 'n orifice upper lobe bronchus	Side curved.	At point.	Extraction. Cure.	4 min.	Oral.	Head liberated by lateral counter-pressure on bronchial wall with lip of bronchoscope.
Fig. 223.	11 Yrs.	Tack (Brass headed).	Left bronchus (Point up) four days.	None.	7 mm.	Head anchored in orifice upper lobe bronchus	Side curved.	At point.	Extraction. Cure.	11 min.	Oral.	Head liberated by lateral counter-pressure on bronchial wall with lip of bronchoscope.
Fig. 224.	1 Yr.	Thumb tack.	Left pyriform sinus, two days.	None.	7 mm.	Disk with perpendicular sharp spike.	Alligator.	Sidewise on spike.	Extraction. Cure.		Oral.	Forceps jaws completely covered point of spike grasped sidewise.
Fig. 225.	5 Yrs.	Nail.	Right bronchus. Point up.	Ether.	5 mm.	"Anchored" by swelling around head.	Side curved.	Point.	Extraction. Cure.	3 min.	Oral.	Head to left, permitted straight line traction

HARDWARE—Continued.

Illustration.	Age.	Foreign Body.	Location.	Anesthetic.	Tube.	Problem.	Forceps	Point of Seizure.	Result.	Time	Route.	Remarks.
Fig. 226.	1 Yr.	Nail.	Trachea and right bronchus, two days. (Pneumonia subglottic edema).	Chloroform.	5 mm.	"Anchored" by swelling around head.	Side curved.	Point.	Extraction.	2 min.	Oral.	Tracheotomy, second day. Died sixth day.
Fig. 227.	10 Yrs.	Nail.	Left bronchus, four years.	None.	7 mm.	Abscess cavity full of pus and granulations.	Side curved.	Point.	Extraction.	27 min.	Oral.	Fatal cerebral embolus about 1 month later.
Fig. 228.	24 Yrs.	Nail.	Posterior branch right inferior lobe bronchus.	Chloroform.	9 mm.	Could not see.	Straight.	On end but not by sight.	Extraction. Cure.	2 hrs.	Oral.	Location by sounding with closed forceps. Early case.

HARDWARE—Continued.

Illustration.	Age.	Foreign Body.	Location.	Anesthetic.	Tube.	Problem.	Forceps.	Point of Seizure.	Result.	Time.	Route.	Remarks.
Fig. 229.	4 Yrs.	Clock leg.	Left bronchus, 25 days. (Pneumonia).	Choloroform.	5 mm.	Impacted in edema.	Straight.	End.	Extraction. Cure.	13 min.	Oral.	Pneumonia resolved in four weeks.
Fig. 230.	76 Yrs	Atomizer tip.	Right bronchus, ten days.	Cocaine. Morphine.	9 mm.	Impacted Hollow end presenting. Edges covered by swelling.	Side curved.	Edge.	Extraction. Cure.	6 min.	Oral.	
Fig. 231.	8 Yrs.	Brass cap.	Left bronchus, forty hours.	None.	5 mm.	Convex end presenting, occluding bronchus.	Side curved.	Flatwise, after tilting with closed forceps used as hook.	Extraction. Cure.	18 min.		Side curved forceps closed serve well as a hook and are at hand for seizure.
Fig. 232.	7 Yrs.	Hinge of carpenter's rule.	Hiatal esophagus, 24 hours.	Cocaine.	7 mm.	Crosswise fixation.	Rotation	Hole in one of longer points.	Extraction. Cure.	45 min.	Oral.	Early case. Cocaine needless.
Fig. 234.	11 mos.	Jack.	Esophagus, below cricopharyngeus. 2 weeks	None.	7 mm.	Tight impaction.	Straight.	Crossing.	Extraction. Cure.		Oral.	

HARDWARE—Continued.

Illustration.	Age.	Foreign Body.	Location.	Anesthetic.	Tube.	Problem.	Forceps.	Point of Seizure.	Result.	Time.	Route.	Remarks.
Fig. 235.	2 Yrs.	Double pointed tack.	Esophagus. High thoracic	Ether.	7 mm.	Tack disappearing. Only 5 mm. of one point remaining.			Recovery.		Oral.	Traction deemed inadvisable. Tack removed from pleura by Dr. J. W. MacFarlane 2 months later.
Fig. 236.	4 Yrs.	Staple.	Trachea. Aortic level. Points up.	None.	5 mm.	Transfixed obliquely. Points buried. Lacerated postero-lateral wall. Mediastinal emphysema.	Rotation.	Curve after turning.	Extraction.		Oral.	Died of vagitis.
Fig. 237.	19 mos.	Staple.	Right stem bronchus. Points up.	None.	5 mm.	Points upward fitting tightly. One point imbedded in swollen mucosa.	Rotation.	Curve after turning with hook.	Extraction. Cure.	½ hr.	Oral.	Coaxed up and turned at orifice of middle lobe bronchus after freeing buried point.*
Fig. 238.	10 Yrs.	Staple.	Tracheal bifurcation. Points up.	None.	5 mm.	Points obliquely upward.	Rotation.	Curve after turning.	Extraction. Cure.	50 min.	Oral.	Turned at tracheal bifurcation.
Fig. 239.	16 Yrs.	Staple.	Esophagus. Below plica cricopharyngeus.	None.	10 mm.	Points upward; not imbedded.	Rotation.	Curve	Extraction.		Oral.	Carried into stomach. reversed and removed. See schema Fig. 212.

*In two other cases turning was accomplished as shown in Fig. 181b.

JEWELRY.

Illustration.	Age.	Foreign Body.	Location.	Anesthetic.	Tube.	Problem.	Forceps.	Point of Seizure.	Result.	Time.	Route.	Remarks
Fig. 240.	19 Yrs.	Shirt stud.	Subglottic.	Cocaine.	Laryngoscope.	Impacted edema.	Alligator rotary.	At serrations.	Extraction. Cure.	1 min.	Oral.	Edema subsided without tracheotomy.
Fig. 241.	17 mos.	Collar button.	Subglottic. 24 hours.	None.	5 mm.	Impacted. In subglottic edema.	Straight.	At post.	Extraction. Cure.	2 min.	Oral.	Digitally impacted by parents. Tracheotomy required for dyspnea.
Fig. 242.	12 mos.	Collar button.	Esophagus below cricopharyngeus.	None.	7 mm.	Impacted.	Straight.	At post.	Extraction. Cure.		Oral.	
Fig. 243.	18 Yrs.	Collar button.	Right stem bronchus. 10 yrs.	Ether.	7 mm.	Fixed in fibrosis below stricture.	Side curved.	End of post, also side of disk after divulsing stricture.	Extraction. Cure.	1 hr.	Oral.	Stricture divulsed. Patient in perfect health 1 yr. later.
Fig. 244.	46 Yrs.	Collar button.	Left stem bronchus 26 yrs.	None.	9 mm.	In abscess below fibrous occluding bronchus.	Straight.	At post, after excision of fibrous obstruction.	Extraction. Cure.	35 min.	Oral.	Longest sojourn of any bronchoscopically removed foreign body.
Fig. 245.	4 mos.	Cuff button.	Esophagus close below plica cricopharyngeus.	Cocaine. 2 per-cent.	7 mm.	Impaction. Post crosswise.	Rotation.	Around post permitting rotation.	Extraction. Cure.		Oral.	Early case. (Before needlessness and danger of cocaine in children were realized).

JEWELRY—Continued.

Illustration	Age.	Foreign Body.	Location.	Anesthetic.	Tube.	Problem.	Forceps.	Point of Seizure.	Result.	Time.	Route.	Remarks.
Fig. 246.	13 mos.	Collar button.	Esophagus below plica crico-pharyngeus, three weeks.	Ether	7 mm.	Impaction.	Straight.	By post after turning.	Extraction. Cure.	11 min.	Oral.	Early case. Respiratory arrest requiring tracheotomy. Author has not used general anesthesia for esophagoscopy in children since.
Fig. 247.	6 mos.	Cuff link.	Esophagus and trachea, 3 mos.	None.	7 mm. 5 mm.	Part in trachea; part in esophagus.	Straight. and side curved.	Small flat part. Shank large part.	Extraction. Cure.	1 hr.	Oral.	Part removed bronchoscopically part esophagoscopically.
Fig. 248.	17 mos.	Cuff link.	Esophagus bronchial crossing, 4 weeks.	None.	7 mm.	Dyspnea. Impacted.	Rotation.	Left end of large part.	Extraction. Cure.		Oral.	Large size of foreign body caused dyspnea. Great caution necessary.
Fig. 249.	10 mos.	Finger ring.	Esophagus. Bronchial crossing.	None.	7 mm.		Rotation.	Presenting. Part	Extraction. Cure.	4 min.		Rotation forceps permitted dangling. Straight forceps would have thrown ring crosswise.

JEWELRY—Continued.

Illustration.	Age.	Foreign Body.	Location.	Anesthetic.	Tube.	Problem.	Forceps.	Point of Seizure.	Result.	Time.	Route.	Remarks.
Fig. 250.	2½ Yrs.	Locket	Esophagus below cricopharyngeus, 36 hrs.	None.	Esophageal speculum.	Impacted. Large.	Rotation.	Ring.	Extraction. Cure.		Oral.	
Fig. 251.	15 Yrs.	Stick pin.	Left main bronchus one week.	Chloroform.	7 mm.	Imbedded point. Pin could not be pushed down.	Side curved.	Point after freeing it.	Extraction. Cure.	15 min.	Oral.	Trachea pushed laterally off point. Counter pressure with forceps.

JEWELRY—Continued.

Illustration.	Age.	Foreign Body.	Location.	Anesthetic.	Tube.	Problem.	Forceps.	Point of Seizure.	Result.	Time.	Route.	Remarks.
Fig. 252.	9 mos.	Open clasp pin.	Right bronchus 36 hours.	None.	5 mm.	Open pin. Point up.	Side curved.	Pin closed with forceps.	Extraction. Died.	6 min.	Oral.	Died of pneumonia. Respirations 52 before operation.

PINS.

Illustration.	Age.	Foreign body.	Location.	Anesthetic.	Tube.	Problem.	Forceps.	Point of Seizure.	Result.	Time.	Route.	Remarks.
Fig. 253.	3½ Yrs.	Pin.	Point up. Left inferior lobe bronchus three weeks.	Chloroform.	5 mm.	Point embedded.	Side curved.	At point.	Extraction. Cure.	30 min.	Oral.	Located "around the corner." See schema Fig. 172.
Fig. 254.	20 Yrs.	Pin.	Point up trachea three days.	None.	Laryngoscope.	Point embedded subglottic.	Alligator.	Below point rotated to sagittal position.	Extraction. Cure.	2 min.		Supraglottic tracheoscopy.

PINS—Continued.

Illustration.	Age.	Foreign Body.	Location.	Anesthetic.	Tube.	Problem.	Forceps.	Point of Seizure.	Result.	Time.	Route.	Remarks.
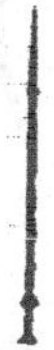 Fig. 255.	19 Yrs.	Pin.	Point up post branch inferior lobe bronchus five days.	Ether.	7 mm.	Failure to find.			Failure to find.			Removed by J. Hartley Anderson by thoracotomy. Recovery.
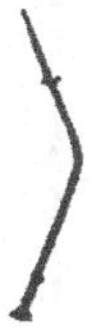 Fig. 256.	7 mos.	Bent pin.	Larynx Point in base epiglottis six days.	None.	Laryngoscope.	Point embedded.	Alligator.	Near point.	Extraction. Cure.	½ min.	Oral.	Easy extraction but great potential danger if dislodged and lost.
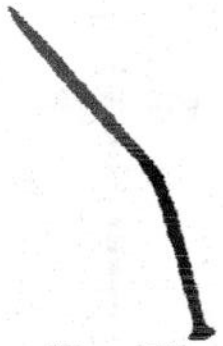 Fig. 257.	9 Yrs.	Bent pin.	Larynx 4 hours.	None.	Laryngoscope.	Point embedded.	Alligator.	In center.	Extraction. Cure.		Oral.	Presenting part seized without study of relations.
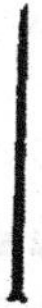 Fig. 258.	16 mos.	Pin.	Post branch left inferior lobe bronchus nine days.	None.	4 mm.	Could not be found.			Failure to find.		Oral.	Died after thoracotomy.

PINS—Continued.

Illustration.	Age.	Foreign Body.	Location.	Anesthetic.	Tube	Problem.	Forceps.	Point of Seizure.	Result.	Time.	Route.	Remarks.
Fig. 259.	16 Yrs.	Pin.	Upper orifice larynx two days.	None.	Laryngoscope.	Point in the aryepiglottic fold.	Alligator.	Near center.	Extraction. Cure.	½ min.	Oral.	Part first seen seized without study of relations.
Fig. 260.	20 Yrs.	Pin.	Point up Middle lobe bronchus.	Chloroform.	7 mm.	Point presenting not embedded.	Side curved.	At point.	Extraction. Cure.	45 min.	Oral.	Early case. Long search before exploration of middle lobe bronchus.
Fig. 261.	17 Yrs.	Double pointed bent pin.	Left pyriform sinus.	None.	Laryngoscope.	Outside of mucosa.	Tissue.	At point.	Extraction. Cure.		Oral.	Elevation of mucosa covering point revealed location. Excision with tissue forceps.

PINS—Continued.

Illustration.	Age.	Foreign Body.	Location.	Anesthetic.	Tube.	Problem.	Forceps.	Point of Seizure.	Result.	Time.	Route.	Remarks.
Fig. 262.	6 mos.	Curved pin.	Post. branch inferior lobe bronchus.	None.	5 mm.	Difficult to find. Point exposed by extreme elevation of patient's head.	Side curved.	At point.	Extraction. Cure.	25 min. 35 min.	Oral.	See schema. Fig. 172. Found at second seance.
Fig. 263.	4 mos.	Hook shaped pin.	Left upper lobe bronchus four days.	None.	5 mm.	Point and head visible, remainder in upper lob bronchus	Hook rotation.	At curve after turning with hook.	Extraction. Cure.	28 min.	Oral.	
Fig. 264.	2½ mo.	Pin.	Point up. Right main bronchus.	None.	4 mm.	Very small infant.	Straight.	Point.	Extraction. Cure.	3 min.	Oral.	
Fig. 265.	4 Yrs.	Shawl pin.	Right bronchus five days point up.	Chloroform. Cocaine.	5 mm.	Transfixion through side holes in bronchoscope	Straight.	On end after breaking.	Extraction. Fragment lost. Cure.	45 min.	Oral.	Pin broken by pushing with forceps. Counter traction with tube.

PINS—Continued.

Illustration.	Age.	Foreign Body.	Location.	Anesthetic.	Tube.	Problem.	Forceps.	Point of Seizure.	Result.	Time.	Route.	Remarks.
Fig. 266.	23 Yrs.	Price tag pin.	Point up right stem bronchus seven years.	Ether.	7 mm.	Fixed in fibrosis below stricture.	Side curved.	On end after divulsing stricture.	Extraction. Cure.	1 hr.	Oral.	Perfectly well, without cough one year later.
Fig. 267.	6 Yrs.	Shawl pin.	Left inferior lobe bronchus. Point up six days.	None.	5 mm.	Point imbedded.	Side curved.	At point after disengaging point by pushing down.	Extraction. Cure.	4 min.	Oral.	
Fig. 268.	2½ Yrs.	Shawl pin.	Left inferior lobe bronchus. 23 hours. Point up.	None.	5 mm.	Point imbedded.	Side curved.	At point after disengaging point by pushing down.	Extraction. Cure.	3 min.	Oral.	

PINS—Continued.

Illustration.	Age.	Foreign body.	Location.	Anesthetic.	Tube.	Problem.	Forceps.	Point of Seizure.	Result.	Time.	Route.	Remarks.
Fig. 269.	12 Yrs.	Shawl pin.	Left bronchus Head in upper lobe bronchus point up two days.	Ether.	7 mm.	Point imbedded.	Side curved.	At point after disengaging point with forceps used as hook.	Extraction. Cure.	18 min.	Oral.	Side curved. forceps serve excellently as a hook for disengaging by rotary movement.
Fig. 270.	23 Yrs.	Shawl pin.	Esophagus. Crossing left of bronchus. Point down one day.	Cocaine.	10 mm.	Pin regurgitated to higher level than shown in radiograph.			Cure		Oral.	Danger of causing perforation because of point down position and regurgitation to higher level than shown in radiograph.

PINS—Continued.

Illustration.	Age.	Foreign body.	Location.	Anesthetic.	Tube	Problem.	Forceps.	Point of Seizure.	Result.	Time.	Route.	Remarks.
Fig. 271.	4 mos.	Shawl pin.	Left stem bronchus. Point up	None.	4 mm.	Point in upper wall of upper lobe bronchus	Side curved.	Center to push down then at point.	Extraction. Cure.			

SAFETY PINS.

Illustration.	Age.	Foreign body.	Location.	Anesthetic.	Tube.	Problem.	Forceps.	Point of Seizure.	Result.	Time.	Route.	Remarks.
Fig. 272.	11 mos.	Closed safety pin.	Trachea. one mo.	None.	7 mm.	Edematous post. wall supraglottic tracheoscopy.	Hook.	Hooked.	Extraction. Cure.	30 min.	Oral.	Supraglottic tracheoscopy.
Fig. 273.	8 mos.	Open safety pin.	Subglottic. Point up 3 weeks.	None.	Laryngoscope	Embedded. point below. Keeper-end above cords.	Alligator.	Keeper for disimpaction and rotation. Point for removal.	Extraction. Cure.		Oral.	Supraglottic tracheoscopy.

SAFETY PINS—Continued.

Illustration.	Age.	Foreign body.	Location.	Anesthetic.	Tube.	Problem.	Forceps.	Point of Seizure.	Result.	Time.	Route.	Remarks.
Fig. 274.	4 Yrs.	Bent, twisted, open safety pin.	Larynx two months.	None.	Laryngoscope.	Extreme dyspnea. Embedded in edema. Protector end presenting.	Alligator.	At presenting part.	Extraction. Cure.	½ min.	Oral.	Antitoxin given. Edema present prior to operation. Subsided without tracheotomy.
Fig. 275.	9 mos.	Open safety pin.	Esophagus; middle third. Point up, one week.	Chloroform.	7 mm.	Open safety pin, point up.	Straight forceps after pin closure.	Protector end after closing.	Extraction. Cure.	35 min.	Oral.	Severe dyspnea at times from compression of trachea by bulk of instruments in esophagus. Not sufficient to interrupt.
Fig. 276.	11 mos.	Open safety pin.	Point up in esophagus. Lower part of middle third. 12 hours.	Ether.	7 mm.	Open safety pin, point up in thoracic esophagus.	Rotation.	Ring of spring end.	Extraction. Cure.	28 min.	Oral.	Carried down into stomach, reversed and withdrawn.

SAFETY PINS—Continued.

Illustration.	Age.	Foreign body.	Location.	Anesthetic.	Tube.	Problem.	Forceps.	Point of Seizure.	Result.	Time.	Route.	Remarks.
Fig. 277.	14 mos.	Open safety pin.	Point up in esophagus above hiatus.	Ether.	7 mm.	Open safety pin, point up in thoracic esophagus.	Rotation.	Ring of spring end.	Extraction. Cure.	22 min.	Oral.	Carried down into stomach, reversed and withdrawn.
Fig. 278.	10 mos.	Open safety pin.	Point down. Esophagus below plica cricopharyngeus 12 days.	Chloroform.	7 mm.	Danger of perforation if pushed.	Rotation.	Ring of spring end presented.	Extraction. Cure.	6 min.	Oral.	Would have been overridden if esophagoscope were passed with mandrin.
Fig. 279.	20 mos.	Open safety pin.	Point up in trachea at bifurcation 1 day.	None.	5 mm.	Open safety pin, point up in a child of 20 months.	Straight after pin closer.	Keeper end after closing.	Extraction. Cure.		Oral.	Pin closed and removed through mouth.
Fig. 280.	4 mos.	Open safety pin.	Point up in trachea at bifurcation two days.	None.	4 mm.	Open safety pin, point up in an infant aged 4 months.	Straight after getting point of pin onto lip of bron. with hook.	Point after getting it onto lip of bronchoscope.	Extraction. Cure.	17 min.	Oral.	

COINS AND OTHER DISKS. (Illustrations of coins made by special permission of United States Government.)

Illustration.	Age.	Foreign body.	Location.	Anesthetic.	Tube.	Problem.	Forceps.	Point of Seizure.	Result.	Time.	Route.	Remarks.
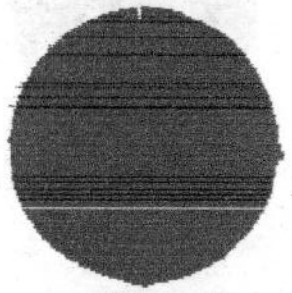 Fig. 281.	3 Yrs.	Coin (nickel).	Trachea, 1 day.	None.	Laryngoscope.	Extreme dyspnea. Coin tilted partially flatwise.	Alligator.	Flatwise after turning.	Extraction. Cure.	1 min.	Oral.	Supraglottic tracheoscopy. Subglottic edema subsided without tracheotomy
Fig. 282.	2 Yrs.	Coin (penny).	Trachea and esophagus; upper third.	Chloroform.	7 mm.	Dyspnea. Coin ulcerated through into trachea.	Side curved.	Flatwise after hooking upward with closed forceps.	Extraction. Cure.		Oral.	Early case. Anesthesia unnecessary. Esophageal extraction.
Fig. 283.	2 Yrs.	Coin (Quarter dol.)	Below plica cricopharyngeus.	None.	Esoph. speculum.	Impaction.	Alligator.	Flatwise.	Extraction. Cure.	3 min.	Oral.	11 physicians told family to "forget about it" or words to that effect. Center third bright. Lateral thirds sulphided.
Fig. 284.	2½ Yrs.	Coin (nickel).	Hypopharynx, three days.	None.	7 mm.	Impaction.	Straight.	Flatwise.	Extraction. Cure.	1 min.	Oral.	Center third dark. Lateral thirds bright. Lateral passage of food in hypopharynx.

COINS AND OTHER DISKS. (Illustrations of coins made by special permission of United States Government.)—Continued.

Illustration.	Age.	Foreign body.	Location.	Anesthetic.	Tube.	Problem	Forceps.	Point of Seizure.	Result.	Time.	Route.	Remarks.
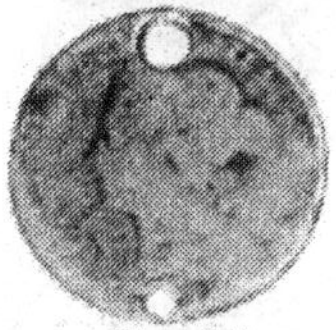 Fig. 285.	2 Yr.	Coin (Canadian quarter)	Esophagus below plica cricopharyngeus, 24 hours	None.	7 mm.	Impaction.	Straight.	Flatwise.	Extraction. Cure.	6 min.	Oral.	Previous failure to push down.
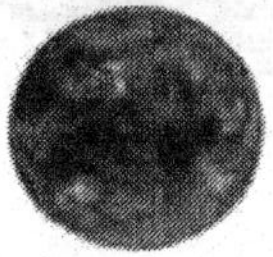 Fig. 286.	1½ Yrs.	Coin (penny U. S.)	Esophagus below plica cricopharyngeus, 1 week.	None.	7 mm.	Below large mass of food.	Straight.	Flatwise.	Extraction. Cure.	2 min.	Oral.	Previous failure to push down with bougie.
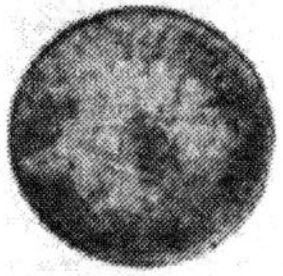 Fig. 287.	11 mos.	Coin (nickel).	Esophagus below plica cricopharyngeus.	None.	7 mm.	Impaction.	Straight.	Flatwise.	Extraction. Cure	1 min.	Oral.	Previous failure to push down with bougie.
Fig. 288.	2 Yrs.	Coin (penny U. S.)	Esophagus. Bronchial crossing. Ten days.	None.	7 mm.		Straight.	Flatwise.	Extraction. Cure.	2 min.	Oral.	Pushed down by previous attempts.

COINS AND OTHER DISKS. (Illustrations of coins made by special permission of United States Government.)—Continued.

Illustration.	Age.	Foreign body.	Location.	Anesthetic.	Tube.	Problem.	Forceps.	Point of Seizure.	Result.	Time.	Route.	Remarks.
Fig. 289.	16 mos.	Coin (Dime U. S.)	Hypopharynx above plica.	None.	Esophageal speculum.		Straight.	Flatwise.	Extraction. Cure.	1 min.	Oral.	Lateral thirds bright middle third sulphided. (Passage of food at sides in upper hypopharynx.)
Fig. 290.	16 mos.	Coin (Penny U. S.)	Esophagus below plica cricopharyngeus.	None.	Esophageal speculum.		Straight.	Flatwise.	Extraction. Cure.	3 min.	Oral.	
Fig. 291.	4½ Yrs.	Coin (Penny U. S.)	Esophagus below plica crico-pharyngeus. (Pneumonia from aspiration of food).	None.	7 mm.		Straight.	As presented.	Extraction. Cure.	1 min.	Oral.	Small coin causing complete esophageal occlusion. Swallowing perfect after removal.
Fig. 292.	2 Yrs.	Coin (nickel)	Esophagus. (Location not recorded).	None.	Esophageal speculum.		Alligator.	Flatwise.	Extraction. Cure.		Oral.	
Fig. 293.	17 mos.	Coin (Penny U. S.)	Esophagus below plica cricopharyngeus, four days.	None.	Esophageal speculum.		Alligator.	Flatwise.	Extraction. Cure.		Oral.	

COINS AND OTHER DISKS. (Illustrations of coins made by special permission of United States Government.)—Continued.

Illustration.	Age.	Foreign body.	Location.	Anesthetic.	Tube.	Problem.	Forceps.	Point of Seizure.	Result.	Time.	Route.	Remarks.
Fig. 294.	3 Yrs.	Coin (Penny U. S.)	Esophagus below plica cricopharyngeus, seven days.	None.	Esophageal speculum.		Alligator.	Flatwise.	Extraction. Cure.	½ min.	Oral.	Tracheotomy previously done by family physician for almost fatal dyspnea due to pressure of coin and lodged food.
Fig. 295.	4½ Yrs.	(Penny U. S.) Coin	Esophagus, below plica cricopharyngeus, 12 days.	None.	Esophageal speculum.		Alligator.	Flatwise.	Extraction. Cure.	1 min.	Oral.	
Fig. 296.	14 Yrs.	Coin (Half dollar).	Esophagus, below plica cricopharyngeus, 17 days.	None.	Esophageal speculum.	Tightly impacted.	Alligator.	Flatwise	Extraction. Cure.	1 min.	Oral.	
Fig. 297.	5 Yrs.	Coin (Half penny British).	Esophagus. Below plica cricopharyngeus. 20 hours.	None.	7 mm.	Tightly impacted.	Alligator.	Flatwise.	Extraction. Cure.	3 min.	Oral.	

COINS AND OTHER DISKS. (Illustrations of coins made by special permission of United States Government.)—Continued.

Illustration.	Age.	Foreign body.	Location.	Anesthetic.	Tube.	Problem.	Forceps.	Point of Seizure.	Result.	Time.	Route.	Remarks.
Fig. 298.	8 Yrs.	Lead disk.	Esophagus. Below plica cricopharyngeus, 3 days	None.	Esophageal speculum.	Tightly impacted.	Alligator.	Flatwise.	Extraction. Cure.	1 min.	Oral.	
Fig. 299.	2½ Yrs.	Double metallic disk from eraser.	Esophagus below plica cricopharyngeus, 5 days.	None.	Esophageal speculum.	Impacted very smooth and resilient when both disks grasped.	Alligator.	Flatwise, edge of one disk only.	Extraction. Cure.	4 min.	Oral.	

BONES.

Illustration.	Age.	Foreign body.	Location.	Anesthetic.	Tube	Problem.	Forceps.	Point of Seizure.	Result.	Time.	Route.	Remarks.
Fig. 300.	2½ Yrs.	Bone.	Esophagus. (Location unrecorded) Five days.	None.	7 mm.	Transfixed.	Rotation.	End.	Extraction Cure.		Oral.	
Fig. 301.	56 Yrs.	Bone.	Esophagus Below plica cricopharyngeus seventeen days.	None.	10 mm.	Boomerang shape. Sharp point.	Rotation.	Sharpest point.	Extraction Cure.		Oral.	

BONES—Continued.

Illustration.	Age.	Foreign body.	Location.	Anesthetic.	Tube.	Problem.	Forceps.	Point of Seizure.	Result.	Time.	Route.	Remarks.
Fig. 302.	80 Yrs.	Chicken bone.	Esophagus middle third twenty-four hours.	None.	10 mm.	Sharp pointed trans-fixed bone punctur-ing walls.	Tissue forceps to cut. Straight forceps to remove	Cut in two, and two pieces removed.	Extrac-tion. Cure.	8 min.	Oral.	Esophageal motility sluggish.
Fig. 303.	44 Yrs.	Beef bone.	Six days in esophagus be-low plica cricopharyn-geus.	None.	Eso-pha-geal specu lum.	Trans-fixed. Very sharp points.	Rotation.	Extreme left point.	Extrac-tion. Cure.	15 sec.		Freedom to rotate prevented trauma.
Fig. 304.	65 Yrs.	Lamb bone.	Esophagus be-low crico-pharyngeus four days.	None.	Eso-pha-geal specu lum.	Trans-fixed. Wide dis tension.	Rotation.	Extreme right end.	Extrac-tion. Cure.	6 min.	Oral.	See schema under "Mechani-cal problems." (Fig. 208).
Fig. 305.	22 Yrs.	Chicken bone.	Esophagus bronchial crossing seventeen hours.	None.	10 mm.	Sharp pointed.	Rotation.	Extreme right edge.	Extrac-tion. Cure.		Oral.	Spasmodic dys-phagia. Body not large enough to occlude.
Fig. 306.	32 Yrs.	Fish bone.	Esophagus be-low crico-pharyngeus four days.	None.	10 mm.	Sharp spicule perpen-dicularly lodged.	Side curved.	Present-ing end.	Extrac-tion. Cure.		Oral.	Danger of per-foration of esoph. if a mandrin were used for introduction.

BONES—Continued.

Illustration.	Age.	Foreign body.	Location.	Anesthetic.	Tube.	Problem.	Forceps.	Point of Seizure.	Result.	Time.	Route.	Remarks.
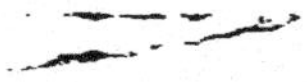 Fig. 307.	57 Yrs	Chicken bone.	Trachea, having perforated from the esophagus in six weeks.	Cocaine.	9 mm.	Point presenting from party wall.	Side curved.	Presenting point.	Extraction. Cure.	3 min.	Oral.	
Fig. 308.	9 mos.	Fish bones. (Vertebra and rib)	Right inferior lobe bronchus.	Ether.	5 mm	Impacted Granulations. Swelling.	Straight.	Presenting part	Extraction Cure.	30 min.	Oral.	
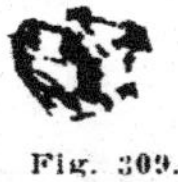 Fig. 309.	17 mos.	Beef bone.	Subglottic 14 days antitoxin given.	None.	Laryngoscope.	Impacted crosswise.	Alligator.	Center and rotated sagitally.	Extraction Cure.	1 min.	Oral.	Supraglottic. Tracheoscopy.
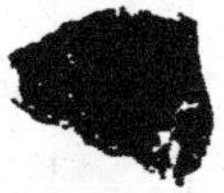 Fig. 310.	39 Yrs.	Beef bone.	Trachea six days.	Cocaine.	Laryngoscope.	Impacted crossing.	Alligator.	Center and rotated sagitally	Extraction Cure.	3 min.	Oral.	Supraglottic. Tracheoscopy.
 Fig. 311	18 Yrs.	Bone.	Right upper lobe bronchus	Chloroform).	9 mm.	Difficulty in finding.	Side curved.	Presenting Part.	Extraction. Cure.	Over two hrs.	Oral.	Two bronchoscopies before found in stem of upper lobe bronchus.
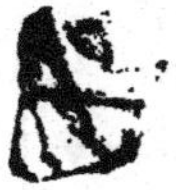 Fig. 312	11 mos.	Bone.	Bifurcation.	None.	5 mm.	Extreme dyspnea.	Straight.	Presenting Part.	Extreme Dyspnea.			

BONES—Continued.

Illustration.	Age.	Foreign body.	Location.	Anesthetic.	Tube.	Problem.	Forceps.	Point of Seizure.	Result.	Time.	Route.	Remarks.
Fig. 313.	43 Yrs.	Pork bone (Part of shaft of long bone).	Esophagus below plica cricopharyngeus.	None.	10 mm.	Transfixation.	Rotation.	Flatwise near end Rotated.	Extraction. Cure.	6 min.	Oral.	Wall of esophagus pushed sidewise to disengage point.
Fig. 314.	27 Yrs.	Chicken bone (Part of rib).	Esophagus at bronchial crossing.	Ether	7 mm.	Transfixation.	Rotation.	Near end	Extraction. Cure.			Early case. Child's esophagoscope used because of tracheal compression by goitre.
Fig. 315.	40 Yrs.	Chicken bone.	Esophagus. Bronchial crossing. (Previously pushed down with bougie).	Ether. (a little Chloroform).	10 mm.	Transfixion. Both points buried.	Rotation	At angle	Extraction. Cure.		Oral.	Point of traction released by lateral counte pres sure with tube mouth. Cervical emphysema from high puncture during previous blind bouginage.
Fig. 316.	24 Yrs.	Pork bone vertebra).	Esophagus above bronchial crossing, ten days.	Ether and Chloroform.	10 mm.	Tightly impacted very large bone in thoracic esophagus.	Rotation	Extreme left end of presenting part.	Extraction. Cure.	20 min.	Oral.	Rotation forceps permitted body to turn in position of least resistance. Ether and chloroform necessary to relax esophagus and thus prevent trauma in withdrawal.
Fig. 317.	52 Yrs.	Turkey bone. (Part of sternum)	Esophagus below plica crico-pharingeus. Perforated. Emphysema neck and chest.	None.	10 mm.	Impacted Point perforated.	Rotation.	Presenting branch.	Extraction.		Oral.	Died of Uremia four days after leaving hospital. Advanced nephritis.

BONES—Continued.

Age.	Foreign body.	Location.	Anesthetic.	Tube.	Problem.	Forceps.	Point of Seizure.	Result.	Time.	Route.	Remarks.
48 Yrs.	Bone (Pork) also chondrial sequestrum.	Hypopharynx, three mo.	Cocaine.	Esophageal speculum.	Buried in perichondrial abscess.	Alligator.	As presented.	Extraction. Cure.		Oral.	Abscess healed in 6 months, leaving slight laryngeal stenosis.
52 Yrs.	Bone (Rib of fish).	Hypopharynx, "Many months."	Cocaine.	Esophageal speculum.	Half buried in perichondrial abscess.	Alligator.	As presented.	Extraction. Cure.		Oral.	Abscess not completely healed when last seen four months later.

MEAT. (Exclusion of those found in cases of diverticulum and hiatal esophagismus.)

Age.	Foreign body.	Location.	Anesthetic.	Tube.	Problem.	Forceps.	Point of Seizure.	Result.	Time.	Route.	Remarks.
54 Yrs.	Meat. (Beef.)	Esophagus. Bronchial crossing, 24 hours.	None.	10 mm.	Friable body.	Mechanical spoon.		Extraction. Cure.		Oral.	Compression stenosis esophagus. Cause undetermined. Meat putrid. Toxic (?) if swallowed.
21 Yrs.	Meat. (Lamb.)	Esophagus filled up from hiatus.	Ether.	10 mm.	Friable. Impacted by previous blind attempts to force downward.	Mechanical spoon.		Extraction. Cure.		Oral.	Ether given because foreign body was supposed to be a large bone. Intoxicated at time of accident.

MEAT. (Exclusion of those found in cases of diverticulum and hiatal esophagismus.)—Continued.

Illustration.	Age.	Foreign body.	Location.	Anesthetic.	Tube.	Problem.	Forceps.	Point of Seizure.	Result.	Time.	Route.	Remarks.
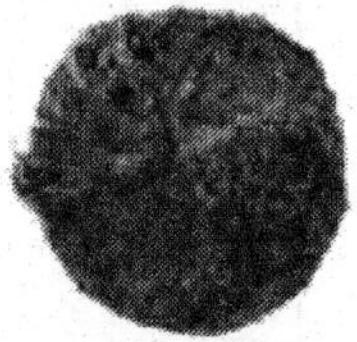 Fig. 322.	75 Yrs.	Meat.	Esophagus. Above hiatal narrowing, one day.	None.	10 mm.	Friable. Impacted by previous blind attempts to force downward.	Mechanical spoon.		Extraction. Cure.		Oral.	Dysphagia since scarlatina in childhood. Esophagus lacking propulsion.
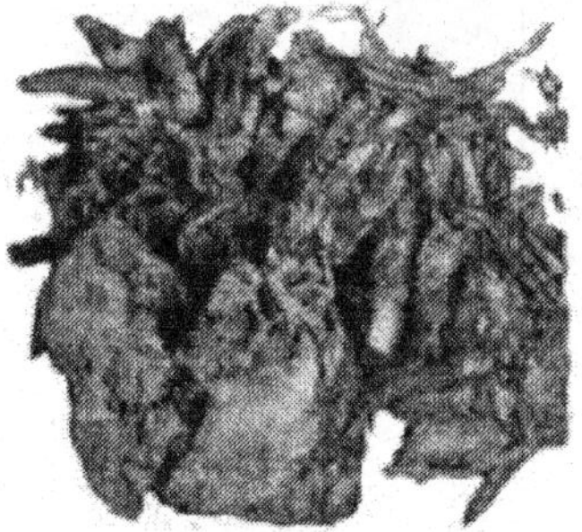 Fig. 323.	60 Yrs.	Meat. (Beef.)	Esophagus. Bronchial crossing to plica cricopharyngeus.	None.	Esophageal speculum.	Friable. Impacted	Mechanical spoon. Alligator forceps.	As presented.	Extraction. Cure.	12 min.	Oral.	Very foul. Toxic (?) if swallowed.
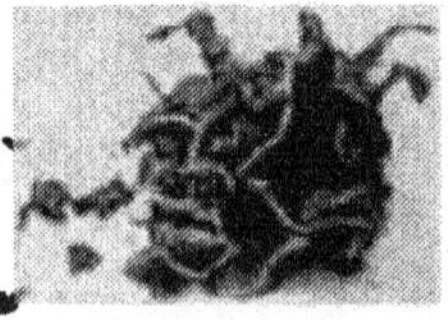 Fig. 324.	60 Yrs.	Meat. (Chicken	Esophagus. Above bronchial crossing.	None.	10 mm.	Friable. Macerated. Shredded.	Mechanical spoon.	As presented.	Extraction. Cure.		Oral.	Absence of impaction raised question of cause of lodgment.

MEAT. (Exclusion of those found in cases of diverticulum and hiatal esophagismus.)—Continued.

Illustration	Age	Foreign Body	Location	Anesthetic	Tube	Problem	Forceps	Point of Seizure	Result	Time	Route	Remarks
Fig. 325.	[illegible] Yrs.	Meat. (Chicken.)	Esophagus. Aortic level.	None.	10 mm.	Tough. Elastic. Impacted in stricture of 5 mm. lumen.	Plain.	As presented.	Extraction. Cure.	[illegible] min.	Oral.	Swallowed lye [illegible] years before. Stricture not [illegible] small lumen.
Fig. 326.	91 Yrs.	Meat.	Esophagus. Bronchial crossing. 3 days (?)	None.	10 mm.	None. Meat waited to be removed. No impaction or occlusion.	Side curved	As presented.	Extraction. Cure.	7 min.	Oral.	Remarkable lack of propulsion. Not true paralysis.
Fig. 327.	68 Yrs.	Meat.	Esophagus. Hiatal level.	None.	10 mm.	Friable. Macerated.	Mechanical spoon.	As presented.	Extraction. Cure.		Oral.	No dilatation nor sign of previous spasmodic stenosis.

SEEDS, NUTS AND SHELLS.

Illustration.	Age.	Foreign body.	Location.	Anesthetic.	Tube	Problem.	Forceps.	Point of Seizure.	Result.	Time.	Route.	Remarks.
Fig. 328.	6 mos.	Hull of beech nut.	Right upper lobe bronchus, 24 days.	None.	4 mm.	Flat hull crosswise.	Side curved. (used also as a hook.)	Flatwise.	Extraction. Cure.	4 min.	Oral.	Side curved forceps used as a hook for turning intruder. Dyspnea relieved by "sponge pumping."
Fig. 329.	26 mos.	Peanut kernel. (Salted.)	Middle lobe bronchus, 19 days.	None.	5 mm.	Friable.	Straight	Delicate by presenting end.	Extraction. Cure.	8 min.	Oral.	Middle lobe bronchial invasion rare.
Fig. 330	2½ Yrs.	Maize.	Tracheal bifurcation, three weeks.	None.	5 mm.	Friable. Macerated.	Straight	Delicate. By presenting conical end.	Extraction. Cure.	11 min.	Oral.	Recovery slow but complete.
Fig. 331.	4½ Yrs.	Watermelon seed.	Trachea, 5 days.	None.	Laryngoscope	Crosswise fixation.	Alligator.	Flatwise Rotated sagittally.	Extraction. Cure.	½ min.	Oral.	Supraglottic tracheoscopy.
Fig. 332.	7 Yrs.	Watermelon seed.	Subglottic larynx, 3 months.	None.	Laryngoscope.	Crosswise fixation.	Alligator.	Flatwise Rotated sagitally	Extraction. Cure.	25 sec.	Oral.	Supraglottic tracheoscopy.
Fig. 333.	3 Yrs.	Maize.	Middle lobe bronchus, two days.	None.	5 mm.	Tight impaction. Friable. Conical.	Straight.	Presenting part.	Extraction. Cure.	18 min.	Route.	Middle lobe invasion rare.

SEEDS, NUTS AND SHELLS—Continued.

Illustration.	Age.	Foreign body.	Location.	Anesthetic.	Tube.	Problem.	Forceps.	Point of Seizure.	Result.	Time.	Route.	Remarks.
Fig. 334.	11 mos.	Walnut shell.	Esophagus. (location not recorded) 48 hours.	None.	7 mm.	Impacted rough body.	Rotation.	At apex.	Extraction. Cure.	3 min.	Oral.	Free rotation permitted prevented trauma.
Fig. 335.	4 Yrs.	Olive pulp.	Esophagus between two strictures above hiatus.	None.	7 mm.	Small foreign body between two excentric strictures.	Plain.	As presented.	Extraction. Cure.	35 min.	Oral.	Upper stricture divulsed.
Fig. 336.	5 Yrs.	Cherry pit.	Esophagus; thoracic: five days.	None.	7 mm.	Smooth round body impacted in stricture.	Plain.	As presented.	Extraction. Cure.	4 min.	Oral.	Almost dead from water starvation when admitted.
Fig. 337.	3½ mos.	Maize.	Left main bronchus, 9 days.	None.	4 mm.	Friable. Complete occlusion.	Strong Expansion.	As presented.	Extraction. Cure.	14 min.	Oral.	Post-operative dyspnea due to "drowning in own secretions" relieved by "sponge pumping."
Fig. 338.	2 Yrs.	Peanut kernel.	Right stem bronchus at orifice inferior lobe bronchus. 3 days.	None.	5 mm.	Impacted. Large amount of secretion.	Straight.	As presented.	Extraction. Cure.	½ hr. twice.	Oral.	
Fig. 339.	9 mos.	Egg shell.	Larynx, 4 weeks.	None.	Laryngoscope.	Fragile. Subglottic edema.	Alligator (Springless).	Delicate.	Extraction. Cure.	1 min.	Oral.	Antitoxin had been given. Subglottic edema present before operation. No tracheotomy.

SEEDS, NUTS AND SHELLS—Continued.

Illustration.	Age.	Foreign body.	Location.	Anesthetic.	Tube.	Problem.	Forceps.	Point of Seizure.	Result.	Time.	Route.	Remarks.
Fig. 340.	4 Yrs.	Gourd seed.	Left main bronchus, 5 months.	Chloroform.	5 mm.	Crosswise. Half in upper lobe bronchus.	Side curved.	Flatwise after hooking upward.	Extraction. Cure.	4 min.	Oral.	Side curved forceps used closed as hook for turning.
Fig. 341.	14 mos.	Glass.	Subglottic, six days.	None.	7 mm.	Fragile. Subglottic edema.	Straight.	Delicate.	Extraction. Cure.	9 min.	Oral.	Subglottic edema present before operation. Subsided without tracheotomy.
	6 Yrs.	Peanut kernel.	Left upper lobe bronchus, 24 hours.	Chloroform.	5 mm.	Fragile.	Straight.	Delicate.	Extraction. Cure.	15 min.	Oral.	Large quantity of pus liberated.
Fig. 342.	5 mos.	"Job's tear." (Coix lachryma Jobi).	Right main bronchus, six days.	None.	4 mm.	Round, smooth, impacted cone, apex presenting. Annular edematous stenosis.	Expansion.	Presenting cone.	Extraction. Cure.	12 min.	Oral.	Large quantity of pus liberated.
Fig. 343.	6 Yrs.	Maize.	Left main bronchus, 5 hrs.	Ether and chloroform.	5 mm.	Impacted. Friable cone.	Straight.	Presenting cone.	Extraction. Cure.	11 min.	Oral.	Broke at glottis. Remainder impacted subglottically. Removed by supraglottic tracheoscopy.
Fig. 344.	3 Yrs.	"Job's "tear." (Coix lachryma Jobi).	Right main bronchus, 20 hours.	Chloroform.	5 mm.	Round, smooth, impacted cone, apex presenting.	Expansion.	Presenting cone.	Extraction. Cure.	4 min.	Oral.	

SEEDS, NUTS AND SHELLS—Continued.

Illustration.	Age.	Foreign body.	Location.	Anesthetic.	Tube.	Problem.	Forceps.	Point of Seizure.	Result.	Time	Route.	Remarks.
Fig. 345.	19 mos.	Peanut kernel.	Right main bronchus, 30 hours.	None.	5 mm.	Friable. Macerated.	Straight.	Delicate	Extraction. Left hospital in ten days	11 min.	Oral.	Some cough remaining 3 months later.
Fig. 346.	5 Yrs.	Maize.	Right main bronchus.	Ether.	5 mm.	Friable. Macerated.	Straight.	Delicate.	Extraction. Cure.	4 min.	Oral.	
A B Fig. 347.	23 mos	Peanut kernel. Necrotic bronchial cartilage Abscess.	Right inferior lobe bronchus, one month.	None.	5 mm.	Friable. Macerated.	Straight.	Delicate.	Extraction. Left hospital.			Abscess evacuated by extraction of foreign body. Died 2 months after leaving hospital.
Fig. 348.	3 Yrs.	Paper pulp.	Esophagus above hiatal level. In previously existing stricture.	Ether.	7 mm.	Foreign body between two cicatricial strictures	Straight.	As presented.	Extraction. Cure.	30 min.	Oral.	Ether given for divulsion of stricture, not necessary. Early case.

BUTTONS.

Illustration.	Age	Foreign body.	Location.	Anesthetic.	Tube.	Problem.	Forceps.	Point of Seizure.	Result.	Time.	Route.	Remarks.
Fig. 349.	16 Yrs.	Button.	Right main bronchus, one month.	Chloroform.	7 mm.	Impaction below annular edema.	Strong expansion.	Flatwise.	Extraction. Cure.	30 min.	Oral.	
	14 Yrs.	Button.	Trachea.	Cocaine.	Laryngoscope	Impacted cross-	Hook. Full curved	Hook in center opening	Extraction. Cure	½ hr.	Oral.	Early case.

BUTTONS—Continued.

Illustration.	Age.	Foreign body.	Location.	Anesthetic.	Tube.	Problem.	Forceps.	Point of Seizure.	Result.	Time.	Route.	Remarks.
Fig. 351.	18 Yrs.	Shoe button.	Right stem (?) bronchus, 11 months.	Chloroform.	7 mm.	Imbedded in granulation tissue.	Rotation.	In loop.	Extraction. Cure.	70 min.		Calcareous incrustations. Early case.
Fig. 352.	7 Yrs.	Shoe button.	Left main bronchus, 3 months.	None.	7 mm.	Impacted Wire loop projecting.	Hook.	Withdrawn by hook inserted in loop.	Extraction. Cure.	6 min.	Oral.	
Fig. 353.	6 mos.	Shoe button.	Right bronchus near orifice.	None.	4 mm.	Impacted. Infant.	Hook.	Withdrawn by hook in loop.	Extraction. Cure.	9 min.	Oral.	Demonstrates possibilities of small tubes.
Fig. 354.	2 Yrs.	Pearl button.	Esophagus below plica cricopharyngeus, 3 days.	None.	Esophageal speculum.	Impacted	Alligator.	Presenting edge.	Extraction. Cure.	2 min.	Oral.	
Fig. 355.	16 mos.	Pearl button.	Esophagus below plica cricopharyngeus, 4 days.	None.	Esophageal speculum.	Impacted	Alligator.	Presenting edge.	Extraction. Cure.	1 min.	Oral.	
Fig. 356.	2½ mos.	Pin button.	Esophagus below plica cricopharyngeus, 3 days.	None.	Esophageal speculum.	Impacted Sharp point laterally imbedded in wall.	Rotation.	Extreme left edge.	Extraction. Cure.	2 min.	Oral.	Point rotated so as to trail behind on withdrawal. See schema under "Mechanical Problems."

BUTTONS—Continued.

Illustration.	Age.	Foreign body.	Location.	Anesthetic.	Tube.	Problem:	Forceps.	Point of Seizure.	Result.	Time.	Route.	Remarks.
Fig. 357. Fig. 358.	2 Yrs.	Pin button.	Esophagus below plica cricopharyngeus, 31 hours.	None.	Esophageal speculum.	Impacted Sharp pointed pin in wall.	Alligator.	Point of pin.	Extraction. Cure.		Oral.	Point protected with forceps.

MINERALS.

Illustration.	Age.	Foreign body.	Location.	Anesthetic.	Tube.	Problem:	Forceps.	Point of Seizure.	Result.	Time.	Route.	Remarks.
Fig. 359.	7 Yrs.	Pebble.	Right main bronchus, 7 days.	Chloroform.	7 mm.	Smooth, hard body impacted below edematous stenosis.	Strong expansion.	By presenting part.	Extraction. Cure.	30 min.	Oral.	
	5 Yrs.	Wooden plug.	Right main bronchus, four days.	None.	5 mm.	Impacted below edematous stenosis. Hard surface.	Strong Expansion.	By presenting part.	Extraction. Cure.	20 min.	Tracheotomic.	Tracheotomy required for dyspnea. Early case.
Fig. 360.	25 Yrs.	Coal (3 gm.)	Left main bronchus, five days.	Cocaine.	9 mm.	Conical. Impacted below edematous annular stenosis. Forceps slipping	Strong expansion.	Presenting cone.	Extraction Cure.	3½ hrs.	Oral.	No sequelae from 3½ hrs. continuous bronchoscopy. Only one reintroduction.

MINERALS—Continued.

Illustration.	Age.	Foreign body.	Location.	Anesthetic.	Tube.	Problem.	Forceps.	Point of Seizure.	Result.	Time.	Route.	Remarks.
Fig. 361	28 Yrs.	Pebble.	Left stem bronchus, 1 month.	Ether.	9 mm.	Hard rounded surface. Forceps slipping off.	Straight.	Presenting part.	Extraction. Cure.	74 min.	Oral.	Early case.
Fig. 362.	10 mos.	China-ware.	Larynx four hours.	None.	Laryngoscope.	Corner in ventricle Extreme dyspnea.	Alligator.	Flatwise, after turning.	Extraction. Cure.	1 min.	Oral.	

DENTAL OBJECTS.

Illustration.	Age.	Foreign body.	Location.	Anesthetic.	Tube	Problem.	Forceps.	Point of Seizure.	Result.	Time.	Route.	Remarks.
Fig. 363.	13 Yrs.	Molar tooth.	Right inferior lobe bronchus, ten days.	None.	7 mm.	Impacted.	Straight.	As presented.	Extraction.	5 min.	Oral.	Typhoid fever. Temp. 103 with positive Widal on admission. Died 10th day after bronchoscopy.
Fig. 364.	30 Yrs.	Artificial denture. Gold.	Bottom of hypopharynx.	Ether.	Esophageal speculum.	Impacted. Sharp serrated edge. (Gold).	Rotation.	At pointed end.	Extraction. Cure.	10 min.	Oral.	Disengagement of point by lateral tubal counter-pressure. Ether necessary to relax esophagus to prevent trauma.

DENTAL OBJECTS—Continued.

Illustration.	Age.	Foreign body.	Location.	Anes-thetic.	Tube.	Problem.	Forceps.	Point of Seizure.	Result.	Time.	Route.	Remarks.
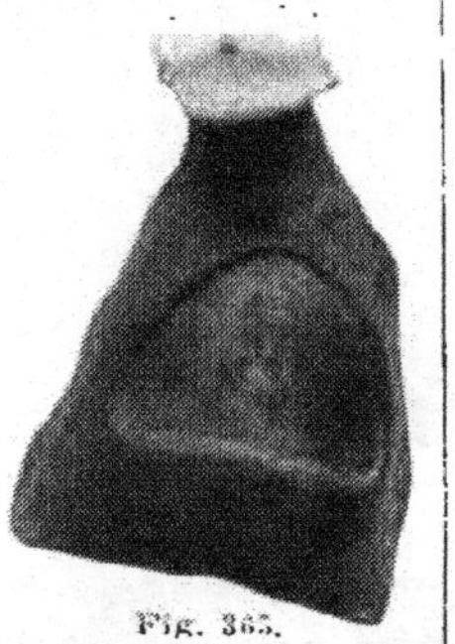 Fig. 365.	80 Yrs.	Artificial denture. Vulcan-ite.	Esophagus below plica cricopharyn-geus, two hours.	None.	Eso-pha-geal specu-lum.	Im-pacted.	Alli-gator.	Teeth present-ing.	Extrac-tion. Cure.	3 min.	Oral.	General anes-thesia not necessary because teeth pre-sharp points to injure eso-phageal walls.
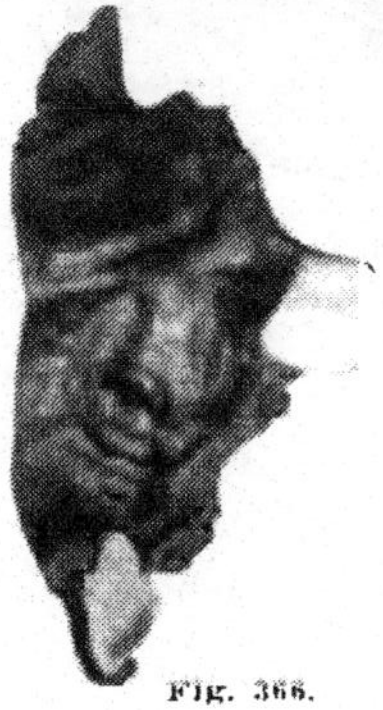 Fig. 366.	32 Yrs.	Artificial denture. Vulcan-ite.	Esophagus at hiatus. (Pushed there by previous operator) 16 days.	Ether.	10 mm.	Tight im-paction from being pushed cross-wise. Sharp wire hook on one end.	Rota-tion.	Extreme right end. (Opposite from hook).	Extrac-tion. Cure.	12 min.	Oral.	Without full relaxation fatal trauma would have been in-flicted.

AMMUNITION.

Illustration.	Age.	Foreign Body.	Location.	Anes-thetic.	Tube.	Problem.	Forceps.	Point of Seizure.	Result.	Time.	Route.	Remarks.
Fig. 368.	6 Yrs.	Shell primer.	Right pleura.	Ether	Eso-pha-geal specu lum.	Foreign body in pleura.	Alli-gator.	One jaw inside.	Extrac-tion. Cure.	3 min.	Oral.	First recorded case of pleuros-copy for foreign body.
Fig. 369.	23 Yrs.	Bullet.	Left bronchial orifice.	Cocaine.	9 mm.	Impacted	Straight.	Sidewise.	Extrac-tion. Cure.		Oral.	Entered by aspiration, not by gunshot.

CHAPTER XXI.

Illustrative Cases of Endoscopy for Foreign Bodies in the Air and Food Passages.

As the factor paramount in peroral endoscopy is the mechanical problem of extraction, and as this problem is dominated by the nature of the foreign body, the following cases are grouped by the character of the intruder rather than by chronological or anatomic data, so that the endoscopist about to deal with a foreign body case may, without unnecessary delay in page-turning for cross-references, see the problem similar bodies have presented, and how they were dealt with, successfully or unsuccessfully. For similar reasons subordinate matters, such as previous bronchoscopies by other operators,* symptoms, and even entire cases of no particular interest have been omitted. The fundamental importance of the duration of the operation being recognized by all endoscopists, it is given under "Time," if recorded. If this were invariably done by all endoscopists, an approximate estimate of the advisable time limit would soon be obtained. The location at the time of removal and the length of sojourn are given together, though it was not always known how long the intruder had been in the particular location stated.

It will be noted that chloroform is mentioned in the earlier cases. This is no longer used by the author, except that if ether fails to produce complete relaxation in the cases of very large and very sharp foreign bodies in the esophagus a little chloroform may be added for relaxation after the stimulant effect of ether makes chloroform safe. All the late cases in children were done without anesthesia, general or local. "Point of seizure" refers to the part of the foreign body seized or the manner of seizing it. The rotation forceps come together only at the points thus permitting rotation to the position of least resistance during withdrawal or such rotation as would facilitate the disimpaction of one point of pointed transfixed bodies, as explained in the two sections on "Mechanical Problems." "Alligator rotation" forceps (Fig. 210) are used through the laryngoscope and esophageal speculum. Where simply "alligator" is given, it refers to an elongated form of Mosher's alligator forceps. The cases include those done by Dr. Ellen J. Patterson as well as those by the author.

As illustrations of modern coins is forbidden by law, special permission was obtained from the United States Government for the making and publishing of the illustrations below.

*In about 45 per cent of the cases here recorded removal had been previously attempted by others. About 15 per cent arrived in a serious state from trauma of rough attempts. In many cases the mechanical problem had been converted from a very simple into a very difficult one. Moribund cases are not included here because no endoscopy was done by the author. All of which may be dismissed from consideration further than to state that if a foreign-body endoscopy cannot be done carefully it had better not be done at all.

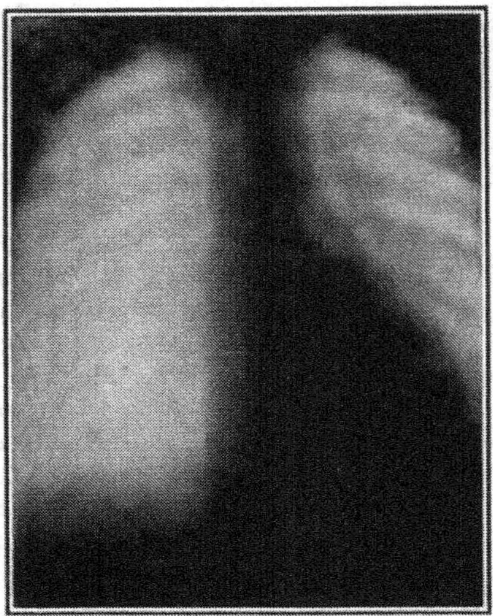

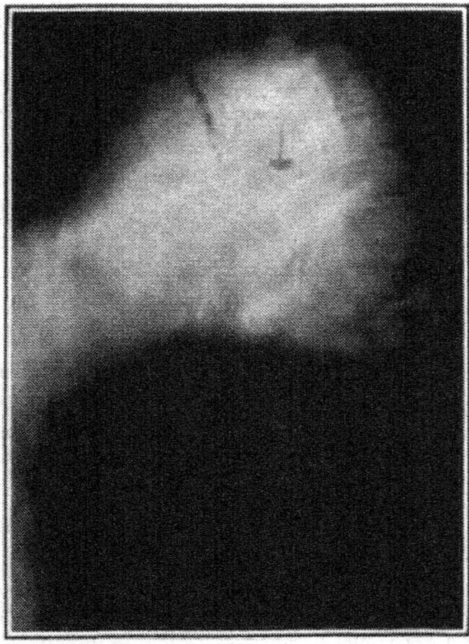

FIG. 370.—Radiographs, lateral and anteroposterior, showing tack in left main bronchus of a boy of eleven years. Tack removed by oral bronchoscopy without anesthesia. (Radiographs made by Dr. George W. Grier. Author's case.)

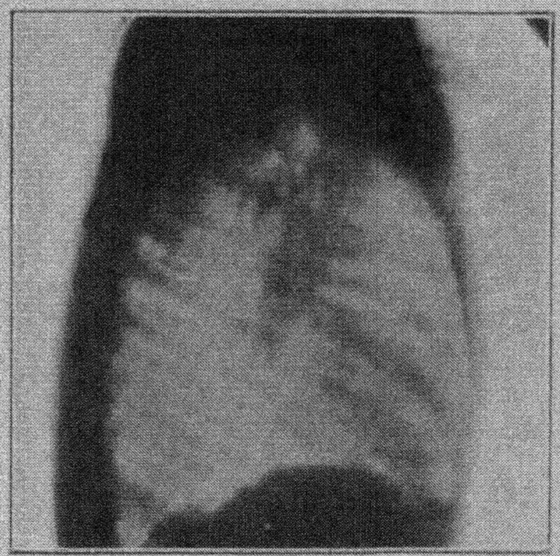

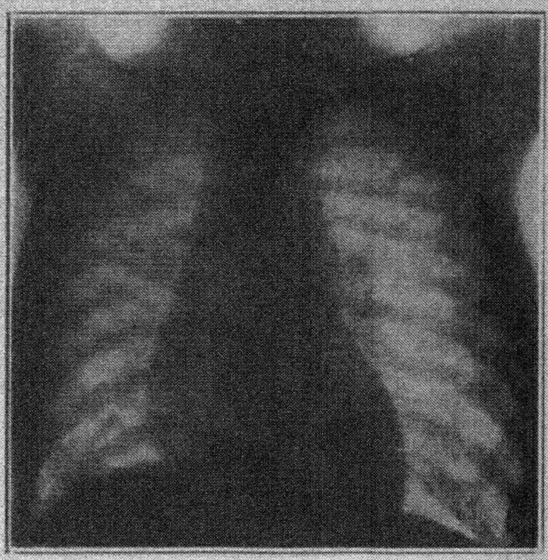

FIG. 371.—Radiographs, lateral and anteroposterior, showing tack in left main bronchus of a boy of eight years. Tack removed by oral bronchoscopy without anesthesia. (Radiographs by Dr. George W. Grier. Author's case.)

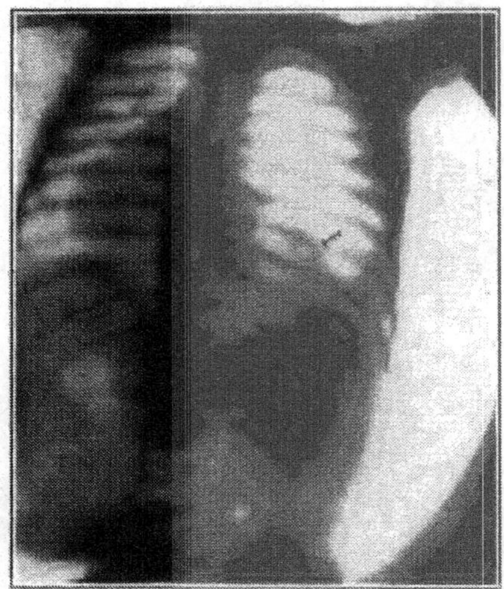

FIG. 372.—Abscess in right lung of a boy 23 months old. The peanut, which caused the abscess, does not show. Peanut removed and abscess evacuated by oral bronchoscopy without anesthesia. Shadow strengthened for photo-engraving. (Author's case.)

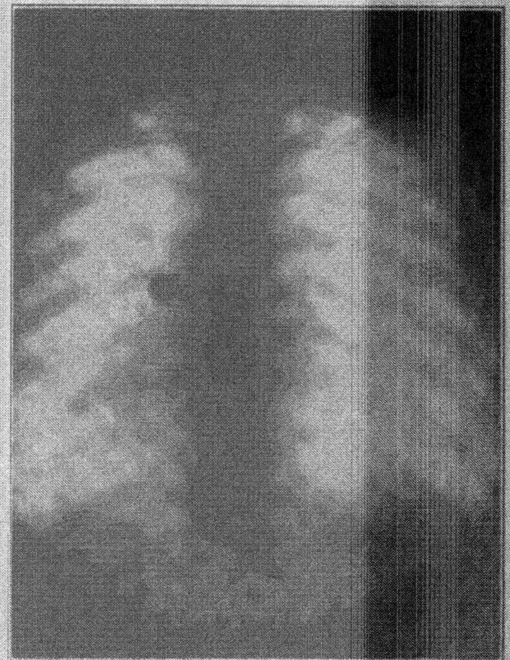

Fig. 374.—Radiograph showing stickpin in left bronchus of a boy of fifteen years. Pin was removed by oral bronchoscopy. Radiograph made by the roentgenologist of the German Hospital, Philadelphia. (Author's case.)

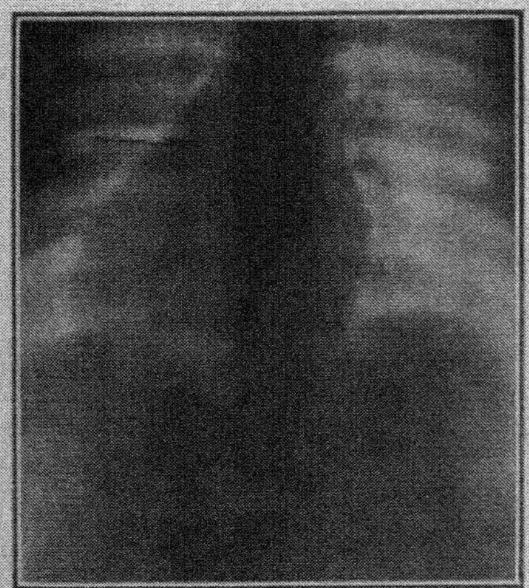

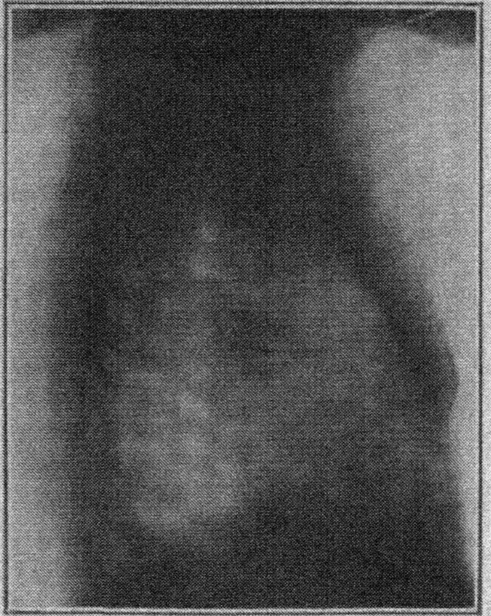

FIG. 374.—Radiographs, lateral and anteroposterior, showing shawl pin in the left main bronchus (head in upper lobe bronchus) of a girl of twelve years. Removed by oral bronchscopy. (Radiograph made by Dr. George C. Johnston. Author's case.)

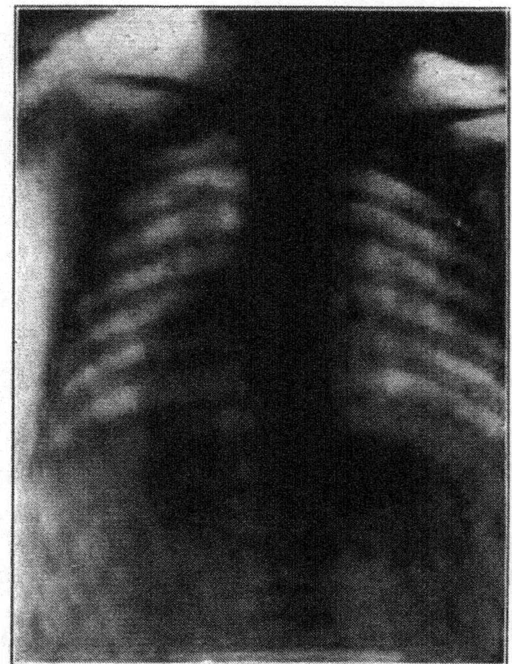

Fig. 375.—Radiographs, showing pin in right bronchus of a boy aged four years. Pin removed by oral bronchoscopy. (Radiograph by Dr. Russell H. Boggs). Pin shadow strengthened for photo-engraving. (Author's case.)

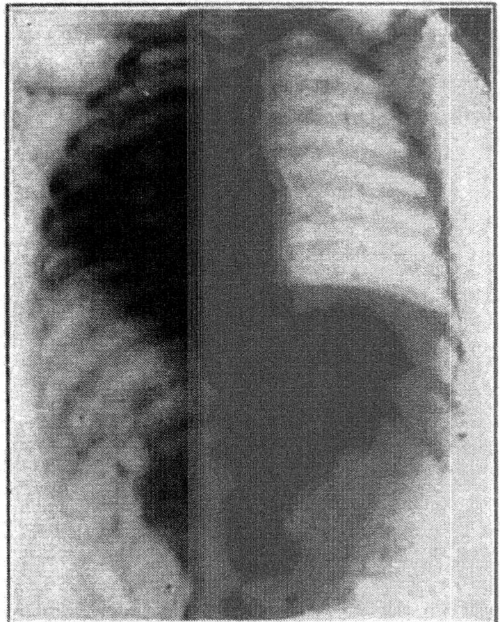

FIG. 376.—Radiograph showing shoe button (only metal part dense enough to show) in left main bronchus of a girl of seven years. Distortion gives appearance of median position. Left lung atelectatic. Compensatory emphysema of right lung. Button was aspirated three months previously. Removal by oral bronchoscopy without anesthesia, a hook being inserted in the eye of the button. (Radiograph by Dr. George C. Johnston. Author's case.)

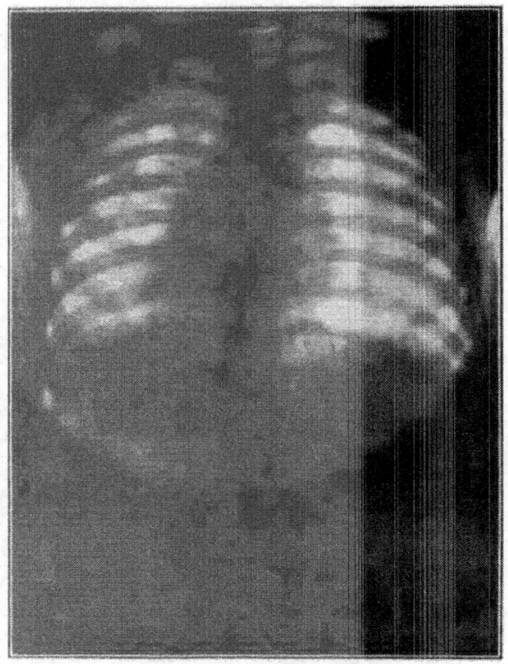

FIG. 377.—Radiograph showing pebble in right bronchus of a girl eight years of age. Removed by oral bronchoscopy. (Radiograph by Dr. George C. Johnston. Author's case.)

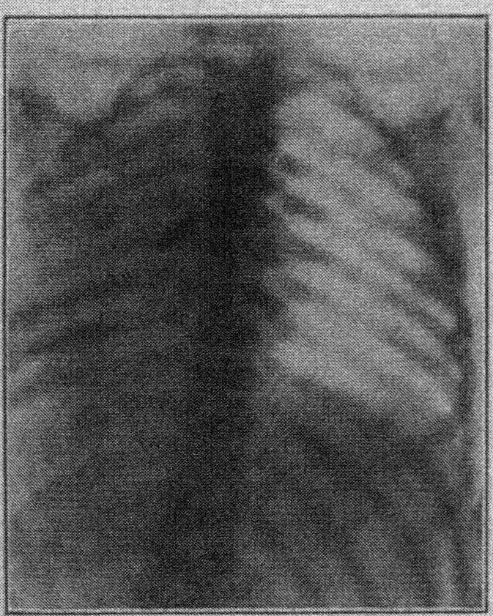

FIG. 378.—Foot of alarm clock in left bronchus of child of four years. Present 25 days. Pneumonic consolidation of left lung. Intruder removed by oral bronchoscopy. Radiograph one month later showed lung normal. (Radiograph by Dr. George C. Johnston. Author's case.)

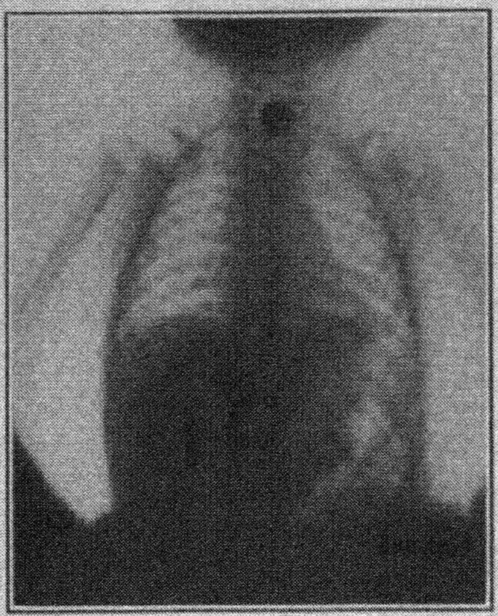

FIG. 379.—Collar button in esophagus of infant twelve months old. Removed by specular esophagoscopy. (Radiograph by Dr. George C. Johnston. Author's case.)

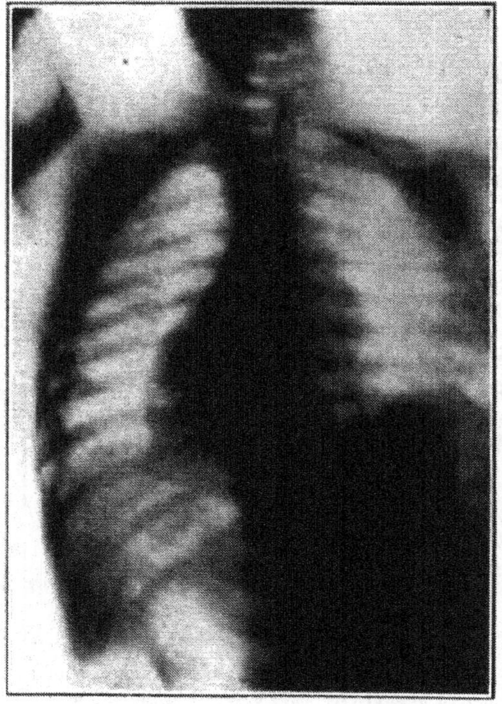

FIG. 380.—Staple (double-pointed tack) in esophagus. Intruder passed into stomach, endoscopically, turned and removed. (Radiograph by Dr. Russell H. Boggs. Author's case.)

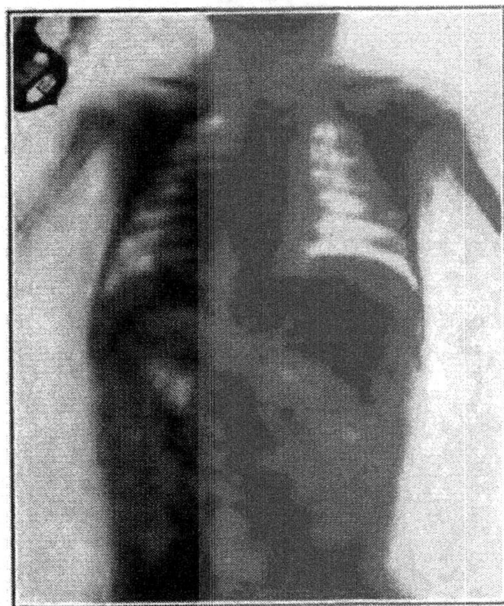

Fig. 381.—Finger ring in esophagus, above bronchial crossing, of a child of ten months. Removed by oral esophagoscopy without anesthesia. (Radiograph by Dr. Russell H. Boggs. Author's case.)

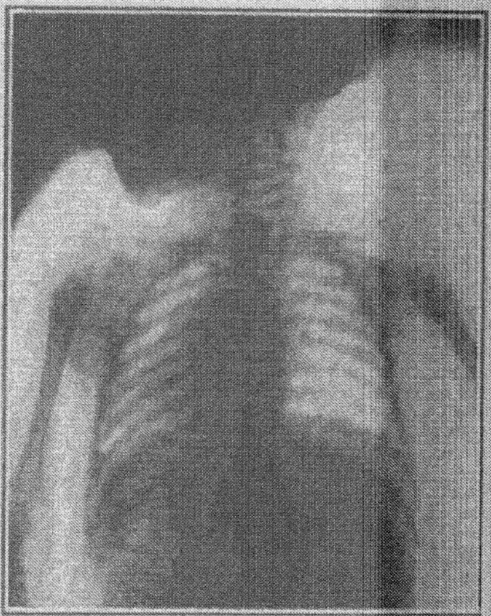

Fig. 382.—Radiograph showing button in esophagus of infant sixteen months old. Removed by specular esophagoscopy without anesthesia. (Radiograph by Dr. King. Author's case.)

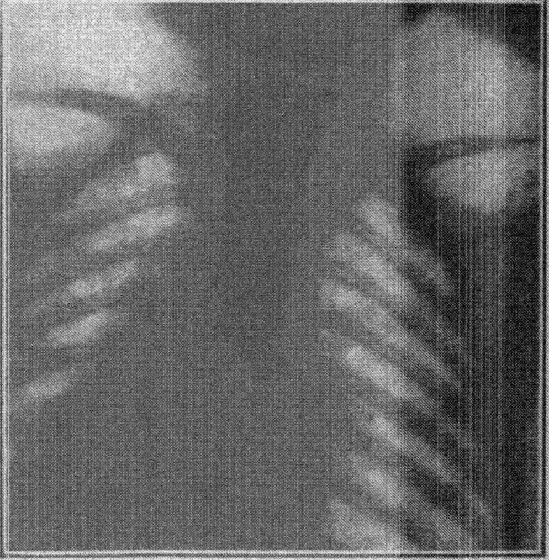

Fig. 383.—Radiograph showing coin (English half-penny) in esophagus of a girl five years of age. Removed by specular esophagoscopy without anesthesia. (Radiograph by Dr. George W. Grier. Author's case.)

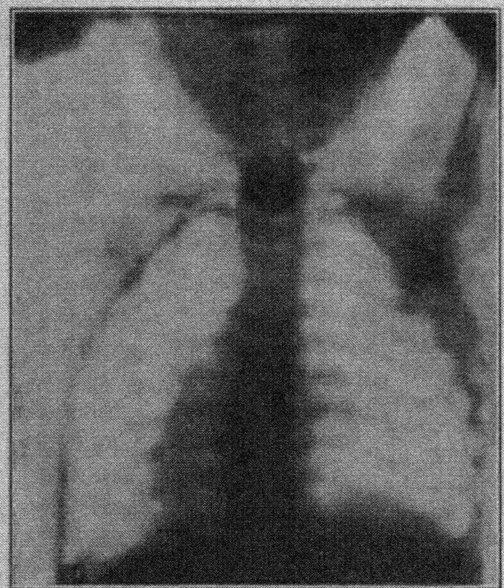

Fig. 384.—Radiograph showing coin (Canadian twenty-five cent piece) in the esophagus of a child of two years. Coin removed by esophagoscopy. (Radiograph by Dr. Russell H. Boggs. Author's case.)

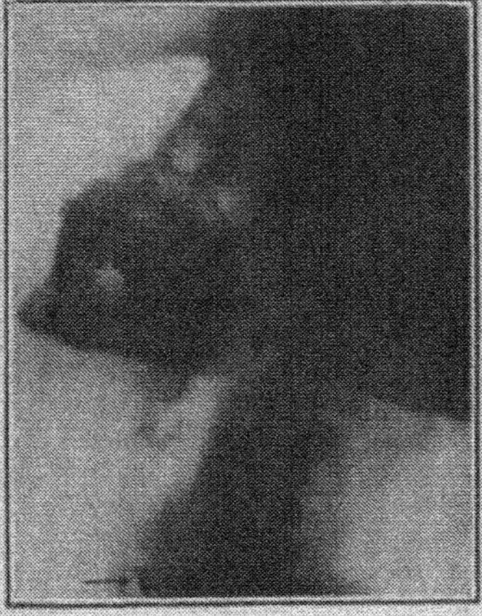

Fig. 385.—Radiograph showing fragment of bone in the trachea of a woman of 39 years. Bones are not likely to show in an anteroposterior view and this radiograph shows how readily a bone low in the neck might be missed in a lateral radiograph. Bone removed by oral bronchoscopy. (Radiograph by Dr. George C. Johnston. Author's case.)

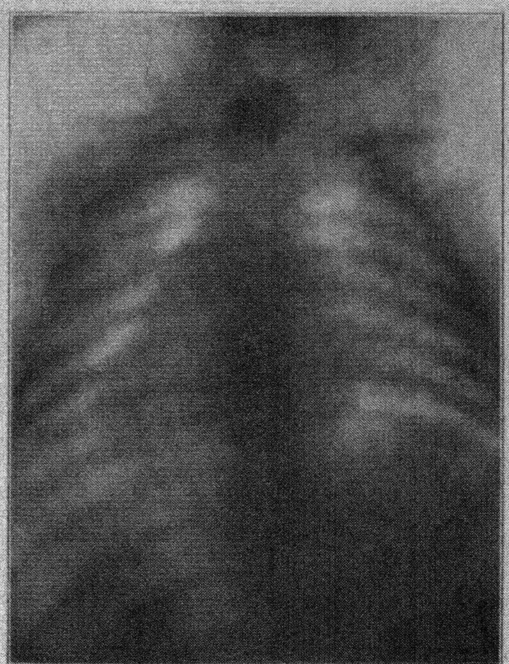

Fig. 386.—Radiograph showing gold locket in esophagus of a girl of 2½ years. Locket removed by esophagoscopy without anesthesia. (Radiograph by Dr. George W. Grier.)

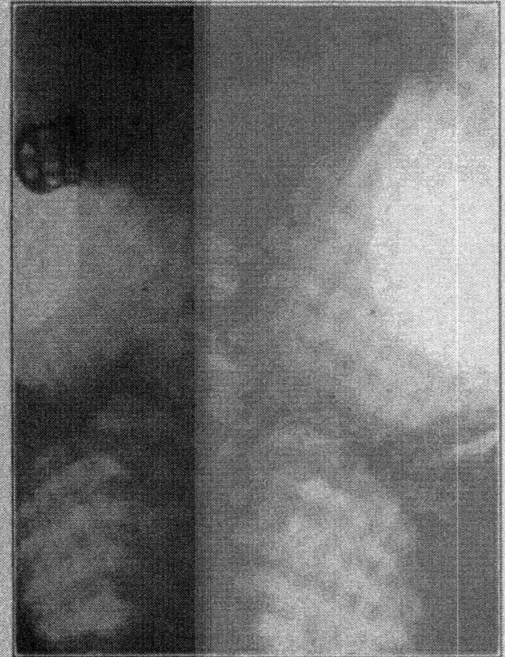

Fig. 387.—Radiograph showing artificial denture in the esophagus of a man aged thirty years. Removed by esophagoscopy under ether anesthesia. (Radiograph by Dr. Russell H. Boggs. Author's case.)

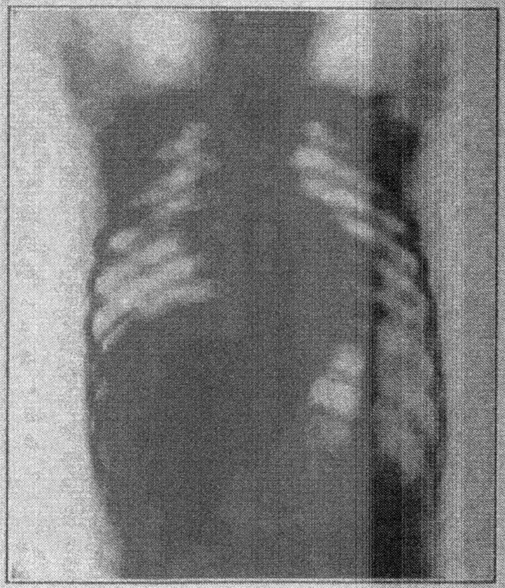

FIG. 387a.—Button with projecting rigid pin in the esophagus of an infant of $2\frac{1}{2}$ months. Removed by esophagoscopy without anesthesia. Laceration of esophagus prevented by the method illustrated in Fig. 209. (Author's case.)

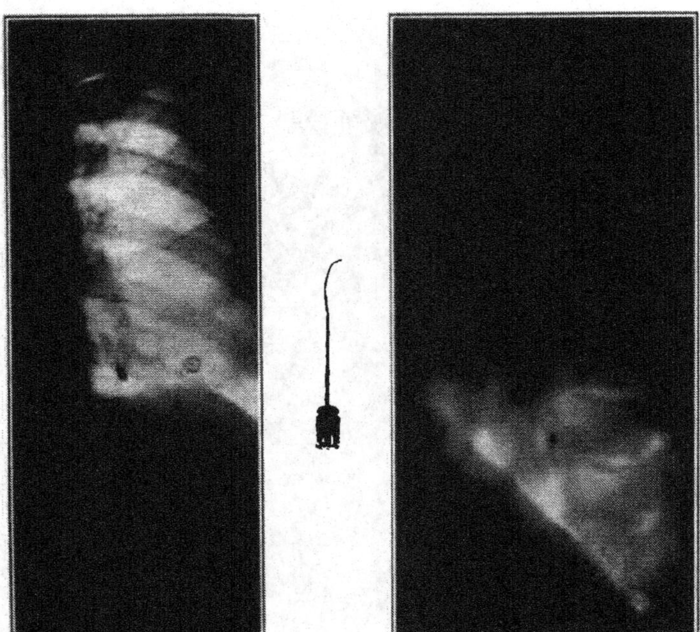

FIG. 387b.—Radiographs showing a dental root-canal broach in a small posterior branch of a larger posterior branch of the inferior-lobe bronchus of a man of 39 years. The foreign body is seen just above the dome of the diaphragm in the anteroposterior radiograph, though really in the part of the lung down back of the dome as shown in the lateral radiograph. Removed through the mouth by bronchoscopy under local anesthesia. This is the lowest position from which a foreign body has ever been removed by bronchoscopy. The full length of a 40 cm. bronchoscope was barely sufficient to reach it (Author's case.)

CHAPTER XXII.

Benign Growths in the Larynx.

The general subject is covered so thoroughly in books upon the larynx that extensive consideration here would be out of place. Only some phases of the subject which have a particular bearing on endoscopic surgery will be considered. The endoscopic appearances are similar to those by the indirect method except as modified by the point of view as explained in Chapter VII. In all adults careful clinical study by the indirect method should precede direct laryngoscopy.

Granulomata in the larynx, while not true neoplasms, in some instances need to be dealt with as such, by extirpation.

Vocal nodules, while not true neoplasms, are occasionally so stubbornly resistant of other methods of cure that surgical measures are needed. When very prominent they may be excised under local anesthesia. Should cocaine cause so much shrinkage as to make accurate excision impossible, general anesthesia will be required. The author has had excellent results in the treatment of sessile vocal nodules by touching them with a fine galvano-cautery point as recommended by Wylie. Sir St. Clair Thomson favors this method in exceptional cases, but points out that extreme dexterity is requisite, a caution that is particularly forceful as we are, in most instances, dealing with a patient to whom the voice is a valuable asset. A form of vocal nodule seen in children and known as "screamers nodes" (Dan McKenzie) may be excised as advised by Albrecht (Bib. 14). Fibromata, while possibly of inflammatory genesis in some instances, are clinically true neoplasms. As a rule direct excision is not followed by recurrence if a goodly portion of basal tissue is removed. A typical case of small fibroma is illustrated in Fig. 79. They are, as a rule, best dealt with by the tissue forceps, Fig. 35. They may be sliced off with the Katzenstein guillotine but the author's personal preference is the tissue forceps mentioned because any desired portion of the normal base can be included in the excision. At times a small granuloma may appear as the healing granulations organize and may persist for a few weeks or even months, simulating recurrence. So long as it does not increase in size, excision is not necessary. Very large fibromata may be excised with the basket punch forceps, Fig. 36. If so large that the base cannot be seen they may be amputated with the snare (Fig. 41), and then the base may be cauterized galvanically, or as the author prefers, excised with forceps. The galvano-cautery is especially useful in destroying the basal vessels of fibro-angiomata. John A. Thompson (Bib. 547) reports an interesting case of removal of fibroma 1x1¼ inches (25x32 mm.) in size, springing from the upper orifice of the larynx.

The depth of removal of benign growths is closely connected with the tendency to recurrence of the particular growth, and some information as to this tendency is obtainable from general laryngeal literature. Benign growths repullulate on the surface and do not infiltrate. Therefore, a less amount of normal is needed than in malignancy. Cystomata have been known to get well after galvano-puncture or excision of part of the sac. In the author's experience recurrence can be avoided with certainty only by complete extirpation of the sac. The same is true of adenomata. Angiomata, which are usually much more extensive and deeper seated than appears, require deep excision, and the galvano-cautery to destroy the vessels at the base, both to arrest hemorrhage and lessen the tendency to recurrence. A diffuse telangiectasis if requiring treatment may be punctured or scarified at a number of sittings with the galvano-cautery. Lymphoma, enchondroma and osteoma, if small, may be excised with the basket punch forceps (Fig. 36), taking as much of normal base as possible without risk of stenosis. Myxomata, other than myxomatous degeneration of fibromata is very rare and there are no data on which to base a rule as to depth of excision necessary to prevent recurrence. Lipomata are also very rare. An interesting resume of the subject will be found in the article by Goldstein (Bib. 171). From the research there reported it is clear that to avoid recurrence it is necessary to remove thoroughly every vestige of the growth. Thyroid gland tumors from aberrant islands of thyroid tissue do not require very radical excision of normal base but should be removed as completely as possible. An excellent article is published by Wells (Bib. 586). The question of the advisability of merely slicing off small benign tumors on the vocal cords or in the neighborhood of the arytenoid joint, and deferring more radical removal of the base until the growth demonstrates a tendency to recurrence is discussed under papilloma. The technic of direct removal of benign growths will be found in Chapter VII and special attention is called to the author's method of operating at the *side* of the tongue instead of over the dorsum. Attention is also called to the recent development of suspension laryngoscopy, the details of which, Prof Killian, the originator, has honored us all by describing in a separate Chapter (VIII). Lynch has devised some excellent instruments for suspension work. As stated by Sir St. Clair Thomson (Bib. 539) external operation is unheard of in the treatment of simple laryngeal neoplasms in adults and should be resorted to only when an expert has failed *per vias naturales.*

PAPILLOMATA OF THE LARYNX IN CHILDREN.

Of all benign growths in the larynx papilloma is the most frequent. It may occur at any age of childhood and may even be congenital. The author has seen one case in which it was undoubtedly congenital and one in which it was probably so. Both cases follow:

Congenital papilloma of the larynx. A male infant, two months of age had had a croupy cry and stridor without cyanosis since birth. It suddenly developed a marked increase in the stridor, with dyspnea and cyanosis. The author was called, but the child was dead when he arrived. Post mortem examination showed a papilloma on the left cord near the anterior commissure. It did not seem sufficiently large to account for death by obstruction even allowing for shrinkage, though the symptoms as described by the parents denoted obstructive dyspnea. The thymus and other viscera were normal. Doubtless indrawing of the upper laryngeal aperture contributed; possibly spasm did also.

In the second case the author was called for direct examination of a new born male infant that was cyanotic and showed deep indrawing at the supraclavicular and suprasternal notches. Direct laryngoscopy, without anesthesia, revealed a large papilloma occupying almost the entire upper laryngeal orifice. It was immediately excised and then the origin was seen to be single on the right cord near the anterior commissure. The patient was about six hours old at the time of operation. It was seen once subsequently (by Dr. L. C. Manchester) about three months after operation. There was then no sign of recurrence, but this is not certain evidence that recurrence did not take place later.

Methods of treatment of papillomata of children. A sharp distinction must be made between papillomata of adults and of children because of the greater difficulty in curing the tendency to recurrence in the latter. In dealing with papillomata of the larynx in children, it is well to remember that we have two classes of case. Those in which the growth gets well either spontaneously or with slight treatment, surgical or otherwise. Second, those which are not readily amenable to any form of treatment and require persistent treatment of recurrences. Sweeping deductions should not be made from reports of isolated cases, even if observed for a year after operation, because of the different behavior of different cases as to recurrence, and cases reported immediately after operation are valueless statistically because of the large percentage of recurrences. If we are ever to arrive at final conclusions, all the cases seen by each observer must be reported, and the report should not be made until after at least one year's observation of cure.

There are nine methods of treatment to be considered.

1. Endolaryngeal applications.
2. Tracheotomy with subsequent rest of the larynx for a period of years.
3. Thyrotomy with radical extirpation of the growth.
4. Fulguration.
5. Radium and mesothorium.
6. Roentgen radiotherapy.
7. Endolaryngeal operation.
8. A combination of two or more of the above mentioned methods.
9. Laryngostomy.

Delavan established the value of alcohol applications in some cases. It is usually best to start with dilute alcohol, say about 50 per cent and increase the strength until absolute alcohol can be used. The applications may be made by the indirect method, using the gauze sponges and sponge holder, Figs. 25 and 26. No anesthetic is needed. The sponges should not be dripping. Spasm usually subsides quickly but this or any other method should not be used without previous tracheotomy if there is stenosis. E. L. Jones has had excellent results from organic salicylic acid saturated solution in alcohol.

Tracheotomy for papillomata. The beneficial effect of tracheotomy has long been noted. It is very marked in some cases, disappointing in others. Apart from its beneficial effect it should always be done as soon as the child develops noisy breathing and restlessness at night. Severe dyspnea with indrawing of the supraclavicular and sternal fossae and epigastrium should not be awaited. The rule should be, here as elsewhere, to do the tracheotomy always early rather than late. Many cases are *in extremis* when they arrive. Ballenger reports the death of a child with papilloma of the larynx on the way to the hospital, and a similar experience is known to almost every laryngologist. In cases of papillomata of large size, completely, or almost completely, obstructing the lumen of the trachea, it is necessary to proceed with extreme caution with the direct laryngoscopy, and not to unduly prolong the examination, because engorgement of the papillomata may very much increase their size and obliterate what little lumen remains. It takes but a moment, without any anesthesia, to get a good view of the larynx; but failing in this, the operator who suspects papilloma in any extremely dyspneic case, is perfectly justified in doing the tracheotomy first and making the diagnosis as to the exact condition afterward. The state of affairs in regard to tracheotomy for dyspnea is precisely the same as gastrostomy for dysphagia.

Thyrotomy for papillomata. Before the days of direct laryngoscopy the author tried thyrotomy for the removal of papillomata in children. The recurrence was so prompt that the author abandoned thyrotomy for this purpose and has repeatedly spoken against it. He is delighted to find that his opinion in this respect coincides with that of the greatest living authority on the larynx, Sir Felix Semon, who mentions one case (Bib. 511) in which seventeen thyrotomies were performed on the same patient with failure to cure. A great deal of damage may be done to the larynx by repeated thyrotomies, and intractable stenosis from deformity is almost certain to result. In these days of quick and thorough removal by direct laryngoscopy, there is rarely justification for doing thyrotomy, because endoscopic removal is just as thorough, no more likely to be followed by recurrence and repeated endolaryngeal removals are harmless if carefully done.

Fulguration for papillomata. Harmon Smith (Bib. 470) has had very satisfactory results with fulguration for papillomata in children and his interesting article should be read for details of the technic.

Radium for papillomata. Thomas J. Harris (Bib. 194) reports very favorable results from the use of radium in one case of his own and in twelve cases in the hands of Abbe, Culbert, Freudenthal, Polyak, Killian and Mazzochi. As stated by Harris, 100 mgm. of radium should be applied. Weaker applications probably irritate. The duration of each application, of course, depends upon the quantity of radium in the container. With 100 mgm. of radium element, or its equivalent in bromide or other salt, a duration of 20 minutes is probably sufficient. From two to ten sittings are usually necessary. A single application in some instances has caused a marked diminution in the growth, but recurrences, as with other methods, will probably require repeated treatments. Some cases do not seem to yield so readily. The future will determine the exact sphere of usefulness, and the dosage and duration of applications. A screening of not less than two mm. of metal and outside of the metal two mm. of hard rubber are essential to protect healthy tissues. The radium container should have an eye by means of which it can be secured in position by attaching it to the tracheotomic cannula above which it is inserted. The capsule may be held in place in untracheotomized cases, but the spasm excited requires a small container with sufficient screening and dosage. Mesothorium has been used by Killian.

Endolaryngeal extirpation of papillomata in children is practically limited to the direct method. No one who has ever worked by the direct method would think of going back to any indirect attempt in children, necessitating as it usually does, general anesthesia. To work with the mirror in an adult under local anesthesia is difficult enough, but to work with a child under a general anesthesia with the mirror presents difficulties that are almost insurmountable, to say nothing of the extreme danger of anesthesia in this class of cases. Worse yet is, as was done in the old days, a finger-guided forceps operation. As elsewhere stated no anesthetic whatever, general or local, is needed in the extirpation of papillomata in children. If, for any reason, a general anesthetic is used, it should be only in the tracheotomized cases because of the danger in dyspnea in untracheotomized patients. If a general anesthetic be used it is absolutely needless to add the risk of a cocaine application in a child. As a matter of fact a general anesthetic has only one excuse, and that is to lessen the spasm of the larynx in order to enable the operator more accurately to apply his forceps. With increased practice the operator will find that even for this purpose it is unnecessary. There is a peculiar sensation of softness to papillomata that, once recognized, is unmistakable and that will prevent the operator from forcibly removing any tissue other than papillomatous because of the firm resistance felt when normal tissue is grasped. In other words, the operator must train himself to apply just the amount of pressure to his forceps which is necessary to remove papillomatous tissue, but which will not bite into normal tissue. It goes without saying that such a degree of tactile sensibility can only be possible with extremely delicate and easy working forceps. Heavy handled, spring opposed, clumsy instruments will bite out anything, even cartilage, before any useful sensation is communicated to even the most delicate touch, because delicacy is destroyed by the opposition of the spring and the crude mechanism. Some authors advise against removal of papillomata in children during the stage of growth, preferring to do a tracheotomy and wait for a period of recession of the growth before extirpation. The difficulty is, as Stucky points out, in determining the period of recession. Papillomata should always be removed and the patient cured of recurrences, because, contrary to statements sometimes made, a child is *not* safe with only a tracheotomy cannula upon which to depend for air, unless under constant care of a physician and an experienced tracheal nurse. Accidental removal of the cannula following indrawing closure of the fistula has caused the death of many children. Others have died of occlusion of the cannula with secretions, dressings, granulations and papillomatous masses. In all cases of papilloma of the larynx the subglottic trachea should be inspected not only once but at every removal of the supraglottic papillomata. Many endoscopists have wondered why they cannot decannulate a papilloma case after removal of apparently all the growth. The reason is that the region between the glottis and the tracheal wound is full of papillomata. For this removal a bronchoscope may be inserted through the glottis, or a bronchoscope not slanted at the end may be used for supraglottic tracheoscopy. The author uses the direct laryngoscope and the tissue forceps, Fig. 35. In some cases the tracheal papillomata can be removed through the tracheal wound. Often it is impossible to distinguish between granulation tissue and true papillomata except by biopsy. It is not necessary, however, clinically to distinguish as it is a good thing to remove granulations which are so exuberant as to simulate papillomata. The technic of direct laryngeal extirpation is considered in Chapters VII and VIII. The special infant-size slide speculum is best for infants under 6 months.

The author's method for papillomata in children. The author has had best results from a combination of the alcohol application of Delavan between excisions by the direct method, and with tracheotomy in all cases that persistently repullulate. No tracheotomy is done at first, if the growth is small and especially if single (they rarely are), because there is a chance of cure by a few extirpations or in a few instances even by a single extirpation. If the child is slightly dyspneic the obstructing part of the growth is first removed directly without anesthesia, general or local, and then the remaining fungations are extirpated at a number of brief seances. The alcohol applications are not used in these cases. When repullations and growths in new locations demonstrate an intractable case, it is treated the same as a dyspneic case. If the child is very dyspneic when first seen the author does a tracheotomy, waits a week or ten days, and then proceeds with the extirpation without anesthesia and the alcohol after-treatment. The child is kept in the hospital under the watchful care of special tracheal nurses. If the growths are subglottic, reactionary edema of this region is very apt to require tracheotomy after extirpation, and therefore subglottic cases, whether dyspneic or not, are tracheotomized unless the growth is single and very small. The effect of the alcohol and the superficial cicatrices is to make an unfavorable soil for the growth of papillomata which, in a sense, resemble venereal warts. Galvano-cauterization is used in the worst cases to destroy the bases and to promote superficial cicatrices. The efficacy of removal and the post operative application of alcohol has been corroborated by Stucky (Bib. 511) and a number of other laryngologists. Its greatest drawback is the length of time required for cure in the very stubborn cases. But it will eventually cure almost all cases, and as the extirpations without anesthesia are not painful (the children do not even cry after the first few treatments) the author feels justified in adhering to it until some equally effective and more rapid method is sufficiently tested.

Laryngostomy. When all else fails in the few most stubborn cases, laryngostomy may be resorted to. Lining the larynx with epidermal epithelium makes a soil upon which papillomata will not grow, notwithstanding the fact that, as occurred in one case of the author, a typical papilloma identical histologically with the laryngeal growths occurred on the normal skin of the neck The after-treatment of laryngostomy extends over months. Unlike thyrotomy, it does not produce stenosis by causing deformity of the larynx. Cases stenosed by injudicious thyrotomy are curable by laryngostomy, which are the only papillomatous cases in which the author advises laryngostomy.

PAPILLOMATA IN THE LARYNX OF ADULTS.

Papillomata in adults are, on the whole, much more amenable to treatment than similar growths in children. Tracheotomy is very rarely required, and recurrences are slower in development. Many more cases are cured by a single extirpation and recurrences at new sites are not so common. In some instances the growths may be single, relatively quite fibrous and pedunculated. This form is beautifully illustrated in an interesting article by Loeb (Bib. 348).

In all forms of papillomata in adults operative removal is so satisfactory that there is little temptation to try other methods.

Depth of removal of papillomata. Should the growth be simply removed from the surface? Or should the basic normal be removed? And if so, how widely? To determine this point clinically, it was necessary to know whether the reappearances of papillomata are repullulations at the site of removal or whether fresh areas became the site of new growths. To determine this point accurate drawings were made by the author, and it was discovered that in eighteen cases out of twenty there was no recurrence at the site of removal if about 3 millimeters depth of normal tissue was removed. That is, there was no recurrence in the scar. In two cases the recurrence was so close as to be doubtful. On the other hand, in this same series of twenty cases in locations where the growths were simply removed from the surface, twenty out of twenty instances recurred. In another series of eighteen cases in which surface removal was done, papillomata appeared in a greater number of new locations after operation. It still remains a question whether the less tendency to recurrence after removal with a normal base was due to extirpation of every vestige of growth, or whether it was simply due to the fact that scar tissue is a bad soil for papillomatous growth. Clinical observation shows that papillomatous growths in the larynx or trachea usually do not spring from a firm thick scar. The author has noted the avoidance of scars by papillomata when extending down the trachea from the larynx toward the tracheotomic wound. In the author's opinion, when the growths are situated on the cords it is usually better to remove them with a very scanty base, telling the patient of probable recurrence. If there is a recurrence, slightly more radical removal is indicated, but under no circumstances should reckless or radical extirpation of normal tissue be indulged in. Cicatricial stenosis and prolonged, possibly permanent, impairment of the voice may result. In case of removals in the neighborhood of the arytenoids, great care must be used to avoid impairment of the laryngeal motility. The growths should everywhere be nipped off with only a small normal base and recurrences should be similarly nipped in the bud. Alcohol applications are useful. In contrast with the prompt and excellent results obtained in most cases, a very stubborn case is occasionally encountered which simulates the conditions found in children. The following is an example:

A single woman, aged twenty-five, was sent to the author by Dr. I. B. Reed for loss of voice of three months' duration following two months of hoarseness. Within the last two weeks dyspnea had been developing and examination by the indirect method revealed a large mass of papilloma occupying the entire right half of the larynx with more masses on the epiglottis and high up on the left ventricular band (A, Fig. 79). These were removed giving complete relief from the dyspnea and permitting some phonation. The patient was not seen for some time and returned extremely dyspneic. A recurrence of larger size than the original growth was found and many new locations were invaded. After removing the upper growth it was found that the papillomata had sprung up in the trachea which at the first operation was entirely free. Patient work and many sittings were necessary until finally at the end of sixteen months the patient was entirely free from any sign of recurrence and has remained so since. A period of four years having now elapsed, the patient may be called cured. The vocal results are excellent, the patient's voice perfectly normal for speaking and quite a good singing voice has also returned. This the author regards as due to the careful avoidance of injury to any of the submucosal tissues. Necessarily a considerable amount of the mucosa itself was removed with the base of the papilloma.

Plastic operation favoring the development of adventitious vocal bands. Some of the cases of papillomata from frequent accidents associated with indirect operations come in with the cords entirely destroyed and the larynx badly damaged. If there is motility in the arytenoids there is good hope of repair by careful work. The following case is an example:

A man, aged twenty-five, had been under the care of one of the oldest laryngologists in the country for two and one-half years for hoarseness. During this time a number of indirect operations upon the larynx had been done for removal of papillomata. The operations were difficult because the patient was insusceptible to anesthesia by cocaine. He was

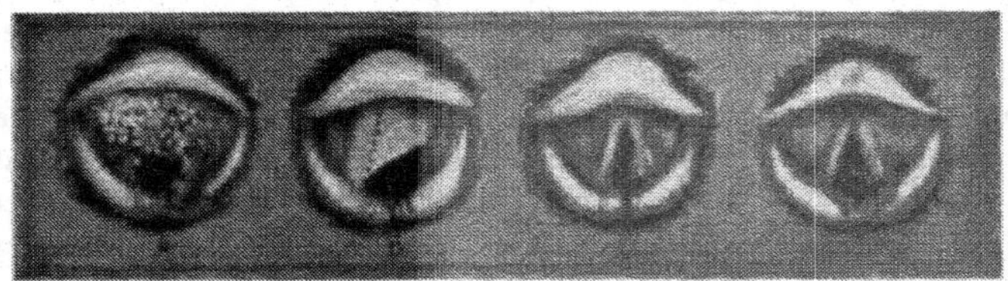

Fig 388.—Illustrating operation favoring formation of an adventitious vocal band in a man aged twenty-five years. A. Papilloma and granulation tissue with destruction of the vocal cords and the tip of one arytenoid eminence as the result of indirect operation. B. Cured of papilloma after many direct extirpations under local anesthesia. A web extended across the larynx from the right side from the neighborhood of the site of the original cord to the remnant of the ventricular band of the left side. Dotted line shows the position of incision for a plastic to assist in forming an adventitious band on the left side. C. Three months later the triangular mass of cicatricial tissue shown in B has become stretched out into an adventitious band. D. Three months later entire stretching out, absorption and disappearance of the elevation, resulting in the normal larynx with good voice. From a crayon drawing by the author. Patient referred to the author by Dr. James F. McKernon.

completely aphonic and could not, with the most violent efforts, phonate in the slightest degree. In this condition he applied to Dr. James F. McKernon of New York City who found the larynx filled with a mixture of papillomatous and granulation tissue. No sign of a cord was present (A, Fig. 388). Part of the arytenoid eminence was gone and its place was taken by a fungating mass of granulation. A part of each ventricular band was gone and granulations covered both bands. On attempted phonation both arytenoids moved, but no sign of anything resembling a vocal cord resulted from the movement. Dr. McKernon referred the case at once to the author for treatment. Under local anesthesia, the author removed all the tissues that looked papillomatous and some of the most exuberant granulations. At intervals during the following year recurrences of papillomata were removed, until at the end of sixteen months the patient returned after a three months' interval completely free from granulation and recurrences. A web extended across the larynx obliterating the entire anterior half as shown at B, Fig. 388. The author then did a plastic operation by making an incision along the dotted line marking out a cord from the cicatricial tissue, the incision extending from the arytenoid clear out to the perichondrium anteriorly. The tissue seemed under tension and the triangular flap after the incision hung almost altogether over toward the patient's left side and away from the adventitious band on the patient's right. The incision was made with the laryngeal knife, Fig. 85. At the end of three months this flap had flattened out and the action of the arytenoid on the cicatricial tissue had formed a very fair adventitious band with a projection simulating a vocal nodule (C). The first impulse was to remove this, but believing that it would furnish tissue to be extended by the combined effects of cicatricial contraction and the arytenoid action nothing was done with it. Three months later the patient returned and examination showed the condition to be as shown in B. The patient at this visit reported that six weeks before, he had astonished himself and his family by speaking. Dr. McKernon, who was kind enough to again examine the patient, in the condition shown at D, stated that he thought the results quite a clear indication of the possibilities of work by the direct method. The patient is now able to do his part of the shouting in a football game. The voice is deep and somewhat rough; but, judging by similar cases, it will become smoother in time.

For the success of the operation it is necessary to wait until the cicatricial contraction has put the scar on tension, otherwise the incision is apt to heal and unite its two edges. On the contrary, if there is tension, as in this case, the incision will gape so widely that there will be no chance of its adhering and the subsequent cicatricial contraction will tend to widen the gap instead of to narrow it. Another factor in the success of this kind of a case is not to remove tissue; differing in this respect from cases of redundancy such as shown in Fig. 15, Plate I. The adventitious bands are always thick at first and become thinned down as the cicatricial tissue contracts and as the effect of the traction of the arytenoid begins to become manifest. The author has used similar operations in cicatricial larynges following conditions other than papillomata, though not always with the same success as in the case above mentioned.

CHAPTER XXIII.

Benign Growths Primary in the Tracheobronchial Tree.

Benign growths primary in the trachea and bronchi. Extension of papillomata from the larynx into the cervical trachea, especially about the tracheotomy wound is of relatively common occurrence, and that form of tracheal benignancy has already been considered in its proper place, with laryngeal growths. Under the present heading will be included only the primary neoplasms of the tracheo-bronchial tree. Papillomata and fibromata are the most frequent of the benign tumors in the trachea. Aberrant thyroid, lipomata, enchondromata, chondrosteomata, adenomata and lipomata occur in the trachea, but not all of these have been reported to have been discovered endoscopically. When the author encountered the first case of primary tracheal benign tumor in the early days of bronchoscopy (Bib. 269) he supposed that such tumors were not uncommon but simply undiscovered. In the nine years that have elapsed since that time he has seen but one other benign true neoplasm in the tracheo-bronchial tree, though he has seen a number of benign "tumors" not truly neoplastic.

Papilloma primary in the trachea. Mann reports two very interesting cases of this kind diagnosticated and removed bronchoscopically. Other interesting cases are reported by von Schrotter and Spiess. The author's previously reported case is as follows:

A girl, aged four years, was brought to the Eye and Ear Hospital Dispensary for cough which had persisted for two months since "strangling" on a crumb of bread that "got down the wrong way." Radiograph by Dr. Russell H. Boggs was negative. Physical examination by Dr. Brush demonstrated a cooing sound all over both sides of the chest. There was no dyspnea or cyanosis. Thinking of the possibility of a foreign body in the bread, the author passed a bronchoscope and found a small pinkish white mass of tissue about six millimeters in diameter, with mammillated surface attached to the left tracheal wall about one centimeter above the bifurcation. Thinking of a foreign body granuloma, the author excised the tissue, leaving a flat surface oozing a trifling amount of blood, but no sign of foreign body. Dr. Joseph H. Barach reported: "Histologic examination of the tissue shows a typical papilloma which could not be confused, histologically, with a granuloma." The child did not return to the clinic. Dr. L. C. Manchester, who kindly went to the child's home to have her brought back to the clinic, failed to convince the parents of the necessity, the cough having disappeared. When seen by him a second time, about three months later, the cough had not returned and there was no cooing sound or other abnormality apparent to physical examination. The child was lost to further observation.

Fibroma primary in the tracheo-bronchial tree. An interesting case of fibroma is reported by Sauer (Bib. 515), occurring in a man, aged 74 years. The growth produced severe dyspnea and was detached by the insertion of the bronchoscope and was coughed up in two pieces. Emil Mayer (Bib. 408) reports the discovery and removal of a soft fibroma from the bronchus of a child bronchoscoped for bronchiectasis.

The author's case of fibroma is as follows: A boy of 16 years was referred to the author by Dr. Henry Eastman for cough which had persisted for six weeks since inhaling an insect thought to have been a fly. The insect had been coughed up and identified in the sputum a few days after the accident but the cough did not ameliorate. Radiographic examination by Dr. George C. Johnston and physical examination by Dr. Henry Eastman were both negative. At bronchoscopy under local anesthesia the author found a smooth, pedunculated and freely movable growth, about six centimeters in diameter attached to the lower margin of the orifice of the left upper lobe bronchus. Traction with straight forceps demonstrated a firm attachment which was excised along with a liberal amount of base by the tissue forceps (Fig. 35). There was blood streaked expectoration for a few days. At bronchoscopy two weeks later there was no sign of recurrence. Dilated capillaries were visible in the neighborhood of the site of removal. Bronchoscopy about eight months later showed no sign of recurrence and the boy seemed normal in every way. Histological examination by Dr. Ernest W. Willetts showed the growth to be a pure fibroma of probably slow formation and long standing.

Enchondroma of the tracheo-bronchial tree. Von Eicken (Bib. 564) reports the removal of an enchondroma of the bronchus by means of biting forceps.

Amyloid tumors of the trachea are reported by Reich (Bib. 463).

Osteomata of the trachea are reported by Mackleston (Bib. 409) and Levinger (Bib. 351).

Echinococcus of the lung in an isolated focus producing dyspnea was discovered bronchoscopically by Kob and the case is reported by Wadsack (Bib. 325 and 587).

Thyroid tumors. (Benign). While not a true neoplasm, the occurrence of aberrant thyroid tissue within the lumen of the trachea may be so regarded and should be so treated. The author has had one such case, as follows:

A woman of 34 years was certain that she had aspirated a fish bone three days before coming to the author. Bronchoscopy revealed a tracheobronchitis. No foreign body was present, but a small pedunculated tumor was found attached to the left anterior wall of the trachea. It was removed with the tissue forceps, Fig. 35, and found by Dr. Willetts to be composed of thyroid tissue. The endotracheal wound healed in a few days, and eight months later there was no sign of any operation having been done upon the trachea and the wall seemed smooth and normal. The thyroid gland and its isthmus were in normal position and of about normal size. It seems quite unlikely that the tumor had any connection whatever with the patient's symptoms, though, as might have been expected, the symptoms subsided and probably would have done so without operation. A very interesting consideration of the thyroid gland in its relations to the trachea has been written by Otto Stein (Bib. 502).

Granuloma of the trachea, the result of perichondritis, has been observed by the author in a number of instances. In two cases it was due to the traumatism of a foreign body aspirated and coughed up three weeks and two months respectively after the accident. In the first instance, the granuloma was found at bronchoscopy two months after the coughing up of the foreign body, and in the second, about four weeks after. In both cases bronchoscopy was done for persistent cough and dyspnea, which led to the suspicion that the foreign body might have been multiple, with consequently one or more still remaining in the air passages. In both instances, removal of the granulation tissue with application of argyrol in 30 per cent solution, resulted in a cure, only one treatment being necessary in one case and three treatments in the other. A very interesting case of granuloma in the trachea is reported by Sir Robert Woods. Extreme dyspnea on both inspiration and expiration had persisted for two months after an attack of bronchitis. Three bronchoscopic removals resulted in a perfect cure. The possibility of a granuloma being tuberculous or luetic must always be kept in mind.

Symptoms of benign tumors of the trachea. Whether or not cough is a usual symptom of tracheo-bronchial benign tumors, it is impossible, to say, because the small number of cases reported form an insufficient basis for deduction, but it seems the most constant symptom. Dyspnea and all of the symptoms of defective drainage of secretions supervene when the growth becomes large enough to be obstructive. Radiography is of service in enchondromata and osteomata, and its routine use in all chronic chest diseases is indicated from many viewpoints. Doubtless the same will be said in the future in regard to bronchoscopy.

Endoscopic appearances of benign growths. The detection of benign growths endoscopically is not at all difficult, but occasionally granulation tissue will be removed under suspicion of being neoplastic. As this is good treatment anyway for exuberant granulation, it is the proper course and the microscope can make the diagnosis. Another possible mistake is a small adherent mass of secretion which sometimes simulates a white growth in appearance. The removal of this clears up the diagnosis. Syphiloma of the trachea, as in the following case, may simulate tumor very closely. A man, aged 40, complaining of severe dyspnea and slight dysphagia, was found to have a sessile tumor projecting from the right posterior wall of the trachea. There was a strong suspicion of malignancy, but as it is the author's rule to apply the therapeutic test to all questionable cases of malignancy no specimen was taken in this case. Four weeks of antiluetic treatment cleared up the tumor completely. In another similar case a specimen was removed because of the exceedingly strong suspicion of malignancy. Dr. Willetts reported the specimen as certainly not malignant and with a strong suspicion of lues. Treatment verified the biopsy. Most important of all is not to mistake an aneurysm which is invading the trachea for a tumor. This is perhaps the one mistake which absolutely must not be made. An aneurysm of sufficient size and duration to invade the tracheal wall can be diagnosticated by the internist, the fluoroscopist and the radiographer. The endoscopic appearances of aneurysm are rather of compression than of a neoplasm involving the tracheal wall. The lumen is apt to be more or less scabbard-like in shape. There may not be an abnormal amount of pulsation. The endoscopic appearances of aneurysm are elsewhere mentioned.

Bronchoscopic removal of benign growths of the trachea presents but little difficulty if proper forceps are used. The author has had great satisfaction in all sorts of removal of tissue from the larynx, trachea, bronchi and esophagus with the forceps shown in Fig. 35. They will bite into the lateral wall if the movable jaw be forced toward the wall. The jaw should be set so as to rise, in the normal position of the handle. In case of large tumors producing great dyspnea quick action may be necessary because the dyspnea is apt to be increased by the spasm incidental to the presence of the bronchoscope in the trachea. Under no circumstances whatever should a general anesthetic be used for such an operation. The larynx may be locally anesthetized and the bronchoscope inserted with an assistant holding the forceps in readiness for immediate removal as soon as discovered. Of course, the presence of tumor may not be suspected, but in every case of dyspnea the endoscopist should be prepared for every emergency. The risks of removal are very slight so far as hemorrhage is concerned if the growth is small, even if it is angiomatous, provided it is not fungations on an aneurysmal erosion. The blood from a slow oozing will be coughed out, before the clots break down.

Edematous polypi in the tracheo-bronchial tree. Edematous polypi and other more or less tumor-like inflammatory sequelae are not infrequently seen in connection with the mixed infections following ulceration from malignant or other diseases.

CHAPTER XXIV.

Benign Neoplasms of the Esophagus.

The author is unable to add anything from personal experience to the single case reported (Bib. 269, p. 113). In the author's experience, therefore, benign tumors of the esophagus are among the most rare affections. He has seen a number of cases of edematous polypi associated with other lesions, benign and malignant, and one without any associated lesions that could be determined at the time of the esophagoscopy. The specimens were reported upon by Dr. Ernest W. Willets as edematous tissue with more or less fibrous connective tissue, and with a layer of squamous epithelium. These, of course, were not true neoplasms, but, like similar tumors in the nose, were the result of prolonged inflammation. The author has also seen a number of cases of granulomata, and in one instance, a mass of scar tissue that resembled a cheloid. A few cases of varicosities resembling angiomata were seen and will be mentioned under Diseases of the Esophagus. Guisez (Bib. 128) mentioned reports of retention cysts by Sargent, Nels and Jahn; epithelial cysts by Wyss; congenital cysts associated with tracheo-esophageal fistulae by Eppinger and Fettner; [illegible] cysts by Wattman; warts similar to dermal verrucae [illegible] by Kelher; [illegible] and lipomata by La-[illegible] [illegible] by [illegible] [illegible] and [illegible]; [illegible] by [illegible] and Mosk[illegible]. The references are not given, but [illegible] cases [illegible] not altogether [illegible] in the pre-[illegible] esophagoscopical findings.

CHAPTER XXV.

Endoscopy in Malignant Disease of the Larynx.

Following the initiative of Sir Felix Semon and Mr. Butlin, the author's thyrotomies for intrinsic laryngeal malignancy of small extent have yielded such a large percentage of cures, that he feels that it would be a step backward to attempt endoscopic extirpation. Therefore, in the author's opinion, the usefulness of direct laryngoscopy is confined to diagnosis of the disease, and, equally important, to assist in deciding the question of operability. As urged by Semon no specimen should be taken in a case clinically malignant, unless the patient has already consented to operation in the event of biopsic confirmation. This applies with especial force to intrinsic disease. The technic of taking a specimen by direct laryngoscopy is given in Chapter VII. Particular attention is called to the author's method of operating at the side of the tongue instead of over the dorsum. The author has had uniformly good results from biopsy in malignancy since taking the specimens by the direct method, which is in marked contrast to prior results from the indirect method. Complications after taking a specimen are rare if the case is malignant. They are the same as might follow any endolaryngeal operation (q. v.). In case of a gumma on the eve of breaking down, the process may be hastened and prompt specific treatment will be necessary.

The decision as to the operability of any laryngeal malignancy depends upon whether the party wall is involved or not. Involvement, no matter how slight, means the patient's chances are slender, no matter how radical the operation, because of the free lymphatic leakage. The degree of involvement can be determined by direct laryngoscopic and esophagoscopic examination of the party wall, on its anterior and posterior surfaces. The esophageal speculum is useful here. In a number of instances the author has found involvement of the party wall below the arytenoids posteriorly in cases free from arytenoid fixation and seemingly intrinsic. In other cases, extrinsic by origin or extension, he has advised against laryngectomy because of glandular nodes observable goscopically in the esophagus, though covered with apparently .l mucosa. In one such illustrative case a series of nodes were it different locations from the left pyriform sinus to the level of pper thoracic aperture, indicating unremovable involvement. The nt dying shortly afterward, enabled autoptical confirmation by Dr. rews (Fig. 389).

Malignant disease of the epiglottis may be, in very rare instances, exception to contraindication of endoscopic extirpation of malignancy.

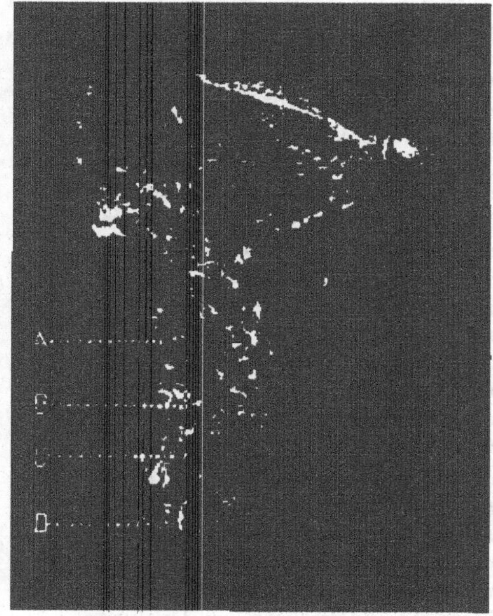

FIG. 389.—Illustrating the possibilities of esophagoscopic aid in decision as to operability of laryngeal malignancy. The author saw esophagoscopically the lymph nodes, A, B, C, D, and others during life and advised against laryngectomy.

In those rare cases of malignancy strictly limited to the tip of the epiglottis and of small extent, endoscopic removal is justifiable provided the amputation of the epiglottis will give a sufficiently wide removal. The author has had two cases of this kind, now well at the age of four years and two years respectively. The method used was amputation as nearly total as possible, of the epiglottis with the heavy snare, Fig. 41. The disease was of very small extent and histologically was found by Dr.

Willetts to be epitheliomatous. Healing was prompt and uncomplicated. Delavan (Bib. 117) reports a cure of epiglottidean malignancy by indirect removal.

Radium for malignant disease of the larynx. As yet radium has not given results that would warrant its use in any operable case in the larynx or elsewhere. In inoperable cases excellent palliative results warrant its use. The dosage and screening required are about the same as will be given later for esophageal malignancy. The container with heavy dosage may be held in place under ocular observation as was done by Dr. Ellen J. Patterson for thirty minutes at each sitting using cocaine anesthesia. Or a tracheotomy may be done, the capsule placed above the tracheotomic cannula to which it is tied with braided silk as is done with the author's laryngostomy apparatus (q. v.). The following is a report of Dr. Ellen J. Patterson's case:

Indirect laryngoscopy showed the condition sketched at A, Fig. 390. The left side was apparently uninvolved, but on the right the entire aryepiglottic fold including the arytenoid eminence was infiltrated, thickened and covered with nodules of a dark reddish color. There was only slight movement of the right arytenoid. The growth seemed to involve the external portion of the ventricular band and there was a slight infiltration at the base of the epiglottis on the right side. A large mass of glands was palpable in the neck low down along the sternomastoid muscle. A large specimen was removed and submitted to Dr. Ernest W. Willetts, Professor Oscar Klotz, Dr. W. Proescher of Pittsburgh, and Dr. Evans of Chicago, all of whom reported the growth to be sarcoma. The patient was not seen again until one month later. Upon indirect examination the growth had almost doubled in size overhanging the glottis as shown at B, Fig. 390. There was now not the slightest motion to the right arytenoid and the left seemed to be slightly impaired. There was a very slight puffiness about the base of the left arytenoid eminence. The disease was clearly inoperable because of the very large mass of infiltrated glands in the neck, the nodes seen esophagoscopically, and the crossing of the process past the posterior commissure. At the request of the patient radium treatment was instituted by Dr. Patterson under the advice of Dr. W. Proescher as to dosage and duration. Radium bromide equivalent to 75 mgm. of radium element was applied daily for thirty minutes, the well screened capsule being placed in contact with the longest diameter of the growth. In addition, the patient was given a capsule containing 50 mgm. of radium element which was bandaged over the infiltrated mass of glands in the neck for ten hours daily. After one month's treatment with the radium the condition, which had been as shown at B, Fig. 390, had entirely disappeared, leaving both aryepiglottic folds and arytenoids almost symmetrical as shown at C. There was quite an improved motility of the right arytenoid, though it was not able to make more than half a normal excursion. The patient was not seen again until two months later when it was found that there was an edematous-looking slight enlargement of the right aryepiglottic fold, though it was not nodular and not of the dark color of the primary condition. Down on the posterior surface of the right aryepiglottic fold there could be seen the upper edge of an ulcer which extended downward into the right pyriform sinus, involving its anterior wall, as shown at D. When the larynx was drawn forward with the direct laryngoscope, the ulcer was seen to extend nearly 2 cm. down into the hypopharynx. Dr. Patterson removed a specimen from the edge of this ulcer. Dr. Ernest W. Willetts reported it to be an undoubted epithelioma with typical epi-

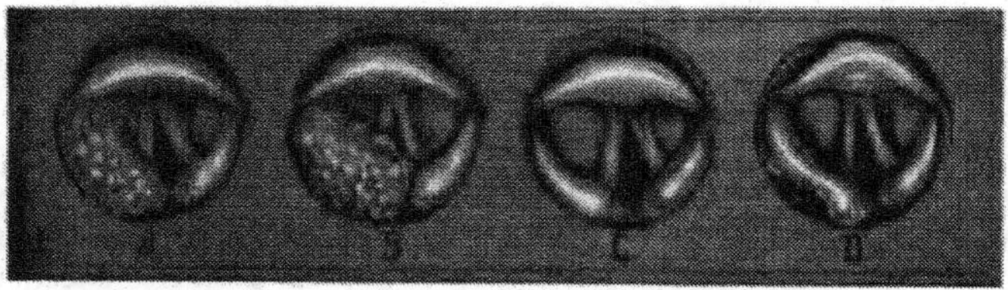

FIG. 390.—Illustrating a case of laryngeal sarcoma in a man of 57 years. The growth (B) disappeared under radium treatment as shown at C. Epithelioma appeared later as shown at D. Heavier radium dosage caused disappearance of the epithelioma. The growth, prior to treatment, had increased from the size shown in A to the size shown in B. Death occurred about a year later of recurrence and metastases (Case of Dr. Ellen J. Patterson.)

theliomatous cell pictures. Drs. Proescher and Klotz concurred unqualifiedly. Under the advice of Dr. Proescher radium bromide equivalent to 200 mgm. of radium element was applied for a half hour on alternate days for five applications. This caused the disappearance of the growth. One year later the patient died of recurrence and metastases.

Remarks. Lues was excluded by a very thorough therapeutic test by Dr. Lawrence Litchfield and Dr. L. C. Bixler. The eminent pathologists mentioned all agreed that there was absolutely no histologic evidence of cancer in the first specimen taken, which was a very large one, and hence fairly representative of the neoplastic process then present. It seems justifiable to suppose that the radium caused the disappearance of the primary condition. The change from a connective tissue type of neoplasm to an epithelial type seems to the author very rare, as he had never before seen such a case. Mr. Walter G. Howarth, who, when honoring the author's clinic with a visit, saw the patient at the stage shown at D, mentioned a case of his own in which there was a change from an epithelial tissue type to a connective tissue type. A papilloma was removed from the uvula of a boy. This was followed six months later by a growth in the velum bulging both anteriorly and posteriorly. Mr. Howarth removed the entire velum with the tonsil, followed by perfect healing. This growth was found to be a fibroma. Four months later a pedunculated mass developed in the scar and was removed by external operation along with involved glands. This growth was found to be a spindle-celled sarcoma. This operation was followed by hopeless recurrence from which the last specimen examined showed a small round-celled sarcoma. All of the specimens were examined by Mr. Shattuck and all of the operations were done by Mr. Howarth. Such cases are exceptions to the law that tissue never changes type. The efficiency of radium in prolonging life in Dr. Patterson's case is undoubted in view of the rapid growth in one month's time prior to treatment as shown by comparing A and B, Fig. 390. That an ultimate cure did not result is disappointing, but the palliative results were well worth while.

Diathermy. Mr. Douglas Harner reports such excellent results from diathermy in the treatment of inoperable laryngeal and faucial malignancy that its use alone or cojointly with radium promises excellent palliative, possibly curative results. (See *Journal of Laryngology, Rhinology and Otology*, October, 1914.)

CHAPTER XXVI.

Bronchoscopy in Malignant Growths of the Trachea.

The author has seen but one case of malignant tumor originating in the interior of the thoracic trachea, at a stage when such origin could be verified. But such cases occurring in the subglottic region of the larynx have been observed by all laryngologists, including the author, and post mortem findings would indicate that endobronchial or endotracheal origin does occur. A case of cancer, probably arising from an endotracheal mucous gland in the subglottic trachea, is reported by Sir Robert Woods. The bronchoscope offers a means for the early diagnosis of malignant tumors of the thorax. As these tumors occur most frequently at the hilus, it is seldom that even an early diagnosis renders surgical extirpation possible, and yet with the rapidly advancing development of thoracic surgery it behooves us, as endoscopists, to develop the early diagnosis of malignancy to the utmost in order to be of assistance to the general surgeon. As is well known, neither the X-ray nor physical signs give any evidence of mediastinal malignancy at a very early stage. Posticus paralysis, it is true. is quite an early evidence, but in most cases it is simply an indication for further investigation in order to determine whether or not the paralysis is due to intrathoracic conditions. The most common form of malignancy in the trachea is a secondary process from a peritracheal growth. As enumerated under the head of malignant disease of the esophagus, the author has seen quite a number of cases where the trachea, or, more often, the left bronchus was invaded by a tumor which also invaded the esophagus. It is not often possible to determine the point of origin of the growth. It may be in the trachea, in the esophagus or, more probably, in the mediastinum. The endotracheal appearances are quite similar to malignant disease elsewhere. In the later stages, which the process has practically always reached by the time it comes to the endoscopist, endotracheal and endobronchial malignancy are characterized by a bleeding mass of fungating tissue bathed in pus and secretion, usually foul. The diagnosis of a malignant process which has already involved the lumen of the trachea is to be made, not so much by the endoscopic appearances as by the removal of a specimen of tissue. No danger whatever attaches to this if carefully done and if aneurysm be excluded. As elsewhere stated, an aneurysm large enough to invade the tracheal lumen can easily be diagnosticated by radiography, fluoroscopy and by the internist. Sarcoma and carcinoma of the thyroid gland when perforating into the trachea, as pointed out by Sir Felix Semon (Bib. 471) usually become pedunculated.

Peritracheal or peribronchial malignancy may cause a compressive stenosis covered with normal mucosa. Endoscopically the wall is seen to bulge in from one side at any part of the lumen causing a crescentic picture, or compression of opposite walls may cause a "scabbard" or pear-shaped lumen. Usually the compression will be found hard and firm and the involved bronchus less easily moved laterally than normal. Deviation of the trachea may be marked in peritracheal malignancy and is to be distinguished from anomalous deviations by the compressive hardness and fixation of the former. Compression by normal or malignant thyroids, especially retrotracheal malignant goitre renders bronchoscopic exploration advisable as a preliminary to operation as mentioned under "Anesthesia." The reader is referred to the beautiful and instructive "Atlas der Bronchoskopie" by Dr. M. Mann (Bib. 361) for pathological studies of cases of mediastinal malignant disease with endotracheobronchial manifestations discovered bronchoscopically; also to the excellent article of Mosher (Bib. 403), Theisen (Bib. 548) and of Ingersol (Bib. 219).

Treatment. Up to the present time but one case of successful extirpation of malignancy has come to the writer's knowledge. This was a case of Kahler, in which a tumor of the right bronchus was removed bronchoscopically, its insertion being afterward cauterized with the galvano-cautery. The tumor was found to be a papillary cylinder-celled carcinoma. At the time of the report the patient had remained free from recurrence at the end of two and one-half years. Ephraim reports the removal of hemorrhagic and obstructive fungations of malignancy with the subsequent application of the galvano-cautery with great relief of pain and the arrest of hemorrhage and the lessening of dyspnea. Until a therapeutic cure shall be discovered most of the cases will be subjects for a palliative tracheotomy and radium therapy. The methods, screening and dosage are probably about the same as those given for esophageal malignancy. In doing a tracheotomy it is necessary not only to open the trachea to put in a cannula, but to make sure that that cannula gets down below the diseased process and pipes the air down to one or both bronchi which are still functionating. In quite a number of the author's cases there has been a mere fistulous tract kept open by the long tracheal cannula long after the tracheal wall has been obliterated by the cancerous process throughout a greater or less portion of its extent. The patient is able to get up secretions better through the long tracheal cannula than he can through the diseased trachea even if he could get air enough down without the cannula, which is seldom the case, so that tracheotomy with the long tube probably prolongs the patient's life by lessening the absorption, as well as by preventing asphyxia.

CHAPTER XXVII.

Malignant Disease of the Esophagus.

Cancerous lesions of the esophagus are usually single. This is rarely discoverable esophagoscopically, because it is rarely justifiable to push an esophagoscope beyond the site of the first lesion. Nevertheless, as a post mortem fact, it has been demonstrated by Seelig (Bib. 469) that implantation metastases may exist in the esophagus below the primary lesion (Fig. 391). Malignant disease of the esophagus is rather more frequent at the upper extremity, next in frequency is the lower extremity near the cardia, the middle portion being least often involved. In all cases of suspected cancer, it is necessary to exclude aneurysm by radiography before making an examination. Then in proceeding with the esophagoscopy it is necessary to exercise great care to pass the tube by sight and not with a mandrin, because the growth may be higher situated than is suspected. Of course this same rule applies to all esophagoscopy, but there has been quite a number of cases reported where the esophagoscope had perforated the very much weakened wall of a malignancy situated close to the cricopharyngeal narrowing. Therefore, it is necessary to be doubly careful, especially as the infiltration may make the passage of the esophagoscope more difficult than usual in this narrow portion of the esophagus. Unfortunately, malignant disease of the esophagus is but rarely seen early. There are two reasons for this. First, the early stages of the disease produce no symptoms. Second, when symptoms begin to appear they are so slight that usually neither patient nor attending physician suspects serious disease, calling for immediate esophagoscopy. With a wider recognition of the usefulness of the esophagoscope for early diagnosis, there will be a change in this respect. It should be an absolute rule that no transthoracic operation for malignant disease of the esophagus should be attempted until after a specimen has been removed and the diagnosis confirmed. For the removal of this specimen, of course, the esophagoscopic method is the only one. The specimen should be ample, and should, if possible, include a little of the adjacent normal, though greater care is needed here than elsewhere as to the amount of normal that may be taken. A little of the mucosa is sufficient. The only contraindication to the taking of a specimen is such a profoundly anemic condition that oozing which may follow may turn the balance against the patient. This anemic condition is usually only found in those cases that have been permitted to become moribund from hunger and thirst from too long delayed gastrostomy. In such cases the gastrostomy should be done at once and the patient fed until the specimen may be taken with safety. Unfortunately, such patients, especially if there have been a few days of water hunger, make exceedingly bad surgical subjects, so that the minor operation of gastrostomy assumes a

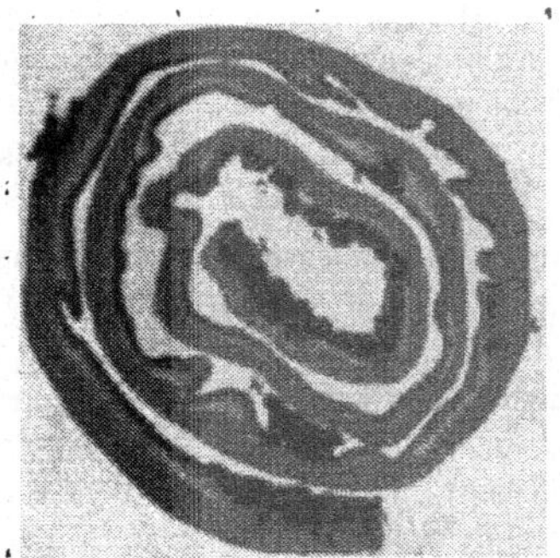

FIG. 391.—Implantation metastases in the esophagus. Diagrammatic representation of a coiled up longitudinal section. The primary lesion at upper end of esophagus is seen at 2; at the lower end at 1. The lesions at 4 and 5 are metastatic. (See article by M. G. Seelig, Bib. 469.)

high mortality. Cases of suspected cancer, like every other esophageal condition, should be examined locally with an esophagoscope before any attempt is made to pass any instrument blindly. The author cannot agree with those who, for any purpose whatsoever prefer to pass a bougie first. There have been too many accidents from this procedure, and the author can see no advantage whatever in it, for there is nothing to be learned by sounding that cannot be learned esophagoscopically, and so far as the patient is concerned, it is no more annoyance to have an esophagoscope passed than to have a sound passed. As for the determining by such a method the length of the tube to be used, which is the last remaining excuse given, it is quite needless. The author's custom is to examine the upper region of the esophagus first with the esophageal speculum and then to pass the 53 cm. esophagoscope, which is the only one needed for adults. Sarcoma is much less frequent than carcinoma but does occasionally occur. It is exceedingly seldom that there is any dilatation above a cancerous stenosis, possibly because the stenosis is seldom sufficiently obstructive until late in the disease. Occasionally, however, quite a considerable dilatation has been observed by the author which leads to the suspicion that there was some spasmodic condition prior to the development of cancer, and possibly the cancerous process was implanted upon the chronic inflammation.

Esophagoscopic appearances and diagnosis of malignant disease of the esophagus. The esophagoscopic appearances of cancer vary greatly, according to the stage in which the disease is seen, and also according to whether the esophagus or neighboring viscera are primarily invaded. The following forms of lesion are those usually seen:

1. Submucosal infiltration covered by perfectly normal membrane, usually associated with more or less bulging of the esophageal wall, and usually associated with hardness and infiltration.
2. Leucoplakia.
3. Ulceration projecting but little above the surface at the edges.
4. Rounded nodular masses grouped in mulberry-like form, either dark or light red in color.
5. Polypoid masses.
6. Cauliflower fungations.

In considering the esophagoscopic appearances of cancer, it is necessary to remember that after ulceration has set in the cancerous process may have engrafted upon it, and upon its neighborhood, the results of inflammation due to the mixed infections. Cancer invading the wall from without may for a long time be covered with perfectly normal mucous membrane. The significant signs at this early stage are:

1. Absence of one or more of the normal radial creases between the folds.
2. Asymmetry of the inspiratory enlargement of lumen.
3. Sensation of hardness of the wall on palpation with the tube.
4. The involved wall will not readily be made to wrinkle when pushed upon with the tube mouth.

In determining deformity of the outline of the esophageal lumen, it is necessary to be careful that the head of the patient is not rotated; because rotation may cause distortion of the esophagus as demonstrated graphically in the radiograph, Fig. 392. In the later stages, when the submucosal growth begins to break through, the mucous membrane becomes nodular, and then is usually darker in color with apparent great increase of vascularity. In the fungating forms of cancer, the fungations may take a polypoid shape, the individual polypi being covered with epithelium and the general color being quite similar to normal esophageal mucosa or to nasal edematous polypi, or they may be quite red. This latter form is rather rare. Much more common are the fungations which look like exuberant granulations in an unhealthy wound. We also occasionally see white grass-like projections such as are seen at times in the

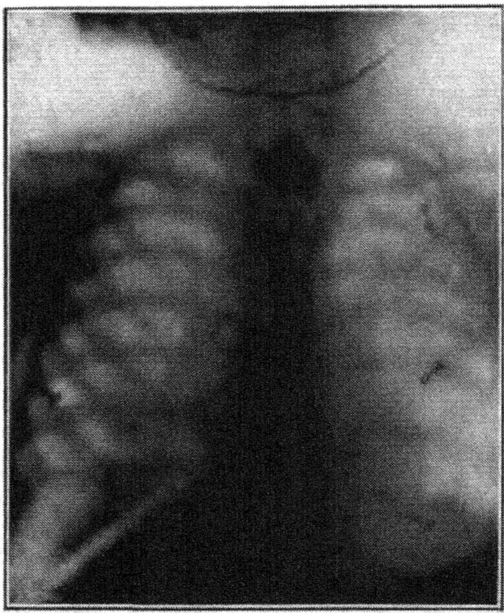

FIG. 392.—Radiograph of a coin in the esophagus, showing the diagonal respiratory esophageal movement with rotated head, and illustrating the necessity of the exact median non-rotated position of the head if any diagnostic importance is to be attached to asymmetrical respiratory esophageal movement in esophagoscopy for suspected periesophageal or submucosal esophageal lesions. Incidentally this illustrates, also, one of the disadvantages of the lateral position for esophagoscopy for disease. Radiograph by Dr. George J. Boyd.

larynx. The ulcerated forms of esophageal malignancy seldom resemble ulceration seen in the mucosa higher up. Part of this seeming dissimilarity is due to the position in which the ulcer lies with reference to the point of view. Ulceration in the esophagus is seen more or less on edge through the esophagoscope, and because of the basal infiltration, it is seldom feasible to turn the ulcer sidewise, as could be done by lateral pressure on the esophageal wall above the ulcer if it were not for the infiltration beneath. If a very large esophagoscope is used, there is more or less turning of the ulcer and then the crater can be seen, and also the distal edges. The edges, in some instances, are under cut, though usually not. In many instances there are smaller budding granulations along the edge of the ulceration. In some instances, the ulcerations are covered with whitish projections, looking somewhat like papillomata, but the individual projections are more pointed. The center may be somewhat lower than the periphery, and in many instances is covered with a layer of exudate, whitish or yellowish in color, the exact color depending, of course, on the degree of illumination. There is almost invariably more or less oozing of blood, even before any instrument or gauze sponge has come in contact with the ulcerated surface. In some instances, the border may be very irregular with a mouse-gnawed appearance to the edges. In one of the author's cases the ulcerated area seemed flat, almost depressed, while on top of it was lying a mass of slough and exudate apparently about ready to detach. All of the foregoing types may occur in the same case, either at different stages or all may co-exist in one lesion. It is quite common to see at least two forms combined in the same lesion. Two things are characteristic of all later forms of lesions. All are bleeding when first seen, or bleed very readily when wiped with the sponges. They all convey the idea of rigidity or fixation of the involved area, which is in marked contrast to the normally thin, easily movable, supple esophageal wall. There is every reason to believe that the very early stage of cancer occurs as leucoplakia in at least a few cases of esophageal cancer. There have, so far, been only a few cases observed, but opportunity for very early esophagoscopies in cancer are so rare that there is no means of determining how frequent such an onset may be. The author has seen three cases of which the following is one:

Male, aged 56, was admitted to the Presbyterian Hospital for difficulty in swallowing of about two weeks' duration. The onset had been quite sudden, at which time he had been unable to swallow anything but liquids. On passing the esophagoscope, we encountered, just above the hiatal level, a white patch about 1 cm. in diameter that looked precisely as if the mucosa had been burned with silver nitrate. The appearance was so much like that of the mucous plaque, and the onset of the symptoms had been so recent, that we ordered the patient at once put upon antiluetic treatment, notwithstanding a negative history and normal glands. At the end of four weeks there was no amelioration of the symptoms, and on passing the esophagoscope I found conditions precisely as before. At neither of these two examinations could I determine stenosis of the esophagus. The 10 mm. esophagoscope passed readily into the stomach without obstruction, so that it was quite evident that the symptoms from which the patient suffered must have been due to spasm, though we were somewhat surprised that the passage of the esophagoscope the first time had not relieved the symptoms, temporarily at least, as is usual in case of spasm. This patient went west and died of "cancer of the stomach." A gastrostomy was done for feeding about two months before his death. No other data were obtainable.

Sarcoma of the esophagus probably resembles in a general way the appearances seen in cancer. The author has seen but one case of esophageal sarcoma. There was a round nodular mass on the posterior esophageal wall, quite dark in color and covered with vessels running in all directions. At the lower border was an ulceration, with elevated edges and depressed center (Fig. 9, Plate III). No fetor was noticeable.

Differential diagnosis. The differential diagnosis by esophagoscopic appearances alone, while not absolutely positive, yet will be rarely in error with any one who is accustomed to seeing malignancy of mucosal surfaces. In cicatricial stenosis, we have a thin, white, web-like band, or thin-edged annular stricture with a dilatation above it. In spasmodic conditions, we have the vertical fold running down into a funnel-shaped point ending in a concentric lumen of minute extent; the mucosa is either normal or pasty and macerated, or in a state of chronic esophagitis. This condition is usually more or less diffused, and there is an absence of that rigidity and infiltration that is seen in malignancy. In the ulcerated type of cancer, it may be exceedingly difficult to exclude lues without a therapeutic test. The differential diagnosis between compression stenosis and cancer of the submucous type, is based upon the rigidity and fixedness existing in the esophageal wall, and the fact that this wall cannot be wrinkled up in cancer while it is freely movable in compression. In compression also we have obliteration of the lumen to a long narrow slit. In the leucoplakia type, mucous patches of lues can be excluded only by the therapeutic test. After all, we must rely mainly upon the histologic examination of an esophagoscopically removed specimen which should, in all cases, be as ample as possible and should include a portion of the adjoining normal.

Treatment of malignant disease of the esophagus. Cancer of the esophagus has, at the present day, 100 per cent mortality, but there is good reason to believe that the surgeon will show a certain percentage of cures as soon as physicians will promptly refer to the esophagoscopist all patients showing the slightest abnormality referable to the esophagus. Thus only can we hope to discover and treat the early cancerous and precancerous conditions of leucoplakia, erosion, maceration, chronic esophagitis, etc. That the physician may do this without hesitation, it behooves the esophagoscopist to so perfect his technic and develop his skill that a patient may be esophagoscoped without distress and without anesthesia, or at most with local anesthesia limited to the pharynx. The work of Henry Janeway, Willy Mayer, Charles A. Elsberg and others has convinced the author that resection of the thoracic esophagus is a practicable procedure and will be frequently resorted to as soon as early esophagoscopies shall make the necessary early diagnosis. The passage of an esophagoscope for diagnosis often gives great relief of dysphagia, and this has lead to advocacy of the old method of bouginage. It is, however, of questionable advisability even for palliation.

Gastrostomy is always indicated sooner or later, and it should always be done before the patient's nutrition fails. Like tracheotomy, we all preach its early performance, but usually do it late. The surgeons who advise against gastrostomy forget that their experience is based on cases operated too late. Granting that the patient is a victim of a fatal disease, there is no reason why he should die in the agonies of thirst and hunger. Death from exhaustion is fairly comfortable, but death from hunger and, especially thirst, is agonizing, and the agony is prolonged by the tantalizingly small amount of fluid that passes the stenosis. If the gastrostomy be done early, there is no unquenchable thirst, no unsatisfied hunger, and most beneficent of all, is the almost invariable improvement in the ability to swallow through the esophagus that follows the esophageal rest after gastrostomy.

Intubation of the esophagus. In the palliative treatment of inoperable esophageal cancerous stenosis, gastrostomy may be postponed by esophageal intubation, in many instances, until very nearly the termination of the case, though by this it is not meant to advise that gastrostomy should be postponed one day after it is clear that nutrition is going to suffer. It is, of course, much more satisfactory to the patient to swallow his food even though it be liquid, than to have it poured in through the abdominal wall. Esophageal intubation has been very satisfactory in the author's hands. All forms of clear liquids will go through esophageal intubation tubes of 4 mm. internal diameter, and raw or very slightly cooked eggs can, with care, be swallowed with much satisfaction by the patient whose esophagus is thus intubated. In fact, any finely masticated food will go through, though occasionally imperfectly masticated particles may lodge in the smallest tubes. The author has had these tubes worn for quite a number of months without exciting ulceration, though, of course, cancerous ulceration was already present in some instances. The tubes should be removed every week or two for cleaning. It is essential to have a duplicate tube for immediate replacement

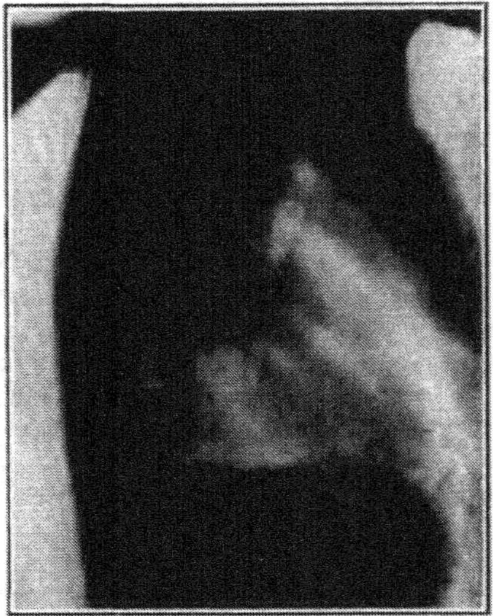

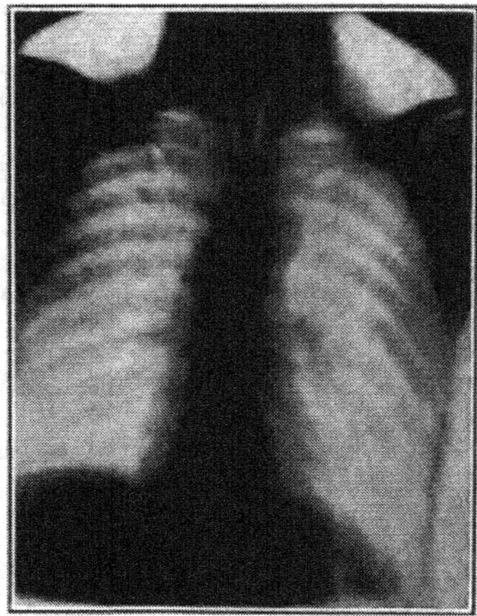

FIG. 393.—Charters Symonds esophageal intubation tubes in situ in a case of esophageal cancer (Author's case).

else the esophageal channel will quickly close so that a smaller tube will be needed. Eventually a smaller and a smaller tube is needed anyway, until none can be introduced. The Charters Symonds tube was intended for introduction with a whalebone stylet, without endoscopic aid. Introduction is greatly facillitated, however, by drawing forward the larynx with the laryngoscope. The thread may be dispensed with and withdrawal accomplished when necessary with the esophagoscope and forceps. In removal of the esophageal intubation tube by the thread without the esophagoscope the funnel-shaped tube will always catch on the cricoid cartilage and serious traumatism may be inflicted if the operator continues to pull. Drawing the larynx anteriorly with the laryngoscope or esophageal speculum, just as if we were exposing the cricopharyngeal constriction, will readily release the tube so that it can be

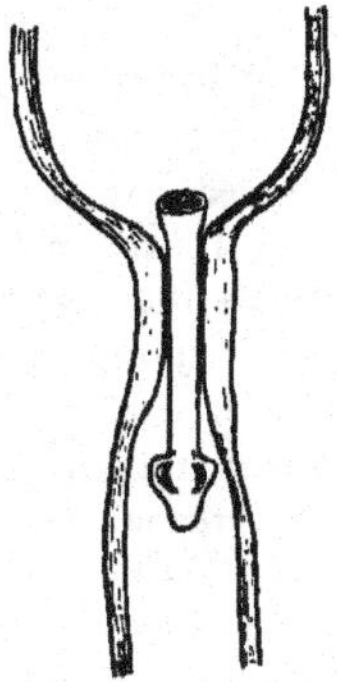

FIG. 394.—Esophageal intubation tube of Guisez.

withdrawn. This is a very important procedure to remember in the withdrawal of any instrument from the esophagus. Serious and even fatal trauma has been inflicted more often in the withdrawal of such instruments as the Graefe basket than in their insertion. The Charters Symonds tube *in situ* is shown in Fig. 393. Guisez has devised soft rubber intubation tubes that seem excellent (Fig. 394).

Radium in the treatment of esophageal malignancy. The author has not yet seen any results with radium that would justify his urging its use in any case that is amenable to operative treatment. He has seen marked effects in inoperable esophageal malignancy, but so far no absolute cures. In none of the cases has sufficient time elapsed to pass final judgment upon the value of radium therapy in neoplasms. The author would prefer to wait for three or four years before giving complete and tabulated data of his results. In order, however, that other workers in this field may have the use of such technic as the author has developed, he deems it best to publish this technic in the hope that it may be helpful to other workers. The chemistry, physics, and, to a still greater extent, the physiologic and therapeutic activities of radium are in such an embryonic state of development at the time this book goes to press, that it is quite impossible, even if the author were capable, to give any final conclusion. For all work with which endoscopy has to deal, the consensus of opinion is that the penetrating or gamma rays are the most effective. To avoid the irritating effect and burns that the softer beta rays would produce, it is necessary to absorb these rays with suitable thickness of metal screen, usually silver or lead of from 0.5 to 2 mm. in thickness. Wherever gamma rays emerge from a metal there are set up secondary radiations, which are soft like the very easily absorbed beta rays. These secondary rays are very irritating and soon produce serious superficial burns. To avoid these deleterious effects, it is necessary further to screen the metal outside with the equivalent of 1 or 2 mm. of rubber, cloth or paper. When so screened with lead and rubber, a quantity of radium equal to 100 mgm. of element can be applied for hours without producing a burn, whereas, 10 mgm. of radium with no more protection than the walls of a glass tube, in contact with the tissues for ten minutes, will lead to serious burns. The shorter the period of application of radium, the larger the quantity that must be used, since an inadequate dose of the radiation merely stimulates a new growth to more rapid proliferation. As the power of the ray diminishes as the square of the distance from the radium, it necessarily follows that the tissues to be acted upon must be as close as possible, and wherever it can be so arranged, the neoplastic tissues should be in contact with the radium container, while normal tissues should be at as great a distance as possible. When we have to deal with a large cancer surrounding the esophagus, as shown schematically in Fig. 395, there is no doubt, as determined by biopsy by Dr. Andrews in consultation with the author, that the periphery of the growth, as shown at P, is stimulated by the attenuated ray that is able to reach it through the thickness of the tissue M. The tissues, H. in contact with the tube, R, should be quickly melted away by large dosage in order to reach the peripheral cells shown at P. before the latter have had too long a time to develop. In the endoscopic application of radium, to obtain results it is necessary to use large dosage for a less time rather than a less dosage for a longer time, because of the discomfort of any esophageal application. By either the larger or the smaller dosage plan, it is necessary that such a degree of radio-activity be developed that it is unwise to have the container in contact with healthy tissue. In esophageal work the only way to be sure that the container is in contact with neoplastic tissue, and no other is to do the work esophagoscopically and to see that the container is placed precisely. The only way to make sure that the container remains where placed, is to see that it is in place by frequent inspection. With all forms of blind introduction there is an uncertainty that renders safety of radium treatment questionable. It has been suggested that a watch on the position of the capsule be kept by the fluoroscopic screen with roentgen rays. The esophagoscope having been removed, the replacement of the capsule, if found displaced, is to be made by a rigid wire carrier attached to the

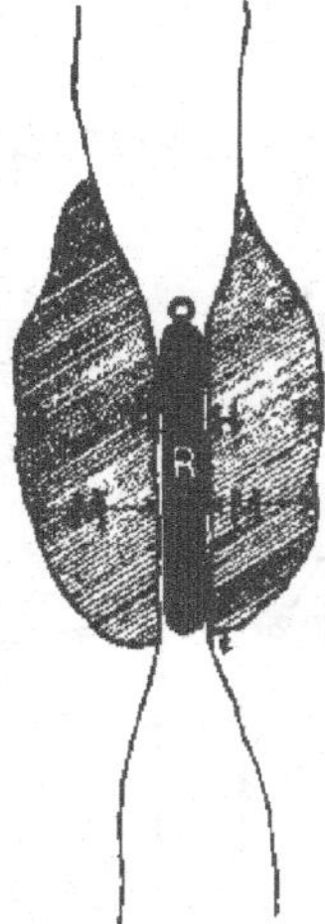

FIG. 395.—Schematic representation of a radium capsule in the center of an annular esophageal cancer.

capsule. This is objectionable because of its inaccuracy, the exact position of the stricture not being visible fluoroscopically without bismuth: and especially because it prevents the use of the flexible joint so necessary for accurate applications to deviated lumina.

The author's method is as follows: The radium salt used is contained in a very small glass capsule, and this capsule is contained in a metal capsule 3 mm. in diameter, the wall of the capsule being 0.3 mm. in thickness. Outside it is covered with a coating of hard rubber vulcanized on (M, Fig. 397). This silver capsule has a solid ring or eye in one end. A long extra drainage tube (B, Fig. 396), which was used by the author in his early work for aspirating secretions from the bronchi before he perfected his "sponge-pumping" method, was found to make the best possible carrier of the utmost simplicity. A small wire is passed through the aspirating tube and brought out at the distal end. A loop of heavy braided silk (not twisted silk) is attached to the wire, and the silk is thus drawn through the tube. To the silk at the distal end, the capsule is attached by means of a loop (P), formed with a bow knot, as shown in Fig. 396. Now by drawing the silk taut, and making it fast around the shoulder of the proximal end of the drainage tube, the capsule is brought firmly into the end of the drainage tube, but not so firmly but that lateral movement is possible. This makes a stiff joint at the

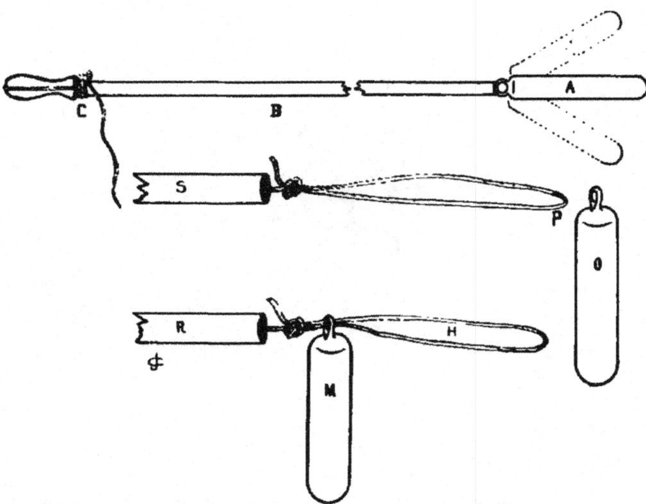

FIG. 396.—Author's method of applying radium endoscopically.

point where the eye of the capsule is drawn into the end of the drainage tube, motion being permitted as shown by the dotted line. For the esophagus a drainage tube of 60 cm. is used, and for the larynx, a 30 cm. length is sufficient, though one of 40 cm. would be needed for the bronchi. Any one who does not have the drainage tube can get the proper length of brass tubing of 3 mm. external diameter from any instrument maker. The purpose of the movement permitted by the joint, is to allow the capsule to be placed flatwise when the axis of application does not correspond with the axis of the endoscopic tube. Thus in treating the laryngeal case before mentioned, Dr. Patterson made the application by placing the capsule along the entire length of the aryepiglottic fold, which would have been impossible had the container been rigidly held in any form of carrier. In the use of forceps, there is always the possibility of the capsule getting lost from the grasp of the forceps during the manipulation, and such an accident might be exceedingly serious. because if not immediately recovered the prolonged activity of the radium would certainly be fatal. For this reason also, the braided silk used should be thoroughly tested. The first two or three applications in each case should be made with the esophagoscope *in situ* for the entire time in order to see whether the container is moved by regurgitant or other movements. For this purpose the esophagoscope should be covered with hard rubber vulcanized on (Fig. 397) in order to prevent irritant secondary rays. The esophagoscope and radium container *in situ* in the living patient are shown in Figs. 398, 399, 400, 401 and 402. When satisfied that the radium capsule will stay where placed the

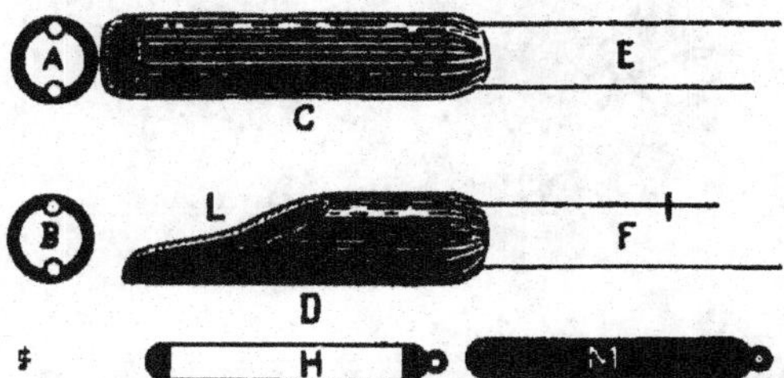

Fig. 397.—Esophagoscopes with hard rubber screens vulcanized on, to cut down irritating secondary radiations.

silk may be untied from the proximal end of the drainage tube and the esophagoscope and drainage tube may both be withdrawn leaving the capsule *in situ* with only a string for later withdrawal (Fig. 400). Anesthesia is not necessary. The best position of the patient for radium applications to the esophagus with the esophagoscope *in situ* is the recumbent, because the esophageal drainage, already defective, is occluded by the radium container, the hypopharynx fills and the overflow into the larynx excites constant cough and strangling, which makes a very trying ordeal for the patient. In the recumbent position the secretions all flow into the fauces and are aspirated through the tube, Fig. 24, attached to the aspirator, Fig. 23. When the radium container is left *in situ* and the esophagoscope is withdrawn the patient may lie face sidewise on the table to permit secretions to drain away.

Dosage is dependent on duration of the applications. The equivalent of 100 milligrams of radium element well screened may be left *in situ*

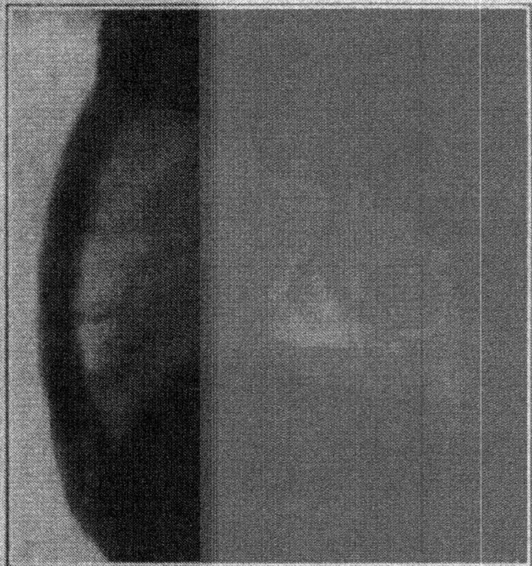

FIG. 398.—Radium container in situ in a case of esophageal cancer. The excessive forward inclination of the capsule is partly due to malignant distortion. (The normal esophagus tends somewhat forward in this location).

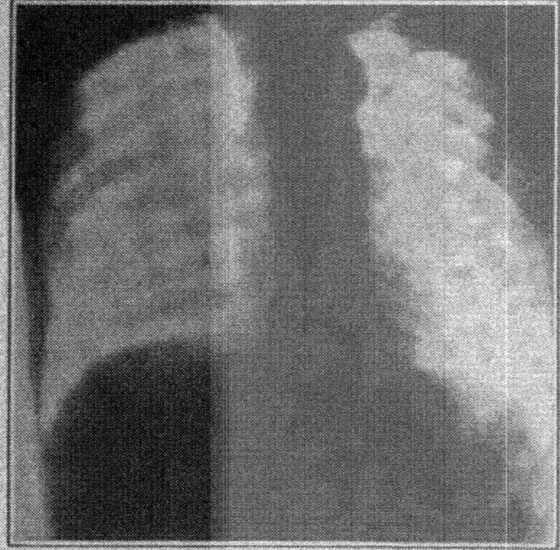

FIG. 399.—Radium capsule in place in a case of esophageal cancer. The esophagoscope, screened with hard rubber, is kept in situ to watch the position of the capsule until certain it will not shift.

for two or three hours, the applications being repeated on alternate days for about ten applications. If excessive local reaction or general toxemia result the treatment should be interrupted for a few weeks. These dosages are given with reservations. The future may determine them to be too large or too small. Mr. Walter G. Howarth has been getting excellent results from the use of 100 mgm. kept *in situ* by means of a wire

[illegible]

[illegible]

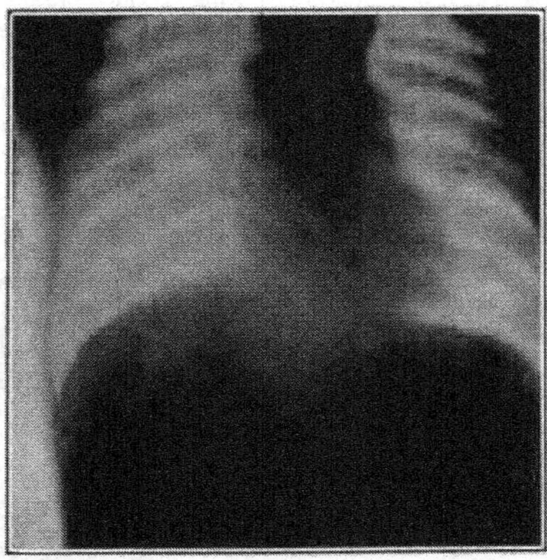

FIG. 401.—Radiograph of radium container in situ showing fogging of the plate by the radium rays, in nine minutes exposure.

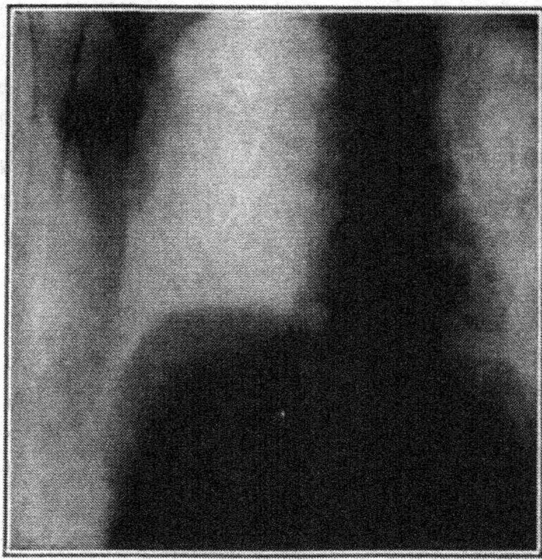

FIG. 402.—Peroral radium application to cancer of the cardia.

CHAPTER XXVIII.

Direct Laryngoscopy in Diseases of the Larynx.

For diagnostic purposes the greatest usefulness of the direct method has been in the laryngeal diseases of children, a field which prior to the development of direct laryngoscopy could not be studied in the living. For treatment, especially surgical treatment, the direct method has placed endolaryngeal surgery on a plane impossible of attainment by indirect methods.

Endoscopic appearances of laryngeal disease. The appearance of the mucosa as to color, edema, ulceration, infiltration and neoplastic processes is so fully studied in books on laryngology that extensive consideration here is needless. Besides the difference in form due to the point of view previously referred to, only one point need be mentioned, namely, the wide variations in color due to engorged vascularity induced reflexly by the presence of the direct laryngoscope so close to the laryngeal orifice. As elsewhere explained, this engorgement varies with the anesthetic used, and is usually greater when no anesthetic at all is used for the examination. It is always wise, therefore, to get, in the first view, an accurate estimate of color. If covered with a mask of secretion this must be quickly and gently wiped away after the first inspection.

Subglottic edema. This has been previously referred to. Because of the easily elevated mucosa and the abundant submucosal cellular tissue it is often the first indication of perichondritis. When the latter has been cured, a chronic edema or hyperplasia should be cauterized as shown in Fig. 87.

Perichondritis, abscess and their sequelae are easily diagnosticated and treated in children on well known principles. Stenosis following these conditions is the subject of a separate chapter.

Tuberculosis. The author is in accord with Kahler, who states that indiscriminate surgical treatment of the tuberculous larynx is a mistake and has led to discredit, whereas properly planned surgical measures in selected cases have yielded excellent results. As stated by Mr. Davis (Bib. 100)—"When the larynx is involved a vicious circle occurs, in which the dysphagia, sleeplessness, and cough produced by the painful lesion markedly increase the rapidity of the progression of the lung condition. The judicious removal by surgical methods of painful lesions undoubtedly relieves pain, and vigorous methods with careful research are needed to attack the much-dreaded laryngeal tuberculosis."

Extirpation of tuberculous laryngeal lesions. When small and isolated, extirpation of the entire lesion may yield excellent results as in the following case:

A girl of eighteen years, referred by Dr. B. L. Calhoun for increasing hoarseness of some months' duration. Indirect laryngoscopy showed a small projection from the right cord (A, Fig. 403) which looked like

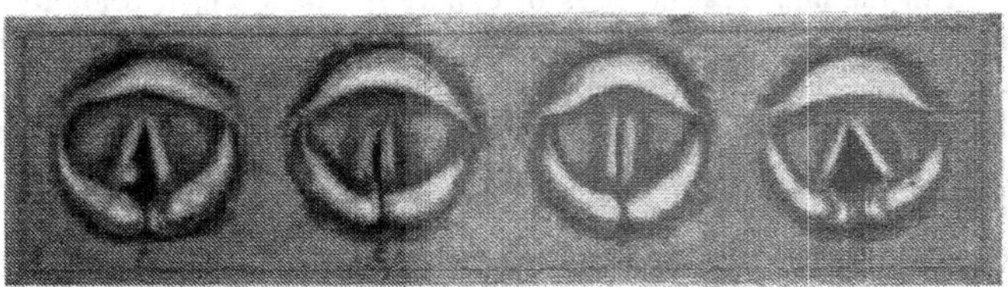

Fig. 403.—Case of extirpation of a small isolated laryngeal tuberculous nodule, in a girl of eighteen years. A Growth on right cord thought to be of inflammatory origin but later proven tuberculous. B. One week after extirpation the cord on the operated side does not seem to be drawn tense in attempted phonation. C. Two weeks after operation phonation is perfect. D. Larynx on inspiration five years after operation.

a singer's node. As a rule the author does not favor the removal of singer's nodules, but as this was one-sided and was clearly the cause of the hoarseness, the author yielded to the patient's demand that the growth be excised in order to restore the voice promptly to enable the patient to finish her year's contract as a singing teacher. The growth was removed by direct laryngoscopy with very happy results as regards voice. Dr. Ernest W. Willetts reported the growth to be undoubtedly tuberculous. This diagnosis was subsequently confirmed by physical examination and by the finding of bacilli in the sputum, which, of course, came from the pulmonary lesion. Rest in bed, open air and a complete antituberculous regime under the skillful care of Dr. Calhoun entirely cured the pulmonary condition, and now, five years later, the patient's larynx is as shown at D in Fig. 403, entirely and completely well. This case illustrates clearly what may be done by direct laryngoscopic excision of tuberculous growths. Manifestly, however, it is only adapted to isolated foci and is not to be applied to the usual massive arytenoid infiltrations. Diffuse infiltrations are not amenable to extirpation, but encroachments on the glottis may be removed with great relief of dyspnea and secondary benefits from improved oxidation.

Amputation of the epiglottis. Tuberculosis of the epiglottis may prove one of the most disastrous lesions that a tuberculous patient can develop, not so much from the toxemia of the lesion itself as from the odynphagia which interferes very seriously with the patient's nourishment; and, unfortunately, nearly all the applications that can be made to lessen the pain of swallowing interfere with the appetite so that food is not relished, and even nausea and vomiting may be induced. If amputation of the epiglottis is necessary, it is very easily accomplished by the method given in Chapter VII.

Galvanopuncture for laryngeal tuberculosis. Of the endoscopic surgical methods galvano-puncture will soon be entitled to first place since the advantages of its endoscopic use have been demonstrated. Deep puncture produces the best results in infiltrations without ulceration, but it is neecssary to avoid puncturing the arytenoid joint. Next to these, fungating ulcerations are most amenable. The fungations after a single application will often disappear and the ulcer will cicatrize. For ulceration superficial cauterizations are preferable. In diffused edematous infiltrations deep punctures are to be preferred. Ulcerative tuberculosis of the epiglottis and lesions involving the posterior surface of the arytenoid and mouth of the esophagus yield readily to cauterant treatment. Excessive reaction sometimes follows the application of the galvanocautery, though rarely. It is best to make only a slight application at first to see how much reaction the particular individual will probably manifest. Deep punctures at a white heat produce less reaction than superficial punctures or those made at a dull red heat. Perichondritis has followed in some instances, but as this is quite a usual complication in tuberculosis of the larynx it could not be determined in any of the cases reported in the literature that the perichondritis resulted directly from the cautery. They would probably have occurred anyway from the mixed infections at work in ulcerated areas. The technic of galvanopuncture is alluded to under the head of direct laryngoscopy.

CONGENITAL LARYNGEAL STRIDOR.

Stridorous breathing may be due to any one of many different forms of obstruction of the larynx and trachea. The text books mention traditional sounds, signs and symptoms by which it was thought distinctions might be made as to the different locations affected. To reiterate these would be useless. A diagnosis based upon anything but looking and seeing is wrong as often as right. Many different conditions were supposed to exist to account for the symptoms of stridor coming on at or shortly after birth and continuing for a year or two. Many of these hypotheses doubtless applied to conditions which really exist in some cases, but it seems best to limit the name to those cases of exaggerated infantile type of larynx, as described by D. R. Paterson, A. Brown Kelly, G. A. Southerland and H. Lambert Lack. Sir St. Clair Thompson's description (Bib. 539) is excellent. "The epiglottis is very long and tapering, and its lateral margins are rolled backward so as to meet, and thus form a complete cylinder above. The greatly reduced entrance to the larynx is bounded by the aryepiglottic folds which are too closely opposed to admit any but the slightest amount of air. The croaking noise is caused by the free and unsupported part of the posterior laryngeal wall and neighboring loose tissue on the summits of the arytenoids which is sucked forwards and inwards during inspiration." This description coincides with three cases seen by the author, one of which is illustrated at D, in Fig. 95. The endoscopic picture varied slightly in the different cases, but the essential form of the exaggerated infantile type was present. The author has seen a case of congenital stridor from other causes. One caused by papilloma was probably congenital, and one was certainly congenital. A marked inspiratory stridor in another case was found to be due to the collapse of the posterior membranous tracheo-esophageal wall into the trachea as a result of the negative pressure in inspiration. This collapse occurs normally to some extent in breathing and markedly in coughing but not so markedly as seen in this case. It was an exaggerated form of the forward movement of the posterior tracheal wall seen in Fig. 144. In one case of thymic stenosis the stridor was marked but was of a less croaking character than in the purely laryngeal form. In a number of cases spasm was present in infants with the history of stridor having been present, "ever since they were born," but as mentioned above, the author considers it best to limit the name congenital laryngeal stridor to the anomalous exaggerated infantile larynx. The diagnosis is very readily made in a few seconds by the aid of the direct laryngoscope without any anesthesia, general or local. In regard to treatment, direct laryngoscopy has nothing to offer save that should asphyxia threaten, a bronchoscopy would sustain life until a tracheotomy could be done. As a matter of fact, however, the author has never seen a case where the symptoms were sufficiently urgent to demand this. If, however, the patient has a history of very severe suffocative attacks with cyanosis and is not so situated that immediate tracheotomy can be done, doubtless it would be very much safer to have the tracheotomy done as a preventive measure. All of the author's cases recovered completely within a year by attention to the general health and especially careful feedings carried out by the medical attendant.

Congenital webs of the larynx and doubtless other malformations may produce stridor. One interesting case of the author is illustrated in Fig. 94. At C is seen a tumor-like mass bulging upward from the vocal cords of a child three months of age, which had had a crowing inspiratory stridor since birth. The child was crying at the moment represented by the sketch. Almost immediately afterwards the child took a deep breath and what seemed to be a tumor was now very plainly seen to be a web stretching across from one vocal band to the other, and while it seemed slightly below the cord in this position yet on phonation the band folded upward into the tumor-like mass seen at C, Fig. 94.

Congenital goitre and congenital laryngeal paralysis of each of which the author has seen one case, may cause congenital stridor but these are better considered under stenosis.

CHAPTER XXIX.

Bronchoscopy in Diseases of the Trachea and Bronchi.

The field opened up by Killian's demonstration of the ease and harmlessness of a careful bronchoscopy is so enormous and so new that thorough, systematic, analytical consideration of it at the present time is impossible. Unfortunately, the trachea is a border line organ to which heretofore relatively little attention has been given. The laryngologist could, with his mirror, see a little of the upper portion but he seldom attempted much in the way of study or treatment. The internist was more interested in the deeper air passages and touched lightly upon it as of little importance. The general surgeon rarely operated upon it except to open it in tracheotomy or to amputate it in laryngectomy. The direct method, however, has opened up a new field of study and the trachea and its diseases will be systematically dealt with in the laryngologic text books of the future. Delavan has called attention to the fact that the earliest use of a direct method of endobronchial medication was carried out by Horace Green in 1841, whose results were published in book form in 1846.

Indications for bronchoscopy in disease. Various indications may be gathered from the hereinafter mentioned bronchoscopic observations in the various diseases. But it may be well to emphasize a few of the most clearly defined and urgently important indications.

1. All cases of bronchiectasis should be bronchoscoped for foreign bodies, for diagnosis and also for local treatment. Emil Mayer found a foreign body in one case of bronchiectasis where its presence had never been suspected. The author has found bronchiectasis present in two cases of prolonged sojourn of a foreign body in the right inferior lobe bronchus, though in both of these cases the foreign body had been discovered radiographically.

2. Every case of dyspnea, except, of course, pneumonia and similar well understood conditions, calls for bronchoscopy.

3. Every case in which tracheotomy does not relieve the dyspnea should be bronchoscoped to determine why the tracheal cannula does not give relief.

4. All cases of hemoptysis which are not definitely proved to be tuberculous should be bronchoscoped for diagnosis, and any severe bleeding may be endoscopically packed as advised by Killian.

5. Every case of paralysis of the recurrent nerve the cause of which is not positively known, calls for bronchoscopy.

6. In any case of thoracic disease in which any element of doubt exists, valuable information may be gained by bronchoscopy.

7. In case of doubt as to whether bronchoscopy should be done or not, bronchoscopy should always be done.

Contraindications to bronchoscopy in disease. The author cannot recall any absolute contraindication to a careful bronchoscopy in any case in which it is really needed. Unless there are urgent indications, however, it had better not be done except for foreign bodies, in case of aneurysm, high blood pressure, advanced heart disease, pulmonary tuberculosis. There are no valid contraindications whatsoever to bronchoscopy in any case of obstructive dsypnea, provided. of course, the bronchoscopist is prompt and certain in his insertion.

Anesthesia. No anesthesia is needed in children. In adults local anesthesia of the larynx is needed. Below this, for scientific study, it is advisable to make at least one examination without any anesthesia, general or local, because of the alteration of the picture by anesthesia. For applications to the tracheo-bronchial tree most operators make an application of a local anesthetic to the larynx. For this purpose, cocaine is used by practically all endoscopists. If applications have to be frequently made, the author would urge the use of extremely diluted solutions and the trial of other local anesthetics and of no anesthetic. In no case should the patient know the drug used for anesthesia. Additional consideration of this subject will be found in Chapter IV.

Position of the patient. The recumbent position is best for children; the sitting position for adults. For examination of a very dyspneic patient, such as an asthmatic during an attack, the sitting position will cause the patient less distress, though for obtaining scientific data, it would be well, when possible, to examine the patient in both the sitting and the recumbent posture. For endobronchial applications, the patient should be in the sitting position in order to get the assistance of gravity in diffusing the medication. For removal of excessive secretions "sponge-pumping" in the recumbent posture is most promptly efficient. (For full consideration of position see Chapter VI.)

Bronchoscopic appearances in disease. The variations of mucosal color in health in different individuals and as influenced by general and local anesthesia, degree of illumination, tubal contact, a film coating of secretions, et cetera, as considered in Chapter IX, must be borne in mind in endoscopy for disease. The first look should comprehend the color as accurately as possible over the entire visible area. With proper illumination the appearances in disease are readily recognized by the rhinolaryngologist who is familiar with the appearance of various mucosal pathologic changes. To appreciate morbid departures in form, it is necessary to be familiar with the normal as seen under widely varying conditions of age, movement, cough, etc. Bronchoscopists have, in the variations of the form and movement of the bifurcation, a very valuable means of contributing to the diagnosis of intrathoracic disease. The carina trachealis in the normal chest moves forward as well as downward during deep inspiration, returning on expiration. The author has noticed in addition to the above mentioned observation of Gottstein, that the descent on deep inspiration is slow as compared to the quick return in the following expiration, and furthermore, after the return there is a distinct interval of repose which is longer than the normal repose of rhythmic respiration. To note this movement, it is necessary that the bronchoscope should not be too near the bifurcation, as the instrument itself will resist movement to a great extent. This normal respiratory movement of the carina is of great diagnostic importance because it is interfered with by various peri-tracheal and peri-bronchial conditions. The fixation is greatest in cancer, somewhat less so in case of masses of tuberculous glands unless these have suppurated, and the movement is only slightly interfered with in aneurysm. In fact, it is not usually noticeable at all, unless the aneurysm is of enormous size.

Exploration of the upper lobe bronchus is limited to the orifice and a short portion of its stem, but useful information may be gained from the secretions seen to emerge.

Endobronchial treatment. Ingals wisely advises caution in the development of endobronchial therapy. As pointed out by Ephraim and others, ordinary oral inhalations of nebulized fluids are practically worthless for the local treatment of disease, for the reason that the nebula does not penetrate even as far as the trachea. This has been proven experimentally on animals. Even where all the air inhaled by the patient is saturated with finely nebulized fluid, it is doubtful whether any appreciable amount reaches the deeper air passages, because of the impinging upon the mucosa at the various turns of the upper air passages. These various surfaces act as baffle plates to remove the minute particles of medication suspended in the air. Intratracheal injections with the aid of indirect laryngoscopy, have slightly better results, but even then the prompt coughing of the patient will remove the fluid before it can reach the deeper passages, even when a large quantity of fluid is thrown in, though of course the larger the quantity the greater the likelihood of its reaching the bronchi. On the other hand, endoscopic applications place the fluid deep down in the bronchi, where all bechic efforts to expel it only serve the better to scatter it over the mucosa. The most commonly used method is with the endoscopic syringe with long metal nozzle inserted through the bronchoscope. Dr. Emma E. Musson of Philadelphia, has been using, with excellent results, a method which she demonstrated before the meeting of the Pennsylvania State Medical Society (Bib. 401). The larynx is exposed with the laryngoscope. A little of a local anesthetic solution is applied to the interior of the larynx, and a long silk-woven tube is passed through the larynx down into the bronchi. The medicated solution is then injected with a syringe, the short nozzle of which is inserted firmly into the proximal, funnel-like, silk-woven tube. The placing of the head to one side will insure the silk-woven tube going into the opposite bronchus, especially if a little curve is imparted to the tube before insertion. This method seems, to the author, the very best, because the application can be made with accuracy and with very slight annoyance to the patient. Of course, skill is required to be certain of the accurate placing of the silk-woven tube in the desired bronchus.

Anomalies of the tracheobronchial tree. Anomalies of the tracheobronchial tree are rare, but variations from what might be considered as an average type are noted by every endoscopist. Kahler (Bib. 300) reports two cases of diverticulum of the tracheobronchial tree consisting of rudimentary bronchial branches. Guisez reports a congenital valve-like web obstructing part of the trachea. The dyspnea was relieved by incision and dilatation. Congenital esophagobronchial and esophagotracheal fistulae have been reported.

Deviation of the trachea and laryngoptosis. An interesting observation of the author is the coincidence, in two cases, of deviation of the trachea with laryngoptosis. The author has seen a third case of laryngoptosis which also had a deviated trachea, but this was a case of cancer. As there was compression of the trachea, as well as deviation, by a mass probably of infected mediastinal lymph nodes with involvement of the esophageal wall, there could be no certainty that there had been a previously existing deviation of the trachea. One case of deviation with laryngoptosis with cervical ribs was reported (Bib. 269, pp. 77, 78). The second patient was a woman of 32 years of age who came to the dispensary for acute laryngitis, which, however, seemed to be in no way connected with the ptosis of the larynx. The woman had never noticed that her "Adam's apple" was any lower than in other people. She had been subject to dyspnea on exertion ever since she could remember; but had not been particularly subject to attacks of hoarseness, such as that caused by the acute laryngitis for the relief of which she applied. A bronchoscopy under local anesthesia showed the trachea deviated sharply backward, as shown at D, in diagram C, Fig. 404. The patient was sent to Dr. Russell H. Boggs for a radiograph of the chest. but unfortunately she did not go and disappeared, no trace of her being obtainable at the address given on the dispensary register. All three of these cases had, in common, the low position of the larynx, the thyroid cartilage being submerged almost to the thyroid notch. The thyrohyoid membrane was of about thrice the normal vertical extent, the necks in the two women, cases A and C, being of usual length, the hyoid bone be-

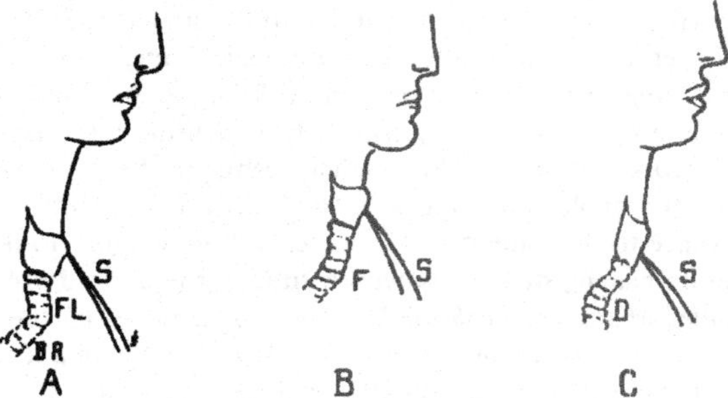

FIG. 404.—Schematic illustration of three cases of laryngoptosis with deviation of the trachea. A and C were probably congenital anomalies. B was associated with mediastinal cancer. In all three cases the larynx was almost entirely below the notch of the sternum (S). FL, deviation forward to the left. BR, deviation backward to the right. F, deviation forward; D, backward.

ing only slightly lower than usual. The man's neck seemed quite short, the increased vertical extent of the thyrohyoid membrane apparently filling up all the space made by the ptosis of the larynx. In all, the trachea was deviated, and in all the esophagus seemed to follow the trachea in the deviation; but it is necessary to eliminate case B from consideration, because of the mediastinal malignancy which compressed the trachea and involved the esophagus. In case A, the deviation was first forward to the left and then backward to the right. In case C, the deviation seemed to be directly backward immediately below the cricoid. The carinal respiratory movements were normal in cases A and C. It is impossible for the author to express an opinion as to whether these deviations were congenital anomalies or not, though the fact of the cervical ribs occurring in one case would rather speak for a congenital condition. It will require a large series of cases to arrive at definite conclusions. The author had the honor of exhibiting case A to Prof. Killian upon his visit to the author's clinic in 1907.

Deviation of the trachea from diseased conditions of surrounding structures is quite common. In nearly every case of very large goitre, there is more or less deviation as well as compression. In substernal goitre, the deviation is, in some instances, even more marked. Malignant growths and glandular masses in the mediastinum are perhaps the most common causes of deviation of the intrathoracic trachea, with aneurysm standing next in frequency, in the author's experience. The differential diagnosis of these conditions cannot be made, as a rule, on the endoscopic findings alone; but when taken in conjunction with the radiograph, the physical examination of the chest and the palpation of the neck, the internist will usually be able to make the diagnosis with great accuracy and will give due weight to the endoscopic findings of the bronchoscopist. While not absolutely diagnostic, it is well to remember that the infiltrations of carcinoma are usually very hard, imparting rigidity to the deformity and compressions of the trachea. It should also be remembered that the level of the arch points strongly to aneurysm, that the bifurcation is usually the seat of the enlarged masses of glands in tuberculous processes, and that an esophagoscopy should always be done in every case of tracheal deviation for the valuable light it will often throw on the case. The author has observed in a case referred to him by Dr. Baetjer of Baltimore, deviation of the trachea in an eight-year-old boy who had a patent foramen ovale.

Compression stenoses of the trachea and bronchi. All of the diseases mentioned as causing deviation may also cause compression. Goitre, cervical or substernal, aneurysm and malignancy are the most common, and may produce severe dyspnea. A goitre together with a mass of mediastinal glands caused a compression of the entire cervical and thoracic trachea (Fig. 405) in a leukemic (leucocytosis 625,000) boy of seven years of age referred to the author by Dr. John W. Boyce for tracheotomy. Not until the long, cane-shaped tracheotomic cannula entered the right bronchus was the dyspnea completely relieved. The boy died two days later, but not for want of air. No post mortem was obtained. Compression stenosis of the left bronchus is a not infrequent condition in hypertrophy of the cardiac auricle. In one such case the author found the left bronchus almost closed and the esophagus so compressed as to interfere seriously with swallowing. There was a posticus paralysis of the left side of the larynx. The author has seen tracheal compression due to mediastinal emphysema caused by a fall down stairs. Compression stenosis of the trachea associated with pulmonary emphysema has been studied in thirty-two cases by Kahler (Bib. 296), who notes that the stenosis becoming much worse on coughing explains the frightful dyspnea from which many emphysematous patients suffer.

The author saw one case of congenital tracheal stenosis due to goitre. That it was an obstructive case of "blue baby" was recognized by Dr. B. B. Wechsler. Prompt tracheotomy by Dr. S. Seegman, and

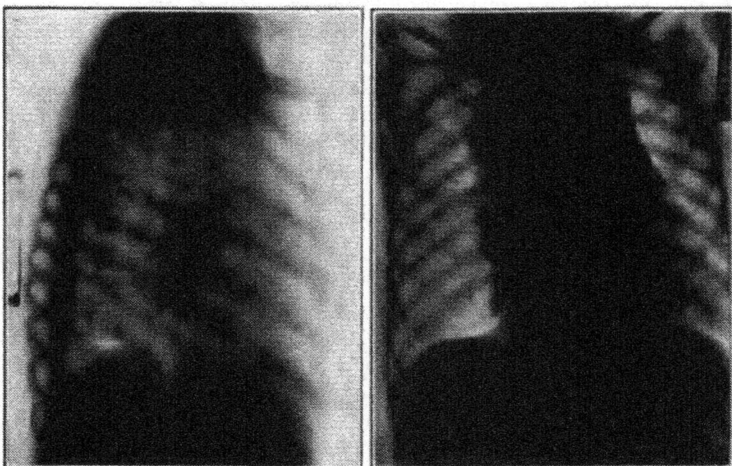

FIG. 405.—Compression stenosis of the entire cervical and thoracic trachea by a goitre and a mass of glands in a leukemic boy, seven years of age. The narrow whitish streak in the lateral view is the compressed trachea and the left bronchus, the latter being displaced backward. The uncompressed right bronchus is seen. Tracheotomy with a long cane-shaped cannula relieved the dyspnea. (Author's case. Radiograph by Dr. George W. Grier.)

the use of one of the author's long tracheal cannulae saved the patient's life.

The recognition of a compressive tracheal stenosis with its elliptical or scabbard shape is quite easy. Of course, it must be recognized that during cough there may be compression of lumen that would be misinterpreted if not compared with the lumen during inspiration or at the momentary rest period between expiration and inspiration. A concentric funnel-like compression stenosis is exceedingly rare and occurs only with annular growths completely surrounding the air tube. To make certain that such a condition is really a pathologic and not a normal narrowing, it is only necessary to remember that there is no narrowing normally in the bronchi between branches. The walls of a suspected narrowing should be searched for lateral branches and if none is given off and yet narrowing exists, we may conclude that it is pathologic, but we must be on our guard not to mistake a perspective foreshortening for a narrowing. In a marked compression stenosis of the trachea the walls will entirely collapse during coughing. Normally the walls of the larger bronchi and especially of the trachea do not collapse though they may narrow slightly. In children they narrow very markedly, especially the membranous posterior wall of the trachea, which advances so far as to take up a considerable part of the tracheal lumen. The bronchi in children narrow very markedly during cough, the narrowing in some situations being concentric, in others scabbard like.

To measure the depth of a compression stenosis the beginning is noted when the tube mouth has reached the first observable narrowing. Then the tube is inserted until it has passed entirely through the stenosed area and arrives at a lumen of normal size and contour. then the depth is again noted. By using very small tubes in tight stenosis it is easy in any case to measure depth in this way, though, of course, if preferred, olivary bougies such as used for esophagoscopic dilatation may be used with the sense of touch as a guide as to the engaging of the olive and its emergence on the other side. By either method the measurement should be repeated on withdrawal. Comparison of the two measurements will minimize error.

Treatment of compression stenoses of the trachea consists in tracheotomy. Literature is full of cases unrelieved by tracheotomy simply because the ordinary tracheotomic cannula of the shops will not reach below an extensive compression. It requires, in most cases, the author's long cane-shaped cannula as described under "Tracheotomy" (See also Fig. 407). The treatment of compression stenosis of the bronchi consists in the use of the long cane-shaped cannula, if the stenosis is near the main bronchial orifice. If deeper the intubation tubes used for cicatricial stenosis of the bronchi may be used (Bib. 269, p. 79). Their use is indicated only when the stenosis is so great as to interfere with escape of secretions from the subjacent air passages.

Permanent cure will, of course, depend upon the curability of the compressive mass.

Thymic compression stenosis. The author has demonstrated bronchoscopically (Bib. 255 and 269) that the enlarged thymus can and does in some instances compress the trachea even to the point of asphyxia. Four cases of thymic tracheostenosis have convinced the author of the purely mechanical conditions present in cases of thymic hypertrophy; and having seen so many illustrations of extreme danger of anesthesia in even the slightest stenosis of the trachea, he feels convinced that the thymus deaths attributed to "status lymphaticus" and "hyperthymization of the blood" are really nothing more or less than arrested respiration, which is, as usual, fatal because respiration when arrested by obstruction cannot be started again without either tracheotomy or bronchoscopic oxygen insufflation. The author would strongly urge that when respiration ceases during anesthesia and cannot be immediately started, tracheotomy should be done, a long cane-shaped cannula inserted, and amyl nitrite insufflated into the trachea. Better still would be the insufflation of oxygen through the bronchoscope, or through the intratracheal insufflation catheter. These are not always promptly available, but tracheotomy can always be done in a few seconds. A slight degree of dyspnea may never be noticed, and may quite readily be at-

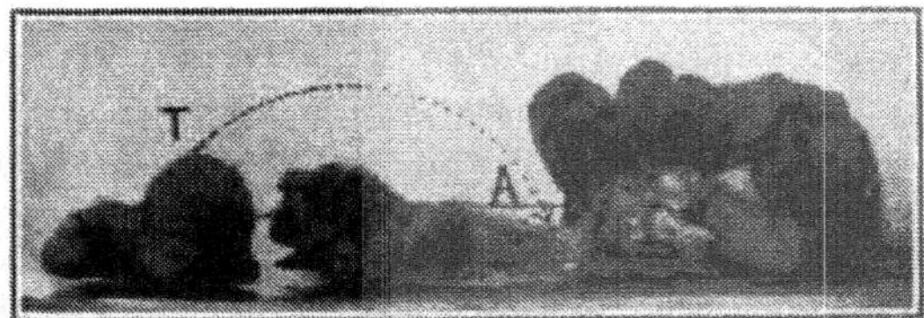

Fig. 406.—From a photograph of a specimen from a new-born infant asphyxiated by compression of the trachea at A by the large fourth lobe, T, of the thymus gland. (Case of Dr. V. L. Andrews.)

tributed to enlarged tonsils or adenoids. The excitement of starting the anesthetic can very readily engorge a vascular structure, like the thymus gland and the increased bulk compressing the trachea produces apnea just as soon as the patient begins to go under the anesthetic. Artificial respiration, as ordinarily done, is absolutely useless in the presence of even very slight degrees of tracheal stenosis. Air can be forced out of the lungs, but it cannot be drawn in. It is a well known fact that engorgement of tissue like the thymus gland increases its bulk. If the hypertrophic gland can compress the trachea, the engorged hypertrophic gland can compress the trachea still more. After death, the congestive part of the bulk may diminish so as not to be noticeable. A beautiful autoptical confirmation of the above mentioned, previously published observations of the author on the purely mechanical nature of thymus death is afforded by Dr. V. L. Andrews' case. A new born child died after making a number of violent ineffective inspiratory movements.

Autopsy revealed a very large four-lobed thymus. The fourth and compressive lobe, T, was compressing the trachea at the end of the dotted line, A, Fig. 406. Dr. Andrews' report is as follows:

"The thymus is short and thick and contains four lobes. It measures 4 cm. in length, 3.5 cm. in width, 1.75 cm. in average thickness. There is a right, left and middle lobe. The left lobe is small. The fourth

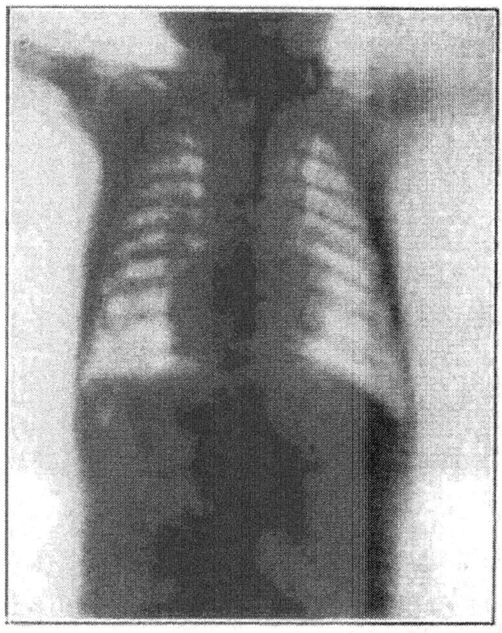

FIG. 407.—Thymic tracheostenosis temporarily relieved with the author's long cane-shaped tracheal cannula. The shadow of the hypertrophied thymus shows to the right of the cannula, and especially strongly at the right of the lower end. (Authors' case.)

lobe extends from beneath the lower ends of the right and middle lobes upward and outward, at an angle of 45°, into the right pleural cavity for a distance of 1.5 cm. The upper end is free in the pleural cavity and is covered by a thin movable membrane (pleura?). The lower end of this lobe lies over the trachea beneath the lower part of the middle and right lobes and at this point, 1 cm. above the bifurcation of trachea, the thymus measures 2 cm. in thickness. Here the trachea presents a flattened appearance antero-posteriorly, more marked on the right side than on the left."

In three of the author's cases the compression was from before backward. In the last case it was lateral the axis of the scabbard-like lumen being from the left posteriorly to the right anteriorly.

As shown by Fetterhoff and Gettings (quoted by H. C. Clark) compression of the trachea may occur from a left innominate vein engorged by an embarrassed right heart, the dilated vein being forced to extend posteriorly because braced anteriorly by the thymus. Treatment of thy-

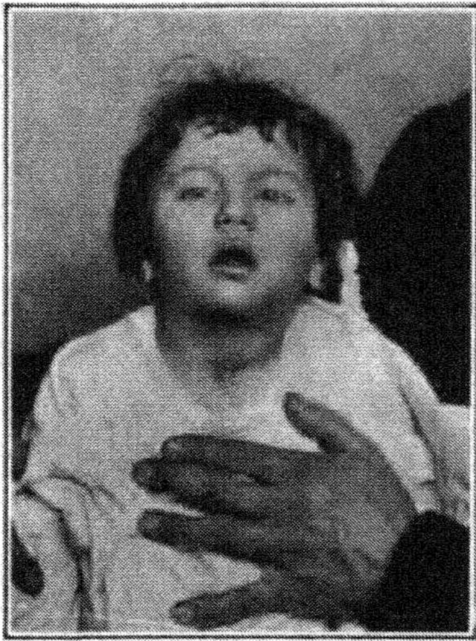

FIG. 408.—Photograph of a child of two years taken six months after thymopexy. (Author's case.)

mic compression stenosis is the same as mentioned for other tracheal compressions, namely the cane-shaped cannula of sufficient length to reach below the compression (Fig. 407). As the author has proven, hypertrophic thymus is dangerous solely from a mechanical compressive point of view. He who will see that a good respiratory channel is mechanically maintained need not worry about such purely hypothetical conditions as "hyperthymization of the blood," etc. Having temporarily cared for the compression stenosis by the insertion of the long cannula, the next step is either thymopexy or thymectomy (subtotal). In the author's first cases all of the gland that could be brought up was shelled out of its capsule and removed. In the last case an equally satisfactory result was obtained by thymopexy. This last case was as follows:

Robert C., aged two years, was referred to the author by Dr. W. H. Wesley for dyspnea and noisy breathing of three months' duration. All of the accessory respiratory muscles were working vigorously. The suprasternal and clavicular fossae were indrawing and there was a typical "trichter brust" at each inspiration. Bronchoscopy revealed a tracheal compression reducing the lumen to a narrow chink whose curved axis was from the left posteriorly to the right anteriorly. Tracheotomy was done under infiltration anesthesia and the enormous thymus bulged largely into the wound. It was drawn upward and stitched with linen to the tendons of sternomastoid muscles and to the skin and tissues at the top of the sternum. The tracheal cannula was removed on the eighth day and the child was discharged well on the fifteenth day. There had been no return of the dyspnea when the photograph, Fig. 408, was taken six months later.

Remarks. The lateral compression visible endoscopically has not previously been observed. From this one case it is not wise to conclude that thymopexy is to be preferred in all cases to subcapsular subtotal thymectomy. Doubtless part of every very large gland should be removed. Total removal is probably impossible even if desirable. An able article with a report of fifty operated cases is written by Parker (Bib. 428). See also a valuable contribution by Schwinn, Bib. 490.

Inflammations and their sequelae. Chronic circumscribed tracheobronchitis is a common affection in adults. Acute circumscribed tracheobronchitis is rather frequent in the course of influenza, (q. v.) as manifested by the dry, barking cough and severe burning pain back of the sternum. In children an occasional interesting complication is seen in the form of laryngeal spasm, doubtless a reflex from an irritated tracheal mucosa, differing from the ordinary diffuse bronchitis in that the important lesion is limited to, or at least most marked in, the trachea and larger bronchi In some instances it is limited to a portion only of the mucosal area of these passages. A case of chronic purulent bronchitis is described in the subsequent paragraph on tuberculosis. Non-tuberculous abscess of the lung has been found and evacuated bronchoscopically (Bib. 271) by the author. The bronchoscope in relation to another case of pulmonary abscess is shown in Fig. 136.* Freudenthal records non-specific ulceration of the bronchial mucosa in one case. Ephraim reports nineteen relative cures of chronic bronchitis out of 23 cases. In many instances, a single application only, was necessary. The applications were followed by increased expectoration and a total change of

*As stated by George L. Richards, a non-tuberculous pulmonary abscess justifies the suspicion of foreign-body origin.

secretions. The solutions used were novocain and suprarenin dissolved in salt solution in some instances, and in others in a five per cent solution of potassium or ammonium iodid. The ammonium iodid was used especially in the dry form of bronchitis, and a few drops of iodine were added to it. In a number of cases he also used weak solutions of argentic nitrate. In two cases of chronic purulent bronchitis, permanent healing was accomplished by repeated insufflation of turpentine emulsion to which suprarenin had been added. In one case each of chronic pneumonia and of double gangrene of the lung, the procedure was ineffective.

Bronchiarctia and bronchiectasis. Bronchial stenoses comprise a number of different lesions. The chief causes of cicatricial bronchial stenosis are traumatism, syphilis and tuberculosis; or, perhaps, more accurately, the secondary infections complicating these lesions. Tuberculous processes are of such slow progress, as a rule, that the lung accommodates itself to the altered conditions, and cicatricial bronchial stenoses secondary to tuberculosis rarely require local treatment, though they do occur as the result of erosion through the bronchial wall. The author has seen six such cases. Cicatricial stenoses, in some instances, may require dilatation in order to secure proper drainage of the infrastrictural bronchiectatic cavity, and thus cure the patient of bronchiectasis with its distressing cough, foul expectoration, dyspnea and lesser symptoms. For syphilitic strictures it may be necessary to use prolonged intubation with bronchial intubation tubes, put in place with the aid of the bronchoscope and left *in situ* for a period of from one to seven days. The tube should be left for a few hours in case of daily removals, or a few days in case of weekly removals. Extubation is performed with an extubator used through the bronchoscope. In order to obtain a sufficient lumen for the insertion of the intubation tube, a laminaria or tupelo tent may be used, placed *in situ* with the author's instrument for the purpose (Bib. 269). The tent is open to the objection, that it obstructs all drainage for the time it is in place, though this need be for only a few hours. Divulsion, as hereinafter described, is the best method by which to obtain a sufficient lumen for intubation, and even if some trauma results from divulsion, cicatricial tissue is not readily infected by the organisms present to which the patient is already more or less immune. Endobronchial neoplasms may cause bronchiectasia. This is an additional reason for bronchoscoping every case with bronchiectatic symptoms. Bronchiectasis and bronchiarctia resulting from foreign bodies are considered in Chapter XVI. Cicatricial stenoses of the bronchi are very readily recognized by the cicatricial nature of their walls with a total absence of rings. This condition, of course, may be more or less confused by inflammatory states which ordinarily mask the view of rings.

In neither of these was he able to make out spasmodic stenosis, and the color of the mucosa was more purple than red. The bronchi were all filled with secretions and the patient's distress was completely relieved by the bronchoscopy with removal of secretions without any application of any kind, the bronchoscopy being done without any anesthesia, general or local. The findings and the results were the same in both instances. Both patients had a recurrence of their attacks at about the usual intervals, no medication having been used. All the foregoing observations by the different observers were during the attacks, and they all go to show that there is a very varied bronchoscopic picture. Between the attacks, the pictures observed by most of the observers have been normal, except in some cases where unusual dilatation of the vessels has been observed. Freudenthal records the appearance of a scar-like mass obstructing the entire lumen of the bronchus. The obstruction was overcome by the local application of a 20 per cent solution of cocaine, liberating an enormous discharge of secretions. In another case adrenalin was used with excellent results after the air passages were cleared of secretion. One of his patients was practically cured, remaining perfectly well and free from attack at the end of six months. In this case, an emulsion of orthoform as follows was used:

Orthoform	6.5
Menthol	0.5
Formalin	0.5
Ol. amygdal. dul.	15.0
Gum acac.	10.0
Aqae ad	60.0
M. F. Emulsio.	

About 10cc. was injected twice weekly for ten applications. Then during an intermission of the treatments, after the great excitement of being exhibited at a medical meeting, a severe recurrence took place. After ten more treatments the attacks ceased and the patient was still well at the end of six months. The patient, a young man of 27, had had asthma since childhood and all of the members of his mother's family were asthmatic. He had never been able to sleep an entire night restfully. In another case, Freudenthal used propaesin instead of orthoform in a like amount. The applications were made in the morning with stomach empty. Out of a total of 13 patients, Freudenthal considered 8 cured, 3 improved and 2 not benefited. Ephraim reports 133 cases of asthma treated endobronchially with a spray of suprarenin with novocain with excellent results. A long-tubed bronchoscopic atomizer was used. In most cases free expectoration resulted within the following twelve hours. The results were not so good in the spasmodic dry asthma, nor in cases in which neurasthenia predominated. Results also were not favorable in cases in which immediate relief of the attack did not follow the application of the solutions injected during the attack. Of the 88 cases in which ultimate results were known, 73 were recorded as good. Of these, 48 were free from recurrence, some of them as long as 1½ years. Most of these were of the most severe type in which scarcely a night in years had passed without an attack. In seven other cases the attacks were notably milder and at longer intervals, the permanent distress less, without, however, permanent cure. Ephraim thought these effects were due to medicinal action of the substance injected, and not to any mechanical effect, because he had observed that the injection of normal salt solution alone produced no objective changes, and a patient showing diffuse bronchial rales before insufflation, showed, after insufflation, a vanishing of the rales on the side which had been treated. In none of the 133 cases had there been any untoward effect. As pointed out by Dr. James Adam in one of the best practical works on asthma that has ever appeared (Bib. 3), asthma in most cases is essentially a toxemia and no treatment can be successful without recognition of this element in the etiology

Influenzal tracheitis. Of all forms of tracheitis, perhaps the least frequently differentiated as a morbid entity is influenzal tracheitis. When the author observed his first cases in the prebronchoscopic days (1889) he believed that he had discovered a new disease. Indirect methods yielded few and uncertain pictures of the tracheal lesions, and, indeed, none in the most interesting class of cases, namely those occurring in infants and children. The advent of direct methods of examination permitted of accurate observation of the clinical appearances of the tracheobronchial mucosa. A very good illustration made from the author's color drawing of one of these cases has been published (Bib. 243). The clinical appearances might be classified under a number of different types, but it has seemed to the author that the differences he has observed are really different stages of the same disease. The first stage has much the same appearance as in influenzal inflammation of the nasal mucosa at the same stage. The tracheal mucosa is reddened. Its color deepens. Swelling of the mucosa begins. Later, an exudate forms, at first serous, then mucoid, then purulent and finally thick, tenacious and exceedingly difficult of expectoration even by the robust adult. In infants who naturally are almost incapable of expectoration, death may occur from inability to rid the air passages of secretion and drowning of the patient in his own secretions (q. v.) may be threatened. The bronchi or even the trachea itself may be occluded by mucosal swelling, or edema, actually causing death by the stenosis. Both these conditions are independent of broncho-pneumonia, which may or may not exist. The author has observed blood-clots on the surface of the inflamed membrane, without true hemorrhage, similar to those in nasal influenza, first described by D. Braden Kyle. Superficial erosions of the tracheal mucosa have been seen by the author in a number of cases. There was in no case any true adherent membranous exudate, on which alone the differential diagnosis rests. Clinically a severe case of influenzal laryngo-tracheitis cannot be differentiated from diphtheria, as it presents the same clinical picture, even to the adynamia. Direct inspection showing abscess of a fibrous exudate will promptly decide, and corroboration by the laboratory from the specimens bronchoscopically removed will follow. A bronchoscope need not be inserted below the larynx. The glottis may be propped open with the tube mouth (supraglottic tracheoscopy q. v.) or often the trachea can be clearly seen by use of the laryngoscope alone. In some instances, there seemed to be but little laryngeal inflammation, the croupy cough being probably due chiefly to spasmodic conditions excited by the inflammation below. The laboratory is seldom of aid if only secretions from the pharynx are sent. If the secretion is obtained by direct methods from the trachea, a reliable report nearly always can be had from specimens taken through the sterile bronchoscope which prevents contamination with organisms. A typical case may be cited:

The author was called to see an infant, aged seven months, suffering with extreme inspiratory dyspnea, with croupy cry and stridulous breathing, but no cough. The onset had been gradual, not nocturnal or sudden, two weeks before. Antitoxin had been given without relief. Pneumonia had been excluded by Dr. Boyce and laryngismus stridulus by an able laryngologist, who, however, pointed out to us evidences of a certain element of spasm in the case. Temperature, 103°; pulse, 130; respiration, 32. The first glance at the larynx through the direct laryngoscope showed it to be free from edema or other obstruction or even active inflammation. When the bronchoscope was introduced, there was absolutely no cough, (no anesthetic used) and during the entire examination, lasting about five minutes, there was not one single effort to cough. The tracheal mucosa was intensely inflammed, and there was a tenacious secretion adherent in scattered locations. This secretion was wiped away readily, leaving no erosion nor bleeding. The bronchial mucosa was intensely inflammed in all the larger tubes; the smaller tubes were obstructed with pus which was moved to and fro in the respiratory current. but there was no coughing effort to expel it. Smears made from the sterile swabs passed through the sterile bronchoscope, showed an abundance of influenzal organisms (Dr. Ernest Willets). There was a little streak of pus extending upward between the arytenoids, and out over the upper edge of the party wall. No anesthetic, general or local, was used and the child seemed in no way inconvenienced by the bronchoscopy. The child made a slow but complete recovery. The interesting points about this case are the inspiratory dyspnea without laryngeal obstruction; the total absence of the cough reflex; the severe tracheo-bronchitis without pneumonia; the ease and certainty with which the laryngeal diagnostic question can be decided by direct laryngoscopy. It is interesting to consider what became of the endobronchial secretion. The interarytenoid streak was evidence of unimpaired ciliary activity, so that it seems probable that a portion of the pus was expelled in this way, the remainder being absorbed. The secretions in some instances require aspiration to save life. Absence of the cough reflex in influenzal tracheitis is seen only in infants, and is not present in every infantile case.

The drowning of the patient in his own secretions. (Bib. 232). When tracheal and bronchial secretions are in excess of the amount required properly to moisten the inspired air they become a menace to life unless removed. Under almost all circumstances the normal activities of the cough reflex, forced expiration, and ciliary action remove these secretions. There are certain circumstances, however, under which these normal agencies are inefficient. Various drugs, especially anti-bechics, hinder the action of the normal agencies; hence should always be avoided. The writer has always opposed their use in all laryngeal and tracheal surgery and in bronchoscopy. Doubtless many of the post-anesthetic pneumonias in surgery remote from the air passages, have been due to the abolition of agencies by which secretions are normally removed from the air passages. Perhaps the most frequent etiologic factor in the failure to rid the air passages of secretion is age. An infant cannot expectorate and is surprisingly inefficient in getting secretions out of air passages even as far out as the laryngo-pharynx. Adults as well as children when dying often fill up with secretions which they are too feeble to expectorate, and in some instances, by the failure of the respiratory blood changes, drowning is the final mechanism of mortality in death primarily due to disease remote from the air passages. The complex physiologic co-ordinated mechanism by which secretions are normally removed is too lengthy to be entered upon here; but disturbances of laryngeal motility and in the author's experience, bilateral cadaveric paralysis especially, are frequently associated with the condition which the writer has termed the "drowning of the patient in his own secretion." One of these cases seen many years ago at the Western Pennsylvania Hospital with Dr. Clarence Ingram was an excellent illustration. A woman, aged forty years, was dying of general lymphosarcomatosis. Pressure from the mediastinal or cervical neoplasmata produced a bilateral cadaveric paralysis. The level of the frothy fluid could be seen rising and falling first in the main bronchi, then higher and higher in the trachea until the level of the upper laryngeal orifice was reached. The woman could not expectorate. Had she not had other conditions and lesions, it would have been easy to have prolonged life indefinitely so far as drowning was concerned by the bronchoscopic aspiration of the fluid. The author has done this in other cases with the result of saving the patients. Before the days of bronchoscopy, he did a few tracheotomies for this purpose with excellent results; secretions could then be readily removed by a nurse trained in tracheal work—secretions that could never have been expectorated. In children, Dr. Boyce's method of assisting expulsion of tracheo-bronchial secretion by holding the child up by the heels has often proved efficient and has tided over a dangerous period. Perhaps the most important class of cases is that in which the secretions due to traumatism or irritation of a foreign body in the lower air passages gradually accumulate and asphyxiate the patient. One of the only two tracheotomies (in previously normal cases) done by the author for dyspnea after the removal of the foreign bodies, would not have been needed had he known what he has since discovered, namely, that children feeble from prolonged respiratory effort, will in some instances and after certain kinds of foreign bodies, fill up with tracheo-bronchial secretions and will die if not relieved. It would seem that some of the instances reported by various writers in which children have died in an unexplained manner after the removal of foreign bodies may be accounted for in this way. The condition was first pointed out to the author a number of years ago by Dr. Ellen J. Patterson. Perhaps the best case to cite as an illustration is the following:

John K., aged six years, referred to the author by Dr. Wagner. Prior to coming under the care of Dr. Wagner, the child had gone through the usual treatment by antitoxin and quarantine for a croupy cough with temperature elevation, due to a beech-nut hull, which had been cast about in the trachea and bronchi for three weeks. A grayish appearance of the skin due to dyspnea favored the diphtheritic diagnosis. The beech-nut hull and a large quantity of secretion were removed at the Presbyterian Hospital, by bronchoscopy. That night the patient became extremely dyspneic and cyanotic. Bronchoscopic removal of a large quantity of thick viscid secretion gave complete relief. There was a less severe recurrence of the symptoms the next night but the child had then rallied enough to rid itself of secretions which were moreover less tenacious. The child made a rapid recovery.

There have been twelve of these cases in the practice of Dr. Patterson and the author. In some the aspiration of secretion was sufficient:

in two instances the administration of oxygen through the bronchoscope after the removal of the secretions saved life. For this the bronchoscope with the anesthetic attachment of Dr. T. Drysdale Buchanan was found very convenient as it permitted of the slightest interruption of the flow of oxygen during the removal of secretions by "sponge pumping." In one instance the swelling of the mucosa, in other words the serous exudate into the mucosal tissue, prevented the pulmonic interchange of gases; the oxygen passed down through the bronchoscope could not be taken up and the child died. This was a case of influenzal tracheo bronchitis complicated by pneumonia. It was not a foreign body case. In one instance the secretions of an influenzal tracheitis were so gelatinous as to require removal with forceps. In some of the cases the secretions were so viscid they could not have been drawn through any form of tubal aspirator.

Bronchoscopy for the relief of patients threatened with drowning in their own secretions is a new and important field of usefulness for the bronchoscope as an aid to general medicine and surgery.

Since the foregoing was written a number of confirmatory observations have been made by others, notably by Carpenter (Bib. 69).

Gangrene of the lung. Guisez reports a case of pulmonary gangrene of very grave prognosis cured by intrabronchial injection of guiacol in oil with occasional injections also of iodoform suspended in oil. Ephraim's results were unfavorable.

Aneurysm. It is probable that bronchoscopy will repeat the history of the Roentgen ray—aneurysms will seldom be overlooked, but will often be diagnosticated when absent. The ordinary normal aortic impulse is most astonishing. It is only after repeated examinations that one grows accustomed to it. Any thoracic tumor compressing the bronchus may show a transmitted pulsation. In one case, that of a woman of [illegible], there was distinct stenosis from external pressure, with an impulse that seemed expansile rather than merely transmitted. Study of the symptoms practically negatived the suspicion of aneurysm. The patient was a neurasthenic and had the palpable relaxed abdominal aorta so common to that class (Boyce). It seems highly probable that her bronchial compression was due to a similar condition in the thoracic aorta. An aneurysmal sac may transmit little or no pulsation. The fact that a bronchoscopically or esophagoscopically visible bulging pulsates is far from conclusive evidence of aneurysm. It is a frequent error to assume that the shape and position of the bulging is indicative of the location of the extratracheal compressive mass. It must not be assumed that because the apparent bulging is from behind that it cannot be an aneurysm of the aortic arch. The compression may be applied in front or at the side, and, yet, because of the posterior deficiency of the tracheal cartilage, the endoscopic appearance may be that of compression from behind. Often lateral compressions may be misleading in the same way. The author has examined endoscopically quite a number of cases of aneurysm, and occasionally has been able to make a diagnosis; but as a rule, he does not regard either bronchoscopy or esophagoscopy, when negative, as reliable a means of diagnosis as the fluoroscope. He does not advocate endoscopy as a means of diagnosis of esophageal disease until after aneurysm has been excluded by the fluoroscope and the well known clinical methods. Kahler advises the relief of dyspnea in aneurysmal compression of the trachea or bronchi, by bronchoscopic dilatation. Von Eicken disagrees with this view, as does also Taunz. Mr. Waggette (Bib. 567) reports the observation of the wall of an aneurysm which had caused absorption of the tracheal rings.

Lues of the tracheo-bronchial tree. Considering the frequency of luetic lesions in the larynx their rarity in the lower air passages is remarkable. Possibly they are more frequent than supposed. The author has seen a few cases (Bib. 243), and other bronchoscopists (Von Eicken, Kahler) many more. The lesions may be gummatous, ulcerative, or inflammatory or may be compressive granular masses. Excision of the margin of ulcers or fungations for biopsy is advisable, and in any event the therapeutic test and the exclusion of tuberculosis will be required for confirmation. Hemoptysis in three cases previously diagnosticated as tuberculous was found by the author to come from a leutic lesion in the lower air passages.

Bronchoscopy in tuberculosis of the tracheo-bronchial tree. It is much to be regretted that tuberculosis has not received the amount of endoscopic study that the scientific value of the data thus obtainable would warrant. The author's own observations lead him to describe the following endoscopic picture below the larynx. The subglottic infiltrations from extensions of laryngeal disease, are usually of edematous appearance but are much more firm than in ordinary inflammatory edema. Ulcerations in this region are rare unless the direct extension of ulceration above the cord. The trachea is but seldom involved compared to the deeper structures, but we may have in the trachea, the pale swelling of the early stage of a perichondritis, the ulceration following the breaking down of such a chondritis and all the phenomena following the mixed infections. These same conditions may exist in the bronchi. In a number of instances the author has seen a cheesy deposit filling the entire lumen of the bronchus which was occluded by cheesy pus and debris of a peribronchial gland which had eroded through. The mucosa of tuberculosis, as a rule, is pale and the pallor is accentuated by the rather bluish streak of vessels where these are visible, as they sometimes are. Erosion from peri-bronchial or peri-tracheal lymph masses may be surrounded by granulation tissue of pale color or occasionally reddish and sometimes streaked with blood. A most common picture in tuberculosis is a broadening of the carina, which may be so marked as to obliterate the carina and to bulge inward, producing deformed lumina in both bronchi. Sometimes the lumina are crescentic, the concavity of the crescent being internal, that is, toward the median line. Absence of the normal, anterior and downward movement of the carina on deep inspiration is almost pathognomonic of a mass at the bifurcation, and such a mass is usually tuberculous, though it may be malignant, and, rarely, luetic. The author had thought that, considering the frequency of involvement of the upper lobe bronchus, pus should be found draining from this bronchus as a rather frequent occurrence; but he has rarely, in a case of tuberculosis, seen any secretion coming from the upper lobe bronchus. Possibly the explanation may be that drainage by cough and gravity had already removed secretion from the upper lobe, or it may be that further observation may prove this experience exceptional. The only lesion visible in a tuberculous case may be cicatrices from healed processes. The author has seen one case of adventitious *diverticulum in the left bronchus* immediately below the bifurcation. The mucosa seemed quite cicatricial and it seemed probable that there had been a suppurative process associated with glands in the mediastium at the bifurcation. There was no active tuberculous lesion at the time, but a radiograph by George W. Grier showed a mass of glands at the bifurcation and calcareous glands in other locations. Tuberculosis may almost entirely destroy the lungs of children without objective signs. In one such case seen with Dr. Baldwin the left bronchus was occluded with cheesy material and autopsy showed extensive tuberculosis of both lungs. Yet the patient, a fourteen-months-old infant with thymic tracheal compression had never been ill, nor had any rise of temperature ever been noted.

Hemoptysis. Endoscopy may afford the only means of locating and diagnosticating the source of hemoptysis. Manifestly endoscopy is not indicated in the hemorrhages of manifest, advanced pulmonary tuberculosis. But in the not inconsiderable number of cases in which persistent spitting of blood occurs in the absence of any objective signs of tuberculosis and there is serious doubt as to the source of hemorrhage, the doubt may be settled definitely by bronchoscopy. If the blood comes from the air passages, it will be noted that there is an interarytenoid blood stream brought by the cilia up along the posterior wall of trachea and out over the interarytenoid space, like the pouring of a narrow stream of water out of the pitcher mouth, giving a curiously appropriate justification for the naming of the arytenoid. This stream can be followed to its source with the bronchoscope. In a number of the author's cases (Bib. 243) the source of the blood has been a tuberculous lesion. In other cases malignancy has been found. Varix of the trachea was the source in one of Ephraim's cases. Aneurysm has been found endoscopically in a number of cases of hemoptysis. The author has found a luetic lesion in three such cases.

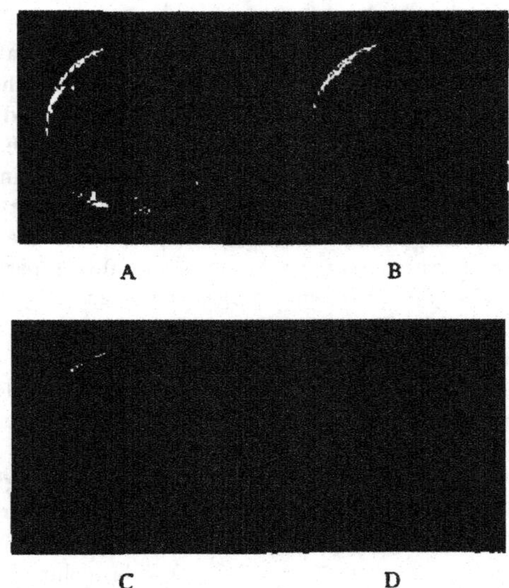

FIG. 409.—Endoscopic views of the bronchi in pneumothorax in a girl of nineteen years. A, left main bronchus. B, same just above the giving off of the upper lobe bronchus. C, inferior lobe (stem) bronchus. D, orifices of inferior lobe branch bronchi.

Pneumothorax. The author has had three opportunities of examining the bronchi in pneumothorax. The endoscopic images in one case are represented by the author's drawings reproduced in Fig. 409. The author can easily understand how such lumina might be produced with the exception of C (Fig. 409), which seems to him unexplainable, unless it was due to absence of cartilage at that point. In the second case a similar concentric diminution of lumen was noted in another location, namely the right inferior lobe bronchus. In the third case no such lumen could be found.

The mucosa in all was dark pink, but not cyanotic, in color. The rings did not show. The main bronchus was collapsed from a point a little below the bifurcation.

Angioneurotic edema. The author has not been so fortunate as to observe a case of angioneurotic edema in the trachea, but it has been seen endoscopically by Halstead and others. In Halstead's case the edema of the bronchial wall produced bronchial dyspnea in a girl of fifteen years. The endoscopic picture was a pale, evenly swollen mucosa producing stenosis.

CHAPTER XXX.

Diseases of the Esophagus.

Prior to the development of esophagoscopy, diseases of the esophagus could be studied only autoptically, little was known and local treatment was ineffective and very dangerous. It is no more justifiable to treat an esophagus, or to ignore esophageal symptoms, without an esophagoscopy, than it is to treat a patient with uterine symptoms without local examination. Until recently the esophagus was being treated like the uterus was in the author's student days, when the family physician regarded local uterine examination as a fussy pretension bordering on quackery.

The classification of esophageal diseases into stenotic and non-stenotic is purely arbitrary, since all diseases of the esophagus may develop stenosis, and stenotic diseases are usually not stenotic in their earlier stages. Paralysis, while not stenotic in the sense of a constriction, is clinically a stenosis because the patient cannot swallow even liquids. Nevertheless the terms "stenotic" and "non-stenotic" are convenient, and with the foregoing limitations on their meaning they will be herein used.

Diagnosis. The deductive methods of pre-esophagoscopic days, being inconclusive and more often wrong than right, are now entirely superseded. Diagnoses are now made esophagoscopically with all the certainty of direct inspection supplemented by biopsy when needed.

Radiography and fluoroscopy in diagnosis of esophageal diseases are of the utmost importance and the roentgenologist and the esophagoscopist are working together, each supplementing the other in many ways, as mentioned under the various diseases. Radiography and fluoroscopy during the swallowing of an emulsion of some substance opaque to the ray are of the utmos importance in the study of diseases of the esophagus and the esophagoscope in no way lessens the necessity of careful radiography and fluoroscopy which should be preliminaries to every esophagoscopy. They should go hand in hand.

Indications for esophagoscopy in disease. Any abnormal sensation, referable to the region or to the functions of the esophagus, noticed by the patient calls for immediate esophagoscopy. Only in this way can we hope to discover diverticula, esophagitis, lues, esophagismus, cardiospasm, superficial ulcer, and other curable lesions in time to cure. Any sensation such as "a lump rising in the throat," the so-called "globus hystericus," calls for esophagoscopy, for the reasons given under "Spasmodic Stenosis." In the absence of any symptoms whatever, it is advisable to make an exploratory esophagoscopy in cases of tracheal or high bronchial or peri-bronchial mediastinal disease for the possibilities of information as to periesophageal diseases. In the absence of any esophageal or tracheobronchial evidence of disease, esophagoscopy is indicated in any case of unexplained mediastinal radiographic shadow. The symptoms of esophageal disease are so often stomachal in character that any obscure stomach case requires esophagoscopy, and there is the added incentive that the left two-thirds of the stomach can be examined at the same time with the same instrument and with no more difficulty, in any case without esophageal stenosis. The pyloric third of the stomach can be examined in only a few cases. The most common form of confusion between gastric and esophageal diseases is for a patient to complain of vomiting when really he regurgitates. Esophageal spasm is often caused by organic or functional disease of the stomach. The gastroenterologist and the endoscopist are working together with mutual benefit.

Contraindications to esophagoscopy are in some instances dependent upon lack of skill on the part of the esophagoscopist. The trained and skillful may examine any case of general or local disease with relatively little risk, while in the hands of the rough, the careless or the untrained, the esophagoscope is a dangerous and frequently fatal instrument. The dangers are in inverse ratio to the skill, and are multiplied by the existence of wall-weakening esophageal disease. While the author would not hesitate to advise esophagoscopy in a patient with aneurysm or very hard arteries, or in one with extensive esophageal varicosities, advanced organic disease, or extensive acute necrotic or corrosive esophagitis, if there were very urgent necessity for it; yet, esophagoscopy can be indicated in such a case only by very urgent conditions, such as the lodgment of a foreign body. If there is anything to be gained by it, a careful esophagoscopy may be undertaken by the trained hand and eye which will stop the procedure when an abnormal tissue which must not be passed or even touched is encountered. In acute esophagitis from the swallowing of corrosives it is better to defer the esophagoscopy until sloughing has ceased and inflammatory infiltration has bulwarked the weak places. Either extreme of age is no contraindication to esophagoscopy. The author has esophagoscoped a number of new-born infants, consequently cannot agree with his distinguished colleague, Guisez, that "esophagoscopy is inapplicable at this age."

Water hunger is one of the most urgent contraindications to esophagoscopy. This condition, which makes the patient a very bad surgical subject, does not seem to be recognized by the profession.

Patients that have been able to get but little liquid down for a number of days, frequently come to the endoscopist and it is the author's custom always to have a surgeon in readiness on arrival of the patient to have a gastrostomy done immediately, should the patient prove to be in a serious state of water hunger. In the less severe cases water is introduced into the circulation by hypodermoclysis and enteroclysis simultaneously, and in the cases on which gastrostomy is done these measures are carried out while the operation is being done. There are few conditions other than spasmodic stenosis and foreign body occlusion that are so quickly relievable that gastrostomy will not be needed anyway, and it is better to do the gastrostomy first and make the diagnosis afterward. Some patients are so far gone when they arrive that they die in spite of prompt enteroclysis, hypodermoclysis and gastrostomy. It seems that when they get beyond a certain point they are hopeless. This point is reached in from three to six days, dependent upon the weather and upon whether the patient had or did not have an abundant supply of fluids prior to the complete occlusion. Of course the time in which death may occur from water starvation may be prolonged by rectal feeding.

Gastrostomy, as indicated above, should always be done in stenotic diseases of the esophagus before the patient begins to suffer for either food or water. Like tracheotomy it should be done early rather than late. If done early, gastrostomy is attended with a mortality of less than one per cent, and as a life saving measure, it is of the utmost importance. Gastrostomy is advisable in some instances, even when the patient can swallow liquids, for the purpose of putting the esophagus at rest. True, secretions will still drain down the esophagus but these do not stagnate and macerate like food, even liquid food, does.

Rectal feeding. The water from nutrient enemeta is absorbed rather readily and, if carefully watched and faithfully and persistently carried out in small continuous dosage, will supply the system with fluids and postpone, for a long time, death by water starvation; but for nutrient purposes rectal alimentation is dangerously inefficient.

Indirect examination of esophageal cases. The larynx and pharynx should be examined in all cases of suspected esophageal disease. Laryngeal disease involving the epiglottis, aryepiglottic folds, arytenoids or party-wall may be thus found to account for all the symptoms and may, in some cases, negative esophagoscopy. It is characteristic of any form of esophageal stenosis, if of a severe type, that both pyriform sinuses will be full of fluid in the erect posture of the patient. The cause of this is that the fluids which normally are continually flowing away through the esophagus, are unable to escape downward in stenotic cases, and thus the pyriform sinuses fill for want of normal drainage. This condition is known as the author's sign and is diagnostic of a high degree of esophageal stenosis. Levy has called the author's attention to an exception to the pathognomy of this sign in advanced cases of laryngeal tuberculosis in which the pain of swallowing is so great that swallowing is deferred as long as possible. Possibly also there is, in some such cases, an esophageal stenosis due to spasm of the cricopharyngeus, a reflex from the painful laryngeal lesion.

Technic of esophagoscopy for diseases. The introduction of the esophagoscope has been fully considered. The esophagoscope should in every case be passed by sight. Danger of perforation and of overriding the disease by mandrin introduction renders the introduction by sight the only method worthy of consideration. No anesthesia, general or local, is needed, as explained in Chapter IV, though local anesthesia of the laryngopharynx is unobjectionable in adults if desired. The position should, preferably, be recumbent as explained in Chapter VI. For the diagnosis and treatment of diseases of the upper end of the esophagus, the esophageal speculum, Fig. 21, is, in the author's experience, the most serviceable instrument. It can be used, if desired, in the recumbent or sitting position of the patient as described in Chapter X.

ANOMALIES OF THE ESOPHAGUS.

Congenital malformations of the esophagus may be divided into imperforation, stenosis, and esophago-tracheal fistula.

Imperforate esophagus. So far, the author has not had an opportunity of passing the esophagoscope on a case of imperforate esophagus, but he has passed the esophagoscope on quite a number of infants, the youngest being two days old. It was suspected in this latter case that an imperforate esophagus existed, but on esophagoscopy, the lumen of the esophagus was found perfectly normal all the way to the stomach. The disappearance, after the passing of the esophagoscope, of the difficulty in swallowing would seem to indicate spasmodic origin. When examined four months later by Dr. Manchester the child was still swallowing perfectly. In view of this case, and of many others on children from a few days to a few months of age, the author must disagree with Guisez in the statment that "esophagoscopy is inapplicable at this age." An esophagoscopy can be done in the new-born with perfect safety, provided a very small tube be used, and, provided, of course, it be with a proper degree of care. The most usual site of the occlusion is in the mediastinal esophagus, the upper esophageal segment ending in a blind pouch, usually more or less dilated. A fistula may exist between the lower segments of the anomalous esophagus, the upper segment being inperforate. (Guthrie and Edington, Bib. 135.)

Congenital esophagotracheal fistulae are the most frequent anomaly. They are due to embryonic developmental errors. So far, no cases of esophagoscopic examination of congenital tracheo-esophageal fistulae have been reported, but as the procedure is safe and simple, doubtless observations will be made. In the case of a nursling of six months of age which fell under the author's care, a tracheo-esophageal fistula, due to ulceration, would never have been suspected had not the parent suspected foreign body, which was found on radiographic examination and was removed by the author. There was no suspicion on the part of the parents, nor of the physicians who examined the patient prior to Dr. Sullivan, of any difficulty in swallowing. The parents were concerned solely with their observation that "the baby coughed until it vomited" and the child undoubtedly had a broncho-pneumonia. In a fistula in the new-born, there might be nothing to lead one to suspect difficulty in swallowing, and doubtless, cases of congenital fistula have been buried under an erroneous diagnosis. Some of the rare cases of tracheo-esophageal fistula without atresia probably live for some time, because some of the food escapes past the fistula into the stomach.

Congenital stricture of the esophagus may be more frequent than heretofore supposed. Cases are encountered by the esophagoscopist where the patient has had more or less difficulty in swallowing which is often described as "not swallowing as well as other people." Very often these cases have more or less frequent intervals of exacerbation of their symptoms when the swallowing difficulty becomes quite troublesome. On esophagoscopy, such cases show a moderate stenosis which does not seem to be cicatricial, and yet is, nevertheless, an organic stenosis not due to compression. There is a strong suspicion that such cases may be in some instances due to the swallowing of caustics in childhood, but in the absence of any such history, the parents being intelligent, it seems justifiable, to class them as congenital. A very interesting suggestion is made by A. Brown Kelly (Bib. 303); namely, that stenosis of the esophagus producing no symptoms until early adult life may nevertheless be congenital, since, as demonstrated by Maylard, congenital narrowing of the pylorus rarely manifests itself before early adult life. The suggestion of Brown-Kelly would explain those rare cases, of which every esophagoscopist of experience has seen a few in which there is an obvious stenosis of the esophagus, non-cicatricial and certainly non-spastic, first producing symptoms after adolescence. Further data are to be hoped for.

Webs in the upper third of the esophagus have been observed. The author has found that in any case where the presence of a web is suspected, the best method of determination is to put the esophagus on the stretch with a very large esophagoscope, or, preferably, with the esophageal speculum shown in Fig. 21. Retraction of the anterior wall of the esophagus will stretch the web quite thin, and it is very easy to pass an alligator forceps through the narrowing and then withdraw the forceps which are spread. This will dilate the constricted lumen due to the web, and if carefully done, the procedure is entirely harmless. It is wise to pass the speculum every alternate day until healing is complete. Smaller webs with larger esophageal lumen may be stretched by passing the esophageal speculum without the use of any other dilating instrument. Unlike cicatricial strictures, the web has very little tendency to vicious cicatrization and reproduction of the stenosis.

Treatment of esophageal anomalies. Unfortunately there is not often an opportunity for treatment. Gastrostomy is indicated in imperforate cases. Esophagoscopy has nothing remedial to offer except in cases of stricture and webs. Strictures can be dilated, but even more care should be exercised here than in cicatricial strictures. The few probably congenital cases the author has seen yielded more promptly than cicatricial stenoses of the same size of lumen and had less tendency to contract. In none of the cases was the full size of the esophageal lumen restored, but the patients remained free from dysphagia. Webs are very successfully dealt with as already mentioned.

Rupture and trauma of the esophagus may be spontaneous or may result from the trauma of an instrument or of a foreign body, or of both combined, as was frequently the case in the old days of blind attempts at pushing a foreign body downwards. MacReynolds reports a case of spontaneous rupture of the esophagus following extensive ulceration of the esophageal wall. The patient had been operated upon for an uncomplicated mastoiditis. The death, some days after operation, was found at post mortem to be due to profuse hemorrhage following rupture, which was in the lower third. No unusual strain had been put upon the esophagus and no solid food had been taken for a week. Rupture of the esophagus is usually attended with mediastinal emphysema, profound shock, a weak rapid pulse, restlessness, fever and rapid sinking. If the pleura has been torn, as is frequently the case, the symptoms and physical signs of pneumothorax are added. In such cases tapping of the pleural cavity will usually obtain a small amount of fluid with fecal odor. Lesser degrees of trauma not perforating all the layers of the esophageal wall, may show slight symptoms of esophagitis (q. v.). The early endoscopic appearances of esophageal trauma are those of a bleeding laceration of the mucosa. Later inflammatory and ulcerative appearances (q. v.) are manifest.

The treatment of trauma without perforation is the same as for acute esophagitis (q. v.). The traumatism due to the foreign body itself is almost invariably exceedingly slight and does not penetrate deeply and heals promptly. Blind methods of removal, however, are often attended with serious and fatal traumatism. The food in any case should be sterile liquids only, and all water should be sterilized and served sterilly. Rupture of the esophagus demands immediate gastrostomy (under local anesthesia) to nourish the patient, to supply him with fluid, and to put the esophagus at rest. If the pleura has been ruptured immediate thoracotomy, with insertion of a drain at the most favorable point of drainage, may save life, which without this procedure, is hopeless. Stimulation, hot-water bags, elevation of the foot of the bed, atropine and other shock combating methods are indicated. The patient's head should be low and the mouth turned toward the pillow to lessen the drainage of secretions into the esophagus.

INFLAMMATION AND ULCERATION OF THE ESOPHAGUS.

Acute esophagitis is usually of traumatic or cauterant origin. If severe or extensive, all the symptoms described under "Rupture of the Esophagus" may be present. The endoscopic appearances are unmistakable to anyone familiar with the appearance of mucosal inflammations. The pale, bluish pink color of the normal mucosa is replaced by a deep red velvety swollen appearance in which individual vessels are invisible. After exudation of serum into the tissues, the color may be paler and in some instances a typical edema may be seen. This may diminish the lumen temporarily. If the inflammation is due to corrosives, a grayish exudate may be visible early, sloughs later.

Ulceration of the esophagus. In the main, the observations of the author in his earlier volume (Bib. 269) have been fully borne out by further experience. While ulceration of the esophagus cannot be said to be a common disease, yet those who examine the esophagus constantly, meet with occasional cases. Superficial erosions are by no means uncommon, and the condition of inflammation, at times associated with erosion and even with ulceration, that accompanies the stagnation of food, is a very important part of the pathology of esophageal stricture. Under the head of spastic stenoses, the author has described the condition as constituting a "vicious circle" wherein spastic stenoses, whether due primarily to esophagitis or other local lesion or not, excite, or at least perpetuate an esophagitis, which, in turn, is a factor in the production of the spastic stenosis. The more constant the spastic condition, necessarily the greater the degree of esophagitis. The author has met with a number of cases of manifestly cicatricial stenosis, which, from the history, seem to have resulted from such a condition. There had been no history of swallowing any corrosives in childhood, and the esophageal trouble came on comparatively late in life so that any accidental cause for the production of a cicatricial stricture would necessarily have been remembered by the patient. One case of ulceration of the esophagus observed by the author deserves special mention:

A girl, aged two years, was brought to the author by Dr. L. C. Manchester for difficulty in swallowing which had come on during an attack of aphthous stomatitis. The child had been listless and had refused to eat. Temperature 102° F. (39° C). It had been thought that it refused to swallow simply because of the pain in the mouth, but after 24 hours without food or water, the child made strenuous efforts to swallow but the milk came back promptly. Upon examination with the child's esophageal speculum, Fig. 21, the cricopharyngeal constriction was seen to be the site of three small ulcerations. The 7 mm. esophagoscope was introduced below these ulcerations, and it was discovered that in the middle third of the esophagus there were two distinct ulcers and one elongated ulceration which had the appearance of two ulcers having coalesced. Just below this were two small vesicles, each surrounded by a red areola. A soft rubber tube was introduced and the child fed. It was given a few drops of an alum, sage and honey mixture, and in about ten days was entirely well of the lesions in the mouth and the swallowing was normal. A second esophagoscopy thirty days after the first, showed a normal esophagus.

Remarks. It was quite evident that the difficulty in swallowing was entirely spasmodic as no stenosis was found and the esophagoscope met with no obstruction in passing all the way to the stomach.

Ulceration may follow trauma of a foreign body, an instrument or a corrosion, and, of course, is part of nature's method of repair. Sloughs may be present, and exudates and exfoliation may modify the endoscopic picture.

Differential diagnosis of ulcer of the esophagus. To recognize the presence of an ulcer esophagoscopically is not difficult if it be not covered with macerated epithelial debris, bismuth, food or secretion, but to determine that it is a simple ulcer, requires the exclusion of lues, tuberculosis, epithelioma, endothelioma, sarcoma, and actinomycosis. Simple ulcer of the esophagus is usually associated with a stenosis, spastic or organic. In the absence of a stenosis, we are usually justified in excluding simple ulcer. This is not absolute (see case above cited), but it arouses a very strong suspicion that the ulcer is either malignant or luetic. The characteristics of the luetic ulcer are the highly inflammatory state of the surrounding mucosa, the thickened elevated edges usually free from granulation tissue, with a somewhat pasty center and not bleeding readily when sponged, though the surrounding mucosa gives one the impression of being intensely vascular. The tuberculous ulcer, if primary in the esophagus, is very superficial and seems to partake more of the character of an erosion than of ulceration. The mucosa is pale and gives one the impression of anemia. It is usually free from granulation tissue, but there may be small granular elevations at different points, usually rather scattered. There may be slight cicatrices. If, however, the tuberculosis is an extension by continuity from periesophageal tuberculous glands, and especially if there is a fistulous communication with a bronchus, we may have quite a cauliflower growth of granulations, though usually they are quite pale. In the cases in which a tuberculous process has invaded the esophagus from either a lung lesion, or a mediastinal adenopathy, there is usually such a manifest tuberculous syndrome that the diagnosis can be made therefrom. The tuberculin test, reverse tuberculin test, guinea pig injection with emulsion of tissue, with the histologic examination of tissue for the bacilli and for the morphology of tuberculosis—all these taken together are almost absolutely decisive; though the remote possibility of a mixed lesion of tuberculosis with lues or malignancy must be borne in mind. The ulcer of sarcoma does not differ materially from the ulcer of carcinoma. The carcinomatous ulcer is usually characterized by the very vascular bright red zone, raised edges, granulation tissue that bleeds freely on the slightest touch, and above all, it is almost invariably situated on an infiltrated base, which communicates a feeling of hardness to the pressure of sponges or of the esophagoscopic tube itself. Another characteristic sometimes seen in carcinoma is the pointed projections springing somewhat like granulation tissue from the ulcer or its neighborhood. A scar may be from the healing of an ulcer of simple or specific character, or, on the other hand, it may be a cancerous process developing on the site of a scar, so that the presence of scar tissue does not absolutely negative malignancy. As a rule, however, we do not see a scar in cases of cancer of the esophagus. In determining infiltration, we must be on our guard not to be misled by the sensation communicated in some cases by the ridge produced by the left bronchus where it crosses the esophagus. In some cases of esophageal disease with dilatation, especially if the stenosis is not far below the bronchus, the ridge protruded by the crossing of the bronchus is apt to be prominent and feels quite resistant to the pressure of the tube. In some instances it is possible to make an accurate diagnosis of a simple ulcer by exclusion through esophagoscopic appearances alone. Usually, however, the aid of the laboratory must be invoked, chiefly because lesions occur more or less mixed in character, owing to the fact that all ulcerations of the esophagus are associated with mixed infections. The resultant infective inflammations give a uniformity in character that interferes seriously with differentiation, because infective inflammation is apt to produce the same esophagoscopic appearance regardless of the lesion which caused the primary solution of continuity. The foregoing remarks apply only to the ulcerated lesions of the diseases mentioned. The differentiation of non-ulcerated lesions is elsewhere herein considered. In any case of ulceration of the esophagus unassociated with stasis, we are justified in pushing the therapeutic test with potassium iodide and mercurial inunctions. We are also justified in sponging the surface of the ulcer with a gauze sponge; but to obtain a specimen, it is seldom justifiable to scrape the ulcer, unless it is on a very much infiltrated base. If the edges are thin and flat, the taking of a specimen of tissue involves some risk. If, however, the ulceration has a thickened elevated edge, this edge may be nipped off with the tissue forceps, Fig. 35. The histologic examination of the tissue and a bacterial examination of the secretions wiped from the face of the ulcer, should give accurate information. If the laboratory report is uncertain, we are justified in repeating the removal of specimens of tissue and secretion a number of times. A positive Wassermann, or luetin, or a positive luetic history only makes the therapeutic test all the more strongly indicated. That the man has had lues does not necessarily mean that the ulcer in question is luetic, for a luetic man may have a malignant growth or be subject to tuberculosis; in fact it is a serious question whether or not lues predisposes to these conditions. Spirochetal findings in a specimen of tissue is decisive, but failure to find is diagnostically valueless.

Treatment of acute and subacute inflammation and ulceration of esophagus. As a rule, a simple ulcer, associated as it almost invariably is with more or less stenosis and stasis, usually yields to the local application of argyrol, with rest of the esophagus. The best way to obtain this rest is to do a gastrostomy for feeding so that nothing but secretions will go through the mouth. The teeth and mouth, of course, should be kept scrupulously clean. If the ulceration heals by these means alone, without any other treatment whatsoever, we may be justified in concluding that the ulceration was of simple character.

In all forms of esophagitis and in the ulcerations consequent upon traumatism, such as that of foreign bodies, the usefulness of bismuth subnitrate has been amply demonstrated by the author. It is given dry on the tongue and swallowed preferably without liquid in order better to adhere to ulcerated surfaces. That it does adhere, the author has noted in a number of cases in which the bismuth had been given therapeutically, and also in cases in which it had been used in order to obtain a ray picture in cases of esophageal stenosis. The combination with a little calomel given from time to time is excellent. Bismuth has quite a good deal of antiseptic action, but whether this be the explanation or not, empirically the author has had abundant evidence that this treatment for inflammation and ulceration of the esophagus is curative. Argyrol in 25 per cent solution locally applied esophagoscopically is also useful in cases of ulceration, and especially those attended with fungations. In three cases where external operations through the neck had involved the esophagus, dysphagia was found by the author to be due to an unhealed wound in the esophagus, and in all three cases, applications of argyrol resulted in healing.

Chronic esophagitis. The appearances of chronic esophagitis will be dealt with in connection with diffuse dilatation and spasmodic stenosis.

Treatment of chronic esophagitis. The best treatment for chronic esophagitis is the correction of stenoses, organic or spastic, which exist below, producing stasis of food. If the stenosis is not completely curable, local remedies are of great aid in limiting the degree of inflammation. Bismuth subnitrate is the best remedy. Calomel may be given also occasionally, both of these being given dry on the tongue. The best local endoscopic application is argyrol in 15 per cent solution.

COMPRESSION STENOSIS OF THE ESOPHAGUS.

Compression stenosis may be the result of any periesophageal disease or anomaly. The most frequent lesions are thyroid enlargement, cervical or thoracic, malignancy, aneurysm, auricular and aortic enlargement, or calcification, lymphatic infiltration, lordosis. Thoracic compressions are usually from mediastinal lesions, though the author saw one case of compression by a cancerous lung that had not yet involved the mediastinum. In another case a walled-off abscess of the upper lobe of the right lung and pleura caused the compression without mediastinal involvement. In two cases of the author compression of the esophagus was due to pressure of a hypertrophied heart. Bassler has reported a case due to hypertrophy of the auricle. Stenoses in the lower part of the thorax are very rarely compressive. The author has seen one such case associated with a pleural fistula which had been discharging for years subsequent to surgical evacuation of an empyema so that the exact nature of the compressive tissue could not be made out. Collier reports a case of compressive stenosis from cancer of the liver and Gottstein one from the pressure of a calcareous area in the pleura.

Differential diagnosis of compressive stenoses of the esophagus. The existence of a stenosis is often indicated by the author's sign of secretion-filled pyriform sinuses. Compression stenosis covered with normal mucosa, can be readily differentiated in most cases from disease of the wall of the esophagus; but the nature of the compressive lesion and its extent outward from the esophagus will usually require the aid of the roentgenologist or fluoroscopist. Compression stenosis is manifested usually by a slit-like crevice which occupies the place of the lumen and which does not open up readily before the advancing tube. The slit may be curved, and its long axis is almost always at right angles to the compressive mass if the esophageal wall be uninvolved. The normal radial creases separating the folds are diminished to two, one at each end of the crescentic slit-like lumen. The covering mucosa may be normal or show signs of chronic inflammation from stasis. If the esophageal wall is uninvolved the esophagus is movable laterally with the tube-mouth and the mucosa can be readily pushed up into folds.

Goitrous compression of the esophagus by a cervical goitre is readily confirmed by palpation of the neck, but with a substernal goitre verification is not so easy. Corroboration is to be had from radiography. The esophagus is not so often seriously compressed as is the trachea.

Aneurysmal compression of the esophagus. Theoretically, one might suppose that the endoscopic picture in an aneurysmal compression stenosis of the esophagus must be expansile. As a matter of fact, however, in all of the cases that the author has observed, the pulsation seems to be simply a transmitted pulsation of the aneurysmal sac acting simply as a tumor might in transmitting the pulsation from the aorta itself. The author has observed, in many instances, in abdominal esophagismus, a very much more marked pulsation with wider excursion in the absence of any lesion, which coincides with the observation of Boyce that cases of abdominal esophagismus are often associated with a very much enlarged aorta. As pointed out by Sargnon (Bib. 491) very slight degrees of aneurysm are extremely difficult to detect either by physical signs or by radiography and may even be overlooked at esophagoscopy unless the most extreme caution is taken. It would be easy to be misled into attempting blind bouginage and doubtless this does happen with those who are not familiar with the uses of the esophagoscope. In using the esophagoscope on such cases it is necessary, as Sargnon points out, not to go below any sort of compression or narrowing until aneurysm has been excluded by all available means including esophagoscopic study.

Aortic compression of the esophagus was alluded to above in writing of aneurysm. In one of the author's cases a compression stenosis was noted at the level of the arch of the aorta. Radiography revealed such a dense irregular shadow of the aortic wall as to render justifiable the opinion that the aortic wall was to a greater or less extent calcified.

The patient was a man 66 years of age. An examination of the literature revealed a number of cases, a most notable one by Anthony Bassler. A number of observers have confirmed observations of Kovacs and Stoerk in regard to the kinking of the esophagus by enlargement of the left auricle. The author has since observed in two cases very marked compressions and deviations from this cause. In both cases there had been no symptoms referable to the esophagus but a large mass of meat had lodged and was removed esophagoscopically.

Carcinomatous and sarcomatous compressions of the esophagus are characterized by their hardness when palpated by the tube mouth or probe.

Adenopathic compression of the esophagus. Minor compressions are often noted, and the diagnostic and prognostic value of the esophagoscopically demonstrable lymph nodes at the sides of the esophagus has been noted in connection with cancer of the larynx. A high degree of stenosis may be due to a large mass of infiltrated glands in the mediastinum especially below the crossing of the left bronchus. Usually tracheal, bifurcational or bronchial stenosis may be found in the same case. In any compressive stenosis of the mediastinal esophagus in an adult, not clearly malignant nor tuberculous, it is wise to give potassium iodid and mercury, which must be pushed to a full therapeutic test without stopping at the first sign of iodism. If this be done, an occasional cure will result, of which the author has seen a number of instances. Lordosis is a not infrequent cause of compression stenosis of the cervical esophagus. The prominence of the posterior wall and the bony hardness render identification easy. It is doubtful if scoliosis produces any compression or deviation of the esophagus. No such cases have been recorded, to the writer's knowledge. The investigations of Hacker and Kollicker render the occurrence doubtful.

The frequency with which posticus laryngeal paralysis is associated with compressive esophageal stenosis should be borne in mind.

Treatment of compressive stenosis of the esophagus. Curative treatment is necessarily concerned with cure of the compressive lesion and hence is not within the province of endoscopy. Unless the diagnosis of the nature of the compressive lesion is certain it is well to give potassium iodid and mercury, as an occasional cure of a gummatous or adenopathic luetic lesion in a supposedly malignant or other case will occur. Palliative treatment by esophageal intubation (q. v.) is indicated in all conditions except aneurysm. This is quite feasible and satisfactory in many cases in which the ordinary stomach tube cannot be passed. Gastrostomy should be done early when necessary.

DIFFUSE DILATATION OF THE ESOPHAGUS.

This is practically always stagnation ectasia. The adherents of the atonic theory of diffuse dilatation are now few and there is little evidence, clinical, anatomical, or physiological, to support their view. In the author's experience, dilatation of the esophagus has been invariably associated with either organic or spasmodic stricture, existing either at the time of the observation or at some time prior thereto. In four cases of dilatation discovered by the author during gastroscopy in patients without esophageal symptoms, there was a history indicating clearly a spasmodic stenosis earlier in life. The action of the stricture in causing diffuse dilatations, whether the stricture be spasmodic or organic, is probably largely due to deglutitory pressure of accumulated food. Though gravitation does not much aid normal deglutition, it probably aids in increasing a suprastenotic dilatation. It is not at all necessary that the food should remain a long time in the esophagus. The esophagus seems to be constituted on the basis of immediately emptying itself of whatever may enter it from either above or below. In other words, it is intolerant of the presence of anything except its own normal secretions and these must be in very small amounts and continually draining away. Stagnation even of secretions will produce not only dilatation, but esophagitis. If a stricture is not very small and yet is sufficient to hold back for a time what has been swallowed, the esophagus acts as a reservoir of a large funnel with a very small opening. When food is swallowed, the esophagus fills and the contents trickle slowly through the opening. This distension is sufficient to result in permanent dilatation, and strange to say, such dilatation always remains once it has been established (Jesse Mayer, Bib. 399), even though the stenosis which caused it has entirely disappeared. It seems likely that the gases due to fermentation of the stagnant food may increase the dilatative pressure beyond what would result from mere gravity, because we practically never see in cases of organic stenosis the enormous degrees of dilatation seen in spastic stenoses. Theoretically it would seem that there existed in cases of hiatal and abdominal esophagismus a spasm also of the cricopharyngeus and associated circular esophageal fibres, preventing ready escape of the gases upward. As a matter of fact many of the patients observe a distress partially relieved at intervals by the escape of gas. That the relief is not complete is probably due to the irritation from food and gases still remaining in the dilated esophagus. A very large dilatation of the thoracic esophagus indicates a spastic stenosis. Cicatricial stenoses do not result in such large dilatations, possibly because of leakage shortening the duration of stasis. Malignant stenoses do not exist long enough to cause very large dilatations, though small ones are common and their size is an index of the duration of the growth; though the possibility of malignancy developing in a spastic case must be remembered.

Treatment of diffuse dilatation of the esophagus. The treatment of diffuse dilatations that produce symptoms consists in dilating the hiatal and abdominal esophagus, even in cases where spasm cannot be demonstrated. This dilatation will relieve the patient of the symptoms and of the stagnation of food, though the increased size of the esophagus after dilatation will never disappear. Treatment is, therefore, the same as if hiatal or abdominal esophagismus could be demonstrated. If chronic esophagitis is present, as it usually is, the administration of bismuth subnitrate with calomel occasionally, and possibly, in some cases, the local esophagoscopic application of argyrol solution, [illegible] per cent, are indicated.

CHAPTER XXXI.

Diseases of the Esophagus. -Continued.

SPASMODIC STENOSIS OF THE ESOPHAGUS.

The author's early urging of endoscopists to make a thorough study of spasm has borne abundant fruit. Esophageal spasm in the early days of endoscopy was considered one of the rarest conditions, while to-day it assumes etiologically and pathologically, first place in importance. The factor of spasm enters into nearly every condition of the esophagus with which the endoscopist has to deal, even in foreign body cases where a foreign body of very small size may excite sufficient spasm entirely to occlude the esophagus, so that even liquids cannot be swallowed. In speaking thus of the importance of spasm and its frequency, the author does not allude to what the beginner in esophagoscopy is likely to encounter. Nearly every beginner thinks in every case in which he has difficulty in introducing the esophagoscope past the cricoid, that the patient has a spasmodic stenosis. It is not until introduction has become easy that the endoscopist is able to determine whether true spasm exists or not, at the upper end of the esophagus. Of course, there is always more or less of spasm of the cricopharyngeus in every case, unless the patient be very profoundly anesthetized; but this does not constitute true pathologic esophageal spasm. Esophageal spasm might be classified into spasms of the upper end and those of the lower end, for it is very rarely that spasm exists in the middle third. The objection, however, to this is that we cannot always dissociate high and low spasms, because they may coexist or may alternate in the same case. A disease of the lower third may cause spasm of the upper end of the esophagus and vice versa. For this reason also, the symptoms and the sensations of the patient are not to be relied upon. The patient may complain of inability to even start food down, when upon esophagoscopy, we find that the lesion is located at the cardia, in which case if we were to rely upon symptoms, we would expect the food to be swallowed and then regurgitated after a longer or shorter time. It is no wonder, then, that little progress was made in the study of the diseases of the esophagus prior to recent general use of the esophagoscope. Without underestimating the very valuable results to be had from radiography, it must be said that only by esophagoscopy can the exact nature of lesions be determined without grave risk of error, as elsewhere mentioned. On the other hand radiography and fluoroscopy render such excellent service that they are indispensable. Consequently the esophagoscopist and the roentgenologist both must labor to obtain the best results for the patient. The best illustration of this is the fact that while the esophagoscope can give all the certainty of actually seeing the spasmodic closure and above all it alone can inform us of the mucosal lesions; yet it cannot, as can fluoroscopy and radiography, inform us of the physiologic functional pathology during the act of deglutition.

Etiology of spasm of the esophagus. It is easy to understand why the esophagus should be especially prone to spasmodic disease. Its entire functional activity is dependent upon reflex action. Each part of the gullet, as the bolus of food reaches and dilates it, is stimulated to contract, thus a peristaltic wave moves with the bolus of food as it is swallowed, and while it is undoubted that the pneumogastric nerves are concerned in the swallowing act, yet it is nevertheless true that the action is excited reflexly, because only the very start of the swallowing motion is voluntary. Once the start is made by the constrictors, the balance of the movement is a reflex peristalsis. Swallowing is impossible if both vagi are cut. The latter experiment would contraindicate the possibility of paralysis or paresis being in some instances the cause of what is known as "cardiospasm," especially as the division of these nerves causes contraction of the esophagus in the neighborhood of the cardiac orifice, as though there were inhibitory fibers supplied only to the region of the cardia. The author, however, esophagoscopically has demonstrated very clearly, by the watching of a few cases where "cardiospasm," so called, has been seen early but for various reasons has remained untreated, that in time dilatation has gradually followed. The etiology of the condition has thus been well established as a dilatation due to pressure above the spasmodic contraction and not to a primary atony of the esophageal wall.

Granting then that spasmodic stenosis is usually a reflex, it becomes interesting to study the sources of the reflex. Hurried gulping of food may cause spasm and thus start what the author has called a "vicious circle" as will be hereafter explained. In the author's experience spasm of the esophagus results in some instances from lesions that themselves produce no sensation. Thus, superficial erosions may excite such severe spasms that nothing can be swallowed and yet the patient have no sensation except on attempting to swallow, and even then the only sensation is one of obstruction not of pain. This is probably to be explained by the fact that the esophageal pain sense is less efficient than the esophageal tactile sense. For, as the author has demonstrated, the esophagus is quite insensitive below the cricoid level. Anyone can demonstrate this insensitiveness by swallowing coffee uncomfortably hot. No sensation is produced after the hypopharynx is passed until the stomach is reached and in the stomach the sensation is so slight as sometimes not to be noticed at all. Clinically, we know that esophageal spasm may be secondary to local diseases of the esophagus, or to disease remote from the gullet. Thus we have esophageal spasm as a result of liver disease, probably superinduced in some instances by engorgement of the veins at the cardiac end of the esophagus. In certain cases, there are undoubtedly lesions of the mucosa in the esophagus and also in the stomach, which could easily excite spasms, and it is equally certain that stagnation due to the spasm and consequent fermentation of food, detention of secretions and maceration could very easily excite or perpetuate the lesions. Thus we have a "vicious circle" in hiatal and abdominal esophagismus. Disease of the stomach may cause severe cases of spasmodic stenosis of the esophagus. The author has seen many cases in which cancer not itself occluding the cardia has produced a hiatal esophagismus that had nearly starved the patient. In other cases observed by the author, gastric ulcer has produced the same condition. Bassler, by post-mortem examination in cases of abdominal esophagismus, has demonstrated the presence of visceral disease above and below the diaphragm.

Spasms of the cricopharyngeus and the adjacent circular fibers of the esophagus are in many instances secondary to chronic gastric disease. They are also associated with rapid gulping of large boluses of food. The latter may be a factor in producing the chronic gastric disorder; but it would seem that it may also be independently causative. The presence of spasm in cases of organic stricture has been seen by all endoscopists, though spasmodic stenosis is rarely seen in a much infiltrated area. A case of spasmodic stenosis from aphthous ulceration was referred to under "Ulceration of the esophagus."

A perpetuating cause in established cases is undoubtedly the "nerve cell habit," and in many cases the presence of an underlying basic neurotic factor is undoubted. In one instance, a patient who was quite hysterical would get an attack of abdominal esophagismus whenever anything did not please her. For instance, she took the notion that the endoscopic divulsions that we were applying to the abdominal esophagus were doing her so much good that they ought to be done every week instead of every two weeks. Regularly the day before the one week was up, her abdominal esophagus would shut up and the dilatation above it would fill. By this it is not meant that she had voluntary control of it, but that the emotions sought their outlet through habitual nerve channels, producing a recurrence of the abdominal esophagismus, which she had had since childhood. This "nerve cell habit" is one of the most frequent causes of recurrences. In the author's opinion the so-called "cardio-spasm" is a pathological prolongation of the physiologic hiatal hesitation in normal deglutition. Esophageal spasmodic stenosis may occur at any age but, in the author's experience, it is rare after middle life, when muscular activity is on the decline. Spasm of the esophagus in the new-born has been observed once by the author. The case was as follows:

Infant M., aged two days, was brought to the author by Dr. L. C. Manchester for inability to swallow. When it would attempt to nurse the lip and mouth motion were correct and the mouth would fill with milk and then the child would choke, cough and strangle and the milk would all run out of the mouth.

These symptoms justified a suspicion of congenital absence of more or less of the esophagus. The endoscope was gently passed. It met with moderate resistance at the cricopharyngeus and again at the diaphragm but the lumen of the esophagus at these points was perfectly normal and the spasmodic constriction gradually yielded to the gentle insinuation of the esophagoscope. Of course the esophagoscopy was done without anesthesia. There was no sign of the slightest trace of blood on the instrument on withdrawal, and best of all, the child immediately took the breast and swallowed perfectly. Four months later when examined by Dr. Manchester it was still swallowing perfectly.

Remarks. This case seems to have been a spasmodic stenosis of the fundiform fibers of the inferior constrictor, and of the diaphragm at the hiatus esophageus. The author has been unable to find any similar case in literature, and feels justified in regarding it as a case of ***esophagismus in the new-born.*** The prompt cure by esophagoscopy we see at times in older patients, so that it is not at all astonishing that the passage of the esophagoscope should cure the spasm in the new-born infant where there has been no time for nerve cell habit to become fixed. Another interesting feature of this case is the demonstration of the harmlessness of careful esophagoscopy with a small tube (5 mm.) in a new-born infant. Guisez and others have stated that esophagoscopy cannot be done in the new-born. While the author has always doubted the correctness of that statement, no opportunity of controverting it by actual experience arose until this case, though esophagoscopy in a number of infants from two to twelve months of age had led me to believe that the procedure could be done without anesthesia, and without harm. A number of esophagoscopies in the new-born have since proven equally harmless.

In addition to the above-considered secondary manifestations of spasm dependent upon demonstrable lesions near or remote, there is a small number of cases in which there is a spasmodic condition which we must consider primary, and which, for want of a better term, must be called idiopathic, objectionable as that term is, until a definite etiologic basis has been discovered. Doubtless at some not very distant day, this class of cases will be eliminated by the results of the present wide-spread interest in esophageal disease. These cases are doubtless in most instances, functional neuroses of such intricate pathology as to be understood only by the trained neurologist.

Globus hystericus is the name given to the sensation described by patients as a "rising of a lump in the throat," or some such expression. In the cases with this sensation esophagoscoped by the author, there was a contraction of the cricopharyngeus muscle. The reflex impulse may be a neurosis of similar etiology to other hysteric phenomena; but quite often it is excited reflexly by local disease in some part of the esophagus, and consequently calls for esophagoscopy in most instances. It seems probable that the choking sensations of grief, and after weeping, and in other emotional phenomena, are due to the same spasmodic condition but, of course, being purely physiological, they do not call for esophagoscopy. The following case illustrates the identity of "globus hystericus" and cricopharyngeal spasm:

A man of 21 years complained that for years he had had a sensation as of a lump rising in his throat at various times, irrespective of attempts to swallow. Within a year he had been unable to swallow anything after twelve o'clock, noon, except on a very few days. In the forenoon swallowing was rarely interfered with. The author observed on one occasion the patient's attempt at swallowing. The water was promptly rejected, coming forcibly out of the mouth and nose, accompanied by cough which persisted for a few minutes. A sensation of a lump rising in the throat was complained of for over an hour. A relative stated that the patient ate ravenously in the early morning and at about eleven o'clock. The patient was well nourished, of rather stupid expression, suggestive of the atypical child. The patient mentioned having been examined a number of years before by Dr. Theodore Diller, the neurologist. The author obtained from Dr. Diller the record of a diagnosis of hysteria though at the time of the latter's examination there was no complaint of a lump in the throat nor of any swallowing symptom.

Examination by the author revealed a typical cricopharyngeal spasmodic stenosis. Swallowing was perfect for a few weeks but the diurnal spasmodic stenosis recurred, and with it came the sensation of a "lump in the throat."

The author has seen a few cases somewhat similar to the foregoing but none of them has been quite so complete.

That the early manifestations of numerous forms of organic esophageal disease have been ignored under the label "globus hystericus" is now unquestionable. These cases may or may not be associated with dysphagia.

Cricopharyngeal spasmodic stenosis. Most cases of cricopharyngeal spasmodic stenosis are unassociated with the sensation of "a lump rising in the throat," known as "globus hystericus," and have no association with hysteria, though they are often erroneously thus diagnosticated. The disease is essentially a spasm of the circular fibers of the inferior pharyngeal constrictor known as the cricopharyngeus muscle. The symptomatic characteristic of this affection is difficulty in swallowing, which consists in a difficulty in *starting* the food downward. Once the food is started it goes downward unimpeded into the stomach. There is no regurgitation of food sometime after swallowing, unless there co-exists in the same case a hiatal esophagismus. These symptoms, however, denote only a high esophageal stenosis. As to whether it is a spasmodic or an organic stenosis, there is only one way to determine, and that is by esophagoscopy It may even be both organic and spasmodic, the latter secondary to the former. Local malignant disease and foreign bodies may also give rise to spasmodic stenosis.

Esophagoscopic appearances of spasmodic stenosis at the cricopharyngeus. High spasm of the esophagus unassociated with diverticulum, may not show a typical form as distinguished from the spasm that always occurs on the introduction of an esophagoscope. In other instances, there will be a slight clamping at the cricopharyngeal level, the pictures then being of a small point of lumen from which radiate slight creases or folds. In other instances, the folds are not so apparent, but the point is in the center of an almost mammilliform projection. In other instances the opening in the projection will be slit-like in form with the anterior and posterior lips meeting in the center line, the slit being more or less transverse. In some instances there is a curved slit, or the lips may bulge upward toward the observer. All of these pictures are occasionally seen in the normal esophagus, during examination without anesthesia. Nevertheless they are spasm pictures, and when they occur in the normal esophagus, they indicate simply the spasm that occurs reflexly from the presence of the tube. When we encounter a patient who says that suddenly while eating he will choke up and food will not go down, and upon esophagoscopy we find any of the above pictures, and especially if the spasmodic picture is shown in connection with a more than usually unyielding closure, and when, furthermore, the spasm gradually yields and the esophagoscope of full size goes through readily without further resistance, indicating a normal-sized esophagus—under such circumstances we are justified in making a diagnosis of spasm of the upper end of the esophagus. It is only the esophagoscopist of large experience who can distinguish between a normal degree of spasm excited by the tube in a normal case, when the tube is passed without an anesthetic, and the case in which there is a pathologic degree of spasm. Furthermore, it is absolutely necessary to be certain that the esophagoscope is properly pointed, that is, that its axis corresponds precisely with the axis of the lumen of the esophagus, and that it is not impinging more upon one wall than upon the other. The closed lumen may open up momentarily when the patient gags or attempts to vomit, or, more likely, when the patient takes a deep breath after a continuous strain of vomiturition. Since there is always more or less spasmodic obstruction to the introduction of the tube at the upper end of the esophagus, the beginner will find great difficulty in distinguishing the difference between a normal and pathologic spasm, and even the most experienced will, in a few cases, be in doubt.

Treatment of spasmodic stenosis of the esophagus at the cricopharyngeal level. All cases associated with a morbid source of reflexes, near or remote, should be cured of the basic lesion. A few of such cases and all of the purely functional cases can be cured by the passage of a large esophagoscope. Recurrences may require similar treatment at intervals for a year or two, but many cases are cured by a single treatment.

Hiatal esophagismus (so-called "*cardiospasm*").* Undoubtedly the old word "cardiospasm," like many of the old words of medicine, covered a number of different conditions of independent etiology and pathology. The word cardia is properly used as the name of the esophageal orifice of the stomach. Spasm limited solely to this orifice, is certainly exceedingly rare, while spasm of the abdominal esophagus and of the esophagus at the hiatus, either separately or together, are relatively common, and should be called by their proper names. The word "cardiospasm" should either be dropped as a misnomer or limited to those rare cases of true cardial esophagismus. Brown Kelley has demonstrated the

*Liberal quotations are made in the following pages from the author's "Rapport" to the International Medical Congress, Section XV, London, 1913.

experimental fact that section of both vagi, without stimulation, is followed by dilatation of the lower part of the esophagus and contraction of the cardia, which he rightly says corresponds to the supposed condition in cardiospasm. But as a clinical morbid entity, such a condition is rarely, if ever, found in the disease commonly known as cardiospasm.

The author's contention in his earlier book (Bib. 269, p. 271) that the so-called "cardiospasm" was in reality, in almost all instances, more properly a hiatal esophagismus or phrenospasm, was based purely upon endoscopic clinical observation. Recently, however, in a very interesting monograph, Liebault (Bib. 329) has furnished the anatomical basis for the observation. From careful dissection he has found the muscular fibers which are so active in a sphincteric action of the esophagus at the hiatal level, as shown in the drawing Fig. 410. On investigation, he found that Rouget had described the local anatomy in essentially the same way. He quotes Rouget's description as follows:

"The muscular fibers of the sphincter, slightly paler than the rest of the muscle, slender and not numerous, leave each crus at the level of the hiatus and pass to the esophagus, with whose fibers they are interlaced terminating by the formation, on the anterior aspect, of loops interlacing with those of the opposite side. The small muscular bundles, more or less developed but constant, ordinarily exist only on the sub-diaphragmatic portion of the esophagus. In one instance, I found a thin muscular lamina 1 cm. in size which extended from the left crus to the cardia, ending by spreading its fibers over the anterior wall of the stomach. I have almost always found the esophagus and cardia united at the external border of the left crus by a lamina of fibrillar appearance but endowed with special elasticity such as characterizes the dartos, and which is found also at the level of the terminal loops of the cremaster in the adult." Liebault adds, "Classically, the hiatus is described as of elliptic form and such, indeed, it appears to be on inspection from above, but on examination of its abdominal aspect it appears rather that the esophagus has insinuated itself between the diaphragmatic fibers, which it has spread apart in order that it may enter the abdominal cavity. It is not an elliptic orifice, but rather a cleft through which the esophagus passes. Liebault agrees with others who have been unable to demonstrate any increase in the circular fibers at the true cardia as compared with the circular fibers of other portions of the esophagus.

In further confirmation of the author's contention (Bib. 269) against the misleading word "cardiospasm," anatomic study, in addition to the demonstration by Liebault above quoted, has also demonstrated the absence of anything that could be called a sphincter at the cardia, and the narrowing at this point that has been shown in so many text books on anatomy is a misfortune. Hill quotes McAllister to the effect that there is no histologically demonstrable sphincter and he states that the circular musculature at this point is weak. Brown Kelly and Williamina Able,

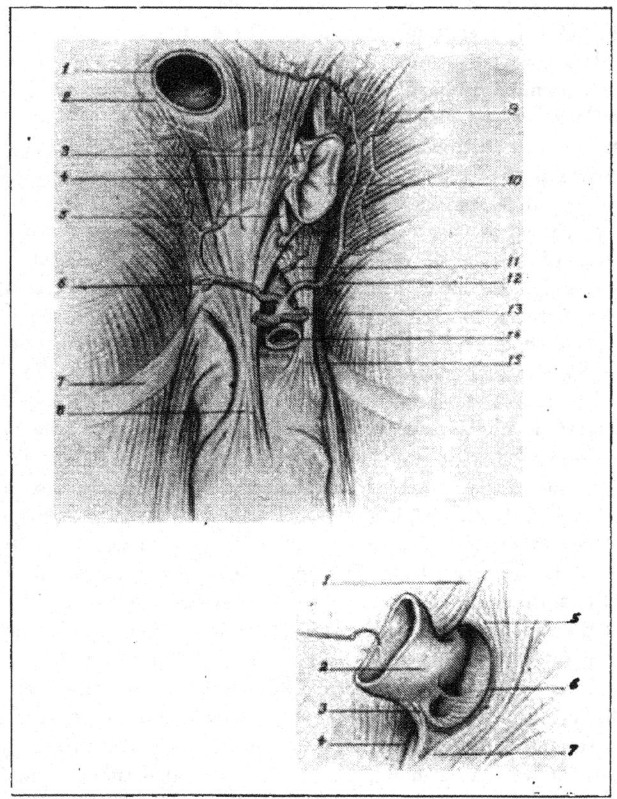

FIG. 410.—Drawing of the under surface of the diaphragm showing the constricting musculature at the hiatus. (After Liebault).

by careful special dissections, have demonstrated that "it is quite apparent to the naked eye that both muscular coats are of uniform thickness, and that no special aggregation of fibers exists at or near the cardia," and that "nothing was found in any of the dissections or in the anatomical works consulted to justify Dr. Hill's statement that the circular fiber musculature was specially weak in this region."

Personally, the author believes that it is only very rarely, if ever, that any spasm exists below the hiatal level, but in order to place the study on a systematic basis, he believes that, as endoscopists, it would be better for us to abandon the word "cardiospasm" and to substitute for it the three clinical types, that may possibly be made out: namely,

1. Hiatal esophagismus.
2. Abdominal esophagismus.
3. Cardial esophagismus.

That the constriction in so-called "cardiospasm" is first encountered at the hiatus no one who knows the hiatal esophagus when he sees it can deny. And no experienced observer can deny that after the tube-mouth has passed the hiatal constriction it goes through the two to four centimeters of abdominal esophagus into the stomach with but little resistance, which lessens as the stomach is approached. The degree of the resistance of this abdominal esophagus varies. In most cases the author has felt inclined to regard it as so slight that he would dismiss it as a factor in spasmodic stenosis if it were not for two things: 1. The possibility of its relaxation simultaneously with the hiatal yielding; and, (2) the radiographic studies. With the question in mind he has watched the yielding of the abdominal esophagus as the hiatus is passed and he feels inclined to say that abdominal esophagismus does not exist except in conjunction with hiatal esophagismus. Further, if cardial esophagismus exists, (the author has observed only three cases which he would feel justified in classing as such) it does not exist except in conjunction with hiatal esophagismus, or as the author first called it, phrenospasm. A study of the radiographs such as Figs. 411 and 412, reveals the possibility of two interpretations. The narrow streak of bismuth shadow below the very evident hiatal constriction might indicate either a spasmodically contracted lumen of the whole abdominal esophagus, or a trickling stream of leakage that was escaping through the almost tightly shut hiatus above. As a matter of fact we know that the food in these cases of spasmodic stenosis does leak through gradually, rarely, if ever, suddenly. Further investigation of this point is needed. From esophagoscopic observations, the author knows that the hiatal esophagus is tightly contracted in the disease known as "cardiospasm."

Hiatal esophagismus, even more than diverticulum, reminds one of the ingluvies of birds, inasmuch as the dilated esophagus fills quickly, and yet there is a constant leakage, which allows a certain proportion of the food to pass on through at a relatively slow rate. In one of the author's patients, the cure of the abdominal esophagismus by divulsion, resulted in food going through so promptly into the stomach, that taking food excited nausea for quite a long time until the stomach became ac-

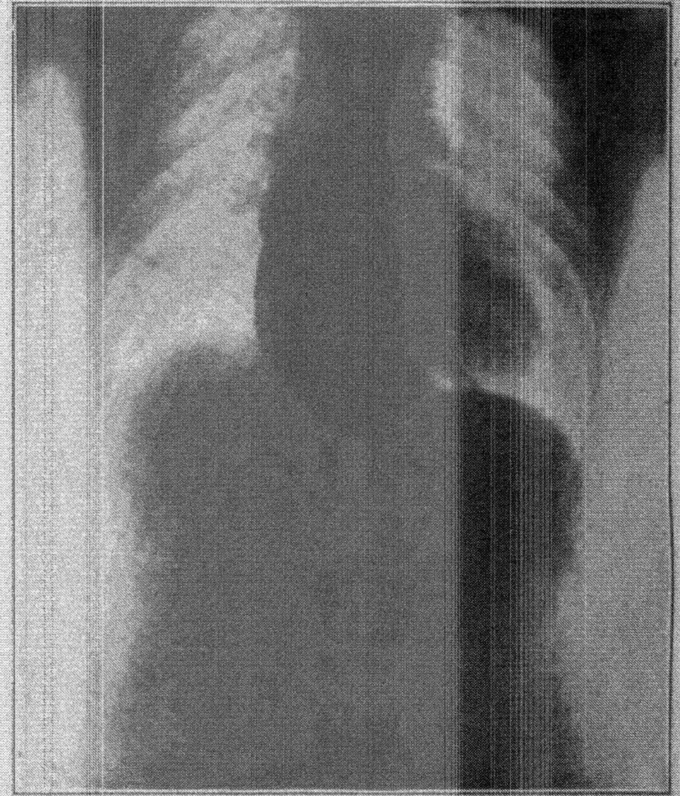

Fig. 411.—Radiograph of a woman of 45, showing an abdominal esophagismus which was afterward cured by endoscopic mechanical divulsion. The "flat floor" of the dilatation shows why previously used blind methods had failed to introduce any instrument through the hiatus.

customed to the unusual sensation of having food go through directly when swallowed. Patients afflicted with spasm of the abdominal esophagus usually complain of distress after eating and regurgitation of food within a period of from a quarter of an hour to several hours after eating. At times, especially if the sac be large, there will be no regurgitation for a number of days, when a large quantity of stale food may come up. In many instances, however, but a very small quantity of food is regurgitated, though the accumulation be large. It will pass gradually, a

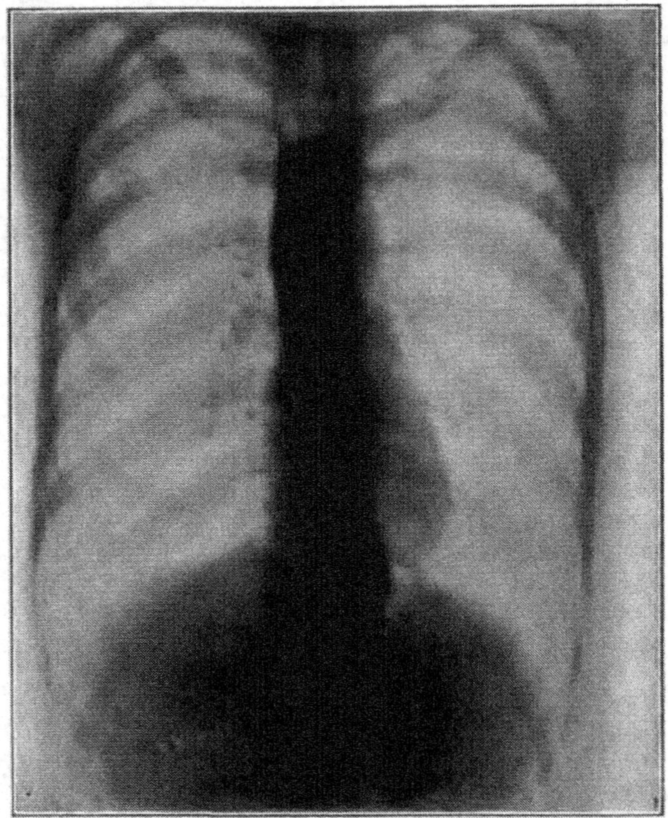

FIG. 412.—Radiograph of a woman of 28, showing an abdominal esophagismus with only very slight dilatation above it. The deviation of the esophagus by the aorta was verified esophagoscopically (Author's case. Radiograph made by Dr. J. C. Bowen).

little at a time, as the spasm relaxes, into the stomach and usually (though not always) before a serious state of inanition supervenes. The symptoms are not meant as in any way diagnostic. There are no absolutely diagnostic signs of esophageal disease, and the author in the present work has referred but little to them. The fact of the matter is that any patient coming in with any symptoms whatever that could be possibly referable to the esophagus, requires an esophagoscopy. Any sort of diagnosis based upon signs and symptoms is so apt to be erroneous, that it is not worth while to more than make a decision that the symptoms justify

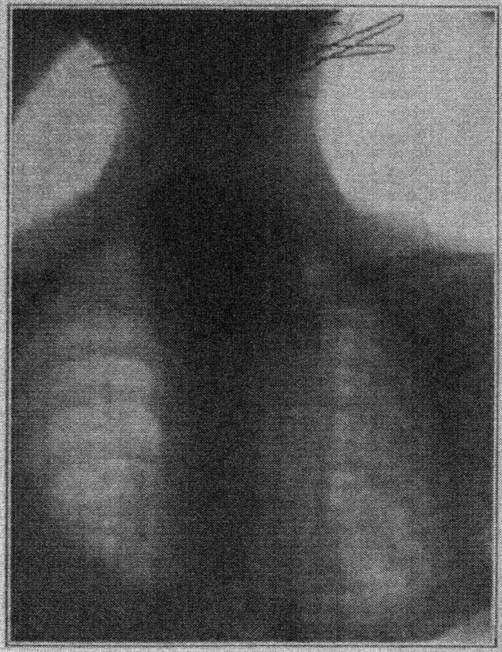

FIG. 413.—Radiograph of a woman twenty-two years of age, affected with hiatal esophagismus simulating diverticulum. The shadow of the bismuth porridge rests upon about 1½ liters of stale food in an enormous dilatation as demonstrated esophagoscopically after emptying. (Author's case).

esophagoscopy. For instance, all the signs of cancer of the esophagus may be present and yet the esophagoscope will show nothing more than spasm of the hiatal esophagus. The exact reverse may be true and the patient may have all the symptoms of abdominal esophagismus for many, many years, and yet esophagoscopy may show an incipient or even well-developed cancer which has arisen upon the site of some inflammatory area within the esophagus.

The diagnosis of hiatal esophagismus is easy in the typical case with an enormous dilatation, a white, pasty, macerated mucosa, and a contracted esophagus which, however, permits a large esophagoscope to pass into the stomach after a delay at the hiatus; but in the early, or in the less typical cases, without dilatation it is often exceedingly difficult to distinguish between purely spasmodic conditions and those of local lesions in the neighborhood of the esophagus but not themselves showing in compressions or very marked deviations of the abdominal esophagus. In such cases, while many esophagoscopists feel sure of their diagnosis, many

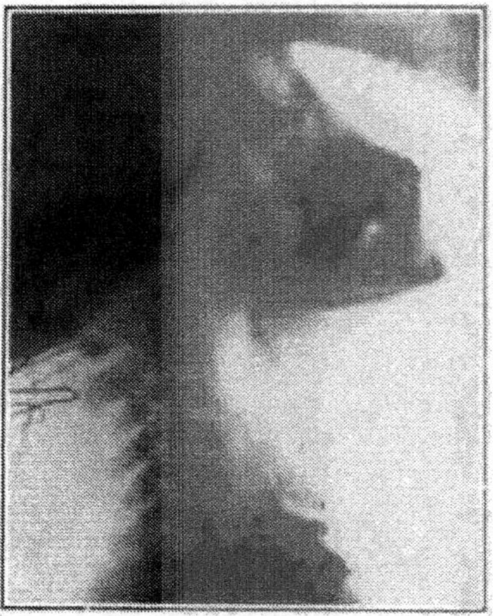

FIG. 414.—Lateral radiograph of same patient as in Fig. 413, the shadow of the bismuth mixture simulating diverticulum. The mass of food after eating protruded in the neck and could be evacuated by external pressure with the patient's hand.

do not agree as to what the endoscopic pictures are, and many endoscopists describe a picture which is seen by other endoscopists in the perfectly normal esophagus abdominalis. It is in such cases that the bismuth radiograph, useful in any case, is of especial value. The best of all methods, however, is by the trained sense of touch which by long experience quickly detects more than normal resistance at the hiatus. This must be determined, and the experience must be acquired by esophagoscopy without general anesthesia because in deep anesthesia there is no resistance, and partial anesthesia introduces a variable element. Local

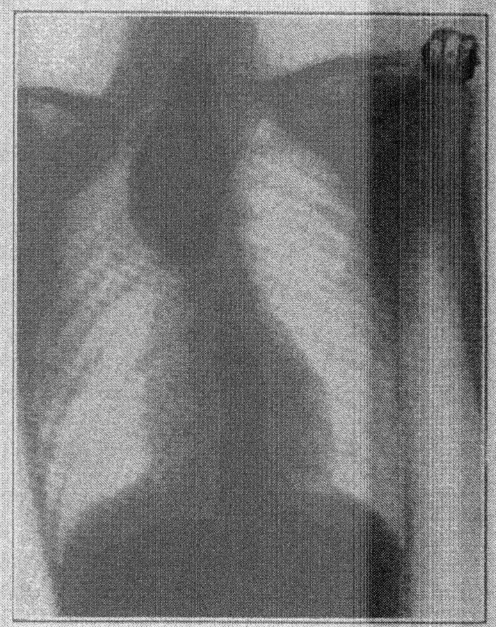

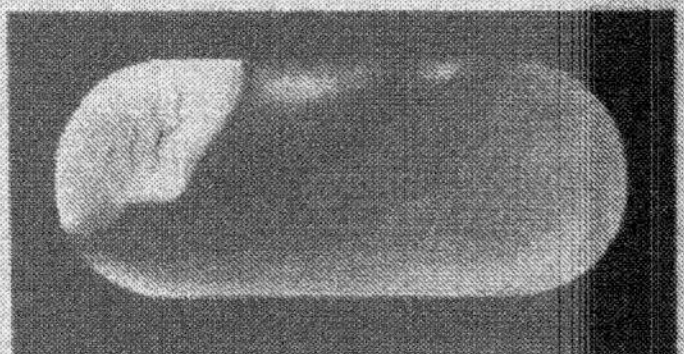

Fig. 415.—Radiograph of a woman of thirty-eight years. The shadow, which so much resembles a diverticulum, was esophagoscopically proven to be a dilatation above a stricture of probably luetic origin. The stricture is behind and above the bottom of the lower border of the shadow of the dilatation. Endoscopic dilatation resulted in a cure, after which a bismuth mixture went through into the stomach so promptly as not to show in a radiograph. Fluoroscopic examination showed swallowing to be normal. (Radiograph by Dr. Russell H. Boggs.) The lower illustration shows the endoscopic appearance of the suprastrictural dilatation. The orifice of the stricture is hidden by the overhanging, whitish, cicatricial fold.

anesthesia has but little and a very uncertain influence on relaxation of spasm. Radiography may lead to error as in the case illustrated in Fig. 413, 414, and 415.

The possibility of the radiograph being taken just before normal physiologic opening of the abdominal esophagus in the deglutitory cycle must be borne in mind in the interpretation of radiographs. It is to be eliminated in each case by the comparison of a number of plates, and by the elapsed time.

Treatment of hiatal esophagismus (so-called "cardiospasm"). Treatment of abdominal esophagismus and hiatal esophagismus, has led to the devising of a number of different water-bags and air-bags, which have yielded good results. In some cases, however, it is impossible to introduce them. The author's personal preference, like that of Brünings', is for a mechanical divulsor inserted through the esophagoscope where the sense of touch and the precision of a steel instrument give one an accurate control. Heavy, spring-opposed handles are a mistake as they prevent the safeguarding of the divulsion by the delicate sense of touch. The author uses the divulsor that Mosher devised for the rapid dilatation of cicatricial strictures, Fig. 48. The method is simple. The 53 cm. esophagoscope is passed into the stomach until it reaches the greater curvature. Then the divulsor, closed, is passed through the esophagoscope until the distal end of the divulsor touches the greater curvature of the stomach. Then the esophagoscope is withdrawn until the slightly expanded expansile portion of the divulsor is endoscopically seen to be all exposed beyond the tube-mouth. The partial withdrawal of the esophagoscope is done under the guidance of the eye so that the largest diameter of the divulsor can be seen to be in the hiatal esophagus. It is then expanded to the full physiological size, about 20 to 25 millimeters in the adult, unless resistance to expansion is felt. Great care is necessary not to use undue force which might rupture the esophagus; but the trained touch will do no harm. The dilator, fully expanded in the living patient, is shown in the radiograph, Fig. 416. The divulsor is allowed to remain in its expanded position for from five to ten minutes. It is then contracted with the screw mechanism, great care being used to avoid pinching the mucosa as the blades close. If there is any tendency to this, the blades should be re-expanded slightly and the divulsor rotated gently. Divulsion is somewhat painful and the use of ether anesthesia is advisable, not only for this reason, but especially to prevent vomiting while the divulsor is fully expanded which might cause trauma. From one to six divulsions at intervals of a week are necessary.

It is necessary after any form of treatment to instruct the patient to eat very slowly and to masticate very thoroughly. It is altogether probable that very rapid eating and insufficient mastication may, in some instances, be one of the factors contributing to the cause of spasm of the esophagus, because we know that in certain instances small foreign bodies will cause a spasm, as evidenced by complete obstruction of the esophagus by a foreign body too small to block up the canal. Liquid foods

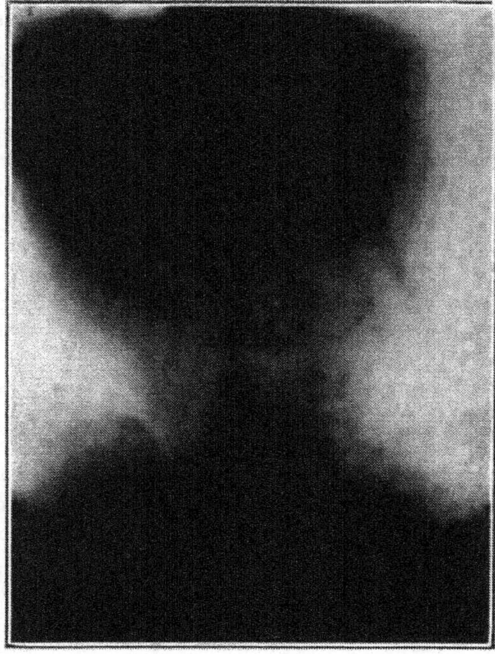

FIG. 416.—Divulser fully expanded (24 mm.) in the living patient, a man of twenty-one years. The double image is due to respiratory movement.

taken in very small quantities frequently repeated are best during the treatments and for a month or longer thereafter in order to permit resolution of the macerated, inflamed esophagus. Undoubtedly there are a few cases that are prone to recur, and the most stubborn are those existing since childhood, with consequent infantile stomach and long-established "nerve cell habit." The neurologist should be called in consultation in cases that do not yield promptly to divulsion.

The foregoing is the method that has yielded the author the best results. There are a number of other methods successfully used by Plummer, Jesse Meyer, Lerche and others, and their writings, reference to which will be found in the Bibliography, should be consulted.

Dilating bags filled with air or water after insertion on the principle of Horrock's maieutic are effective if accurately placed. It is so difficult, however, to place them accurately by blind methods, that esophagoscopic placing seems preferable to the author, who, however, may be biased. Gastrostomy through the abdominal wall with retrograde dilatation of the cardia has been done quite a number of times, but in view of the beautiful results that are obtainable endoscopically, such procedure seems unjustifiable, until endoscopic methods have utterly failed to cure. It is difficult to see how any more thorough stretching can be done from below than could be done from above. Gastrostomy for feeding is, usually, contraindicated because a stomach tube can be placed with the esophagoscope, if a case is encountered where the spasm is so severe or the superjacent diffuse dilatation is so great that the stomach tube cannot be passed otherwise. The author has seen a number of cases where the stomach tube could not be passed because the patient could not aid by swallowing efforts, and the stomach tube would strike the flat floor (See Fig. 411) of the dilatation and had no tendency to enter the hiatal esophagus. In all such cases the author has found it exceedingly easy to introduce the gastroscope and through it to pass a soft rubber stomach tube for feeding. The gastroscope was withdrawn, leaving the feeding tube in situ. In case an endoscopist is not available, gastrostomy for feeding is, of course, advisable before the patient's nutrition has suffered too much. Duodenal feeding through the duodenal feeding tube has been used with excellent results by Clement R. Jones, T. Wray Grayson and others.

CHAPTER XXXII.

Diseases of the Esophagus.—Continued.

CICATRICIAL STENOSIS OF THE ESOPHAGUS.

*Etiology.** The most common cause of cicatricial stenosis is the swallowing of corrosive poisons, especially caustic alkalies. It is a pitiable thing to see little children threatened with starvation because of a cicatricial esophageal stenosis due to the swallowing of some form of caustic alkali to which the laxity of our laws permitted them to be exposed. The law requires that the druggist shall label corrosive poisons "Poison" and the careful druggist adds antidotal advice. Next door to the druggist, the grocer sells corrosive poisons having on the label no hint of caution, but having directly misleading statements, such as "Will not hurt the hands," "Will not harm the most delicate fabric," etc. It is the general impression that concentrated lye is a relic of the old days of home-made soaps, but investigation shows that it is in common use in the household for labor-saving cleansing of all kinds. Its harmful effect on the hands conveys to the thoughtful some hint of the caustic nature of its contents. But the frequency with which patients with esophageal stricture, following the swallowing of concentrated lye, come in an almost fatal state of inanition to the esophagoscopist, is an index to the thoughtlessness of the users of concentrated lye, and an urgent call for legislation that shall compel the manufacturer to label concentrated lye containers "Poison" and to state a few antidotes, even if this does diminish slightly the sale of such products. Esophageal stricture from the swallowing of commercial lye has been for many years a lesion of common observation by those interested in the esophagus. The frequency declined with the more general substitution of cheap commercial soaps for the home-made products; but concentrated lye is still in extensive use for general

*Part of this section on etiology is revised, with additions, from the author's "Chairman's Address" to the Section on Laryngology of the American Medical Association, 1910. (Bib. 241.)

scrubbing and cleansing purposes. Furthermore, strictures of the esophagus are again on the increase owing to the flooding of the market with a large number of proprietary "cleansers" for household use and "washing powders" for laundry use. The author has seen three cases of the most severe ulceration and sloughing of the esophagus from the swallowing of strong solutions of three of these proprietary preparations. The author has had the preparations analyzed and all contained similar ingredients: an abrasive, a strong powdered soap, and a caustic alkali: namely, soda ash. The proportions varied from eight per cent in the "cleansers" up to forty or fifty per cent in the laundry powders; but in none was the corrosive alkali so diluted as not to be caustic to the delicate esophageal mucosa of a child. And, worst of all, the mixture was not thorough; therefore some portions were more concentrated than others, so that under certain conditions it would be possible for a child to get a concentrated dose of caustic. Another thing which doubtless contributes to the danger is the insoluble nature of the abrasive and the slower solubility of the soap. Thus, a little water dissolves out the alkali in strong solution. The accident in a number of cases occurred through the child's swallowing the rinsings of the almost empty can. The economical mother was endeavoring to extract the dregs for use; and, totally unsuspicious of a preparation which could not "injure the most delicate fabric," did not place the can out of reach of the child. In another instance the cleansing powder had been sprinkled on the dishes in the dish-pan. From one cup it was not removed by rinsing, the powdered soap in its composition making it adherent, and from this cup the child drank. In the third instance the child drew water from a faucet into a cup that had been used to measure out a quantity of a proprietary washing powder for laundry use. On not one of the containers of these three widely advertised proprietary caustic preparations was there one hint of the dangerous nature of the contents. Ammonia, "salts of tartar" (potassium carbonate), mercuric bichloride, strong acids, etc., are less frequent causes of cicatricial stenoses. It was at one time supposed that cicatricial stenosis of the esophagus was invariably due to the swallowing of corrosives. It is quite well established now, that tuberculosis, lues, scarlatina, diphtheria and various pyogenic conditions can produce ulceration followed by cicatricies in the esophagus. MacReynolds reports the discovery at autopsy of a large area of ulceration in the esophagus of a patient who died of spontaneous rupture of the esophagus, complicating mastoid disease. Chronic esophagitis from spasm with stagnation of food and secretions, as seen in abdominal and hiatal esophagismus, (erroneously called "cardiospasm") may result in superficial erosions which when the pyogenic infections become engrafted upon them, may result in serious cicatrices. Thus we have an organic stenosis following upon a spasmodic stenosis. Every esophagoscopist of large experience has seen cases of cicatricial stenosis of the esophagus in which he is utterly at loss to discover the original cause of an undoubted cicatricial stenosis. The so-called "peptic" ulcer of the lower portion of the esophagus may be a cause. Observations by Guisez, MacKinnie and also some observations of the author point clearly to the fact that spasmodic lesions can produce organic stricture by the erosions due to the accompanying esophagitis. Decubitus ulcer of typhoid fever has caused cicatricial esophageal stenosis. The author has previously pointed out the occurrence of an ulcer in the esophagus from sphacelus of the esophageal mucosa in the low vitality of profound typhoid toxemia. Since that time five cases of post-typhoid stenosis from cicatricial contraction have been sent to the author. In four of these cases the cicatrix was at the cricoid level, evidently due to the pressure of the cricoid against the vertebral column, pinching the esophageal wall, the vitality of which was lowered by the typhoid toxemia, ending in sloughing and ulceration. In the other case the cicatrix was at the level of the crossing of the left bronchus. Whatever be the nature of the original lesion the stenotic cicatrix is usually the result of the inflammatory infiltration resulting from the prolonged ulcerative processes due to the secondary mixed pyogenic infections. Any sort of stenosis of the esophagus, if long continued, may, by the stagnation of food and secretion, set up esophagitis and ulceration resulting in cicatrices. In view of this, slight degrees of congenital stenosis may be considered, possibly, a contributing cause. As pointed out by Brown Kelly (Bib. 303) slighter degrees of organic stenosis, in some instances possibly congenital, may have existed for years unnoticed by the patient. Cicatricial stricture of the esophagus may follow prolonged sojourn of a foreign body. The presence of a foreign body results in a localized ulceration with hyperplasia. During a prolonged period, this round-celled infiltration increases and later, after the foreign body is removed, the contraction of the cicatricial tissue results in a greater or less stenosis of the esophageal lumen. In one case of this kind, seen by the author, in a child four years of age, a coin had been removed by a general surgeon by external esophagotomy after the coin had been *in situ* for nearly one year. After the wound had healed, the child could swallow quite well, but in a few weeks difficulty in swallowing began to appear, becoming gradually worse until at the end of two months a very severe degree of stenosis was present, permitting only liquids to pass. The author cured the stricture by forcible dilatation and continued bouginage *per tubam*. It seemed to be very much more amenable to treatment than the stricture cases following the swallowing of lye, and the stricture was only single, while those following the swallowing of caustic alkalies are usually multiple, the openings not being concentric.

Site of cicatricial stricture of the esophagus. The author's experience has been quite at variance with that of Guisez. The latter reports that out of 38 cases due to corrosives the site of predilection for the cicatricial stricture was at the cardia, and when there were more than one, the next most frequent site was the upper orifice, the tightest being at the cardia. In the author's experience, he has never seen a case of stricture due to caustic situated at the cardia. Out of a total of 27 of this class of cases, 18 were in the middle third of the esophagus, 6 at the level of the hiatus, 4 near the cricopharyngeus. Where the strictures were multiple they were usually quite close together, though in three cases there was a stricture just below the cricoid and another in the middle third. Of the cases in the midlle third, the most frequent site was at about the crossing of the left bronchus. Stricture of the pylorus as well as of the esophagus following the swallowing of a corrosive has been reported by Bruel. (Bib. 50.)

Prognosis. Untreated, the mortality of cicatricial strictures of small lumen is very high. Slighter degrees of stenosis are prone to increase from stasis, esophagitis and secondary ulceration. By early gastrostomy with proper feeding through the tube, life may be prolonged indefinitely. As a matter of fact, however, old people who have worn a gastrostomy tube since childhood are never seen. Statistics from which the causes of death might have been determined are lacking. Doubtless mortality would have been less if gastrostomy had been done earlier. Under blind methods of treatment the patient was almost certain, sooner or later, to succumb to perforation by the bougie, the danger increasing as the superjacent dilatation increased, rendering more and more difficult the finding of the strictural orifice. The prognosis of cicatricial stenosis of the esophagus untreated is unfavorable so far as recovery is concerned. There probably is never a complete spontaneous recovery. Occasionally slight strictures may become temporarily stenosed with food, or the stenosis may be increased by swelling, producing, for a short period, a very severe stenosis. This may subside and a condition of relative cure so far as dysphagia is concerned may result, and the patient may be quite comfortable; but this is only the disappearance of a relatively temporary condition. In regard to danger to life, the prognosis in cicatricial stenosis of the esophagus is good if an early gastrostomy is done and the feeding is carefully followed out according to a well planned dietary. The foregoing represents the prognosis of cicatricial stenosis before the development of endoscopic treatment. Under modern methods the prognosis is favorable as to ultimate results, though some of the cases require a long period of treatment, the duration depending upon the number of strictures, the presence or absence of pouches between the strictures and the previous duration of the condition, as well as upon the tightness of the stricture. In recent cases where there is but a single stricture or two strictures, the lower one of concentric lumen, the cure is rapid and the results excellent. On the other hand, in multiple strictures, not concentric, and of long-standing, with extensive fibrotic changes in the esophageal wall, due to

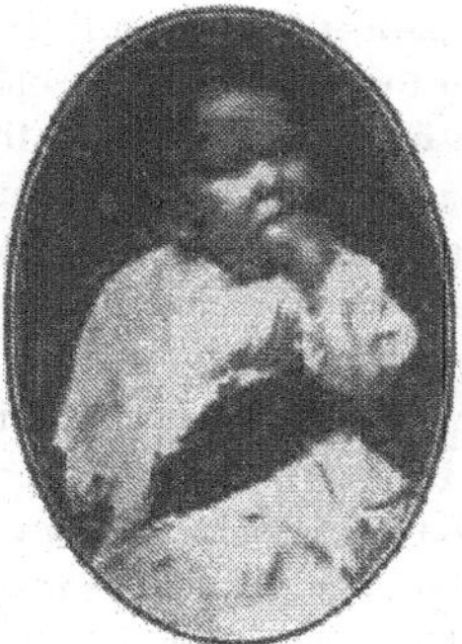

FIG. 417.—Photograph of a child, twenty months old, a victim of cicatricial esophageal stricture. It is in the act of inducing vomiting by the insertion of its fingers to the fauces, a self-discovered means of relief, quite remarkable, considering the age. Referred by Dr. F. LeMoyne Hupp.

prolonged chronic esophagitis, and especially if the lumen of the stricture is exceedingly small—in all such cases, the treatment is very much more difficult, and though the ultimate prognosis is not unfavorable, the treatment will be prolonged by recurrences. As to mortality under endoscopic methods, the author has never yet lost a case. The only death occurring in his clinic was from blind bouginage before his present endoscopic technic was developed.

Symptoms. Lengthy consideration of the symptoms is not now necessary, as it was in the days of the often erroneous deductive diagnosis. If a patient has any trouble in swallowing or regurgitates or "vomits" his food or chokes or coughs when attempting to swallow, esophagoscopy is indicated and deductive or blind instrumental attempts at diagnosis are time-wasting, misleading and utterly useless. It requires but a few minutes without an anesthetic, general or local, to look at the esophagus with the esophagoscope and make a positive diagnosis of cicatricial stricture. Radiography is useful in excluding aneurysm and in determining the presence of a stenosis and the extent of the dilatation above it. That the stricture is cicatricial can be determined only by esophagoscopy. The most usual complaints of the patients are difficulty in swallowing, cough, and regurgitation. Distress after eating, to be relieved only by regurgitation is seen in low strictures (Fig. 417).

Esophagoscopic appearances and diagnosis of cicatricial stricture. The endoscopic picture in a typical case is easily recognized, but it may be masked by various conditions other than the cicatrix. If there is complete stagnation, or if the patient has recently eaten, fragments of food may be noticed adherent to the walls of the esophagus, or lodged in the pockets existing below the first stricture, or in the case of a recent and illy-masticated meal there may be quite an accumulation above the stricture. Often it will be found that the patient has come for a complete stenosis, which, upon examination is found to be due to the lodgment of a particle of food acting as a cork in the lumen of the stricture. This does not occur as often as might be supposed for the reason that the patients usually learn that, by inserting their finger back of the tongue and causing a regurgitation, food particles can be, in most instances, dislodged and regurgitated. If the food has remained for any length of time in the esophagus, decomposition has occurred and in case of nitrogenous food, the odor may be very foul. In case of starchy foods and sugar, there will be usually a sour odor. This is not the normally sour odor of stomach contents, but a peculiar odor due to the fermentation of starches and sugars. All food and secretions must be removed and the mucosa sponged clean. If there has been no stagnation the color of the cicatricial portions of the esophageal wall is usually paler than normal, and may be decidedly white and blanched. Vessels are often visible in this white tissue. In certain cases there may be patches of reddish, acutely inflamed mucosa, and if there is very much dilatation above the stricture, there may be a macerated condition of the esophageal mucosa. Where the mucosa has been uninjured by the caustic, the epithelium may be furred up and pasty in appearance from maceration. The epithelium covering the cicatricial tissue does not usually fur up to the same extent and may be quite smooth and shining in marked contrast to the furred epithelium in the portions undamaged by the corrosion. Whitish spots of erosion and even ulceration may be visible at certain points (Fig. 12, Plate III). It is quite likely that these erosions play an important part in the increase of the stenosis and the diminution of the strictural lumen through contraction and fibrosis of the round-celled inflammatory infiltrate, constituting what the author has called a "vicious circle." The scars from the swallowing of caustics in some instances are linear and seen in perspective, they appear wedge-shaped from foreshortening (Fig. 12, Plate III and Fig. 4, Plate III, Bib. 269). They are in some instances depressed below the surface of the mucous membrane, though in other instances they may project toward the lumen in a more or less cord-like way. In other cases they are flush with the neighboring mucosal surface. In passing down a cicatricial esophagus very often there is a very noticeable absence of the normal radial creases. The cicatricial tissue in a cicatricial stenosis may take the form of a band running across in any direction and causing more or less flattening of the circular outline of the lumen at that point Exactly annular strictures occur and occasionally they are most beautifully symmetrical and funnel-shaped. As a rule, however, they are more or less eccentric, and their outline is more or less oval, or angular. Where the amount of cicatricial tissue is small, the outline is not fixed but changes with the respiratory movements and even with the transmitted cardiac impulses, antiperistalsis and movements imparted by the esophagoscope. If the first stricture encountered is not very small, the view through the stricture usually is that of a cavity below. In this cavity it is very rare to see the lumen of strictures which usually exist below, because the lower ones are not concentric with the upper ones, nor are their lumina easy to find. If the upper stricture is not very tight and the lower one is smaller, there is a strong tendency to pouch formation from the pressure of food accumulating between the two strictures.

Differential diagnosis. In a typical case, a cicatricial stenosis is readily recognizable by the descriptions already herein given, but there are cases in which a diagnosis is extremely difficult because of associated lesions. When inflammatory conditions and ulceration are present, they must be first treated by a rest in bed, very careful restriction of the diet as to quantity, and all food should be liquid. Bismuth and calomel taken dry on the tongue in small quantities at frequent intervals, with liquid diet, will cure, in most cases, the esophagitis with erosions and ulcerations that accompany stenotic conditions. In addition to this, local application of argyrol to ulcerations and to granulation surfaces will aid in clearing up these lesions. The cicatricial nature of the stenosis then becomes quite apparent. Cancerous stenosis is accompanied by infiltration and a distortion of the shape of the lumen of the esophagus, which, even in the absence of open ulceration, is quite different from the thin [illegible] almost membranous cicatricial stenosis. Impermeable cicatri- [illegible] hard, but cancer rarely is impermeable until late.

and in cancer, there are usually projecting fungations and edematous polypoid masses, when the disease has reached a condition of severe stenosis. Prior to this time, infiltration of the esophageal wall is quite apparent to palpation with the tube and probe Moreover, in cancer there is more or less of fixation of the entire esophagus, which does not yield readily laterally to manipulations of the tube. It is necessary, however, to remember that cancer may develop at the site of a cicatrix, as evidenced by the following case:

Robert M., aged 58 years, applied for admission to the Western Pennsylvania Hospital for difficulty in swallowing, which had persisted with variations in degree since the healing of a bullet wound 20 years before. Within the last few months, there had been a steady increase until only liquids could go down. There was a depressed wound in the neck on the right side, and a scar three inches in length on the left side corresponding, according to the patient's statement, to the site of an operation to remove the bullet which had not emerged. The patient stated that immediately following the injury, he had noticed no bleeding, but he had vomited material like coffee grounds not long after. On passing the esophagoscope, I found a pharyngeal pouch or diverticulum. The subdiverticular opening was in the usual location, anterior to the pouch. This opening was large, admitting a 10 mm. esophagoscope for about 5 cm. At this level, the esophagus deviated very markedly to the left, the walls were tightly adherent and there was a stricture of oval outline with a flat ulceration of about 1 cm. in diameter, just touching the right strictural margin. I excised the edge of this ulcer, including a portion of the stricture. Examination of this tissue by Joseph H. Barach, showed it to be a squamous-celled epithelioma.

Remarks. It is quite clear from the foregoing history that a cicatricial stricture existed for 18 or 19 years, and that the cicatricial tissue became the site of the implantation of the cancerous process. Whatever may be our ideas concerning irritation as a factor in the development of carcinoma, there can be no doubt that cicatricial tissue and chronic inflammatory conditions offer a favorable soil for the development of cancer. The development of a diverticulum from cicatricial stenosis is worthy of note as a very rare observation.

In compression stenosis of the esophagus, the lumen does not taper down to a point as in strictures, and the outline of the lumen is linear and more or less crescentic, from the bulging inward of one wall convexly from one side (Fig. 7, Plate III, Bib. 269), though occasionally it is seen as a flattening of the walls with a more or less straight long diameter. Unless the compression is from a very firm growth, a small esophagoscope can usually be insinuated through the compression, and the mucosa below will be found to be normal. The mucosa above in cases of severe compression, may show the signs of chronic esophagitis which accompany stasis and maceration. Ordinarily, however, compressions are characterized by normal mucosa, which is in marked contrast to the thin white appearance of the strictural margin. Spasmodic stenoses are characterized by a wrinkling of the esophageal lumen which throws the membrane into folds, and the crevices between these folds taper down to a vanishing point, as shown in Fig. 7, Plate III. Moreover, gentle pressure continued for a time will cause the spasmodic stenosis to yield and the esophagoscope will pass on through. The mucosa below is usually normal, while that above may be more or less altered by chronic esophagitis; but the diagnostic point is the opening up of the constricted area to the full lumen as soon as the spasm yields to pressure. General anesthesia may be used to overcome spasm, but this is rarely, if ever, necessary for the skilled esophagoscopist, though until skill is acquired, great caution is necessary in applying any pressure on the supposition that a condition is spasmodic stenosis.

Treatment of cicatricial stenosis of the esophagus. In dealing with the esophagus, it must always be remembered that it is one of the most intolerant organs with which we have to deal surgically. Shock is out of all proportion to the extent of the operation or of the lesion, as shown in ordinary acute esophagitis from traumatism. Therefore, we must not undertake treatment without due preparation of the patient as regards everything that concerns his strength and endurance. If the patient has not already been gastrostomized, it is wise to keep a very close watch on the state of his nutrition during any form of treatment. It is always possible for local reaction to entirely shut up the esophagus, and the patient will very quickly suffer. Procedures are so much simplified by having the patient regularly fed through a gastrostomic tube and the putting of the esophagus at rest is so beneficial that there should be no hesitation in advising it in the worst cases. In most instances, however, a lumen for liquids remains, and with care in diet, gastrostomy will rarely be necessary. The general preparation of the patient, as mentioned on a preceding page, should be carried out as a preliminary to any operation or examination on the esophagus. In addition thereto, absolute rest of the esophagus to reduce the esophagitis, is an essential operative preliminary. Absolutely nothing but water, milk, ice cream and consomme should be allowed, and bismuth subnitrate with a little calomel from time to time should be swallowed dry, in small doses at frequent intervals. Patients in a state of water hunger make exceedingly bad surgical subjects, and absolutely no attempt at endoscopy should be undertaken until the patient has fully recovered from food and water starvation as before mentioned.

The question arises: To what extent shall dilatation of a stricture be carried out? This must be determined by the functional result. In some cases it is necessary to produce a very large opening because of the sacculation almost amounting to a diverticulum above the stricture. In one of the author's cases, this was so great that it pressed on the lumen of the esophagus below the stricture and interfered with swallowing to such an extent that it was necessary to bite out the spur with forceps so as to obliterate the bottom of the sack. In this case, the stricture was in the neck. It is questionable whether such a procedure would be justifiable in the thorax. In another case a valve-like fold overhanging the lumen of the stricture required removal. In cases in which there is very little sacculation, a relatively small opening will give an excellent functional result, and if an opening of six or seven millimeters can be maintained, the patient will have no trouble functionally, if food is perfectly masticated. Imperfectly masticated food of any kind, of course, becomes a foreign body. The author has had cases that would swallow all kinds of food when properly masticated but their esophagus would become occluded from the swallowing of the pulp of a grape containing the seeds. A number of times when this has occurred, maceration and softening of the pulp of the grape has allowed the seeds to go through and the stenosis to be relieved, but of course foods of this kind should not be partaken of. In two other instances, an orange seed lodged between the upper and the lower stricture in a patient that for many months before had been having no trouble whatever with eating all kinds of food. After the author removed the orange seed, no further trouble was experienced, though two years have now elapsed in one case, and a year in the other, during which time the patients have been partaking of all kinds of food thoroughly masticated. These cases show how small a lumen may suffice. It may be said, then, that the degree of dilatation should be determined altogether functionally. Having obtained good useful swallowing, it is questionable in some cases whether it is wise to persist in an attempt entirely to obliterate the stricture and restore full lumen, which involves more risk to the patient than is involved in the obtaining of a useful lumen. A good functional result is better determined by a bismuth radiography or fluoroscopy than by the sensations of the patient. The stomach should be empty of food (it is never entirely empty of secretion) and the bowels should be freely emptied by an enema before any operative procedure upon the esophagus. There is a disposition on the part of the profession to disregard this common preoperative precaution in patients who have been unable to swallow any food for several days. No anesthesia, general or local, is needed and as any form of treatment has to be frequently repeated, all forms of anesthesia are contraindicated. The problem is to determine the best method of getting a start in the dilatation of strictures of exceedingly small lumen, say one or two millimeters in diameter. There have been many dilators and divulsors devised, most of which can only be used in stricture of such large lumen (say six or seven mm.) that they do not urgently need dilatation. Such instruments are of use in hiatal and abdominal esophagismus, but cicatricial esophageal strictures of large lumen, or those in which a good start has been obtained, are of easy management, and the choice of methods is of little moment. Small almost impermeable strictures on the contrary are extremely difficult to dilate in the first stages of the work. Personally the author has found nothing equal to bouginage per tubam.

Bouginage per tubam. The author uses the double olive bougies (Fig. 61, p. 108, Bib. 269) only in the most minute strictures and then only to get a start. In almost all cases the start can be made and the treatment continued with the filiform bougie permanently mounted on the steel stem (Fig. 53). Three or four successively larger sizes can be used at one seance. The last and largest bougie that can be safely inserted is left in for about twenty minutes, the esophagoscope being withdrawn, if desired, after the bougie is placed. At the next treatment about two days later the start can usually be made with a bougie one or two sizes larger than the starting size at the previous treatment. Treatments are continued at intervals of a few days until the largest size that can be inserted through the esophagoscope can be inserted and withdrawn without resistance. The patient is then ready for the daily swallowing of a common bougie of the old type. Under no circumstances should he push it. It should be preceded by the swallowing of about 10 cc. of olive oil for lubrication. After three or fourth months the interval may be lengthened to a week or two, but must not be abandoned for a year. Even then a monthly passage is advisable for the early detection of any tendency to recurrence. In children the size must be increased from year to year proportionate to the normal esophageal growth and development. The foregoing is the author's method in all cases where the stricture is single and also in all cases of multiple stricture in which the lumina of the lower strictures are concentric with the upper one. The most difficult cases to treat are those in which there are many strictures, and especially where the lumen of the stricture is not concentric nor in line with each other. In addition, there may be more or less sacculation between the strictures rendering it extremely difficult to find the aperture of the strictures below the first as shown in Fig. 418. The author's method of dealing with these strictures is to dilate first the upper one forcibly and widely, then take the second one which now comes into view because a small tube can be put through the first one, which has been dilated. For this purpose none of the divulsors to be had are of any use. They do not stretch at the very end, so that they must be inserted far beyond the stricture to obtain any divulsion. Such insertion is impossible in the most difficult class of cases with which we have to deal; namely, multiple eccentric strictures, because the second stricture will prevent the insertion of the instrument far enough to obtain any divulsion on the first stricture. For this reason, the author has de-

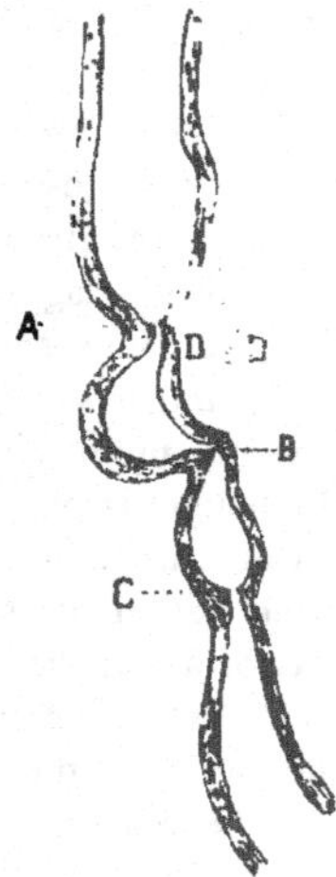

FIG. 418.—Schematic illustration of a series of eccentric strictures with interstrictural sacculations, in the esophagus of a boy of four years. Divulsed seriatim from above downward with the divulsor (Fig. 52), the esophageal wall, D, being moved sidewise to the dotted line by means of a small esophagoscope inserted through the upper stricture, A, after divulsion of the latter.

vised the divulsor shown in Fig. 52. With this instrument, we can divulse the first stricture, even though it be less than 1 cm. away from the second stricture. This is a safe procedure, because between the two strictures there is always more or less of a pouch. In using the word "safe," the author, of course, means relatively safe, because any esophageal instrument must be used with care and tactile appreciation of the exact amount of force applied.

Since the stagnation of food is the greatest factor in the production of esophagitis in these cases, it is necessary that the diet shall be carefully regulated. Food should be taken in minute quantities at a time, allowing a long time for a meal to be ingested. Liquid foods only are to be permitted in certain cases. In other cases, and later on in all cases, solids may be used, provided they be thoroughly masticated. Semi-solids, and especially very soft boiled eggs, custards and the like usually go down about as well as liquids, even in small strictures. The patient

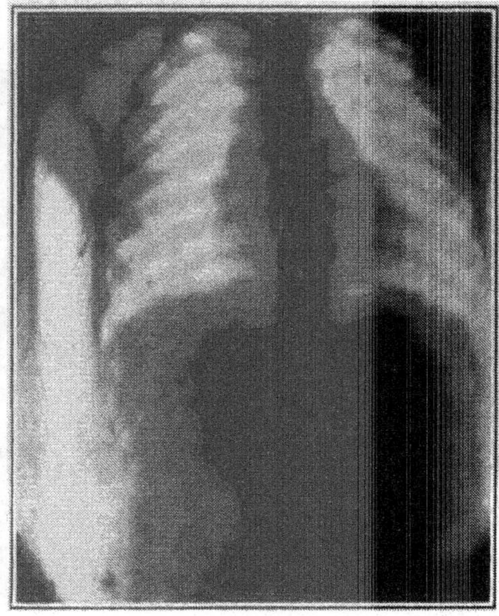

FIG. 419.—Radiograph showing complete cure of a cicatricial stenosis. The bismuth mixed with bread and milk went through into the stomach so promptly and completely as not to show in this radiograph made immediately after taking the mixture. The gastrostomy tube shown in the radiograph was immediately abandoned. (Radiograph made by Dr. George W. Grier. Author's case.)

must be instructed that should any accumulation of food be felt it must be regurgitated and followed by a glassful of a weak solution of sodium bicarbonate. If this sodium bicarbonate does not go through promptly, it should be regurgitated also, thus accomplishing a lavage of the esophageal mucosa. Ice cream is a very valuable food in all forms of stenosis and in all stages of after-treatment, not only because of the cold, but because it is always ingested slowly. Of course there is nothing to prevent a patient taking any liquid food slowly by the teaspoonful, but as a matter of fact, once the patient gets away from the hospital it is exceedingly difficult to enforce the rule of teaspoonful taking of fluids.

Numerous cases illustrative of the success of this treatment could be cited, but a few will suffice:

A boy of three years, consulted Dr. E. L. Jones of Cumberland, for inability to swallow even water or saliva for eight days. The child had swallowed lye eight months previously, and the inability to swallow had come on gradually. Dr. Jones immediately referred the case to the

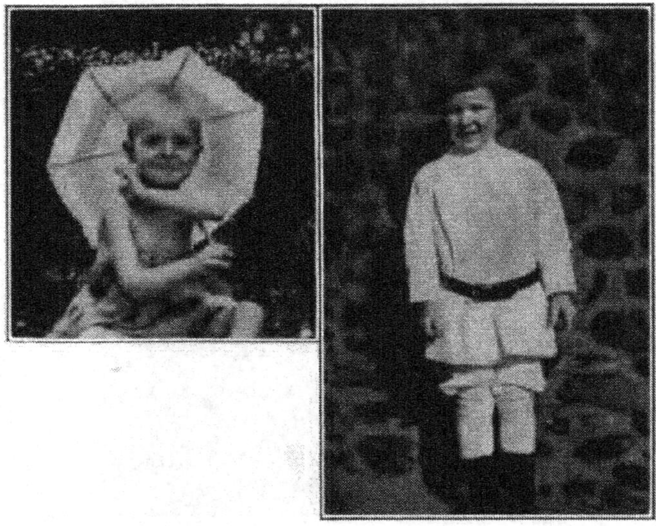

Fig. 420.—From photographs of a boy of four years. Weight when first seen 26 pounds. After 28th endoscopic bouginage, 42 pounds. Patient referred by Dr. H. T. Price.

author. The child was *in extremis* and its life was saved only by a prompt and skilful gastrostomy by Dr. James W. MacFarlane. One week later the author passed an esophagoscope and found at the cricopharyngeus a tight stricture (1 mm.) which was divulsed with the divulsor, Fig. 52. A second eccentric stricture about 1 cm. lower down was similarly divulsed and bouginage per tubam completed the cure. Six seances were required to restore normal swallowing (Fig. 419). The gastrostomy tube was abandoned. No anesthesia was used for the treatment. The child now, one year later, is able promptly to swallow any normally masticated food.

Remarks. The statement of the parents that the child had swallowed no water for eight days is probably inaccurate. Some little fluid must have leaked through the stricture or the child could not have survived.

A girl of two years was referred to the author by Dr. Abraham of New York City for inability to swallow which came on a few weeks after swallowing a solution of a washing powder. A general surgeon failed to pass a bougie under chloroform anesthesia. Esophagoscopy by the author revealed a tight stricture (1 mm. diameter) at about the crossing of the left bronchus. A double olive bougie could be felt to engage in

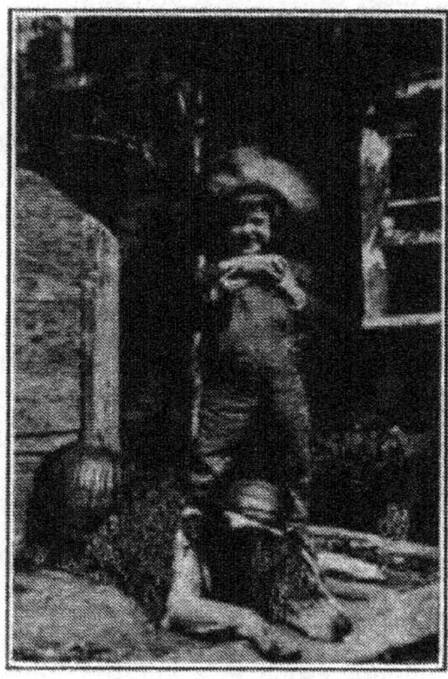

FIG. 421.—Same patient as in Fig. 420. Two years later.

two strictures below, making three strictures in all. Bouginage per tubam in about fourteen treatments cured the child completely. She swallows food the same as any child. Now, five years later (seven years of age) she can swallow a silk-woven bougie, 12 mm. diameter, without the slightest check to indicate where the stenosis had been.

A boy, four years of age, was referred by Dr. H. T. Price for inability to swallow. Immediate gastrostomy by Dr. R. E. Brenneman saved the child's life. Esophagoscopy by the author revealed a stricture 1 mm. in diameter. The smallest double olive bougie would pass through but was stopped by occlusion below. Bending the stem between the two olives, enabled the author by rotation to find the lumen of the stricture below, when a third obstruction was found (Schema Fig. 418). All three eccentric strictures were treated by the author's method before described, resulting in an ultimate cure. (Figs. 420 and 421).

Having described the method by which the author has been able to restore normal swallowing to almost every patient with a permeable esophagus, some other esophagoscopic methods may be described. Blind methods are not within the scope of this book.

Internal esophagotomy is, in the opinion of Killian and of the author, an extremely dangerous procedure. If justifiable at all it is only so in the hands of the most experienced and skillful esophagoscopists. It is necessary ocularly to recognize and cut cicatricial tissue only, never the normal esophageal wall. This recognition is not always easy and may be impossible. Personally, the author does not use internal esophagotomy because he deems theoretically that dilatation subsequent to incision would be very apt to result in a tear taking its start from the incision. In the absence of an incision forcible dilatation carried out with reasonable care and especially with an acute tactile sense, need never tear cicatricial tissue. The author used, endoscopically, in a number of cases (Bib. 257) the string-cutting esophagotome, Fig. 51, without mortality or serious symptoms, but the above outlined methods are so satisfactory as to leave little to be desired. The author's esophagotome (Fig. 51) can be turned so that the cutting by the to-and-fro motion of the string will be only on the manifest cicatricial part of the stricture. Guisez (Bib. 178) reports excellent results from internal esophagotomy.

Electrolysis has yielded excellent results in the hands of Guisez (Bib. 178).

String swallowing. So far the author has never yet encountered a case in which he could not esophagoscopically find the lumen in any stenotic case that had a lumen. If the lumen could not be found, doubtless the string swallowing method of Sippey could be adapted to esophagoscopic use, the esophagoscope being threaded over the proximal end of the string, the distal end having been swallowed some days before.

Retrograde esophagoscopy. The first step is to get rid of the gastric secretions. There is always fluid in the stomach, and this keeps pouring out of the tube in a steady stream. Fold after fold is emptied of fluid. Once the stomach is empty, the search begins for the cardial opening. When it is desired to do a retrograde esophagoscopy and the gastrostomy is done for this special purpose, it is wise to have it very high. Once the cardia is located and the esophagus entered, the remainder of the work is very easy. Bouginage can be carried out from below the same as from above. It has been claimed that bouginage from below is easier because there is never any dilatation below the stricture to contend with, and strictures are much more apt to be concentric as approached from below because there has been no distortion by pressure dilatation due to stagnation of the food operating through a long period of time. This does not coincide with the experience of the author, who has found peroral treatment of cicatricial stenosis easier and much more satisfactory in every way.

Impermeable strictures may be classified under three heads.

1. Strictures of the cervical esophagus.
2. Strictures of the middle third.
3. Strictures of the lower third.

The cervical strictures are readily amenable to external esophagotomy with a plastic operation for the opening up and reformation of the esophagus. The esophagus can be built up if necessary out of skin flap turned inward provided such flap can be procured from a location free from hair. Such a flap must, of course, be turned in without severing its attachment totally from the skin and rather a broad pedicle will be required to make sure of the nutrition of the flap until it becomes anchored in its new position and vitalized by a new blood supply.

Impermeable strictures of the middle third of the esophagus are not amenable to treatment by any means at present known, and the patient will have to be satisfied with a gastrostomy, unil transthoracic esophagotomy has been fully developed. J. W. Murphy and Samuel Iglauer have done an internal esophagotomy, the peroral esophagoscopist using the transillumination of the light of the retrograde esophagoscopist as a guide for incision. The patient in this instance did not survive, but success seems possible. Esophagoplication as done by Willy Meyer and others will ameliorate the patient's condition.

In case of impermeable stricture of the lower third the patient can be cured by an operation by the Brenneman method. The general surgeon makes a new opening into the stomach, above the gastrostomic opening, and as high up as possible. The surgeon then inserts his finger into the esophagus up to the point of stricture while the esophagoscopist, working from above, inserts his esophagoscope down to the stricture. Under these circumstances the surgeon can feel the end of the esophagoscope with the finger and is reasonably safe in cutting through into the lumen of the esophagoscope. A soft rubber stomach tube is then passed down by the esophagoscopist, and seized by the surgeon from below or vice versa. This stomach tube is left in situ for a few days and is replaced by attaching with stitches a freshly sterilized one to the old one, which serves to pull the fresh one down into place. Tubes must be used for three or four weeks or longer until the inner surface of the divided stricture is epithelialized. Then bouginage *per tubam* must be used to maintain the opening. In the author's case of this kind a very promising result failed of ultimate cure because of neglect of the patient to return regularly for bouginage. The really difficult part, the esophagotomy done by Dr. R. E. Brenneman, was an unqualified success.

Intubation of the esophagus has been very successful in the hands of Guisez, whose excellent soft rubber tube for the purpose is illustrated in connection with esophageal intubation. (q. v.) Brünings uses a urethral bougie passed with a stilette having a thread, on which travels a nut, which thus makes an adjustable shoulder preventing the stilette reaching the extreme end of the bougie. A hole is burned with a hot wire in the proximal end of the bougie for the insertion of a silk thread for the withdrawal The bougies are allowed to remain *in situ* about an hour.

CHAPTER XXXIII.

Diseases of the Esophagus.—Continued.

Diverticulum of the Esophagus.

Diverticula have been classified, according to their supposed etiology, into traction and pulsion diverticula. The traction variety is situated usually within the thorax and is due to the adherence of cicatricial tissue; the pulsion diverticulum is situated in the neck but may extend to the upper thoracic aperture.

Traction diverticulum of the esophagus is a rare condition and still more rare is its endoscopic discovery, because it usually causes no symptoms.

The etiology of traction diverticula is very concisely stated by Arthur Keith, as follows: "1. A localized adhesion of the esophagus to the surrounding part, usually due to inflammation of one of the bronchial glands. 2. Traction of this adhesion which occurs during coughing, deep inspiration and deglutition. In these acts the trachea and the esophagus move independently and elongate the adhesion formed between them with the result that traction diverticula of the esophagus are formed."

Traction diverticula are very much less likely to be discovered than pulsion diverticula because they are, as a rule, much less in depth and constitute really a localized one-sided enlargement of the tube, scarcely amounting to a true pouch. Unless the esophagoscope is kept moving laterally from one side to the other, they may easily escape discovery in the folds of mucosa, unless a very large esophagoscope be used, so as to dilate the esophagus nearly to a full normal lumen. Once the diverticulum is found, unlike in pulsion diverticulum, the sub-diverticular lumen is easily found and followed, because it gapes on inspiration and it is not slit-like, because there is not the same subjacent orbicular muscular contraction, nor is there resistance to movement of the esophagoscope in any direction. In some instances lateral movements of the tube will discover that the esophagus is adherent to a peri-esophageal mass. The mucosal appearances may be the same as in pulsion diverticulum. The author has seen but one case which was as follows:

A man of 48 years was referred by Dr. MacCandless for choking on swallowing, which symptom was of two months' duration. There was profuse and foul expectoration. The left vocal cord was paralyzed, and the left arytenoid was atrophied. Bronchoscopy showed a mass of granulation tissue in the left bronchus and a traction diverticulum in the esophagus with a mass of granulation tissue on the border of an ulcer through which air leaked into the esophagus when the patient coughed. The diverticulum consisted of a pouch-like dilatation of the anterior wall of the esophagus above the crossing of the left bronchus. There was no stenosis below the diverticulum. No spasm was apparent at esophagoscopy, and the esophagoscope of full adult size could be introduced all the way to the stomach. A specimen of the granuloma was removed through the esophagoscope. Milk was found bronchoscopically in the bronchi after swallowing. The patient died of exhaustion three months later at his home. Autopsy was not permitted. Evidently the symptoms were produced by leakage of food into the bronchi. Examination of the removed tissue by Dr. Ralph Duffy showed it to be tuberculous. There is no available treatment for traction diverticula. Fortunately they rarely require treatment, because they rarely produce symptoms.

Pulsion Diverticulum of the Esophagus.

Pulsion diverticula of the esophagus are usually small and may not be larger than 1 or 2 cubic cm. capacity. On the other hand, they may be quite large and may bulge out the neck like a large and low goitre, especially when filled with food. See Fig. 425. They may be centrally located behind the cervical esophagus, but usually their bulk is to one side, more often the left side.

Etiology. Pulsion diverticulum is essentially a hernial sac caused by pressure of the food bolus at a point where the wall is weakly supported, as will be understood from the schema, Fig. 422. The firm contraction of the cricopharyngeus may be realized by the firmness with which the cricoid cartilage is pulled backward against the vertebral column, as is familiar to every esophagoscopist, and as shown graphically in Fig. 423. Zenker recognized the effect of pressure in the causation of pulsion diverticulum, but it remained for Killian to demonstrate the anatomically weak point in the support of the wall and the spasmodic resistance ahead of the bolus. Congenital diverticula have been reported. It might be supposed that an especially weak wall might exist from birth were it not for the fact that the greatest of all predisposing factors seems to be age. Pressure diverticula are never seen in young people, very rarely before middle life. Possibly crude boluses from imperfect mastication by defective teeth may contribute, but considering the rarity of diverticula and the general prevalence of imperfect mastication this alone could not be causative. Sir Felix Semon reports a very interesting case of diverticulum of the esophagus occurring in conjunction with a congenitally deformed larynx. Undoubtedly cicatricial stenosis, in fact,

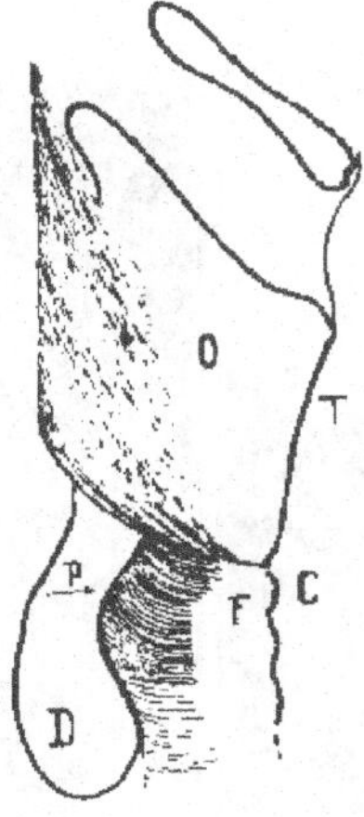

FIG. 422.—Schema illustrative of the etiology of pressure diverticula. O, oblique fibers of the cricopharyngeus attached to the thyroid cartilage, T. The fundiform fibers, F, encircle the mouth of the esophagus. Between the two sets of fibers is a gap in the support of the esophageal wall, through which the wall herniates owing to the pressure of food propelled by the oblique fibers, O, advance of the bolus being resisted by spasmodic contraction of the orbicular fibers, F.

any sort of stenosis below the level of the inferior constrictors, may, in rare instances, contribute to the formation of a diverticulum. Some of the author's cases of diverticulum have been somewhat cicatricial at the sub-diverticular orifice. This, of course, in a long-standing case, might easily have resulted from erosion and ulceration following the esophagitis due to stagnation. Undoubtedly after a diverticulum has developed to a certain degree there exists "a vicious circle," that is the food in the pendulous portion presses on the subdiverticular portion of the esophagus and thus increases the difficulty of swallowing, and consequently increases stenosis, with consequent increased pressure upon the pouch. From excessive activity the oblique fibers may hypertrophy. It is thus clear that all that is needed is to get a start; later, even though the causes which originally started the trouble should disappear, the diverticulum will perpetuate itself and continue to increase in size. (Fig. 424 and 425).

Prognosis. Untreated pressure diverticula because of the above mentioned "vicious circle" probably always increase steadily in size and consequently in distressing symptoms. This is shown in the two radio-

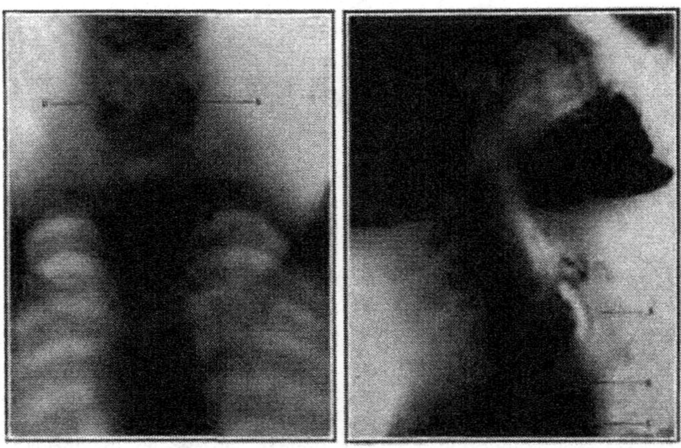

Fig. 423.—Bismuth radiograph illustrating normal swallowing. The bismuth mixture is seen in the pyriform sinuses, D, E. At A and C is seen the bismuth mixture in process of swallowing while the cricoid cartilage is in close contact with the posterior pharyngoesophageal wall.

graphs of one of the author's patients who declined operation. (Figs. 424 and 425). The history of this case follows:

Male, aged 46 years, referred to the author by Dr. T. D. Davis. Patient stated that trouble in swallowing and spitting up of food began suddenly after he "felt something give way" during a violent attack of coughing. Cough had persisted since. Loss of weight six pounds. Esophagoscopy showed a small pouch extending outward slightly to the left. The cricopharyngeal fold was quite acutely inflammatory and the pouch showed chronic esophagitis. The subdiverticular opening was a narrow slit. It admitted a 7 mm. esophagoscope readily, but the adult size (10 mm.) fitted very tightly. Chronic laryngitis was manifest but laryngeal motility was normal. The patient declined operation. Four years later he was found under the care of Dr. Marks. Operation and esophagoscopy were both declined by the patient, but Dr. Marks very kindly had the radiograph, Fig. 425, made by Dr. George C. Johnston. The prognosis of radical operation will depend partly upon the condition of the patient. If feeble from malnutrition and advanced age the prognosis is more grave than in a vigorous person of middle age. Stettin collected statistics of sixty radically operated cases with ten deaths (16.6

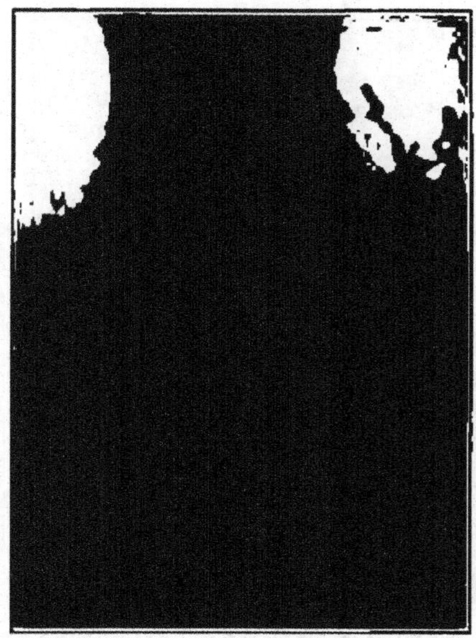

Fig. [illegible].—Pulsion diverticulum filled with bismuth mixture in a man aged [illegible] years. (Radiographed by Dr. Russell H. Boggs. Author's case.)

per cent). As the duration of the operation is lessened by one-half by esophagoscopic aid, the mortality in the future will be diminished, especially in the aged and feeble.

Symptoms. The chief symptoms are cough, regurgitation of food, gurgling sound and subjective sensation on swallowing, a peculiar sour odor to the breath, and difficulty of swallowing. Boyce's sign can usually be elicited immediately after swallowing. It consists in a gurgling sound produced by pressure of the hand on the side of the neck. A fresh swallowing movement without food or water is needed for each test.

The sound is probably made by forcing out of air and bubbles of secretion from the sac. All symptoms are valueless diagnostically but they are urgent indications for esophagoscopy.

Diagnosis. A radiograph is very valuable and should always be made, but to rely upon it to the exclusion of esophagoscopy is to take a chance of serious or fatal error as mentioned in connection with spasmodic and organic stenoses and malignancy. (See also Fig. 415.) Various blind methods have been brought forward, with a great deal of

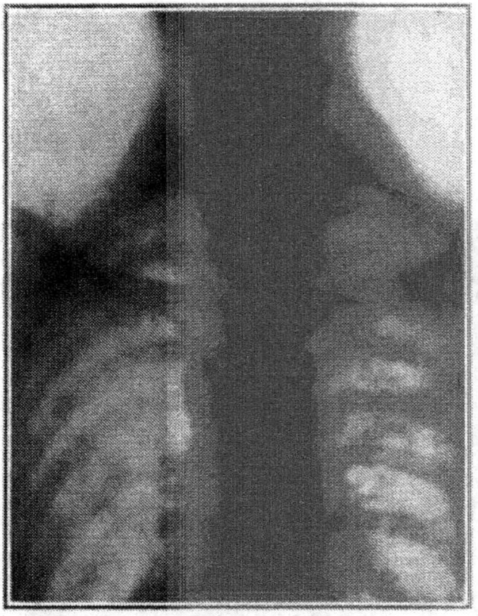

Fig. 425.—Same patient as in Fig. 424, four years later, the patient having declined operation. The great increase in size is usual in untreated cases. (Radiograph made by Dr. George C. Johnston. Author's case.)

enthusiasm, for the diagnosis of esophageal diverticulum. They are very ingenious and would be perfectly justifiable in the days when esophagoscopy was crude or unavailable. It is hard to eradicate traditions in medicine, and text books are still being published stating that the first step in the diagnosis of diverticulum is to pass a sound; and then follow descriptions of various other blind methods in groping for a frequently erroneous diagnosis. These are all wrong. They annoy the patient and are inconclusive. The published statement of one surgeon that he made an erroneous diagnosis of carcinoma of the esophagus and did a gastrostomy in a case of diverticulum in which he "decided to dispense with the esophagoscope because he did not wish to subject the patient to the risk and great annoyance" leads one to suppose that the surgeon did not have available the services of a skilled esophagoscopist, or possibly he had only seen the crude work of the early days. There is neither risk nor great annoyance connected with modern esophagoscopy. The first step in the diagnosis should be a radiograph and the next step should be esophagoscopy. The diagnosis will then be made positively or negatively with a certainty that will render further diagnostic procedures superfluous. As a large quantity of bismuth is required for

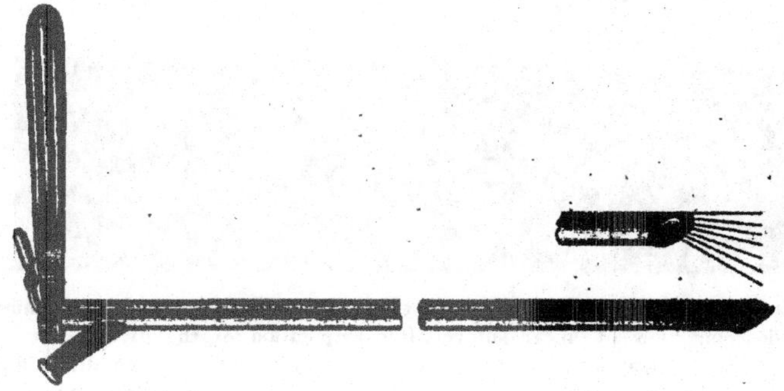

FIG. 426.—The author's esophagoscope with slanted end, facilitating introduction in any case and especially useful in entering the subdiverticular opening in cases of diverticulum. The drainage canal facilitates aspiration of secretions without interruption of the work. Though similar to the bronchoscope, this esophagoscope differs in having no lateral openings, and in the branch tube entering an auxiliary drainage canal ending at the tube mouth, like the regular esophagoscope which it has superseded. The lip is also useful in foreign body work.

radiography of a large diverticulum or in the case of dilatation bismuth subcarbonate should always be used rather than the subnitrate. Zirconium oxide, though somewhat expensive, is strictly non poisonous. As pointed out by Kahler, if there is reason to suspect a tracheoesophageal fistula the swallowing of bismuth emulsion had better be avoided. In one such case a radiographic picture was obtained of the entire tracheobronchial tree filled with bismuth which had found its way in through such a fistula. Malignant, spasmodic, cicatricial and compressive stenoses are to be excluded by the esophagoscopic appearances Aneurysm is to be excluded by radiography and fluoroscopy.

Esophagoscopy in cases of suspected diverticulum. Until a number of cases have been explored the esophagoscopist will find some difficulty in locating the subdiverticular esophageal opening. The insertion of the tube into the pouch is usually very easy. Its running into a blind end or sort of pocket beyond which it will not go, and in the bottom of which there is no opening, is almost diagnostic of pressure diverticulum. If in addition to this on withdrawing the esophagoscope a little distance, we are able to find on the anterior wall, a narrowed, usually slit-like opening into the lower esophagus, and we are able to enter this opening with either a very small tube or a probe, which passes down readily, the diagnosis is absolute. The author uses the slanted-end esophagoscope (Fig. 426) to enter this slit and explore the subdiverticular esophagus. True malignancy may exist below, and this the author has seen

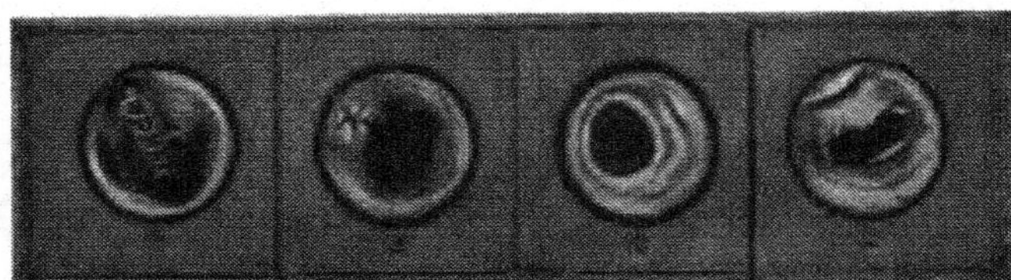

FIG. 427.—Esophagoscopic views in cases of diverticulum. Patient recumbent. A, endoscopic view of linear suture after amputation of the diverticulum. B, after suture by ligation and transfixation in another case. Crayon drawings by the author, after operation by Dr. Otto C. Gaub. C, view looking into pouch after partial withdrawal of the esophagoscope in a man aged 67 years. Slit-like orifice of subdiverticular esophagus seen in upper right quadrant. D, view of diverticular orifice in case of a woman of 58 years of age. Subdiverticular orifice overhung by a fold in upper left quadrant. The ledge between the orifice and the diverticular opening, supported by the orbicular fibers of the cricopharyngeus, is cicatricial.

in one case, though, in his opinion, the development of malignancy was secondary to the diverticulum and to the subsequent pathologic changes; because ordinarily malignancy does not last sufficiently long for a diverticulum to develop from malignant stenosis. It is quite characteristic of high diverticula due to pressure that the pouch seems to be the continuation of the pharynx, and it is only with the most minute care and skillful work that the subdiverticular opening can be found. Great care must be used not to perforate the bottom of the pouch and not to use any pressure upon it. When the esophagoscopist finds that the tube has entered a blind cavity and cannot be introduced further, he should withdraw the tube while keeping a close watch on the anterior wall. Careful search on this wall will discover an opening, sometimes slit-like (C, D, Fig.

427) sometimes very small, rarely stellate, and very frequently overhung by a somewhat projecting fold. Some esophagoscopists have failed to find the opening and have advised the swallowing of a thread with which to guide the esophagoscope. Such an expedient is quite unnecessary though there is no objection to its use other than the delay and the annoyance for twenty-four hours or longer when, instead, but a few minutes of esophagoscopy should suffice. The subdiverticular opening is apt to gape during swallowing. Therefore, it is often advantageous to get the patient to make the swallowing movement if he can. This is one of the advantages in making the examination without general anesthesia. The best way of conducting these examinations is to use the esophageal speculum Fig. 21, and after having discovered what seems to be the cleft, to insert a child's size of the esophagoscope with a slanted end, Fig. 426, through the speculum. When it is certain that we really have discovered the subdiverticular opening, the slanted-end esophagoscope can usually be entered without difficulty and without the speculum, provided there is no stricture. If there is a stricture, it should be divulsed with one of the divulsors previously mentioned, or an adult esophagoscope (Fig. 426) can be forced into it, using the slanted end as an entering wedge. The square-ended esophagoscope, which is so safe and popular for general use, is here at a disadvantage because of the difficulty of insertion into the cleft-like orifice along the anterior wall of the orifice of the diverticulum. One would suppose from the name diverticulum, that in passing down the esophagus one would notice a little side opening leading off into the pouch. This, however, is far from the case. Usually in pharyngeal diverticulum, the whole hypopharynx ends in a blind sac. The upper orifice of the diverticulum is seemingly just simply the entire pharynx. The subdiverticular esophageal opening, on the contrary, is a minute cleft up above the bottom of the diverticulum, and usually on the anterior wall of the diverticulum, often close against the cricoid cartilage. The ledge between the orifice of the diverticulum and the subdiverticular orifice of the esophagus is supported by the orbicular fibers of the cricopharyngeus (often hypertrophied), whose contraction ahead of the downward propelled bolus has been the prime factor in the production of the hernia known as diverticulum. It is not so much this ledge that interferes with exposing the subdiverticular orifice as it is the pressure of the cricoid cartilage which pushes the esophagoscope backward and outward into the large and unobstructed diverticular orifice. It requires firm anterior pressure with the tube mouth to expose any orifice of the subdiverticular lumen and then it will be found to be the merest slit and not a gaping orifice.

In the very early stages of diverticulum, there is sometimes not a true pouch. In such instances, the subdiverticular opening is easy to find. The color of the mucosa lining a diverticulum may be reddish or it may be macerated with a grayish color almost resembling an exudate. That it is not a true exudate is manifest by the impossibility of removing it, and it seems to be simply macerated epithelial cells furred up but not detached. In other cases the diverticulum is rather paler than usual. and there being no pasty exudate on the surface, minute vessels are plainly visible in every direction. There may be superficial erosions and patches of inflammation. Cicatrices were noted by the author in one case. The depth of a pulsion diverticulum may be from one to ten

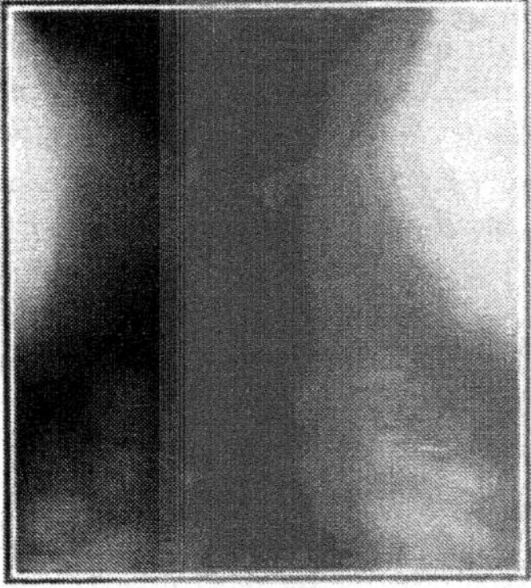

Fig. 428.—Beginning recurrence of esophageal diverticulum in a man aged 53 years, within a year after removal by a very skillful surgeon.

centimeters, though usually they are not over 4 centimeters in depth, as determined esophagoscopically, which means in a more or less collapsed state. When full of food, they are, of course, dilated to a very much greater extent. In one of the author's cases the diverticulum filled with air every time the patient swallowed without food or drink. Its normal state seemed to be air dilatation. The same condition was suspected in other cases but not proven.

Recurrence of esophageal diverticulum after operation. Pulsion diverticulum has been known to recur after thorough removal by the most skilful surgeons; and surgeons who have no record of recurrences possibly have not had opportunities of following their cases. In a case esophagoscoped for the exclusion of malignancy by the author in consultation with Dr. George W. Crile and Dr. George E. Brewer there was a large diverticulum which had formed during the twelve years following a resection of the first diverticulum by Dr. Morris Richardson, whose operation was, of course, thorough and complete, and had given perfect relief for years. The recurrence brought back all of the old symptoms. The patient recovered absolutely normal swallowing after a very skilful operation by Dr. Crile, and now, at the end of four years, is swallowing normally without signs of recurrence.

Recurrences are doubtless due to the same causes as produced the original diverticulum. The author has thought that, as the original cause is the weak point in the support of the esophageal wall, a leakage after operation, with consequent localized inflammation, far from being undesirable, might be a great advantage in bulwarking the weakly supported area of the wall, which is necessarily right at the point of amputation of the sac. As yet, the number of cases that have been followed have been too small to yield any data. One case observed by the author tends to confirm this theoretical conclusion. Figure 428 shows a beginning recurrence within a year after thorough removal by a very skilful surgeon. There was no leakage after the operation.

Treatment of pulsion diverticulum. No endoscopic treatment is of any avail in esophageal diverticulum, so far as the removal of redundancy is concerned. If the diverticulum is very small, the lower opening may be freely dilated. This accomplished a cure in one case of the author, but the diverticulum was very small. There was no organic stricture, only spastic stenosis. In another case the subdiverticular orifice was small and cicatricial. Divulsion resulted in relief of the symptoms, but the diverticulum remained. Both cases had refused external operation. When there is any degree of redundancy present, in the author's opinion, it is very much better to have an external operation done by the general surgeon. The author has devised an operation where, by the use of the esophageal speculum, Fig. 21, the bottom of the sac may be grasped by forceps and drawn in, encircled by a ligature and the end cut off and sealed over with a touch of tincture of iodine, about half strength. As yet no suitable case for this operation has come under the author's observation. Glottic spasm resulted every time traction was made, in the two cases tested. In the event of radical operation being contra-indicated because of advanced age or of organic disease present in quite a proportion of cases, the best palliative treatment is to keep down the chronic inflammatory state by preventing the entrance of food, or by evacuating and cleansing the sac. The best method of doing this is that of Starck as follows:

"The aim should be to prevent food from getting into the diverticulum, and, if it does, to clear it out. This can sometimes be accomplished by reclining in a certain position, by stooping over or by pressure on the throat from without or other maneuver. This should be studied until some measure is found which will relieve. If nothing of the kind can be discovered, then the diverticulum tube must be used. It may be necessary during the meal, as the filling of the diverticulum may com-

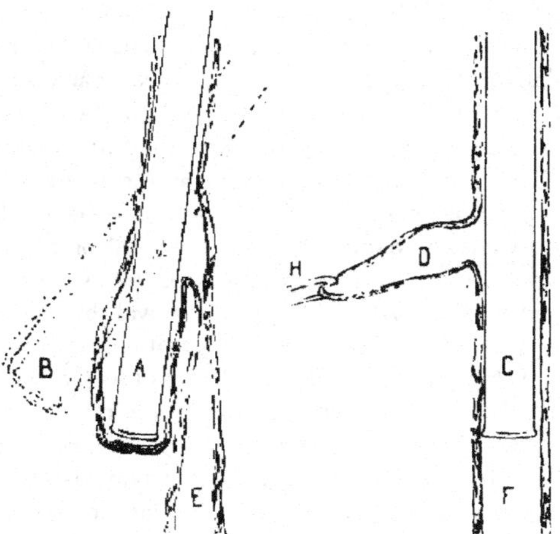

FIG. 429.—Schematic representation of esophagoscopic aid in the excision of a diverticulum. At A the esophagoscope is represented in the bottom of the pouch after the surgeon has cut down to where he can feel the esophagoscope. Then the esophagoscopist causes the pouch to protrude as shown by the dotted line at B. After the surgeon has dissected the sack entirely loose from its surroundings, traction is made upon the sack as shown at H and the esophagoscope is inserted down the lumen of the esophagus as shown at C. The esophagoscope now occupies the lumen which the patient will need for swallowing. It only remains for the surgeon to remove the redundancy, without risk of removing any of the normal wall.

press the esophagus so that its lumen is obstructed; in any event the toilet of the diverticulum should follow the meal. Nearly every patient has his own method of eating to prevent annoyance from the food getting into the diverticulum; one can swallow better when he looks at the ceiling, another when he bends his head to the right or left, another as he stoops his body forward, or presses on the trachea from the front or the side or from behind the sternocleidomastoid muscle. Neukirch had a patient who could swallow best when he reclined, lying on his right side. The various postures should be tried until the one giving the most relief is discovered."

The excision of a diverticulum in the neck, one would suppose from the description in the text books to be an exceedingly easy procedure, and so it may be in the case of a large diverticulum in an emaciated long-necked person. On the contrary with a short thick-necked individual and a small diverticulum, it may be exceedingly difficult; so much so that it has happened to a number of very competent surgeons that after the operation the diverticulum remained as before. If a diverticulum at operation were full of a solid as it is when the radiograph is taken, finding it would be easy, but the sac is extremely elastic and when empty, as it must be for operation, it shrinks up to small dimensions. It lies back of, or close alongside the esophagus, and may be indistinguishable from a fold of the esophageal wall, and it may be on the opposite side of the neck at the time it is sought. Free dissection of the esophagus clear from all surrounding structures and bringing it out for examination as one would an intestine is, of course, impossible. All of these considerations render the operation as ordinarily done a lengthy and a tedious one that is quite an ordeal for old debilitated patients. The duration of the operation is lessened by a half or two-thirds and the difficulties for the surgeon are greatly diminished if he have the cooperation of an esophagoscopist as originally proposed by Dr. Otto C. Gaub. A description of the esophagoscopist's part of Dr. Gaub's operation is all that is within the province of this book. This will be fully understood by reference to the schema, Fig. 429. In these operations it is, of course, absolutely necessary that the surgeon have his sterile tables, nurses and assistants entirely independent of the esophagoscopist who has his sterile organization at the head of the table with the anesthetist. Two cases in which the author thus assisted Dr. Gaub may be cited.

Mrs. D., aged 58 years, referred by Dr. R. W. Fisher, for increasing difficulty in swallowing solids. Foul breath and a cough were annoying at times. Had "ulcerated sore throat" four years before. Swallowing symptoms were of one year's duration. No regurgitation. Examination with the esophageal speculum (Fig. 21), without anesthesia, general or local, showed a small diverticulum to the left side. Withdrawal revealed the orifice of the subdiverticular esophagus anteriorly to the right covered with a fold. The ridge between this orifice and the diverticular orifice was cicatricial (D, Fig. 427). The subdiverticular orifice was easily entered with the beak of the slanted-end esophagoscope (Fig. 426) but would not permit the entire end to enter readily. Enough pressure was used to stretch the cicatricially contracted orifice and permit the esophagoscope to enter freely. At esophagoscopy, seventeen days later, without anesthesia, the esophagoscope entered readily without any sign of recurrence of stenosis. Radiography by Dr. George C. Johnston showed the diverticulum (Fig. 430). External operation was quickly and skillfully done by the Otto C. Gaub method in which the esophagoscopist with esophagoscope inserted through the mouth into the bottom of the pouch presents the sac in the wound to the surgeon after the latter has dissected externally down to the esophagus (Fig. 429). After

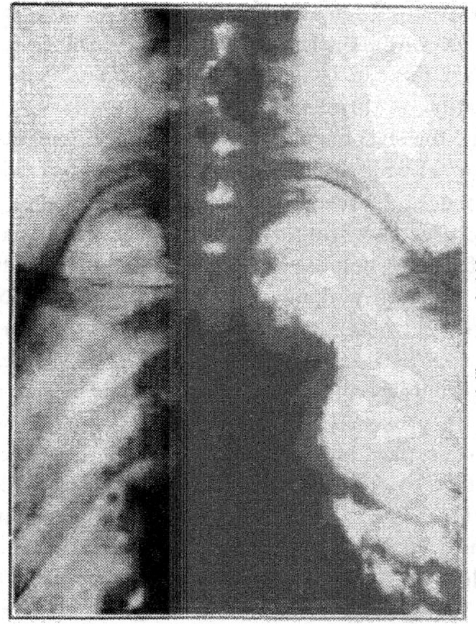

Fig. 430.—Radiograph by Dr. George C. Johnston showing diverticulum in case of a woman, aged 58 years. Diverticulum afterwards removed by the Otto C. Gaub method.

Dr. Gaub had laid bare the esophagus by external dissection he asked the author to insert the esophagoscope and present the pouch in the wound. When Dr. Gaub had seized the bottom of the sac with forceps and made traction the esophagoscope was withdrawn to the hypopharynx and the orifice of the diverticulum disappeared while the subdiverticular orifice opened up ahead of the tube-mouth in full lumen. Inserting the esophagoscope in this lumen as far as the crossing of the left bronchus the surgeon amputated the redundancy while the esophagoscope indicated the normal lumen. The neck of the sac was ligated and transfixed.

When the esophagoscope was withdrawn a neat puckered spot of suture was seen by the author who made the sketch, B. Fig. 427. The stump externally was lightly touched with pure carbolic acid, and supporting sutures were used. Feeding was by catheter inserted at esophagoscopy. Primary union and prompt recovery followed, and one year later the patient was still swallowing perfectly.

Remarks. In this case Dr. Gaub made traction on the bottom of the sac with forceps and the author withdrew his esophagoscope to the

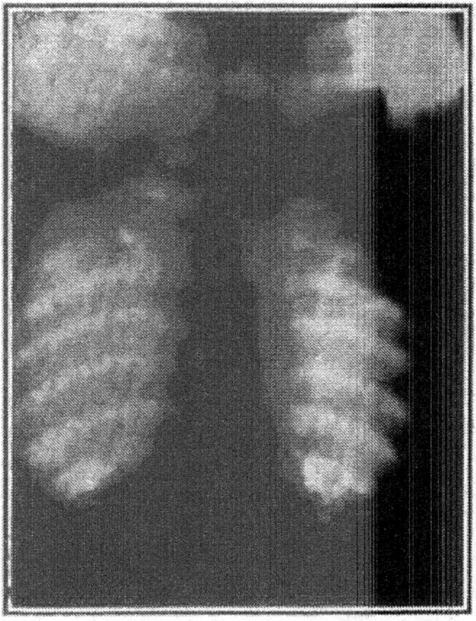

FIG. 431.—Radiograph by Dr. Pancoast of Philadelphia, showing a diverticulum in a man of 67 years. Diverticulum removed by the Otto C. Gaub method.

hypopharynx and noted that the traction by Dr. Gaub caused the subdiverticular esophagus to gape widely, bringing it into a straight line with the esophagus below. This manipulation demonstrated clearly that the difficulties in swallowing and in finding the subdiverticular orifice at diagnostic esophagoscopy are largely concerned with the pouch and its position, and not alone with the spasm of the orbicular fibers of the cricopharyngeus.

Mr. F., aged 67 years, was referred by Dr. David Riesman and Dr. Walter J. Freeman of Philadelphia. They had made the diagnosis of diverticulum. Severe cough, purulent expectoration and difficulty in swallowing had made the patient's life miserable for the past year. Regurgitation and foul breath had been noticed for six months. Examination with the esophageal speculum, using a little 8 percent cocaine solution to the laryngopharynx, showed a large pouch confirming the radiograph by Dr. Henry K. Pancoast, Fig. 431. The subdiverticular orifice (C, Fig. 427) was easily entered with the slanted-end esophagoscope, Fig. 426. There were no signs of cicatrices or inflammatory processes. The orifice of the pouch just as the esophagoscope emerged from it was circular in outline and rolled over at the margins (C, Fig. 427). The Gaub operation with esophagoscopic aid was done by Dr. Gaub, the steps being the same as in the preceding case, and the same observation

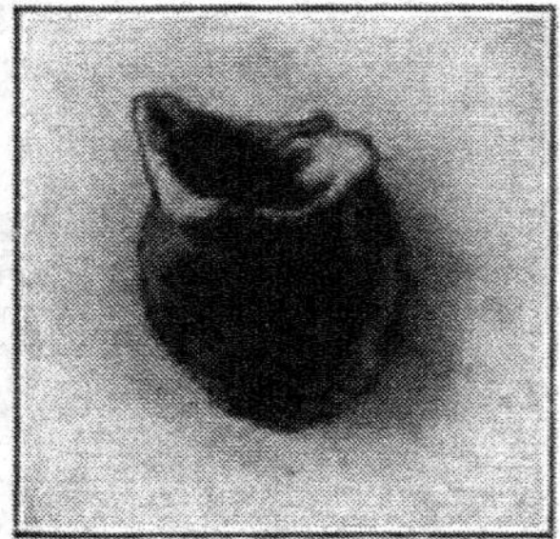

Fig. 432.—Pulsion diverticulum of the esophagus removed from a man aged 67 years, by Dr. Otto C. Gaub.

as to opening up of the subdiverticular esophageal lumen was made as in the preceding case. The pouch after removal is shown in Fig. 432. The recovery was rather tedious. Leakage of about one-third of swallowed liquids gradually improved as the fistula closed. Healing was complete and swallowing perfect in about four weeks, the patient returning to Philadelphia six weeks after operation.

Remarks. This patient was regarded by Dr. J. M. McKelvy before operation as an unfavorable surgical subject because of feebleness, advanced age, impaired vessels, and chronic purulent bronchitis. The post operative condition verified the opinion: and it was only by the attentive after care of Dr. Gaub and Dr. McKelvy that the patient made such an excellent recovery. Intratracheal insufflation anesthesia with the Elsberg apparatus was used in both the foregoing cases. The insufflation method not only removes the anesthetist from the operator's way, and avoids infective risks, but also insures safety of respiration and a quiet peaceful anesthesia, in spite of tracheal pressure from the esophagoscope or glottic spasm from the surgeon's dissection.

After-care. As the primary cause of the diverticulum was high pressure of swallowed food and drink held back by the spasm of the orbicular fibers of the cricopharyngeus at the bottom of the hypopharynx, naturally it follows that swallowing will put great strain on the stitches. For this reason it is wise to place a feeding catheter of small size in the esophagus at the time of operation, preferably through the esophageal speculum. If put in afterward it may catch at the point of suture. Should leakage start and the leakage through the neck wound be so great that enough food and water do not reach the stomach, fluid food can be carried safely past the wound by feeding through the catheter. If this be done an abundance of sterile water must be drunk in addition in order to flush out the wound. Usually by this time granulations afford some protection against serious infection and the channels to the mediastinum are sealed. The wound, in case of leakage, is already infected with the esophageal and buccal organisms, but to these the patient is more or less immune. The water must be sterile to insure exclusion of virulent infections from without. If offensive odor develops, frequent irrigation by swallowing sterile water will quickly cause it to disappear. Mr. Walter Howarth made the excellent suggestion, apropos of the case of Mr. F., that hydrogen peroxid be added to the water. In order to determine the amount of fluid that goes into the stomach, the method of Dr. Otto C. Gaub is useful. When the patient swallows water the leakage is caught in a curved pan held at the external wound, and the quantity is measured. Subtraction of this from the total quantity swallowed necessarily gives the amount that went to the stomach. As oral sepsis is one of the greatest dangers, cleanliness of the mouth must be insured by brushing the teeth every few hours, and by the rinsing of the mouth with alcohol 1 part to 5 of water. After operation it is wise for the surgeon to have a bismuth radiograph taken and to have an esophagoscopy, both as a matter of record and to make sure that everything is anatomically as well as functionally normal in the esophagus.

CHAPTER XXXIV.

Diseases of the Esophagus.—Continued.

PARALYSIS OF THE ESOPHAGUS.

Paralysis of the esophagus may be motor or sensory.—Motor paralysis of the esophagus is perhaps more frequently seen as a glosso-labio-pharyngeal paralysis of either toxic origin as in diphtheria, or of central origin. In any case, swallowing is apt to be seriously interfered with, and, strange to say, esophageal drainage is interfered with also. This is manifest by the filling of the pyriform sinuses with secretion (author's sign of esophageal stenosis) until the secretion overflows into the larynx, just as in an esophagus occluded by cancer or organic stricture. This is apparent on indirect as well as direct examination. It is a remarkable thing that though the normal esophagus can swallow "up hill" with ease, food, either liquid or solid, will not go down the paralyzed esophagus by gravity alone. The act of deglutition is a purely muscular process and the food is forced down by coordinate muscular activity. Normally the esophagus empties itself promptly of everything which is put into it. It abhors the presence of anything except secretions, and even secretions are promptly gotten rid of in a state of health. Phylogenetically, the erect posture was developed late, therefore, there has been no opportunity for the development of deglutition with the assistance of gravity. Muscular action is depended upon entirely. Therefore, it is well to mention here again what was stated in the first volume (Bib. 269): namely, that the first symptom of paralysis or paresis of the esophagus is inability to swallow. That *paralysis of sensation* in the esophagus may result in inability to swallow because of the lack of the necessary serial reflex impulse is proven by the following case referred to the author for esophagoscopy by Drs. E. B. Howarth and Robert Milligan. A man of forty-eight years had difficulty in swallowing for eight weeks, culminating in absolute inability to swallow. On indirect laryngoscopy laryngeal motility was found to be perfect. The pyriform sinuses were full of secretion. A bronchoscope was passed to the bifurcation of the trachea without anesthesia, general or local, and there was not the slightest sign of a cough reflex. Esophagoscopy showed presence of cricopharyngeal and hiatal contractions, though very weak and unlike normal spasmodic resistance to the advance of the esophagoscope. A 10 mm. x 53 cm. esophagoscope passed readily into the stomach. There was no gagging, retching or attempted vomiting. The author made a diagnosis of sensory paralysis, with consequent absence of the normal serial deglutitory reflex, and turned the case over to Dr. C. C. Wholey for neurologic analysis and treatment. The following is Dr. Wholey's report:

"Patient's mental condition is good, but he shows some anxiety regarding his condition. There is noticeable dilatation of the venules over cheeks. E. J.'s (biceps), W. J.'s, and muscle tap (biceps) all plus and equal on both sides. K. J.'s (taken in bed) absent—also absent when sitting. Plantars lively. No Babinski. No Oppenheim. Tongue protrudes slightly to the left. *Eyes.* Pupils—Rt.—4 x 4, irregular (wider below.) Lft. 3½ x 3½, irregular (wider above). Both pupils react promptly to light with fair excursion; both react to accommodation. Patient shows slight Rhombergism; is able to pucker lips and protrude tongue. Abdominal reflex absent. Cremasteric present but slow in response. *Sensation*: Patient's sensation to touch, heat and cold normal over entire body, but sensation for pain is diminished from the hips to soles of feet. Increasing analgesia as soles of feet are approached, being very marked in soles of feet. For the last one and a half to two years patient has complained of sensation of pins and needles in thighs, of impairment of the sense of taste, of anorexia from time to time during the past few months, and obstinate constipation (loss of sensation in rectum). Desire has been present, but patient has been impotent sexually during the past 1½ years. Patient says he has been unaware of any desire to urinate or to defecate during the past month; simply goes mechanically. Patient coughs a great deal, brings up thick mucous, but his expelling power seemed to be largely from the diaphragm and abdominal muscles. Examination of urine is negative, except for the presence of a reducing agent present in small amount and found to be glucose. No T. B. found in sputum. Blood picture is negative, except for very slight leucocytosis. Wassermann negative. The spinal fluid shows 5½ lymphocytes per cmm. Globulin positive. Wassermann negative. Radiographer after examination of lumbar region reports osteo-arthritis of vertebrae. Radiograms of lumbar and cervical regions show numerous small spicules projecting from bodies, and lateral processes of vertebrae.

During the week subsequent to above examination, patient had several periods during which he developed Cheyne-Stokes respiration, and seemed in imminent danger of dying. Mercurial inunctions have been given after above examination, and during the week subsequent to the attacks, patient has become much better, coughing much less, respiration easier and there is less difficulty in taking the stomach tube. Sensation over thighs and legs more acute. Area about rectum and over buttocks supplied by the sacral nerves remains without any sensation for pressure or pain. Radiogram shows enteroliths in rectum. *Diagnosis.* The case presents the characteristics of a disseminated myelitis, located mainly in the lumbar and cervical regions. It is apparently due to pressure and irritation of the spinal nerves and their root zones (especially sensory) by bony inflammatory products, and to the same pressure upon the medulla, affecting the vagus noticeably after the union of its sensory and motor bundles. It is possible that the same underlying cause has brought about both the myelitis and the osteo-arthritis, and in view of the fact of the patient's improving so noticeably since being upon mercury, I should regard syphilis as the causative agent. The affection is largely sensory in character and the parallelism between the symptoms affecting the centers in the medulla (deglutition, coughing, respiration, etc.) and those in the lumbar region (sacral segments), is very striking, it being observable that only voluntary activity is possible, such as starting the act of deglutition or of micturition, but all those reflexes depending upon sensory stimulation are either abolished or greatly crippled." The following is an illustrative case of esophageal *motor paralysis*:

Nellie S., aged 21 years, referred by Dr. J. E. Gross for gradually increasing difficulty in swallowing. Difficulty in speech had lasted three weeks. There was no nausea, no regurgitation of food, but on attempting to swallow, choking and coughing promptly followed and the food came back immediately. The patient had not been able to swallow liquid for the last four days, and was in an extremely serious state of water hunger. On examination, the movement of the palate was defective, but there was a slight movement of irregular character. Pus was streaming down from the sinuses posteriorly. The pyriform sinuses were full to overflowing with secretion. The movements of the tongue were sluggish. Enunciation was very imperfect and difficult to understand. The patient was languid, extremely feeble and emaciated. Esophagoscopy caused no inconvenience after draining out all of the fluid in the pharynx. The esophageal mucosa was exceedingly pale, and no sign of cricopharyngeal contraction was apparent. The intra-thoracic portion was enlarged by the negative pressure of inspiration rather more than usual. Hiatal contraction was about normal for a feeble person relaxed by water hunger, and examined without anesthesia. Dr. W. K. Walker, after a careful neurologic examination, reported as follows:

"The patient presents dysarthria and dysphagia, with paresis of the muscles of the lips, tongue, palate and pharynx. Closure of the eyelids is weakened. Though there is general weakness, it is not more than can be accounted for by weeks of deprivation of nourishment and fluids, through inability to swallow. There are no sensory disturbances; hand-grasp is of fair strength; gait is normal. Deep reflexes of upper extremities are normal. Knee jerks, right and left, are absent. Respiration is entirely costal and there is marked breathlessness and tachycardia after esophageal tube feeding. There is no marked weakness of the jaw muscles; neither is there involvement of the bladder or rectal muscles. The mind is clear. Diagnosis: Myasthenia gravis or asthenic bulbar palsy." The patient was given water and liquid food with a stomach tube and gained slightly in weight, but died after about two months from paralysis of respiration. Dr. Edward E. Meyer, the neurologist, under whose care she was at this time, was unable to obtain an autopsy.

Endoscopic appearances of paralysis are characteristic if the paralysis is complete. There is noted an absence of the spasmodic contraction, which usually characterizes an esophagoscopy without anesthesia. This is most noticeable at the cricoid. At the hiatus, no lessening is usually noticed in the degree of contraction, probably because these contractions are dependent largely on the diaphragmatic musculature, which may not be involved. The esophagus is apt to be quite flaccid and it is also unusually insensitive to the introduction of the tube, even though the paralysis be purely motor. If the patient has been able to take any food, particles adherent to the esophageal wall may be noted. Their absence, however, is not to be taken negatively.

Etiology. The causes of esophageal paralysis may be classed under four heads. 1. The toxic type, such as diphtheritic paralysis. 2. Purely functional paralysis, as in hysteria. 3. Peripheral paralysis as from neuritis. 4. Central paralysis is usually from a bulbar lesion, as in glosso-labio-pharyngeal paralysis. The latter condition may be luetic as may also the neuritis.

Diagnosis. The most common diagnostic error is to mistake esophageal paralysis for hysteria. When a patient is starving for food and water and complains of inability to swallow and the esophagus is seen on esophagoscopy without anesthesia to be free from spasm at the cricopharyngeus, and is patulent to a large esophagoscope, the diagnosis of hysteria must not be made until paralysis is excluded. Flaccidity may readily be mistakenly attributed to weakness from inanition. But if the possibility of paralysis is kept in mind the total absence of the normal spasmodic constriction at the cricopharyngeus when the esophagoscope is passed without anesthesia will be conclusive. Paralysis of the esophagus is practically always accompanied by other paralyses about the upper air and food passages that are distinctive and easily recognized. Difficulty of swallowing with a history of recent diphtheria should always bring esophageal paralysis to mind, and immediate esophagoscopy should be done. In paralysis of esophageal sensation, the reflexes of coughing, vomiturition and vomiting are absent or deficient at bronchoscopy and esophagoscopy, and the muscular contraction of the cricopharyngeus is feeble or absent.

Treatment. There is no form of endoscopic treatment that is of any use. Esophagoscopy is of value in determining whether or not there is any lesion in the esophageal lumen that would contraindicate the passing of the feeding tube. If there is any lesion, such as sloughing or erosion, gastrostomy should be done. In the absence of such lesions, which are rare, the patient can be nourished effectually with milk put in through the ordinary stomach tube. The treatment will then depend entirely upon the internist and the neurologist.

LUES OF THE ESOPHAGUS.

Luetic disease of the esophagus is, relatively, a rare disease, though it is not as rare as the standard literature on the subject would seem to indicate, for two reasons. 1. Prior to the days of esophagoscopy, but little was known of esophageal disease, except what happened to be found at post mortem. 2. The esophagus is rarely explored at autopsy. Prior to the days of esophagoscopy, a few diagnoses of luetic disease of the esophagus were made solely upon the fact that difficulty in swallowing disappeared upon the administration of specific treatment. Necessarily, this leaves a large possibility of error. Such cases might be spasm or compression. The esophagoscope, however, has demonstrated that luetic disease of the esophagus may show itself either as a mucous plaque, a gumma, an ulcer, or a cicatrix. In the absence of associated lesions, it is not possible to make the diagnosis on the esophagoscopic appearances alone. They must be taken along with the history, the concomitant lesions, the therapeutic test, the Wassermann test, the luetin test, the examination of tissue and a search for spirochetes. In the cicatricial form, the absence of any other cause for a cicatrix coming on late in adult life, should arouse a strong suspicion of lues. Where there is a history of difficulty in swallowing in childhood, there is always a possibility that the swallowing of some caustic, or the traumatism of a foreign body may have been overlooked, and as suggested by Mr. Tilley, the possibility of the late manifestation of congenital stenoses must be borne in mind.

Esophageal luetic stenosis, like the same condition following any other form of ulceration, is very apt to give the history of difficulty of swallowing, which improves as the ulcer heals and then comes on with renewed severity as the scar contracts.

Esophagoscopic appearances. In considering the esophagoscopic appearances of lues, it is necessary to remember that the appearances in ulcerative stages are due largely to the mixed infections and the resultant inflammatory condition. The same is true of tuberculosis and of cancer when these have reached the ulcerative stage. The differential diagnosis of the various ulcerative lesions in the esophagus is considered under "Ulceration of the Esophagus." The mucous plaque of the esophagus looks quite similar to that seen in the fauces. It may be slightly elevated in one part, and simply a bluish white cloudiness in another part. The lesion is typically inflammatory in character. The cicatrix of luetic esophagitis does not differ from other cicatrices. The esophagoscopic picture of a scar which involves only a small portion of the ring of the esophagus, is very apt to present a linear appearance on esophagoscopy for purely mechanical reasons, inherent in the inspection of the interior of a collapsed tube, which is explored by an endoscopic tube (see Fig. 14, Plate III). The gumma of the esophagus does not differ materially in appearance from gumma seen anywhere else in the mucosa, except in so far as it is an endoscopic instead of a right-angled view. The foregoing is a brief description of the various lesions as seen by the author. No one has seen a sufficient number of cases to be able to classify the endoscopic pictures, and even though it were possible to do so, the diagnosis would necessarily, here as elsewhere, rest upon the laboratory findings, the therapeutic test and the concomitant lesions.

Treatment. The treatment of luetic esophagitis, as with the same infection elsewhere, is altogether systemic and not local. One point, however, is of great importance, and that is to prevent the cicatrices from contracting after the healing of ulceration, should the esophagoscopist be so fortunate as to encounter the case in the ulcerated stage. Unfortunately, however, he is much more apt to see it in the cicatricial stage when the mechanical treatment required for cicatricial stenosis must be instituted. In the stage immediately following the healing of the ulcer, the scar can be prevented from contracting if a silk woven bougie is passed every day, and left *in situ* for a half hour or longer. The bougienage should be done by the esophagoscopist himself under the direct guidance of the eye. Once established, cicatrices of luetic origin are exceedingly stubborn to treat, and may require the string-cutting esophagotome or other form of internal esophagotomy, followed by daily dilatation. Complete cure, as in the case illustrated in Fig. 415, will reward patient, careful work.

TUBERCULOSIS OF THE ESOPHAGUS.

Tuberculosis of the esophagus while relatively much more rare than the same process in other viscera, nevertheless is probably not so rare as the literature on the subject would seem to indicate, because in all probability it usually occurs in patients with advanced pulmonary lesions in which the difficulty in swallowing is but a minor addition to the rapidly fatal stage of the disease. The difficulty in swallowing is often considered to be a part of the laryngeal trouble. In some instances the larynx is not even examined by the internist, and in other instances it is probable that laryngeal tuberculosis coexists with the esophageal, and is considered to account fully for all dysphagic symptoms. Furthermore, the disease has received such scant consideration in medical literature that it is not likely to be thought of, even in a manifestly tuberculous patient. The disease may occur as a primary infection, or, more frequently, as an extension from a tuberculous process in the larynx, mediastinal lymphatics, pleura, the larger bronchi, or even the lung itself. When seen as an extension from the larynx, especially as "party-wall" lesions, the esophageal lesions present much the same picture as the laryngeal disease. When, however, they are primary in the esophagus, the endoscopic appearances are rather those of superficial ulceration or a simple erosion and there may be yellowish or whitish granules in the neighborhood of the erosions or ulceration, or the granules may exist alone. Open ulceration means, necessarily, secondary mixed infections, which modify the picture. Cicatrices have been observed only twice by the author, once in connection with ulceration, and once in connection with an invasion of the esophagus by peri-bronchial tuberculous glandular processes. When the disease invades the esophagus from the surrounding tissues in the mediastinum, there is more or less compression of the esophagus, and rigidity and fixation with very much impairment of the normal esophageal movements and the transmitted respiratory and pulsatory movements. The tuberculous process may have been found to be completely healed and the result of the cicatricial contraction may be in rare cases, a traction diverticulum. The author has seen one such case esophagoscopically. The mucosa did not differ much from the normal, except that it was whiter in color with vessels visible, and did not have the velvety appearance of normal mucosa. The fixation was very marked and could easily be demonstrated by traction upon the opposite wall with the distal end of the esophagoscope, demonstrating clearly that the involved wall was partly adherent to the peri-esophageal structures. In one of the author's cases a fistula existed from the esophagus through into the left bronchus. The esophageal end of the fistula was covered with reddish granulations, which bled freely when touched, while the bronchial end of the fistula, on bronchoscopy, was seen to be surrounded with a pale mucosa, with small whitish granular elevations in groups at various points. The granulations were pale and did not bleed. They were limited to the margin of the fistula, and did not seem so exuberant as in the esophagus. The ulcerations of esophageal tuberculosis usually are more superficial and less inflammatory in appearance than either cancer or lues. Some points of difference from these and simple ulcer are given under the head of inflammation and ulceration, but the diagnosis of tuberculous lesions here, as elsewhere, will rest largely on the laboratory findings. Esophagoscopy renders its greatest service in being able to obtain with precision, ample specimens from the lesions. Actinomycosis has occurred in the esophagus, though the author has never seen a case. The possibility should be borne in mind in the examination of specimens of supposed tuberculosis. In considering the esophagoscopic appearances of tuberculosis, it is necessary to remember that after ulceration has set in that the mixed infections are apt to run riot and that the appearance may be largely due to the secondary processes resulting from this inflammation. One characteristic of the few tuberculous lesions that the author has seen in the esophagus, is the marked absence of vascularity. The mucosa seems pale and the patches whitish, with minute dots of raised whitish color. In one of the author's cases there was so much stenosis of the esophagus that the entire mucosa for some distance above the tuberculous lesions was so pasty from maceration that it was difficult to outline the lesion, and it was not until after three or four weeks of absolute rest of the esophagus, following a gastrostomy, that the esophagoscopic appearances of the tuberculous lesion itself could be determined. This patient, a man of 34 years, referred by the Presbyterian Hospital Dispensary, improved very much after gastrostomy and a feeding of large quantities of milk and eggs through the gastrostomy tube, together with absolute rest in bed. There was a fibroid phthisis in the lung, but no involvement of the larynx. The view, Fig. 15, Plate III, is made from a drawing by the author and represents conditions after the swallowing had very much improved and there was practical freedom from dysphagia. The mucosa surrounding the tuberculous lesions is seen to be normal, while the lesion itself is of a dull grayish color and there is a total absence of visible vessels. A specimen of tissue examined by Dr. Willetts showed the lesion to be tuberculous.

Treatment. Local treatment is useless. A general anti-tuberculous regime is needed, and above all, if there is any serious difficulty in swallowing, gastrostomy should be done at once for feeding in order not to let the patient's nutrition suffer, for above all things, nutrition must be kept at the highest possible point of efficiency. Feeding with a stomach tube can be done, but it is exceedingly dangerous in the presence of ulceration, and is in some cases painful to the patient. Above all, a gastrostomy puts the esophagus at rest, which is beneficial to any form of esophageal disease. Orthoform in doses of half a gramme swallowed dry on the tongue may be used if there is pain, though none of the author's cases of tuberculosis of the esophagus, where the larynx and epiglottis were uninvolved, have had pain.

VARIX AND ANGIOMA OF THE ESOPHAGUS.

Varix and angioma of the esophagus rarely produce symptoms, and are not ordinarily of very much importance unless they are wounded or they spontaneously bleed. Occasionally a case is encountered where there is considerable bleeding, the patient complaining of regurgitating blood, which is bright red and not of the dark or "coffee ground' character of blood that has been in the stomach. Varicosities in the esophagus may coexist with "cardiospasm." Which was the primary lesion has not yet been determined. In one of the author's cases hemorrhoids and varicosities on both legs were enormous. Varicosities are usually in the lower third of the esophagus, probably because the veinous system is more developed there than higher up. These veins empty chiefly into the portal vein and a number of cases have been reported where the condition seemed to depend upon obstruction of the portal circulation, as in hepatic cancer or cirrhosis. Careless esophagoscopy producing undue pressure against one lateral wall will cause an exudation of blood into the submucosal tissue forming a hematoma (Fig. 153) which has been mistaken by a number of esophagoscopists for a varicosity or an angioma. The author has had no experience in treating varix or angioma because the few cases seen by him did not require treatment. Guisez reports the cure of a case of angioma at the cardia by means of radium, and this method seems to be particularly appropriate.

ANGIONEUROTIC EDEMA.

The author has not been so fortunate as to see a case of angioneurotic edema, but a very interesting observation of this disease is reported by Arrowsmith (Bib. 8), who is an expert endoscopist of large experience. A woman, aged 50 years, complained of difficult and painful swallowing of a few weeks' duration, with history of previous similar trouble of indefinite duration. Esophagoscopy by Dr. Arrowsmith showed "a mass just below the cricoid cartilage, filling two-thirds of the lumen of the esophagus, with its attachment centered on the left side. Allowing for the distension of the esophagus by the tube, this mass undoubtedly almost occluded it, when mechanical stretching was absent." The mass was also seen by Drs. F. C. Paffard and L. Grant Baldwin. Lues being excluded the logical diagnosis of neoplasm, probably malignant was made tentatively, and the case referred to the author who found the esophagus normal and hence concluded the stenosis must have been spasmodic. On further investigation of the case, including the testimony of the patient's previous medical attendants clear history of angioneurotic manifestations were discovered by Dr. Arrowsmith to have preceded the esophageal symptoms and later to have accompanied the attacks of dysphagia and odynphagia. These manifestations were as follows:

"Commencing with frequent and painful urination and vesical tenesmus, there would be an extreme irritation of the urethra and meatus, with external appearances suggesting urethral caruncle; *always* followed by symptoms of marked gastrointestinal disturbance and of pronounced pylorospasm. Edema of the larynx placed her in a very critical condition for forty-eight hours. Two months later she had a similar, though milder, attack."

Subsequent attacks of angioneurotic manifestations were characterized by pruritic cutaneous wheals, urethral, vesical and gastric symptoms accompanying the attacks of dysphagia and odynphagia. No esophagoscopies were obtainable after the two mentioned, one showing the angioneurotic eruption in the esophagus and the subsequent one showing the esophagus to be normal.

Treatment, if any, for the condition would be general not esophagoscopic. Passing of a feeding tube with esophagoscopic aid might be needed if the attack were very prolonged.

ACTINOMYCOSIS OF THE ESOPHAGUS.

Actinomycosis the author has never seen. Its possibility should be borne in mind, but the diagnosis doubtless will rest upon the histologic examination of a specimen removed esophagoscopically. Reports of cases so far have been autoptical.

DEVIATION OF THE ESOPHAGUS.

Deviation of the esophagus is seen not infrequently in cases of mediastinal tumors. The author has encountered one very interesting case of esophageal deviation associated with a spine deformed by a previously healed vertebral tuberculosis (Fig. 132a). The patient, a woman aged 46 years, was referred to the author by Dr. J. W. Fairing for the removal of a chicken bone from the esophagus. The author readily found and esophagoscopically removed the chicken bone without any problem of interest; but the marked deviation was so rare that the patient was sent for a radiograph from which to make an illustration (Fig. 432a). Fluoroscopy with bismuth, by Dr. Boyce, showed the deviation; but the bismuth bolus went down so rapidly that a stomach tube was used by

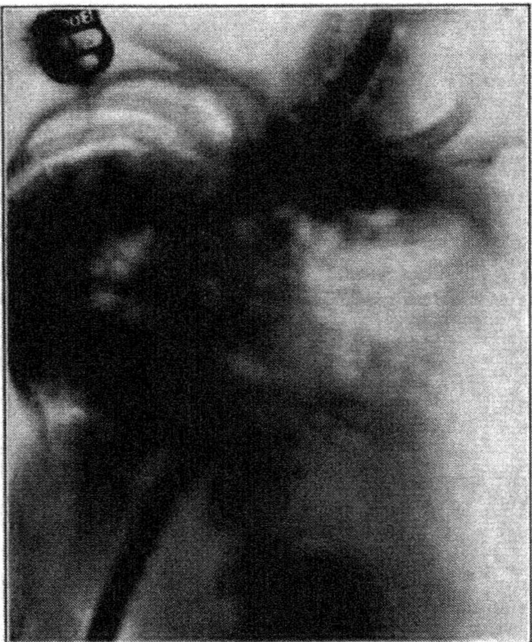

FIG. 432a.—Radiograph of a woman, aged 46 years, showing a deviation of the esophagus, that produced no symptoms. A stomach tube was inserted for demonstration. (Radiograph made by Dr. Russell H. Boggs. Author's case.)

Dr. Boggs for radiography. Doubtless the esophagus had been dragged aside by the deviating spine; the dragging being facilitated by the longitudinal esophageal redundancy caused by the shortening of the straight distance from the hypopharynx to the hiatus. The patient had never had any esophageal symptoms and the deviation would not have been discovered had it not been for the foreign body accident. It is interesting to note that beyond the following of the deviated lumen there was no difficulty in esophagoscopy notwithstanding a marked anterior, as well as lateral, spinal deviation.

CHAPTER XXXV.

Gastroscopy.*

The interest awakened by the author's work (Bib. 269, 237, 239) has borne good fruit. In different parts of the world, earnest workers have been perfecting technic and instruments. The author's early contention that safety demands that introducing shall be with a tube devoid of a lens system, in order that lesions may be detected and avoided, and that the axis of the instrument may be readily kept in line with the esophageal axis, has now been universally accepted. After the distal end of the tube has reached the stomach, a plug with a window has been used in the proximal end of the tube so that positive pressure from an oxygen tank (Janeway) or a hand bulb (Mosher) may be used to push away mucosal folds, and when a lens system is inserted in the tube in the form of a long tube with a window in the side of the distal end, an excellent view of the distended stomach is obtained. The author personally can testify to the beautiful view of the gastric mucosa obtained in the Janeway gastroscope, and while the use of inflation and of a lens system for gastroscopy is at least thirty years old, yet the optical formula and the particular combination of illumination, lenses, inflation apparatus and tubes in the Janeway gastroscope make it a highly efficient instrument. Excellent results have also been obtained by Moure (Bib. 392), Hill (Bib. 200), Elsner (Bib. 128) and others, and all of these instruments are now doubtless developed to a point where the personal skill of the operator counts for more than the particular instrument. The usefulness, safety and practicability of the gastroscope is an accomplished fact. The need now is for careful, skillful men interested in the stomach who will use it. The laryngologist's field is already too large without adding the stomach. The value of gastroscopy in establishing a diagnosis

*In this chapter liberal quotations are made from the author's Rapport at the International Medical Congress, London, 1913, and from his paper read by invitation before the New York Academy of Medicine, Jan. 23, 1907.

in severe and obscure stomach disease has been abundantly proved. The tendency, however, to resort to it only in very serious conditions often prevents one of its greatest achievements, which would be in the early diagnosis of cancer and of pre-cancerous conditions. When endoscopists who have developed the gastroscopic technic, are sufficiently numerous and sufficiently skilful so that the physician or the surgeon may feel justified in sending them cases before the patient's condition becomes desperate, gastroscopy will be of great use to the physician and surgeon, but gastroscopy probably will never be done by the physician or the surgeon himself. He will take the endoscopist's report along with that of the radiographer and analyst and decide as to the best handling of the case, just as the otologist in a brain case takes the report from the internist, the laboratory, and the ophthalmologist. Unlike tracheo-bronchoscopy and esophagoscopy, it may be said of gastroscopy that while its positive reports are extremely valuable, its negative reports are less so, just as with ophthalmoscopy in brain disease, the Wassermann reaction, and many other of our most valuable aids in medicine and surgery. A very important point in increasing the range of mobility of the distal end of the gastroscope in the stomach has been demonstrated by Henry Janeway. It consists in an elevation of the knees of the recumbent patient to the vertical or flexed position, as this relaxes the abdominal wall.

Seven years' additional experience have shown the correctness of the statement (Bib. 269) that there is no human being with a normal spine and a normal esophagus into whose stomach a straight and rigid gastroscope cannot be readily and safely introduced, provided: (1) The patient is fully anesthetized. (2) An open tube of light construction is gently passed by sight. (3) The patient's head is held in the Boyce position. (4) The operator is a skilful esophagoscopist.

Statements to the contrary are the result either of inexperience or of experience with gastroscopes that cannot be passed by sight. Flexible guides are unnecessary, rarely of aid, and are dangerous. The inexperienced will have trouble at the cricopharyngeus, but surely no esophagoscopist will. It required only thirty-eight seconds, in the author's clinic, for Professor Killian, in his careful, skillful way to pass the author's gastroscope from the mouth to the greater curvature of the stomach. The writer cannot understand why so many authors have stated that they had difficulty in passing a rigid instrument through the cardia. All difficulties are overcome by carefully following the directions given under "Introduction of the Esophagoscope."

It is true that we do not always get a complete view of the gastric mucosa, but as Halstead has pointed out the same may be said of the nasopharynx. Indeed the author knows of no case of gastroscopy where he has failed to get a view of the stomach, which is more than can be said of the nasopharynx by ordinary methods of examination.

Some recent experiments by Rosenow in the production of gastric ulcer by the injection of streptococci opens up a wide field for gastroscopic study on the dog.

Mortality of gastroscopy. That there is practically no mortality from gastroscopy in very careful hands has been shown by the replies to the author's circular letter of inquiry. Out of 110 cases done by eight different endoscopists there was no mortality from any cause within two weeks after gastroscopy. The author has now examined the interior of 238 living stomachs with the peroral gastroscope, and so far only one patient has died from any cause whatever within one month after the gastroscopy. As previously reported, this patient was moribund from a bleeding ulcer of the stomach when admitted to the hospital. But, taking the figures just as they stand, the mortality is only a fraction of one per cent.

Technic of gastroscopy. In the main the description of the technic in the earlier publication (Bib. 269) is correct and has stood the test of further experience. Introduction with mandrin and finger, however, was abandoned by the author before the book was off the press and the gastroscope was passed by sight as described in Chapter X. The author still uses the open tube gastroscope, but believes that, after all the data thus obtainable have been noted, the use of a lens system in the open tube will in a proportion of cases yield additional information, and is a valuable acquisition. The advantages of the open tube are the undistorted image, the facility of probing, removal of a specimen of tissue or fluid, sponging away a coating of secretions, etc. When one dilates the stomach he pushes its walls far away from the reach of the tube; walls which otherwise would collapse over the tube mouth, to be examined and palpated by the probe and tube. The portion of the stomach nearest the centre line of the body is the most easily examined. The collapsed stomach is relatively small, and much of it is near the middle line (Fig. 133). When one distends the stomach he pushes most of the otherwise explorable area away from the central line and thus laterally out of range. The diaphragm is rendered much less movable when the stomach is distended, and, furthermore, thus is rendered impossible the practice of a most valuable part of the technic, namely, the manipulation of the abdomen externally by an assistant, which brings into view the fundal and pyloric ends. A lens system and an inflated stomach prevent sponging away of secretions with which many lesions are covered. The position and shape of the stomach in the living subject has been most curiously misunderstood. Fig. 434 is traced from one of the classical text-books on anatomy. Whatever may be the position and shape of the stomach in the cadaver or in the living subject after the abdomen is opened, it was certainly not in any such position in any of the 238 cases examined gastroscopically by the author and it may be said that the stomach is of such shape as to fit whatever space is available at the particular moment. The author's method of outlining the stomach is to find a given boundary with the extremity of the tube. The

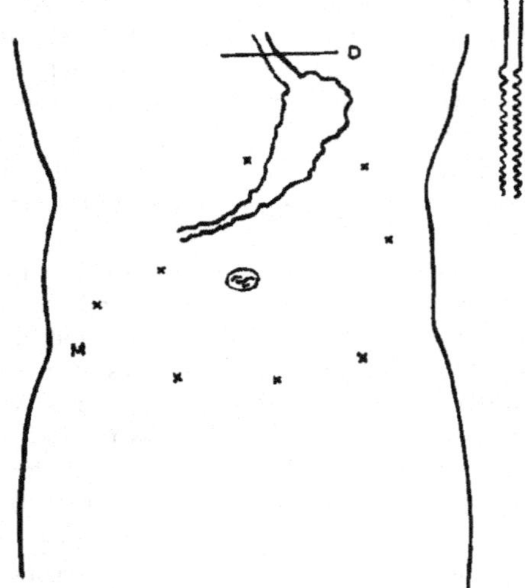

FIG. 433.—Position of the stomach in the case of Isabel A. Crosses show where the wall of the stomach was intentionally pushed by the gastroscope. The schema in the upper right hand corner shows the other plane of the stomach.

distal end of the tube is felt by the abdominal palpator, who makes a mark on the patient's skin with a skin pencil. Another position on the boundary is then found and marked, and thus a series of marks dot the skin of the abdomen corresponding to the stomach outlines. An obvious source of error is the drag of the tube, which may displace the stomach. This can be avoided by a careful watch through the tube and care to make a vertical insertion for each mark. This gives the position of the stomach when empty. The radiograph, which is more generally useful, gives the position when containing fluid or food. The stomach wall can be pushed into almost any position, as shown in Fig. 433, which illustrates the position of the stomach in the case of Isabel A. (Bib. 239). The stomach gave the impression of a loose bag dangling on the end of the gastroscope, freely movable in all directions, by either the movement of the gastroscope or the manipulations of Dr. Harold A. Miller, who was palpating the abdomen externally. The diagram at the upper right hand corner of the illustration shows schematically the other plane as it appeared to be when gastroscopically examined. Passing down the esophagus, as soon as one passes the cardia, folds and wrinkles are encountered, a slight deflection bringing either the anterior or the posterior wall into view. The degree of motion shown in Fig. 433 is obtainable

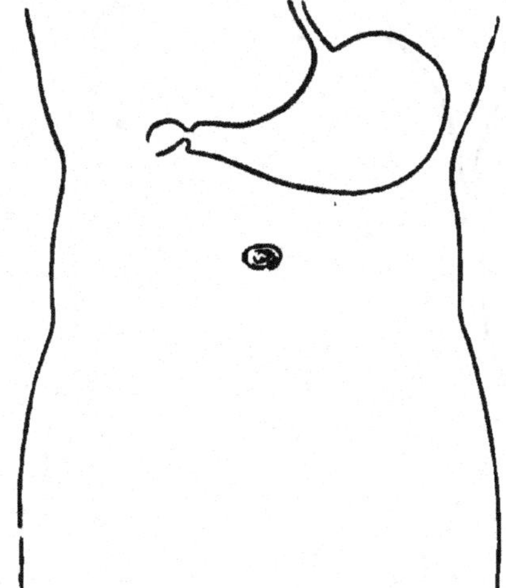

Fig. 434.—Position of the stomach as shown in a classical text-book on anatomy.

only under the relaxation of deep anesthesia. When gastroscopy is attempted, under morphine narcosis, as Mikulicz attempted it, the musculature of the diaphragm pulls upon the central tendon, so that the gastroscope is guyed rigidly like a tent pole, and if the stomach can be entered at all, only such portion can be inspected as lies in a line with the axis of the entry of the tube. When relaxed under deep anesthesia the hiatus esophageus does not relax or enlarge so as to permit of motion: but the entire dome of the diaphragm can be moved sidewise because it is of dome-like form. If it were a tightly stretched membrane, as shown by the dotted line in Fig. 435, there would be no yield in any direction;

but being arched (as shown in Fig. 435) its "slack," as one might say, permits of a range of motion of from 10 to 15 cm., provided the central tendon is so relaxed by deep anesthesia as not to be pulled upon from all sides by the diaphragmatic musculature. A range of lateral motion of seventeen centimeters was observed by Dr. J. Hartley Anderson in the opened abdomen of a living patient. This movement was imparted solely by the gastroscopist manipulating the gastroscope by its proximal end. Dr. Anderson with gloved hands grasping the gastroscope could place it anywhere in the unopened stomach, and any part of the wall could be moved to the tube mouth. One of the most promising fields for

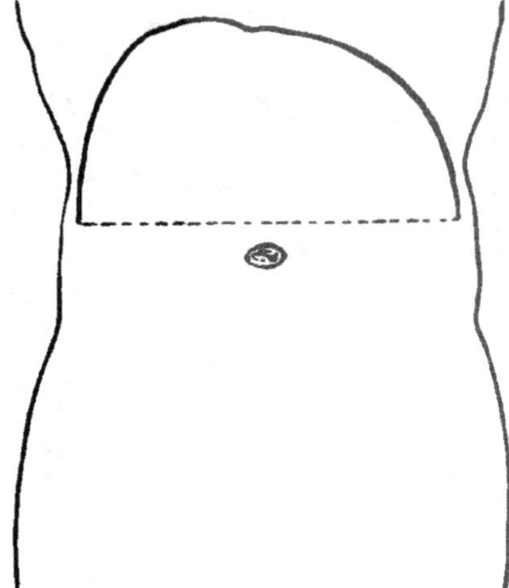

FIG. 435.—Illustrating the anatomical reasons for the wide range of mobility of the gastroscope in the stomach. If the diaphragm were a plane or tightly stretched membrane as represented by the dotted line a gastroscope in the hiatus could not be moved laterally. The dome shape permits of a wide lateral range of movement because of redundancy, provided the diaphragmatic musculature is relaxed by deep anesthesia.

open tube gastroscopy is the aid rendered by the endoscopist as an assistant of the abdominal surgeon, who will assist the surgeon not only in diagnosis, but in the operating room during the operation, by working through the mouth in conjunction with the surgeon whose hand is in the opened abdomen. The endoscopist, of course, has his own instrument nurse and sterile organization at the head of the patient, entirely separate and apart from that of the abdominal surgeon, to whom the endoscopist can give a prompt report on the interior appearance of any suspicious portion of the stomach wall palpated and presented at the tube mouth by the surgeon. The suspected tissue is placed in front of the tube mouth by the surgeon whose hands are in the opened abdomen palpating the, as yet, unopened stomach. Extensive citation of cases would unduly expand this book. A few will serve for illustration.

Case LXIX. Daniel B., aged sixty-two years, was admitted to the Western Pennsylvania Hospital to the service of Dr. John W. Boyce, complaining of feeling weak, and of loss of appetite, emaciation, and headache, all these symptoms appearing gradually about one year previously. There was no nausea or vomiting. The temperature was normal, the pulse 96, and the respirations 24. After the mouth of the gastroscope passed the cardia, in the first 4 cm. of the passage, the anterior and posterior walls of the stomach opened up in normal folds ahead of the tube mouth. Below this, however, the tube mouth entered a cavity with smooth unwrinkled walls. At the bottom of this cavity was a crescentic slit-like depression looking somewhat like the primiparous os uteri (C, Plate V). When the mucosa was sponged clean of bubbly secretion, the slit-like depression was found to have a considerable depth, which, however, was not probed, although to have done so would have been technically easy and probably harmless. The surrounding mucosa was of pale pink color, without rugae, and when the tube mouth was withdrawn the depression was still visible in the same position in a cavity, the wall of the stomach at this point being evidently held open by adhesions to the abdominal parietes or viscera. Fully to appreciate the picture, it is necessary to realize that the empty stomach is collapsed. When examined gastroscopically, it opens up ahead of the tube and collapses after its withdrawal, in a manner similar to that of the vagina upon the introduction and withdrawal of the vaginal speculum when used upon a patient in the dorsal position. But here was a case in which the anterior wall of the stomach was adherent, so that it was held up (dorsal decubitus); thus the posterior wall dropped away by gravity and left a cavity. The cicatrices and adhesions were such that no mucosal folds could be produced in the neighborhood of the slit. When Dr. Ogilvie tapped upon the abdomen the vibrations were seen to be beautifully transmitted in waves over the upper (anterior) wall of the stomach. The picture was beautifully clear, and the author and his colleagues, who saw for themselves, felt justified in pronouncing the lesion the cicatrix of a healed perforating gastric ulcer. Had it been an operable lesion, it could have been precisely located by holding the tube mouth against it while the abdominal surgeon cut through the stomach wall from the celiotomic wound.

Case XX. Margaret Z., a servant at the Western Pennsylvania Hospital. Six months before, gastrojejunostomy had been performed by Dr. George L. Hays. Complete symptomatic cure had followed. Under general anesthesia, the author passed the gastroscope, and readily found the anastamotic opening in the form of a slit, which, when pulled open by the instrument, showed a slightly puckered border, below which could be seen the mucosa of the jejunum (A, Plate V).

Dr. W. L. Rodman, with my assistance, examined gastroscopically a gastrojejunostomy wound two weeks after the operation, and saw the opening and the non-absorbable sutures in situ. His report on the examination is as follows:

"The patient was etherized, brought before the class, and the gastroscope introduced. It was surprising to me how well the interior of the stomach could be inspected. The gastroenterostomy opening was plainly visible, was found to be patent and working perfectly, and the Pagenstecher or linen thread used as a suture material was plainly seen. I see in gastroscopy a valuable addition to our diagnostic resources in gastric diseases, provided the instrument can be employed by one skilled and deft in its use. Particularly will it be valuable at the time of an exploratory laparotomy, inasmuch as the gastroscope can be so guided that even the pyloric end of the stomach can be brought clearly in view. The case above referred to was discharged from the hospital as cured a few days later. He was a very intelligent Englishman and was comforted by the assurances given him by Dr. Jackson after an inspection of the gastric mucosa. The patient had suffered long, had become addicted to morphia, and feared that he had carcinoma. This was the first time that gastroscopy was practiced in Philadelphia. I may add that a letter received months after his return to England stated that he was enjoying perfect health."

The author has discovered great advantages in placing the patient face downward with a pillow under the chest, and in some instances under the pelvis also, in order to get the assistance of gravity in dropping forward the abdominal wall. It is not generally realized the extent to which the spine curves forward and projects into the abdomen as well as into the thoracic cavities. This anterior projection into the abdominal cavity interferes seriously with gastroscopic examination of the pylorus, because in the dorsal position there is a tendency for the pylorus to drop backward and reach a plane posterior to that of the middle portion of the stomach that is prevented from dropping backward by the anteriorally projecting spine. In the use of lens systems, the gastroscopists have been misled into thinking they were looking at the pylorus, when really they were looking at only a more or less funnel-shaped cavity formed by the limited area of the stomach wall that was inflated. This gives in miniature, the same general shape as the pyloric antrum, and it is the tendency of all lens systems to deceive one as to the actual size of the visual field.

Presbyopic gastroscopists should have a special pair of glasses with a 60 cm. focus, as the glasses for ordinary reading distance will blur the more distant gastroscopic image.

Gastroscopy for foreign bodies. The esophagoscopist is often consulted in regard to foreign bodies that have reached the stomach. The author's opinion is that the great danger in the swallowing of foreign bodies is that they will lodge in the esophagus, where serious, even fatal, ulceration may occur. Once they have reached the stomach they are relatively safe. This does not mean, however, that it is ever justifiable to attempt to push a foreign body down by the blind methods, or by esophagoscopic methods, because it is his belief that any foreign body that has gone down through the mouth can be brought back the same way. Nor is it to be taken that once a foreign body has reached the stomach that the patient can be told to pay no more attention to the matter. On the contrary, every foreign body that is known by the ray to have reached the stomach, should be watched. So long as it remains in the stomach, it is relatively safe. When it reaches the intestines, as it usually does within from one to three days, it should be watched every alternate day radiographically, in order to make sure that it is moving. Should it lodge in one position for five days, a laparotomy should be done at once for its removal, as it will certainly perforate. Quite a number of perforations of the ileum have been reported, some recent cases by Steiff, Ross and Hodge. The author had one case in which consent to esophagoscopy was refused when the needle was in the esophagus. Later when lodged for five days in the intestines, the family was urged to allow a general surgeon to do a laparotomy. Consent to this was also refused and the child died of a septic peritonitis following perforation.

In all cases, great care should be taken to avoid cathartics. Very bulky foods, such as potatoes, bread, oatmeal and the like, should be given freely in order to distend the bowel and embed the foreign body. The insane and the intoxicated, and also some performers, swallow very large and sharp objects, such as open pocketknives, glass, etc. A large number of such objects have been removed from a single stomach. All such cases demand immediate external operation by a general surgeon. In case of such a body as an open safety pin, the author would advise laparotomy by the general surgeon rather than take a chance of its not perforating in passing through the intestines, because of the combination of the point and the spring. It is quite possible that it might pass harmlessly, but on the other hand the risk of perforation is great. Assisted by a fluoroscopist using the Grier double-plane fluoroscope, the gastroscopic removal of foreign bodies is easy, with the author's gastroscope.

Open-tube gastroscopes (such as the author's esophagoscope Fig. 19) are the only forms available for the removal of foreign bodies. Forceps cannot be used through lens-system gastroscopes.

Gastroscopy through the celiotomic wound. For this purpose a thick short tube should be used. A very ingenious speculum for the

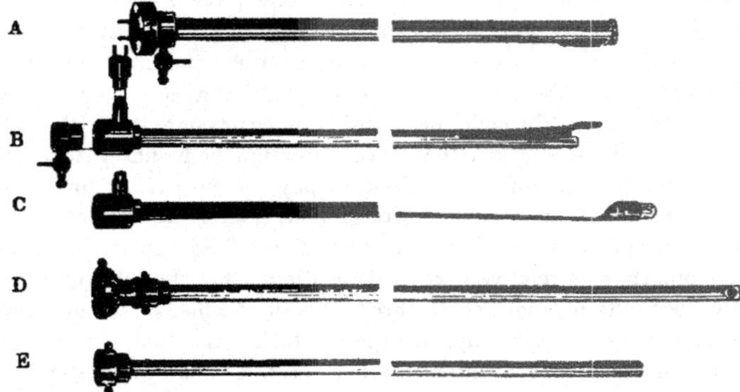

Fig. 436.—A, open tube. B, light carrier to be used during introduction. C, large lamp needed with lens system. D, lens system. E, open tube for use with large lamp.

purpose has been devised by Robert Rendu. It is expansile at its distal end and gives a large visual field.

Lens-system gastroscopy. After having obtained all possible data from open-tube gastroscopy, a lens system may be introduced. The Janeway gastroscope is shown in Fig. 436. The introduction of the open tube is by the author's method as described in Chapter X. Then the small lamp carrier, B, is withdrawn and the large lamp carrier, C, is introduced. Next the lens carrier, D, is pushed inside of the hollow large lamp carrier. The lens carrier displaces the large lamp sidewise, permitting the window of the lens system to project beyond the distal end of the open tube. Oxygen from a tank, or air from a compression tank or hand ball, is then used to distend the stomach while the degree of distension is watched through the tube. It seems probable that, as suggested by Janeway, the air or oxygen that escapes around the tube in the esophagus would prevent an injurious degree of pressure. This must not be relied upon, however, and caution against over-distension is advisable. The distended area in the stomach assumes a funnel-like form ending at the apex in a depression with radiating folds that leads the observer to think he is looking at the pylorus. This illusion is contributed to by the foreshortenings of the image of the lens system. Proper comprehension of the image necessitates familiarity with the particular instrument used. This must be acquired by practice on a manikin which can be readily devised from an open box, which permits comparison of the image with the corresponding naked eye view.

A good illustration of endoscopic views of the stomach through the Janeway lens system is shown in Plate VI.

Part II.

Laryngeal Surgery.

INTRODUCTION.

It is not intended here to teach the fundamentals of modern aseptic surgery. The reader is supposed to have had a number of years of practical training in a good clinic under a master of surgery.

Operating room organization. Modern surgery is not the work of one man but of an organization. It is impossible for one man to attend to all the details of the modern operating room, and he is dependent upon the conscience, skill and ability of his assistants, nurses, radiographers and others. The organization does not need to be large, but it must be harmonious and each must work for the common good rather than to satisfy personal ambitions. There must be no failure upon the part of any nurse, instrument or apparatus at a critical moment, in short it is in every sense of the word, "team work" and practice together is essential for the best results, as in a football team.

CHAPTER XXXVI.

Acute Stenosis of the Larynx.

For the present purpose any condition that narrows the lumen ot the larynx and immediately subjacent trachea in a relatively short time may be considered an acute stenosis. Such narrowing may be due to a foreign body; to accumulation of secretions or exudates; to distention of the tissues by air, inflammatory products, serum, pus, etc.; to displacement of relatively normal tissues as in abductor paralysis, congenital laryngeal stridor; to neoplasms; to granulomata. Two or more of the foregoing may be combined. In fact, the stenosis in almost all cases, whatever the cause, is mechanically increased by the presence of secretions, temporary inflammatory conditions, etc., in the already narrowed lumen.

Edema of the larynx is the most frequently heard of acute stenotic condition. The name, however, has been used too generally in the absence of means of accurate diagnosis especially in children, prior to the advent of direct methods of examination which have recently rendered accurate diagnosis possible. Edema may be glottic, supraglottic or subglottic. Strictly speaking, the name glottis refers to the chink or lumen. and cannot be affected with edema. Nevertheless the bordering tissues can be edematous, and "glottic" in this case is used to mean a region. As a pathologic fact, however, the vocal bands are rarely, themselves, acutely edematous, though they are frequently pushed inward by the edema of the basal tissues, and thus the cordal edges encroach on the glottic lumen, though not themselves edematous. As shown by Logan Turner (Bib 542) the loose cellular tissue is most frequently concerned in laryngeal edematous processes. Acute inflammatory stenosis may be associated with relatively superficial mucosal and submucosal inflammation or with perichondritis. These processes may be primary or may complicate many general diseases, especially typhoid fever.

Acute laryngeal stenosis complicating typhoid fever deserves especial consideration, as it is frequently overlooked and the patient is permitted to die without a suspicion of the laryngeal stenosis, because these patients, in many instances, make no fight for air and often are only slightly, if at all, affected by hoarseness as shown by the author in an extensive study of the larynx in typhoid fever (Bib. 252). A typical case of acute stenosis complicating typhoid fever reported by J. H. Bryan (Bib. 56) is particularly valuable as giving an accurate description of the living laryngoscopic picture by a keen, experienced observer. A

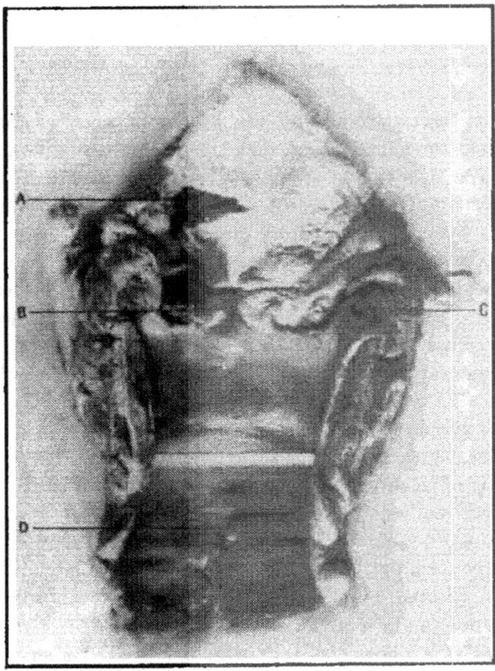

FIG. 437.—Photograph of specimen of larynx acutely stenosed by perichondritis complicating typhoid fever in a man aged forty years. A, gap where specimen was excised post-mortem. B, necrotic left arytenoid cartilage hanging by a shred. C, necrotic area from which right arytenoid cartilage necrosed and disappeared before death. D, interior view of tracheotomic wound. Specimen lent by Maj. Frederick Russell, U. S. A. Patient of Dr. Joseph H. Bryan.

photograph of the autoptic specimen is reproduced in Fig 437 by courtesy of Maj. Frederick R. Russell, Surgeon, U. S. A., who kindly lent the author the specimen from the Museum of the Surgeon General's office. Acute laryngeal stenosis in typhoid fever may be due to cordal immobility from either paralysis or inflammatory arytenoid fixation in the absence of edema.

Laryngeal stenosis in the new-born. Another class of cases is the children born with laryngeal stenosis of anomalous morbid or traumatic laryngotracheal stenosis. Examples of these are not common compared to the number of births, but doubtless are usually overlooked when they do occur because they are simply put down as a "blue baby." The distinguishing feature is that whereas a "blue baby" from failure of the foramen ovale to close is pumping the air in and out regularly, and a "blue baby" from apnea does not make the respiratory movements, the laryngeally stenosed baby is making the respiratory movements but little or no air is passing in or out, and there is indrawing at the suprasternal notch, around the clavicles, and, in some cases, even in the epigastrium. The following case communicated to the author by Dr. Freeland is so complete and accurately observed that it may be taken as typical.

"Female; full-term; 7 pounds; lived twenty-four hours. Easy forceps delivery. Mother had right-sided pyelitis with temperature 101 to 103, pulse 110 to 130, for three days before delivery. Cords pulsating strongly and regularly and child had a good color on delivery. Made occasional voluntary efforts at inspiration, but gradually passed into condition of white asphyxia. Resuscitated by hot bath and mouth to mouth artificial respiration. After ten to fifteen minutes was breathing regularly and had a good color. *Never cried.* Respirations shallow. From this time on there were repeated attacks of secondary asphyxia from which the child was revived with oxygen and mouth to mouth insufflation. After four to six hours these attacks of asphyxia were accompanied by the excretion of frothy brownish mucus from the throat and lungs. Respirations were always shallow and labored and the accessory muscles contracted strongly with each inspiration, even after resuscitation from attacks of asphyxia. The lungs were full of moist rales, the respiratory murmur was very short and much less pronounced than the usual infantile type. Except for some retraction of the head there was no evidence of cerebral hemorrhage. The child died in twenty-four hours in an attack of asphyxia, having been kept barely alive for some hours by constant watching, oxygen, removal of mucus from the throat and mouth to mouth artificial respiration. It never cried, a point that did not receive much attention until the autopsy was performed. The clinical diagnosis was atelectasis. Autopsy was performed by Dr. Andrews, who found: Malformation of larynx, sub-dural hemorrhages, bilateral. Hematoma of scalp, right side. Subserous hemorrhages of lungs and heart. Inflammatory foci in right lung. Subcutaneous hemorrhages. Anemia. Larynx; cricoid and arytenoid cartilages are much thickened and firmer than normal. The glottis is very small, just admitting the head of a moderate-sized probe. The vocal cords are shortened, thicker and firmer than normal. Remarks: The pathology found was doubtless all secondary to the laryngeal stenosis. Death was by asphyxia.

The author has seen three cases of acute laryngeal stenosis from perichondritis in infants a few weeks old. The thymus gland was large in all three cases, probably due to the vascular engorgement of dyspnea, and, had the children died, the death would have been attributed to status lymphaticus. In each of the cases direct examination revealed laryngeal stenoses and a total absence of thymic or any other tracheal compression, and, most important of all, tracheotomy completely relieved all the symptoms, the children recovered and were decannulated after the cure of the laryngeal stenosis. As to the cause of the perichondritis the author is unable to say positively. The cases were all forceps deliveries, and traumatism either during accouchement or clearing the mouth and pharynx afterward might have been a factor. The father of one of the patients was luetic, but neither lues nor tuberculosis has appeared in any of the three children though they are now two, three and six years of age respectively. The stenotic symptoms began in all three of the cases between the second and the fourth week. The author at present, has another similar case of stenotic laryngeal perichondritis, starting three weeks after delivery and reaching the almost fatal point in the eighth week. The laryngeal nature of the trouble was recognized by Dr. William Kirk who sent the case to the author. The child was moribund from starvation and loss of sleep. It had been so busy fighting for air that it had no time for eating and sleeping. The left side of the subglottic region was bulged in until there was only a slight crevice left through which to breathe. The swelling was firmer than an edema and contained pus. The author did a tracheotomy with complete relief of the dyspnea after which it nursed and slept normally. A quantity of mucopus escaped from the trachea as soon as the tracheal incision was made. Like all the other patients, it gave the usual tracheotomic sigh of relief and respiratory pause after the trachea was opened.

The glottis normally is relatively narrow in the new-born.

Surgical treatment of acute laryngeal stenosis. Multiple puncture of acute inflammatory edema is readily accomplished with the knife, Fig. 85, used through the direct laryngoscope, Fig. 14. As a rule, however, this is by no means certain to be helpful for any length of time and recrudescence of the edema may be fatal in the absence of a tracheotomist. In view of this, and especially in view of the great therapeutic effect of tracheotomy in all inflammatory states of the larynx, tracheotomy should, in most cases, be done in preference. Intubation is treacherous and unreliable in all except diphtheritic cases. In the latter, O'Dwyer's intubation is ideal, if the patient be carefully watched.

CHAPTER XXXVII.

Tracheotomy.

INDICATIONS FOR TRACHEOTOMY.*

As a therapeutic measure in diseases of the larynx, tracheotomy should occupy a more prominent place than has ever been accorded to it. Whether the therapeutic effect is due to rest of the larynx or not, the author is unable to say, but the effect in many diseases is abundantly proven according to his experience. Inefficacious antiluetic treatment of luetic laryngitis has immediately produced results after tracheotomy. A number of writers have discredited tracheotomy in tuberculosis. The author's experience has been quite the reverse. In a number of cases with advanced laryngeal tuberculosis, but with relatively slight lung lesions, marked improvement and relative cures have followed tracheotomy, combined in some instances with the healing of ulcerations and the reduction of infiltrations by the galvano-cautery. These procedures enabled the patient to be nourished systematically in cases in which the patient was rapidly declining because of inanition, owing to the odynphagia. Tracheotomy was done in these cases only partly for the purpose of rest of the larynx, but mainly to permit of perfect ventilation of the lung, which was but inefficiently carried on through the narrowed glottic chink. Perichondritis and other inflammations of any etiology are often very promptly benefited by tracheotomy.

Tracheotomy for foreign bodies is no longer indicated either for the removal of the intruder or for the insertion of the bronchoscope. In the absence of a bronchoscopist the surgeon is perfectly justified in relieving dyspnea in a foreign body case by tracheotomy. Tracheotomy may be urgently indicated for foreign body dyspnea, but not for foreign body removal.

Tracheotomy for respiratory arrest. In the absence of any stenosis of the larynx, tracheotomy may be urgently indicated in respiratory ar-

*This chapter is a revision of a lecture delivered by the author, by invitation, before the Philadelphia Laryngological Society, Sept. 23, 1913.

rest for the insufflation of oxygen and amyl nitrite. Ordinary Sylvester artificial respiration is much more efficient if a tracheotomy has been done because it eliminates the pharyngo-laryngeal "death zone." The pulmotor and similar apparatus are fairly efficient. Bronchoscopic oxygen insufflation is better than either, if available. Paralysis of respiration in bulbar palsy, cerebellar abscess and the like may produce intense cyanosis, for which tracheotomy may not be indicated. But unless the diagnosis is certain from previous study of the case, arrest of respiration with cyanosis is always an indication for tracheotomy. The cause can be ascertained later. Many times more people have died for want of a tracheotomy than have ever died from the operation.

There comes a time when a patient may die because he can no longer stay awake to breathe. When he attempts to doze, the loss of the accessory muscular activity deprives him of air and he is wakened by threatened asphyxia. We all preach early tracheotomy, but practically always do it late—dangerously late. Rarely indeed is it justifiable to wait for cyanosis, or still worse, ashy gray "cyanosis." When respiratory arrest comes from laryngeal or tracheal obstruction it comes abruptly. Five factors contribute to relatively sudden death in dyspneic cases.

1. The patient from want of sleep reaches the point where he cannot longer stay awake to breathe.

2. Secretions accumulate rapidly toward the last because the laryngeal condition interferes with expectoration.

3. The patient worn out by his fight for air gives up from exhaustion.

The foregoing three factors apply with especial force to dyspnea of gradual onset and especially in children.

4. Venous engorgement suddenly increases in increasing progression as dyspnea increases. Thus a vicious circle is established.

5. Any excitement or struggle increases dyspnea, hence the first steps of an operation or of attempted application of an anesthetic inhaler, precipitates respiratory arrest.

It is particularly dangerous to postpone tracheotomy over night unless a good experienced tracheal nurse is watching the patient. Too often nurses who are ordinarily good and well-trained, but inexperienced in tracheotomy, will think the patient is "sinking" when really he is asphyxiating. Death for want of a tracheotomy has resulted from the failure to recognize that a patient with a monolateral paralysis is in constant danger of asphyxia in two ways: (1) The paralysis may become bilateral. (2) There may be bilateral adductor spasm (or spasm of the mobile cord). The first of these is more often recognized than the latter, for it does not seem to be generally known that severe and dangerous bilateral spasm even in a palsied cord, may be caused from a mediastinal pressure effecting both the afferent and efferent vagal fibers. The author has seen such cases. If a patient with monolateral recurrent paralysis goes where he cannot be watched, he does so at his peril. Tracheotomy may be indicated as a preliminary procedure to laryngectomy and other procedures. It is sometimes needed to relieve bechic air pressure in order to obtain healing of the plastic flap, in the closing of tracheal fistulae. Angioneurotic edema of the larynx is usually an urgent indication for early tracheotomy.

Subcutaneous rupture of the trachea from external trauma may necessitate tracheotomy as shown in the following case. The author was called to the Presbyterian Hospital to examine a case of extreme dyspnea and cyanosis. He found a boy of fifteen years admitted with a history of having fallen down a flight of steps, striking his neck across the arm of a chair that stood at the foot. Apparent unconsciousness for a few minutes was followed by pain on swallowing, and in a few hours by an emphysematous swelling of the neck which gradually extended over the entire body from the edges of the scalp to the soles of the feet. Severe dyspnea began about 24 hours after the accident. Occasionally coughing brought up a considerable quantity of bloody mucus. Indirect laryngeal examination was negative. Introduction of the bronchoscope showed the trachea full of bubbling bloody secretions which, when cleared away, showed a horizontal wound in the tracheal mucosa extending from the front of the trachea around the left side about the level of the second ring. Below this the trachea was compressed to a scabbard shape. Pushing the bronchoscope on downward completely relieved the dyspnea. The bronchoscope was left *in situ* while a long incision was made in the front of the neck. When the trachea was reached the point of rupture was found to be between the first and second rings. The usual vertical tracheotomic incision was made quite low down and a long tracheal cannula inserted which relieved the breathing completely on removal of the bronchoscope. The emphysema subsided in a few days, the patient was decannulated without difficulty and a prompt recovery ensued.

Subcutaneous rupture of the trachea is a very rare accident but there are a number of cases scattered through the literature. The author believes, however, that this is the first case observed bronchoscopically. It serves to demonstrate the usefulness of the bronchoscope in the diagnosis of the exact mechanical cause of dyspnea and also demonstrates the advantage elsewhere mentioned of using the bronchoscope temporarily to relieve dyspnea and to furnish useful, though not essential aid in tracheotomy.

Acromegalic stenosis of the larynx as shown in Fig. 438 is a rare but urgent indication for tracheotomy. Glottic spasm in a case referred to the author by Dr. M. L. Stevenson was severe at times and would have been fatal without tracheotomy. The acromegalic overgrowth of the larynx was so great that the slightest spasm would shut up the already narrowed glottic chink.

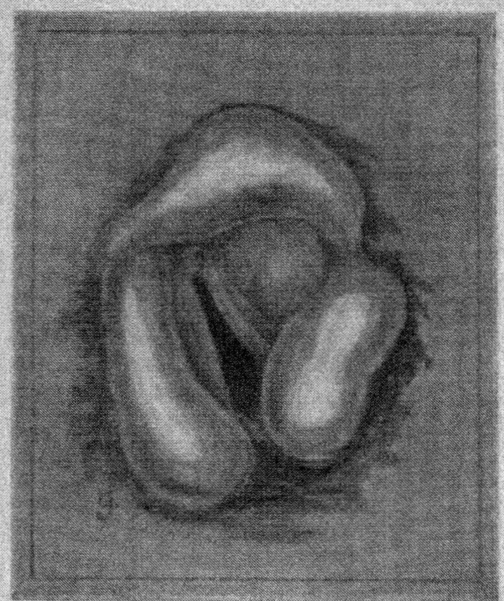

FIG. 438.—Acromegalic stenosis of the larynx in a man forty years of age. The thyroid cartilage was shown by a radiograph to be enormously overgrown. The massive contour of the laryngeal landmarks corresponded to the massive facies. Frequent glottic spasm, with the narrowed chink, required tracheotomy.

CONTRAINDICATIONS TO TRACHEOTOMY.

There are no contraindications to tracheotomy.

MORTALITY OF TRACHEOTOMY.

The mortality of tracheotomy must be distinguished from that of the lack of promptness in performing it, and especially from that due to inefficient after-care. We frequently save life when the patient is unconscious, limp and relaxed, with the respiration entirely abolished, and the pulse nearly or quite imperceptible. In the experience of all of us, many times has the result of quick work seemed like quickening the dead. In one of the author's cases the heart, as well as the lungs, had ceased to act, the pupils wide open and fixed, according to Dr. Clarence Ingram and Dr. Thomas T. Kirk, who were watching the patient. The operation should be done in all patients apparently dead of asphyxia. Under local anesthesia and at the proper time, tracheotomy should be free from dangers of shock, hemorrhage, or consecutive broncho-pneumonia. Between the skin and the trachea, in the middle line, there is no large vessel, and no important structure. There should be no more mortality from the operation, *per se,* than from the opening of superficial abscesses by an incision of equal length. The shortened route, with consequent deficiently warmed, moistened and filtered air, does not seem to be injurious to the lower air passages. Mortality during tracheotomy is usually caused by general anesthesia. Mortality after tracheotomy is usually due to want of proper care and watchfulness. No tracheotomic case should draw an unwatched breath so long as his larynx is tightly stenosed.

Of 472 tracheotomies done in the clinic and elsewhere by Dr. Patterson and the author, there has been a mortality of 6 (1.27 per cent). This includes all cases that died from any cause whatever within a week of the operation. These statistics show that the operation is much less dangerous than is generally supposed. It is to be noted that in many of the cases the operation was done later than it should have been, and if the series had shown even a ten per cent mortality, it would not have changed the author's opinion that the operation is an entirely safe one when performed at the first indication.

INSTRUMENTS.

For a tracheotomy the essentials are a knife and a pair of hands. Even eyesight is not essential, and the author twice has been quite successful in a dark room with nothing but a knife. Such performances, while life-saving and justifiable in emergencies, are to be avoided, when possible, by early operation with proper preparation. In all surgery it is wise to have the armamentarium as simple as possible. It is especially necessary in operations which, like tracheotomy, are, in some instances, extremely urgent. The following list contains all that should ever be needed:

TRACHEOTOMY INSTRUMENTS.

Headlight.	Curved needles.
Scalpels.	Needle holder.
Retractors.	Tape (good white linen).
Tenaculum.	Gauze sponges.
Trousseau dilator.	Sand bag.
Hemostats.	Catgut ligatures.
Scissors.	Silk worm sutures.
Tracheal cannula.	Tubing for oxygen tank.
Infiltration solution.	Hypodermic syringe for local anesthesia.

Tracheotomic cannulae. The cannulae of the shops are very defective and have been the cause of death in many cases. In all the adult sizes they are too short to reach the trachea after the reactionary swelling has reached its maximum. This swelling, in some instances, doubles the distance from the trachea to the skin, and thus withdraws the cannula from the trachea. The thin stream of air hissing through the tracheal incision deludes the nurse and the patient slowly sinks. Such cases (Fig. 441) have been recorded as "edema of the lungs" or "dyspnea only temporarily relieved by tracheotomy," etc. Cases of compression and other forms of tracheal stenosis require a cannula still longer and in some instances it must reach to the bifurcation (Fig. A, 439 and Fig. 442). A fenestrum in a cannula is a great mistake. The patient can get plenty of air past the unfenestrated cannula and the latter avoids the troublesome ulcerations, fungations and cicatricial mischief set up by a fenestrum; which, moreover, is seldom in position to do any good. Tapered cannulae are due to a curious misunderstanding of physics. To overcome the deficiencies found in all the cannulae in the shops, the author has had made by Messers Pilling a full set of cannulae (B, Fig. 439) of sufficient length to reach the trachea in every instance, no matter how great the swelling, even in cases of Ludwig's angina. Later when the reactionary swelling subsides, the space between the shield and the neck is taken up by additional dressings (Fig. 441), propping the shield out to the proper point so that the inner end of the cannula does not turn forward and press against the trachea. This extra length, with proper curvature enables the operator to fit the tube exactly to any case, and in no instance is the cannula accidentally withdrawn from the trachea with consequent asphyxia of the patient. These tubes are made to the author's scale (Fig. 440). If these tubes are found too long, the chances are the tracheotomy has been done too high. For stenosis deep down beyond the point where a tracheotomy wound can get below it, the long cane-shaped cannulae shown at A, Fig. 439 are to be used. With the aid of the bronchoscope to determine the condition, no patient should die for want of air as long as he has the lung tissue to utilize it. These long cannulae may, in some instances, require cutting off to the proper length. Under ordinary circumstances, they should never touch the carina at the bifurcation of the trachea, though in some instances it is necessary to extend them into one or the other bronchus, as in the case illustrated in Fig. 405. The usefulness of these cannulae in thymic stenosis has already been herein illustrated (Fig. 407). A cane-shaped cannula completely relieving the dyspnea of compressive malignant retrosternal goitre

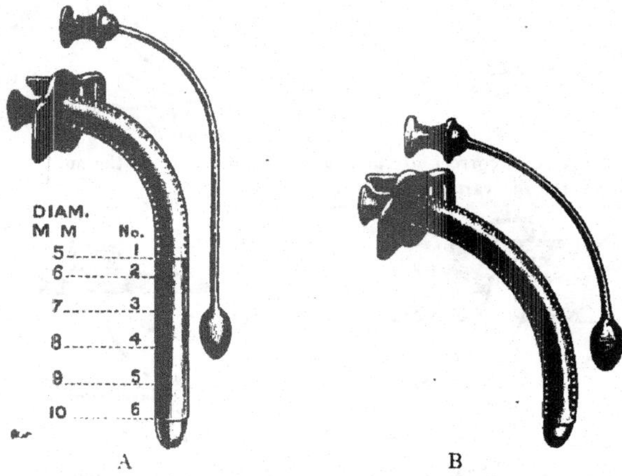

Fig. 439.—Author's tracheotomic cannulae. A shows cane-shaped cannula for use in intrathoracic compressive or other stenoses. B shows full-curved cannula for regular use. Pilots are made to fit the outer cannula; the inner cannula not being inserted until after withdrawal of the pilot.

is shown in Fig. 442. To prevent trauma to the tracheal cartilages or to the walls of the fistula, as well as to facilitate introduction when the fistula tightens from cicatricial contraction pilots are necessary with any kind of cannula. It is unnecessary to have the pilots fenestrated and hollow, because the introduction of the cannula involves but a moment and it is easy for the patient to get along without breathing, or even to hold his breath, for such a brief time.

Some patients with more or less chronic conditions which interfere with inspiration, but having expiration free and easy, can be relieved of the necessity of closing the tube during expiration when they wish to speak, by the valve cannula of DeSanti. The inspiration is through the cannula in the ordinary way, but on expiration a valve closes off the opening to the external air through the neck and thus the air is forced through the larynx, which the patient uses for phonation. The author prefers, however, the finger for temporary occlusion, and a cork for prolonged occlusion, as mentioned in connection with chronic laryngeal stenosis.

An emergency may occur away from home when a tracheotomy has to be done, and there is no cannula at hand. Under such circumstances, it has been customary to recommend the suturing of the edges of the

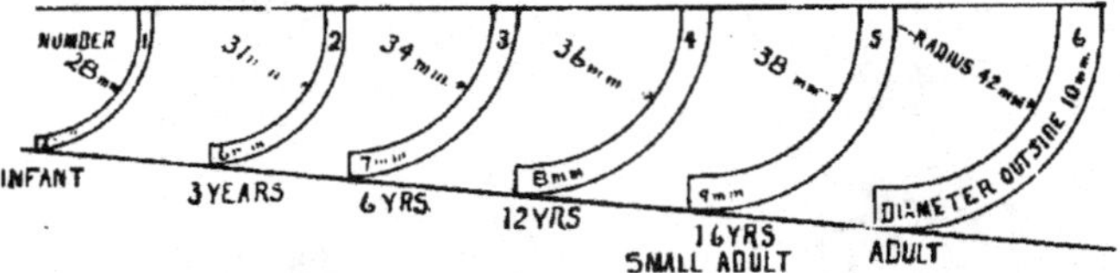

Fig. 440.—Scale of correct size and radius of curvature of the author's tracheotomic cannulae for the various ages.

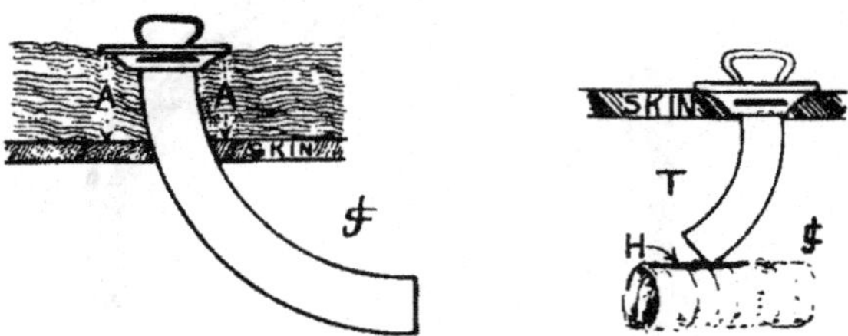

Fig. 441.—Schema showing thick pad of gauze dressing, filling the space, A, and used to hold out the author's full-curved cannula when too long, prior to reactionary swelling, and after subsidence of the latter. At the right is shown the manner in which the ordinary cannula of the shops permits a patient to asphyxiate, though some air is heard passing through the tracheal opening, H, after the cannula has been partially withdrawn by swelling of the tissues, T.

trachea to the skin. This is quite unreliable, because no such sutures can be relied upon to hold the trachea very long. A makeshift cannula formed by slitting one end of a short piece of rubber tubing and attaching strong cord to each half of the slit end, may be used, but if the patient is left in inexperienced hands, the chances are that he will asphyxiate from an accident to such a contrivance. Of course, if he is in charge of anyone who understands spreading the tracheal wound, he will be safe if closely watched; but the sooner a proper cannula is obtained the better. No hospital or surgeon should be so poorly equipped as to be compelled to resort to a makeshift so hazardous to human life. Cannulae should never be made of aluminum. This metal is corroded by boiling, and often by wound secretions. It loses its polish quickly and soon becomes very rough. Hard rubber is very objectionable because it loses shape on boiling, and its walls are so thick as to leave too little lumen. If made thin it may break. Soft rubber is open to the same objection and besides is very irritating to the wound. Either sterling silver, or "German silver" (neusilber) plated with pure silver should be used.

High or low tracheotomy. Which? It is very unfortunate that there ever was made the distinction between operations above and those

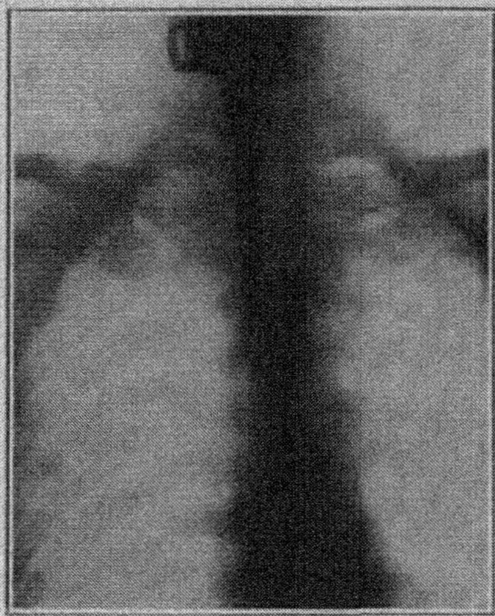

Fig. 442.—Radiograph of a man of fifty years with a substernal goitrous compression stenosis, the dyspnea of which was completely relieved by the author's cane-shaped tracheotomic cannula.

below the isthmus of the thyroid gland. Usually three separate operations are described under tracheotomy; namely, intercricothyroidotomy, high tracheotomy, low tracheotomy. Intercricothyroidotomy should never be done, unless the operator does not feel competent to do a quick tracheotomy below the cricoid. Obviously, anything is justifiable to save life, but the risk of subsequent stenotic troubles is very much greater after a stab operation through the cricothyroid membrane. Only a small cannula can be inserted. To enlarge the incision the cricoid must be cut which is a thing to be avoided when possible. Furthermore, one may not know the lower limits of a stenosis, which may be too low to be relieved by the cricothyroid operation. It is unfortunate that any distinction has ever been made between high and low tracheotomy because most operators when a low tracheeotomy is decided upon proceed to make a low incision. No wonder they consider it a difficult operation. A low incision means a short incision and consequently they are working at a great disadvantage down in a deep narrow wound full of blood. If there was no division into high and low operations the trachea would always be exposed high where it is superficial and followed down to the point at which it is decided to open it. The inexperienced operator will find it easy to lay bare "Adam's apple." He should not incise it, but simply follow it down until he comes to the first tracheal rings. If he makes a long external incision, allowing himself plenty of room for the separation of the tissues, the trachea can be very quickly followed from above downward, and incised at any point desired. If the thyroid gland is very much hypertrophied, it may be necessary in some instances to cut through the isthmus, retracting each lobe, though ordinarily this is not required, because the isthmus is freely movable upward or downward, and room enough can be obtained for the insertion of the cannula either above or below. Cricothyroidotomy should not be the operation of choice. It or anything else is justifiable for the saving of life but cutting through the cricothyroid membrane means invasion of the subglottic region of the larynx by inflammatory reaction, and this is almost certain to be followed by more or less laryngeal stenosis and perichondritis. Dr. Patterson and the author have noticed that a very large proportion of the cases coming to our attention for the relief of post tracheotomic laryngeal stenosis has been in the cases where the operation has been done through the cricothyroid membrane. Every one of these cases was an emergency operation and saved the patient's life, many of them being done practically in the dark and were perfectly justifiable, yet the author deems it his duty to call attention to this matter because of the prevalent opinion among laryngologists and general surgeons that the high tracheotomy, even as high as the cricothyroid membrane, is an operation of choice when quick work is needed. Division of the thyroid gland is a trifling matter and should in no case influence the operator to make the mistake of doing tracheotomy higher than the second ring of the trachea. When done for subglottic edema, the opening should be made below the third ring of the trachea, not but that a higher tracheotomy with a properly fitting cannula would relieve the dyspnea, but the reaction around the tube, plus the subglottic inflammation already present, is very apt to lead to stenosis. Particularly pernicious is it to incise the cricoid cartilage. Stenosis is almost certain to follow.

The author has been called upon to do a tracheotomy in a case of *laryngoptosis* in a man 54 years of age affected with cancer of the larynx. As almost the entire thyroid cartilage was below the sternal notch, as shown in another case (Fig. 404), a subhyoid pharyngotomy was done and a cane-shaped tube, Fig. 439, was inserted down through the larynx into the trachea. When the cannula was removed for cleaning, the growth would push out and close up the lumen within about one minute's time, but by having two cannulae, as is our regular custom, and with the obturator, with which these tubes are fitted, the nurse could very readily make the change. All forms of trapdoor, transverse and other special plans for the tracheal incision are often followed by stenosis (Fig. 12, Plate I) especially if the tube is worn for a long time.

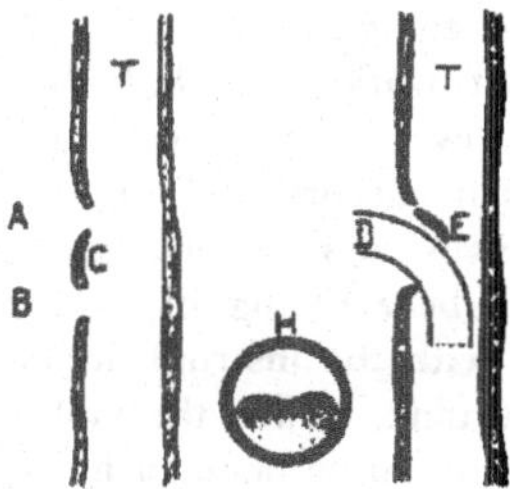

FIG. 443.—Schema showing the necessity for avoiding making two tracheotomic openings close together. A represents the old tracheotomic wound and B the new one, leaving one or two rings in the island of cartilage, C, undivided. When a tracheotomic cannula, D, is inserted the island, E, is pressed back into the lumen of the trachea, T, resulting eventually in a permanent stenosis as shown in the schematic endoscopic view, H, which represents the view down the trachea at the point, E, when the tracheotomic cannula was temporarily removed for oral tracheoscopy.

When necessary to do a tracheotomy below one not already healed, it is necessary to work without leaving an island of cartilage between the old and the new wound as will be understood by reference to Fig. 443. It is not that the island of cartilage in this instance would be apt to die, but a ring or two of cartilage has very little resistance to pressure and one or two rings will be easily pressed in by the cannula as shown in the illustration, and to become fixed there by inflammatory tissue as happened in the case from which the drawings were made.

When a tracheotomy is urgently needed before a diagnosis has been made in a case suspected of being luetic, cancerous or tuberculous, it is best to commence the incision high up so that the thyroid cartilage can be exposed and examined. Very often in laryngeal lues and tuberculosis that has progressed so far as to need tracheotomy, perichondrial involvement of a plainly inflammatory character is manifest.

Asepsis. In emergencies, the saving of life may demand the disregard of all the rules of modern surgery, not only as to the preparation of the patient but even as to the sterilization of a knife and the hands. It has happened to every surgeon not to see the patient until after the breathing has ceased. Except under such extreme circumstances all the aseptic precautions should be carried out with the same care as if the brain, abdomen or thorax were to be opened. Such a statement may seem superfluous to the surgeon, who, of course, expects to do all his work thus. But it is necessary to be especially disciplinary, as there is a natural tendency upon the part of nurses, internes and others to permit laxity because the patient coughs through the wound and, in some instances, the surgeon must work through both mouth and wound. It must be remembered, however, that the patient is more or less immune to the organisms he himself harbors, while he may be extremely susceptible to organisms, nominally and morphologically the same introduced from another source. Rubber tubing of proper size for the oxygen tank should be sterilized with the instruments and one end attached by the unsterile nurse to the tank. Then the tank should be covered with wet sterile towels so that it can be handled by the sterile assistant. All confusion and septic risks are thus avoided when oxygen is needed in a hurry. The author's tank holder illustrated on a previous page, is a life-saving convenience.

Preparation of the patient. All the precautions mentioned in Chapter III must be carried out, except in great emergencies. In addition, it would be wise to extract carious teeth, or have them filled and to combat oral sepsis in all the ways mentioned. If any operation on the larynx is contemplated, it becomes absolutely imperative to get rid of every dead tooth or root and to clean up and fill every spot of caries. The face and front of the neck should be shaven in case of a man. The skin of the neck and chin should be prepared by iodin solution, used on the dry skin, in the case of adults. The more tender skin of children should be scrubbed with a gauze sponge, using soap and water, followed by dilute alcohol. It is especially necessary to avoid causing a dermatitis by a too irritant preparation of the skin. In surrounding the field with towels, the upper part of the face should be left bare for observation.

Position of the patient and assistants for tracheotomy, and for artificial respiration. The patient should be recumbent. The head of the table should be lower than the foot. The neck of the patient should be extended and rendered prominent by a sand bag under the shoulders and neck, not extending further toward the occiput than the prominent seventh cervical vertebra. If this extreme extension too greatly increases dyspnea, the sand bag may be moved a little more toward the head. One assistant or nurse should kneel at the head of the table so as to be out of the way while attending strictly to the very important duty of holding the patient's head exactly in the middle line without permitting rotation. The operator should be on the patient's right, the first assistant in charge of sponges and hemostats, on the left; the second assistant, who holds retractors, stands at the patient's head, sharing the space with the nurse who kneels. The patient, if a child, may be wrapped in a sheet to restrain the arms and legs, but it is far preferable to have both legs held by a nurse and both arms held by a physician who can watch the pulse at the same time. If breathing ceases the assistant at the head of the table takes the two elbows of the patient for calm orderly artificial respiration, 20 times a minute, compressing the chest with the patient's elbows at the end of the down stroke, raising the ribs by the pull on the elbows at the end of the up stroke. Thus done, the arm movements do not interfere with the oxygen tubing held by the assistant at the side opposite the operator.

Anesthesia for tracheotomy should be local. General anesthesia is not only unnecessary but introduces an enormous element of danger out of all proportion to the anesthetic risk in the general run of surgical work. The danger may be primary from asphyxia or secondary from aspiration of infected blood, pus or secretions. The cough reflex is the watch-dog of the lung, and when the trachea is to be opened should be preserved or stimulated, rather than drugged asleep. Aside from this, general anesthesia, strange as it may seem, often renders our technic more hasty and careless than local anesthesia, for the following reasons: When tracheotomy is decided upon, there is usually sufficient dyspnea to demand some voluntary use of the accessory muscles of respiration. As complete anesthesia approaches, this voluntary action ceases, cyanosis increases until the respiratory center is paralyzed from over-stimulation, and the patient makes no further breathing effort. He never will make another breathing effort unless the trachea is opened widely and on the instant. For with an obstructed larynx, artificial respiration is never efficient for complete oxygenation of the blood. The trachea under these circumstances is by some operators opened by a stab, rather than by an incision, and it is small wonder if the percentage of mortality is almost as high as of stab wounds, inflicted with homicidal intent. In the hands of the most skilful and experienced, the incision may be badly placed: (unless the author's method is followed); in the hands of the unskilled or the excitable, serious accidents have occurred, such as the opening of the esophagus or a large vessel. A collection of tracheotomy specimens shows incisions at all sorts of positions and angles (Fig. 444). There is no time for hemostasis; the opening is made at the bottom of a pool of blood, and the first inspiration necessarily aspirates clots, and possibly pus, or infectious secretions, into the bronchioles, where it remains, because the cough reflex is absolutely abolished by the cumulative action of general anesthesia, deep cyanosis, and shock. There is, therefore, a large mortality from shock, hemorrhage, sepsis, and bronchopneumonia. How prone the profession is to underrate the dangers of general anesthesia is shown by the continued succession of case reports

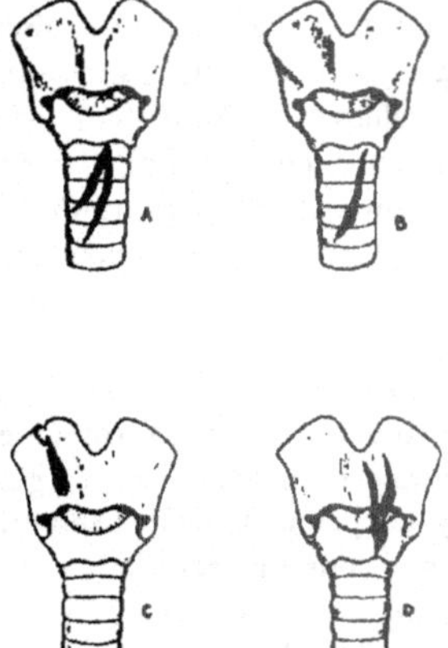

Fig. 444.—Schematic illustration of faulty incisions of the trachea due to faulty technic. (From observations of Laurens).

in which respiration has ceased on the table and a stab operation is done. Our general conception of the operation is a composite picture of many such instances, because we are all disposed to defer it until dyspnea and cyanosis are extreme. Particularly fatal is the common error, permitted by nearly every surgeon, of starting tracheotomy without anesthesia and then giving the anesthetic after the patient has manifested evidences of pain. The administration of ether, or still worse, chloroform, after the subject has suffered for sometime, will hasten dangerous or fatal apnea. If morphine also has previously been given, we have a combination peculiarly synergistic in killing the patient. In the dog, bronchoscopic oxygen insufflation has maintained life with a total absence of respiratory movements for as long as 18 minutes, when respiratory movements were resumed. With the human being, however, the operator will prefer to institute artificial respiratory movements rather than wait for them to be spontaneously resumed. In most instances, also, inasmuch as tracheotomy is to be done anyway, the surgeon, will prefer the insufflation of oxygen into the tracheal wound, and the addition of a few nitrite of amyl "pearls" to the insufflated vapor will save life.

The foregoing comments on respiratory arrest and its treatment are made here, under the heading of anesthesia, in order to emphasize the

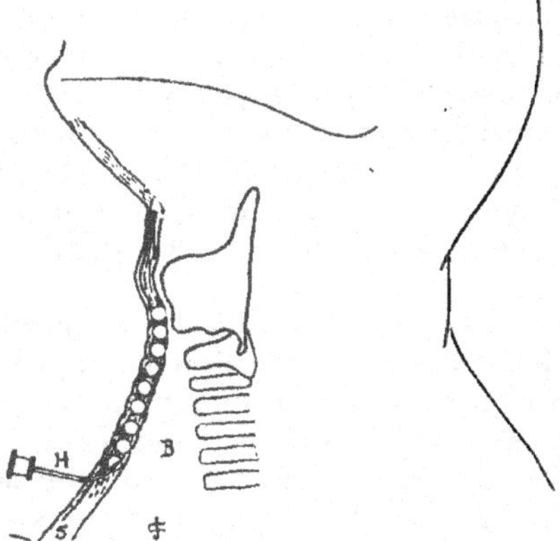

Fig. 445.—Schema illustrating intradermatic infiltration anesthesia for tracheotomy. The infiltration is between the layers of the skin, not under the skin. The infiltration needle, at H, is in the position of making the first injection. The needle is withdrawn and inserted at the upper border of the white wheal made by the first injection. Then the needle is withdrawn again and inserted at the upper border of the second wheal, and so on upward until the region of the thyroid cartilage is reached. The full length of the incision is thus anesthetized, with no pain whatever except the single prick of the first injection. The reinsertions are at the upper edge of the anesthetized area each time. If now it is desired to infiltrate the deeper tissues at B, one or two insertions through the anesthetized lines may be made for deep injection. Deep injections are unnecessary, however, as the subdermal tissues are not sensitive

too often unrecognized fact that it is usually the attempt at general anesthesia that precipitates apnea.

Not only is local infiltration anesthesia safer but it is much quicker and less troublesome. Not more than a minute is required for the injection and the operation can follow immediately.

Local anesthesia for tracheotomy The solution should contain a minute quantity of cocaine. Salt solution alone will cause slight anesthesia, but the addition of cocaine, no matter how little, obtunds the nerve ending better than the pressure of salt solution alone. In the author's clinic, a one-tenth of one per cent cocaine solution is used. The salt solution is sterile and cocaine tablets, which are kept constantly in formaldehyd vapor, are added, just before operation, the solution always being freshly prepared. It is essential that the injection be intradermatic, not hypodermatic. The method will be understood by reference to the schema, Fig. 445. The author has in a great many instances dispensed with even the local anesthesia in patients that were not unconscious. The pain was said by the patient to be trifling, as in the following instance: In a tracheotomy done for post-typhoid laryngeal perichondritis, at the Allegheny General Hospital, upon a patient referred by Dr. McNaugher, the operation required 32 seconds by the watch and was done without any anesthesia whatever, general or local. The patient, a woman of thirty years, said "ouch" twice, and stated afterwards that the operation was no more painful than the accidental pricking of one's finger by a pin.

Anesthetizing a tracheotomized patient. No hesitation need be felt in anesthetizing a tracheotomized patient so far as the tracheotomic wound is concerned. Such patients are far safer than one not tracheotomized, and there is no trouble with the tongue or the tissues attached to the hyoid bone falling backward and downward, obstructing breathing. They take the anesthetic quietly. It has been necessary many times for Dr. Patterson to remove tonsils from patients under treatment in the clinic for laryngeal stenosis. In every instance the patient went under ether quietly and was kept fully under until the operation was completed, all vessels twisted and oozing stopped. The technic is simple. A fold of gauze is laid over the tracheotomic cannula and, if the laryngeal stenosis is not complete, another over the mouth. The ether is dropped upon both pieces so that no matter which way air is taken in, it carries the ether vapor with it. It is necessary before starting to see that a good stout tape is securely attached to the cannula and tied back of the neck in the regular way. One assistant or nurse trained in tracheal work should be stationed to give undivided attention to the cannula and secretions coming from it. A Trousseau dilator should be at her hand should anything happen to the cannula. If insufflation anesthesia is to be used, in a tracheotomized case, it is usually preferable to insert the catheter through the larynx provided there is a widely open wound for escape. Presumably the larnyx is stenosed, but, if not, of course insufflation through the larynx is the same as if no tracheotomy had been done.

Technic. The classical descriptions of the steps in tracheotomy are very faulty. The division of the tissues after identification, layer by layer, on a grooved director is a needless, time wasting encumbrance. The skin and subcutaneous cellular tissue should be cut at the first stroke of the knife. This incision should be in the median line and should extend from the thyroid notch to the suprasternal notch. The deeper tissues are then divided by shallow incisions, the vessels being drawn aside with retractors held by an assistant; or seized before division as may seem best. The back of the point of the knife may be used or a blunt dissector if desired. The trachea is to be bared above the cricoid first and then followed downward. When the entire trachea from the cricoid to about the fifth ring has been bared of overlying tissues, the thyroid being retracted upward or downward, all bleeding having been arrested, the trachea may be incised at the desired location. In making the tracheal incision three things must be carefully guarded against.

First, incising the posterior tracheal wall by allowing the knife to go in so deeply as to cross the trachea and cut the posterior tracheo-esophageal "party-wall." This is especially likely to happen during the forward protrusion of the posterior wall during cough, and in the small trachea of infants.

Second, a badly directed incision (B, Fig. 444.).

Third, a double incision, from making two incisions instead of one. (A, Fig. 444). If the first incision is not long enough, the knife should be accurately inserted in the first incision and this incision elongated. The island of cartilage between two incisions, as at A, Fig. 444, is almost certain to die and even if it does not, stenosis is apt to follow, from displacement of the island and cicatricial contractions of the tracheal wall. Badly directed incisions are most apt to occur from a twisted position of the patient's head distorting the position of the trachea, or with those operators who do not follow the author's two-step finger-guided method of emergency tracheotomy.

Whatever be the plan of operation, one very common error must be avoided. Almost every operator is tempted to terminate his incision of the trachea just as soon as he hears a hiss of air. The Trousseau dilator or a hemostat is then inserted through a very small wound, and, when spread, it rips the trachea open sidewise, tearing the interannular membrane. It is far better to feel the knife go through three separate rings, each of which will communicate a separate and distinct sensation to the finger, and they can be easily counted though not seen. This insures a sufficiently long incision for the easy insertion of the cannula without tearing the interannular membrane. For the elongation of an insufficient tracheal incision the probe-pointed bistoury is safest, but with care to avoid deep insertion the ordinary scalpel is safe. When there is time, it is, of course, wise to stop all bleeding, ligating when necessary, and to have the wound perfectly dry and hemostats removed before the trachea is opened. Having incised the trachea the Trousseau dilator is gently used to spread the lips of the tracheal incision. Great care is needed to avoid damaging the annular cartilages or the interannular membrane. Either accident may cause chondrial necrosis and subsequent stenosis. If the patient has been very dyspneic, he will take a deep breath, as soon as the trachea is opened, and then will cease breathing for a few seconds. This in our clinic is called the "tracheotomic sigh of relief" and is present in almost every previously dyspneic case, especially in children, and is, really, just a moment of rest and relaxation after the prolonged fight for air. This apnea is readily distinguished from respiratory arrest of apnea vera by the difference in color of the patient's cheeks. If there has been much glottic obstruction a quantity of pus may escape. After the patient has had a few deep inspirations, the cannula is inserted and the wound dressed. The upper and lower ends of the incision may be drawn together with a few stitches, but as a rule the incision should not be closed close to the cannula, because of the likelihood of making a false passage when the cannula is changed. For this purpose, a large open wound in which the trachea can be promptly located and its incision spread is imperative. It is necessary for safety as well as to prevent trauma to the cartilages. Patients have been known to die "unrelieved by tracheotomy" because the interne inserted the cannula down between the layers of the tissues of the neck where it was left under the supposition that it was in the trachea. Injury of the cartilages or their perichondrium may result from forcing in a cannula. The old advice to suture the trachea to the skin in tracheotomies for foreign bodies, instead of using a cannula, in the hope of bechic expulsion of the foreign body has had a most pernicious influence, in as much as it has led to the habit in various cases of such stitching which is a frequent source of tracheal stenosis because of the damage done to the interannular membrane and to the perichondrium of the tracheal rings. Only in the operation of laryngostomy is such a procedure justifiable and even here the author has found it best to dispense with it as unnecessary. Many operators elevate the trachea with a tenaculum before incising it. In the deliberate operation with a dry wound, in which the trachea can be seen, this is an excellent way to fix and elevate the trachea for the incision. The author, however, prefers to incise the undisturbed trachea.

As mentioned in connection with some of the cases a bronchoscope in the trachea greatly facilitates a tracheotomy and, while the author would not advise a preliminary bronchoscopy as a routine procedure, yet in all cases where bronchoscopy is done for conditions requiring immediate tracheotomy the bronchoscope should be left in position and cut down upon from the outside. Not only does the bronchoscope serve as a staff for guidance, holding the trachea up clear of the lateral danger zone, but it also insures plenty of air for the patient with admixture of oxygen if desired so that the tracheotomy can proceed in an orderly way with thorough hemostasis before the trachea is opened.

In tracheotomizing patients wearing an intubation tube, it is better to substitute a bronchoscope for the intubation tube before commencing the tracheotomy.

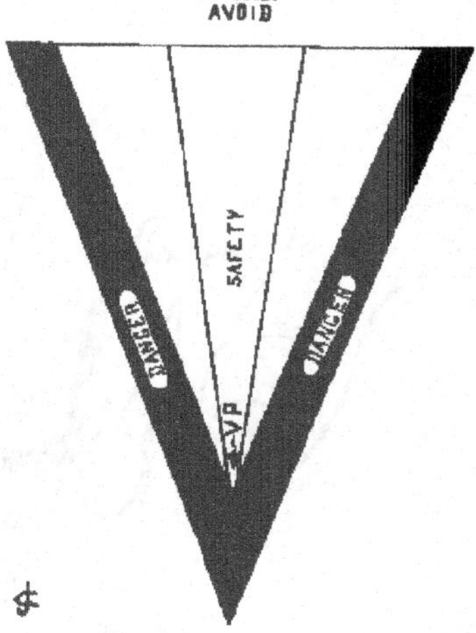

Fig. 446.—Schema of practical gross anatomy to be memorized for emergency tracheotomy. The middle line is the safety line, the higher the wider. Below, the safety line narrows to the vanishing point VP. The upper limit of the safety line is the thyroid notch until the trachea is bared, when the limit falls below the first tracheal ring. In practice the two dark danger lines are pushed back with the left thumb and middle finger as shown in Fig. 447, thus throwing the safety line into prominence.

Emergency tracheotomy. The stabbing of the cricothyroid membrane, or an attempted stabbing of the trachea, so long taught as an emergency tracheotomy is a mistake. The author has always taught his "two-stage, finger-guided" method as safer, quicker, more efficient and not likely to be followed by stenosis. To execute this promptly, requires the operator to forget his text-book anatomy and memorize the schema, Fig. 446. All of the important vessels and nerves are at the sides of the trachea. The thumb of the left hand pushes back the vessels and nerves on the patient's right and the middle finger of the same hand pushes back the left side vessels and nerves. (Fig. 447). The purpose of using the middle finger is to leave the left index free for its duties in the second stage. The pressure backward forces the center safety line into prominence. Now a long incision is made from the thyroid notch almost to the sternal notch, and deep enough to reach the trachea. This completes the first stage.

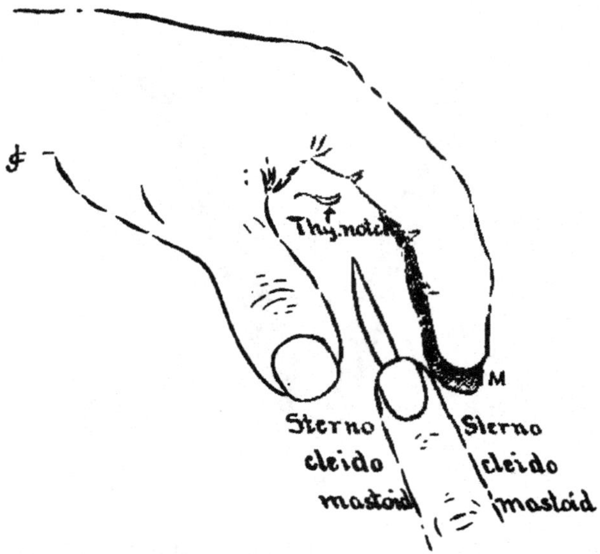

FIG. 447.—Schema showing the author's method of rapid tracheotomy. First stage. The hands are drawn ungloved for the sake of clearness. The upper hand is the left, of which the middle finger (M) and the thumb are used to repress the sterno-cleido-mastoid muscles, the finger and thumb being close to the trachea in order to press backward out of the way the carotid arteries and the jugular vein. This throws the trachea forward into prominence, and one deep slashing cut will incise all of the soft tissues down to the trachea.

Second stage. The entire wound is full of blood and the trachea cannot be seen but the trachea is to be found very readily by the tip of the index finger which detects the ridges of the tracheal rings feeling like a wash board. The left index is moved over a little bit to the patient's left side in order that the knife shall come precisely in the middle of the trachea, and the trachea is steadied by the left index so that the incision can be made quite accurately in the middle line. notwithstanding it lies buried at the bottom of a pool of blood. The head of the table should be lowered, just as soon as the incision in the trachea is completed and a hemostat or the Trousseau dilator, if it be at hand, is used to spread the lips of the tracheal wound, then the patient is turned over on the side, provided the patient is breathing freely, in order that the blood may run away from the wound and less of it may be aspirated. In cases, however, where respiration has ceased, it is necessary to keep the patient on the back so that efficient artificial respiration may be kept

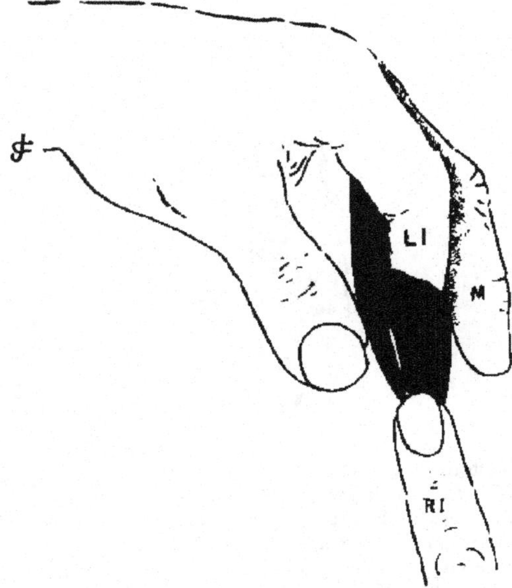

FIG. 448—Illustrating the author's method of quick tracheotomy. Second stage. The fingers are drawn ungloved for the sake of clearness. In operating the whole wound is full of blood, and the rings of the trachea are felt with the left index which is then moved slightly to the operator's left, while the knife is slid down along the left index to exactly the middle line when the trachea is incised.

up. In doing a tracheotomy after respiration has ceased, it must be remembered there will be no hissing in or out of air. Strange as it may seem, many an operator has been misled into thinking he has not opened the trachea by the absence of this sound which is so reliable if the patient is breathing. During artificial respiration, the air should hiss in and out and this is the test of the efficiency of the artificial respiratory movements. Of course, if the wound is properly spread with the Trousseau forceps or a hemostat or the cannula is inserted there is no hissing sound but the air passes in and out and there are always thin-blown bubbles of blood and secretion to indicate that the artificial respiration is forcing the air to move in and out. The use of oxygen and amyl nitrite at this stage has been referred to above.

If the operation has to be done in the dark as has happened twice in the author's experience, the left index finger feels the thyroid notch

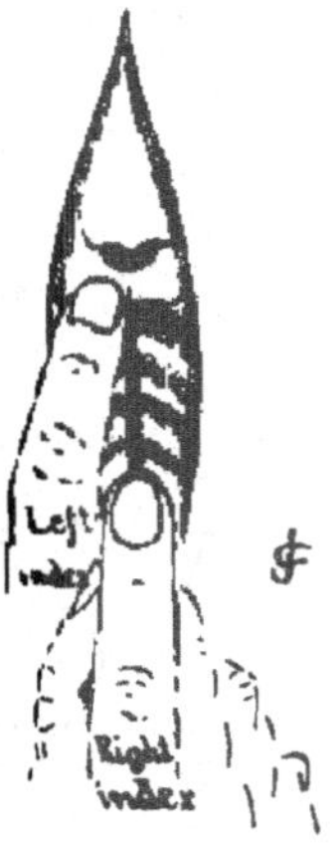

FIG. 449.—Substitute second stage of the author's two-stage finger-guided emergency tracheotomy. This plan for the second stage is easier for many operators, than that shown in Fig. 448. In practice the whole wound is a pool of blood, in which the trachea cannot be seen. The trachea is here shown free of blood to illustrate how it is found by palpation with the left index, which also serves as a guide for the knife that is slid down along the index in making the tracheal incision. The author prefers the second-stage position shown in Fig. 448

in the first stage (Fig. 447). The incision is guided along the prominent central safety ridge by the fourth and fifth fingers of the *right* hand of which the thumb and first two fingers are holding the knife. The second stage is the same as if there were light.

The author has found in teaching his method of emergency tracheotomy to others, that some persons are unable to use the index freely and independently for palpation while fixing the trachea with the thumb and the median finger. For them the second stage is easier executed as shown in Fig. 449.

RULES FOR EMERGENCY TRACHEOTOMY.

1. A stabbing operation is to be avoided.
2. Two incisions are better than one.
3. Press back the neck each side of the trachea with the thumb and middle finger of the left hand to throw the median safety ridge into prominence.
4. Make a long deep incision from the thyroid notch almost to the suprasternal notch. Working down in a small deep wound is difficult. This first incision should lay bare the thyroid and cricoid cartilages and a few upper rings of the trachea, but you cannot see them for blood.
5. Feel for the corrugated, wash-board-like trachea in the wound.
6. Incise the trachea while feeling it with the index.
7. Make the incision below the cricoid—preferably below the first ring of the trachea.
8. Don't expect a hiss of air if the patient is not breathing. Slip in a cannula and start artificial respiration.
9. Artificial respiration should force air in and out of cannula if everything is right.
10. Amyl nitrite blown in with oxygen, is the best restorative in respiratory arrest. Both may be drawn in by artificial respiration by the method described in a preceding paragraph headed "Position of assistants for tracheotomy and artificial respiration."

AFTER-CARE OF TRACHEOTOMIZED CASE.

A laxative, as after any other operation, is usually advisable. In regard to diet, if there be no contraindication pertaining to the condition for which the tracheotomy has been done, and the temperature be normal, there is no reason why the tracheotomized patient should not have a light tray. Occasionally a patient is encountered who will have some difficulty with food finding its way into the larynx, but this is exceedingly unusual. Ordinarily, tracheotomized patients are able to swallow after the operation just as well as before. Cleanliness of the mouth must be insured by brushing the teeth after taking food, and by the frequent rinsing of the mouth with alcohol 1 part to 5 of water. As the cough reflex is the watch dog of the lungs, antibechics, especially bromides and all the opium derivatives, should be particularly forbidden. The old-fashioned croup tent is of no value, and possibly is injurious to tracheotomized patients. It certainly deprives them of the copious ventilation which is necessary. There is, however, in our clinic, abundant evidence proving that vaporization of compound tincture of benzoin from hot water in the room is beneficial. Plenty of fresh air is absolutely essential. At least one window should never be closed in any weather, except during bathing or sponging.

A good nurse experienced in tracheal work is vital. In the author's work the special tracheal nurses have saved hundreds of lives that would have been lost under any good capable nurse with general training, but without special training in tracheal work. They know how to sponge away secretion before it is drawn in again. All these nurses know by the sound when the breathing is clear and they are competent to remove the outer cannula and replace it with a clean one. Without special training and experience, the nurse or even the interne should not be permitted to change the outer cannula. The inner cannula should be removed by the nurse as often as necessary. In certain cases of very thick secretion, the cannulae may become gummed together and occluded so much that though air still comes through, it is not in sufficient quantity, and, worst of all, the secretions cannot get out. Such cases often require the removal of both the cannulae, every hour, for evacuation of secretions that will not come out through the tube. In ordinary cases, however, the removal of the outer cannula once daily is sufficient. It is most astonishing to see the statement in print, and to hear surgeons advise, the cleaning of the outer cannula at such intervals as a week or even a month. Daily cleansings of the outer cannula are imperative. The nurse must be trained to dress the wound, for the dressing must be done very frequently, even every half-hour, if secretions are abundant. The old surgical rule to disturb the wound by dressing as seldom as possible, is one of the causes of the high mortality of tracheotomy under routine surgical regime. Conditions here are entirely different from anywhere else in the body. The air-infected secretions and discharges must be absorbed and removed by very frequent dressings. Gauze, wrung out of mercuric chloride, 1:10,000, is used in three pieces.

a. A large, thick, folded piece to pack around the cannula. (Not a narrow strip.)

b. A bib piece on the surface surrounding the stem of the cannula under the tape-holders.

c. A filter piece to lay over the entire front of the neck.

This latter piece should be changed as often as soiled, even if every ten minutes. Both the filter and bib pieces should be fastened by small safety pins, at the side of the neck, to the tapes which hold the cannula. Thus no bandage is needed. Duplicate cannulae for each case facilitate dressings and permit of repairs. If only one cannula is available, the cleaning is apt to be done hastily resulting in imperfect cleansing or in damage to the cannula. Dinged edges are certain to cause erosions and cicatrices. Tracheotomic cannulae when worn for a long time, no matter of how good construction, nor how carefully cleaned, become damaged and should be carefully watched for beginning breakage. The most common accident is the breaking off of the tube from the tape holder with resultant escape of the tube down the trachea. Before the days of bronchoscopy this was a very grave accident. Hunt (Bib. 211) reports a very interesting bronchoscopic removal of a very large cannular tube. Coolidge removed one in 1899, one of the earliest bronchoscopies.

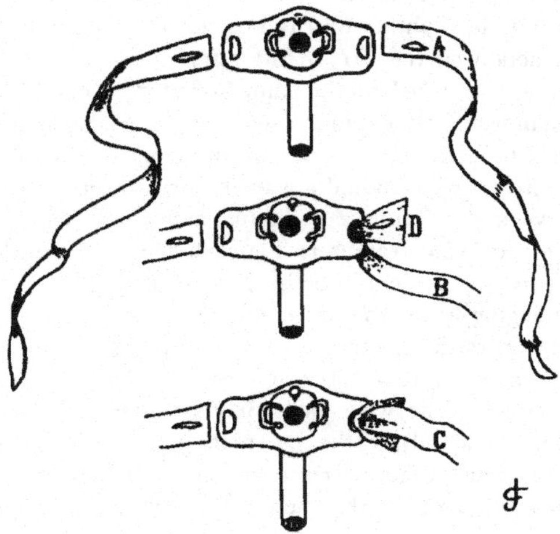

Fig. 450.—Schematic illustration of Dr. Ellen J. Patterson's method of attaching the tapes to tracheotomic cannulae. Near the end, A, a slit is cut in the tape with scissors, the tape being folded for cutting. The end, A, is then passed through the slot in the tape plate from the under side as shown at D. The end, B, is then pulled through the slit in the tape, and drawn taut as shown at C. The tape must be of good strong linen and must not be less than 19 mm. (three-fourths inch) wide.

Many parts of the cannulae have been removed since, and while almost all have been successful, yet the patient may asphyxiate, and every care should be taken to see that the cannulae are in perfect condition. Cannulae, especially inner ones, require careful cleaning. It is quite common to find nurses, unless specially taught, failing to get out all the mucus from the central part of the tube. This is boiled in place, and hence the cannula gets obstructed soon after replacing. The pipe cleaners sold by tobacconists are excellent for cleaning tubes, two or more being used at once, in a bundle.

The cannula may be obstructed by exuberant granulations. These should be removed with forceps, which method is preferable to caustics in our experience. Tracheal papillomata may obstruct the cannula and may appear in great abundance in the trachea after they are removed from the larynx. They should be searched for with a small bronchoscope and removed with forceps and pure alcohol may then be applied carefully to the points from which they spring, being especially careful not to allow any to get down into the trachea. Obstruction of the cannula by membrane in diphtheritic cases is not at all uncommon, and requires prompt action on the part of the nurse.

The tapes are attached to the cannula before the cannula is introduced. The manner of attaching the tapes to the tube, clearly illustrated in Fig. 450, has been in constant use in our clinic for many years with great satisfaction. A pilot should always be used to prevent trauma, and for the first week the Trousseau dilator must be used to spread the tracheal incision to avoid trauma to the cartilages. The little bent wire loops that are usually attached to the inner cannula, are very much in the way in sponging away the secretions, and considerable practice on the part of the nurse is necessary in order quickly to wipe clean the coughed out secretions from between these loops before the secretions are drawn in again. The wire loops may be done away with and the finger nail used to withdraw the inner cannula. But if this is done, there may be serious delay in removing the inner cannula in case it becomes obstructed, and as this might be such a serious matter, the author has preferred to leave on the wire loops and to train the nurses to wipe between them. There should be no breathing sound audible with a properly fitted cannula. The classical "stridor serraticus" which used to be considered as properly pertaining to the cannulated patient is noticeable by its absence with a proper cannula, except, of course, when the cannula is obstructed with secretion or when the patient coughs. A sterile "tracheotomy tray" should be in the room of every tracheotomized patient.

A tracheotomy tray should contain:

Tracheal cannula, duplicate of one patient wears.

Trousseau dilator.

Dressing forceps.

Scissors.

Sterile vaseline.

Tape.

Gauze sponges.

Gauze squares.

Sol. mercuric bichloride--1-10,000.

In the after care of tracheotomized cases, it is necessary to remember that edema of the lungs, pneumonia, broncho-pneumonia and fatal bronchitis are the rarest of complications following tracheotomy. Many patients die from unrecognized purely mechanical conditions and very few from the just-mentioned diseases. When a patient is not doing well, the trachea should be examined. It is necessary to remember that dyspnea or obstructed breathing or simple "sinking of the patient" apparently of exhaustion and without dyspnea may be due to

(a) Obstruction of the cannula by dried, cooked, thick or even thin secretion.

(b) Obstruction of the trachea itself by the same substances below the cannula.

(c) Obstruction of the trachea by compression.

(d) Cannula not reaching into the trachea.

Decannulation. The cannula should not be abandoned until the patient can sleep quietly with the outer cannula in place, the inner cannula being removed and a tight fitting cork placed in the outer orifice of the outer cannula. If the patient cannot do this, the larynx is stenosed and special work will be needed to decannulate the patient as will be explained in a future chapter. When the cannula is no longer needed the wound must be packed so as to heal from the bottom outward. There will never be cartilaginous union, but fibrous union of the divided edges of the tracheal incision must be complete before the outer tissues are allowed to close. Healing cartilage is prone to be associated with exuberant granulations and these may occlude the trachea and require a new tracheotomy for dyspnea. A number of such cases have been sent to the author, who located the trouble bronchoscopically. (See Fig. 12, Plate II, in the earlier volume. Bib. 269.) In order to keep the wound open, it is necessary to pack it firmly, not with a strip of gauze an end of which might get into the trachea, but with a small firm roll of gauze wedged into the depression corresponding to the wound, which latter is first overlaid with a large piece of gauze that covers the entire front of the neck, including the wound, as will be illustrated in connection with thyrotomy.

Complications. Erysipelas, diphtheritic and severe pyogenic infections of the wound ought to be exceedingly rare if a very careful aseptic technic is carried out. Even streptococcic and pneumococcic infections from the air passages in previously purulent cases, are exceedingly infrequent if the author's method of frequent dressings, (every one to three hours), be followed, especially when the dressings are wrung out of one to ten thousand bichloride solution. Tracheal ulcerations from pressure of the cannula are exceedingly rare if the cannula fit properly.

Such ulcerations may be followed by cicatricial contractions resulting in stenosis. The most serious of all complications is necrosis of more or less of the cartilaginous rings, and this is sure to result in more or less stenosis. This complication is best avoided by the directions given for preserving the perichondrium and the inter-annular membrane, and by careful selection of the cannula to fit the patient. Open air treatment is one of the best prophylactic and therapeutic measures for all infective complications.

Hemorrhage after tracheotomy may occur especially during the straining of coughing A vein or artery may lose its ligature, but as it is exceedingly rarely that vessels of any size are cut through, it is not usually a serious matter, unless a great quantity of blood should get down into the air passages. The best way to arrest it is, of course, to open up the wound and search for the bleeding points with hemostats. If the vessels have retracted into the soft tissues, it may take some little search, but they can always be found. Ordinarily, subcutaneous emphysema following tracheotomy is of little consequence and soon disappears. It is much more likely to appear if the tracheal wound is sutured, but occasionally happens, though rarely, with wounds packed open.

CHAPTER XXXVIII.

Chronic Stenosis of the Larynx and Trachea.*

Chronic stenosis almost invariably comes to the surgeon in the form of a tracheotomized or intubated patient who cannot abandon his cannula or intubation tube because of the laryngeal stenosis. Therefore, it will contribute to clearness to consider the subject from this viewpoint. The different forms of laryngeal stenosis associated with difficult decannulation or extubation may be classified into the following types:

1. Panic.
2. Spasmodic.
3. Paralytic.
4. Ankylotic (arytenoid).
5. Neoplastic.
6. Hyperplastic.
7. Cicatricial.
   (a) Loss of cartilage.
   (b) Loss of muscular tissue.
   (c) Fibrous.

Panic. Breathing through the neck with a properly placed tracheotomic cannula is so much easier than breathing through the mouth that, once the patient becomes accustomed to tracheotomic breathing, for quite a while he does not feel that he is getting enough air through the mouth, even though the larynx is perfectly patulous. In addition to this there is a "nerve cell habit" arising from previous experience with the stenosis that terrorizes the patient, especially a child, the moment he feels the slightest dyspnea. In children crying tends to increase stenosis (by disturbance of respiratory rhythm and by venous engorgement), and fright is very apt to do so in either adults or children. Glottic spasm may or may not contribute. All these things taken together

*Revised, with additions, from the author's paper read before the American Laryngological Association, 1913. (Bib. 263. Interesting discussion.)

may be called "panic" and constitute quite a formidable obstacle to decannulation even where there is no real stenosis of the larynx.

Spasm. Spasmodic stenosis may be associated with panic, or may be excited by subglottic inflammation. It is usually overcome by the same means as those suggested for panic, together with the treatment of the inflammatory condition that may be present. Doubtless one of the chief causes of adductor spasm is the prolonged wearing of an intubation tube, especially a large one, which prevents activity of the adductors, and of the abductors; because the action of these two sets of muscles is reciprocal, and the normal balance is, of course, interfered with by the presence of an intubation tube for a long period. Three methods of treatment may be used in these cases to get the patient permanently extubated. 1. Replacing the intubation tube with a special one, which has a very narrow neck with a long anteroposterior lumen in order to allow free glottic action for a time, until muscle balance is restored. 2. In a few cases of not very severe type it is possible to get them well by a patient extubation with replacement as soon as the child begins to get blue. This requires a facile intubator who has plenty of confidence in his ability to slip in the intubation tube promptly and without trauma. This method will not succeed in a violently spasmodic type, where the symptoms are so urgent and severe that the tube can be left out for only a few seconds. But in the less severe type of cases it is quite often successful. 3. Tracheotomy for extubation is the quickest method of cure in purely spasmodic cases without organic stenosis. The wearing of a tracheotomic cannula for a week or two will permit the restoration of muscle balance, and by corking the cannula with a slotted cork, as elsewhere herein mentioned, the child can be gradually weaned away from the cannula, and thus permanently extubated and decannulated.

Paralysis. Bilateral laryngeal paralysis causes a severe stenosis of the larynx, provided the paralysis is not cadaveric. In cadaveric paralysis there is usually sufficient breathing space, and this has led to operative nerve division to relieve stenosis. The author agrees with Charles H. Knight that nerve division has been a failure, but the author has thought that nerve excision might yield better results. In the one case in which the author tried nerve excision, it was a failure. In decannulation in paralytic laryngeal stenosis three methods of treatment may be followed. Cordectemy has yielded good results in rare instances, the cords being excised either by thyrotomy or endolaryngeally. The author had one success after evisceration of the larynx endoscopically by the direct method. The results of thyrotomic evisceration (Fig. 451) are absolutely ideal in cases where there are no lesions other than the bilateral paralysis. Formerly, when it was thought that excision of the cords meant permanent loss of voice one might hesitate to recommend evisceration. In two cases operated upon by the author a fairly loud, though very rough phonation, mostly in a monotone, was obtained by both the patients. It was a good useful voice, in both instances, though, of course, it did not have the flexibiltiy that we see after thyrotomy for conditions in which there is unimpaired mobility of the arytenoid joints. In both of these cases, however, the author did a careful dissection, taking out all the soft tissues and not simply the cords alone. The technic was the same as for thyrotomy (q. v.) except that the perichondrium was not removed, and the dissection was done on both sides instead of only one. Both patients were permanently decannulated. Great care is necessary to make sure that all of the sub-glottic tissue is dissected out. Of course the operation is only to be recommended when the paralysis is unassociated with essentially fatal conditions, such as aneurysm and malignant mediastinal tumors. George L. Richards reports a case in which spontaneous recov-

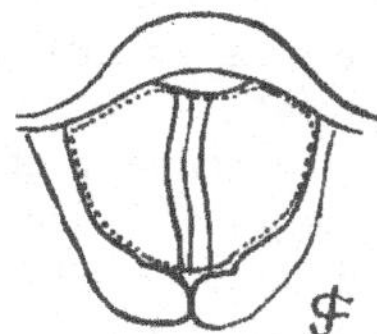

Fig. 451.—Schematic representation of evisceration of the larynx for chronic paralytic stenosis. The dotted line represents the line of dissection, endoscopic or thyrotomic.

ery from a laryngeal paralysis occurred, but that was in a child and was for a short time only. As a rule, it may be said that when bilateral paralysis remains twelve months it will never be followed by recovery, because of muscle atrophy or joint stiffening. Therefore, the operation is justifiable, if the patient wishes to be decannulated and considers some impairment of voice more than outbalanced by the getting rid of the cannula and by being made absolutely safe from asphyxia. It is rather appalling to note the number of patients with bilateral laryngeal paralysis that have died as a result of accident to the intubation tube or cannula. In bilateral recurrent paralysis of recent occurrence it may be worth while to attempt suturing the recurrent to the pneumogastric, provided the paralysis is recent, even if it is not peripheral. Monolateral paralysis does not usually cause sufficient dyspnea to call for a tracheotomy, but it is worthy of note that excision of a scar and suture of the recurrent laryngeal after injury has been successful in restoring motion to one cord (J. Shelton Horsley and Clifton M. Miller).

Ankylosis. Bilateral ankylotic conditions of the cricoarytenoid joints may prevent decannulation until the laryngeal stenosis is relieved. In one case of this kind, thyrotomic evisceration of the larynx, as mentioned above for paralysis, completely cured the stenosis in a man forty years of age. (Fig. 451.) Of course, evisceration is not to be advised, except in such cases as have remained rigid for a period of twelve months or more, and it is not meant to include the fixation that is associated with malignant, tuberculous or leutic infiltrations. Endoscopic evisceration (Fig. 452) is preferable to thyrotomic evisceration. (For technic of endoscopic evisceration, see Chapter VII.)

Neoplasms. Decannulation in neoplastic cases will, of course, depend, so far as stenosis is concerned, upon the nature of the growth and its curability. In malignant conditions after thyrotomy, stenosis practically never occurs. After hemilaryngectomy, stenosis may follow from a flaccid condition of the side wall of the larynx, or there may be a cicatricial contraction diminishing the stenosis. As a rule, in these cases, the author believes the best treatment is continuous dilatation from the prolonged wearing of a large intubation tube, though it is better to defer intubational dilatation until quite certain that the malignancy is not going to recur; because if the malignancy recur re-operation for malignancy can be so planned as to take care of the stenosis, by evisceration of the normal half of the larynx. In cases of stenosis associated with benign tumors other than papillomata, decannulation rarely presents difficulties. The removal of the tumor usually restores the laryngeal lumen.

Papillomata. Papillomata present quite a different problem, inasmuch as the growths persistently recur, though, of course, unlike malignancy, they do not infiltrate. Their removal usually restores the lumen and the patient may be thus readily decannulated; but recurrence must be carefully watched for and removed before the stenotic stage is reached. As a rule, it is better to wait for at least six months after discontinuance of recurrence before beginning decannulation as hereafter described. If papillomata have been carefully removed, and no injury has been done to the motor area of the larynx, there will be no cicatricial stenosis. Unfortunately, quite a number of cases are seen in which direct or indirect operations have removed masses of normal tissue, which has been followed by severe cicatricial stenosis. In some instances, the motor area has been damaged so as to lead to ankylotic stenosis.

Compression stenoses of the trachea. Peritracheal neoplasms occasionally cause compression stenosis as do also hypertrophy of the thymus and thyroid glands. Decannulation in a thymic compression (q. v.) case is very readily accomplished by either thymopexy or a subtotal thymectomy. A struma can be dealt with by the usual well known methods.

Hyperplastic and cicatricial chronic stenoses preventing decannulation may be classified etiologically as follows:

1. Tuberculosis.
2. Lues.
3. Scleroma.
4. Acute infectious diseases.
   (a) Diphtheria.
   (b) Typhoid Fever.
   (c) Scarletina.
   (d) Measles.
   (e) Whooping Cough.
5. Decubitus.
   (a) Cannular.
   (b) Tubal.
6. Trauma.
   (a) Tracheotomic.
   (b) Intubational.
   (c) Operative.
   (d) Suicidal and homicidal.
   (e) Accidental (by foreign bodies, external violence, bullets, etc.)

Most of the organic conditions, outside of the paralytic and neoplastic forms, are almost all the result of inflammation, often with ulceration and the secondary tissue changes. In the infective granulomata, such as lues and tuberculosis, and in the acute infectious diseases, it is practically always the mixed infections from oral sepsis running riot that do the harm. The chief exception to this is diphtheria, which in many cases is distinctly a necrotic process, wherein the replacement of the lost tissue by cicatricial tissue causes the stenosis either by cicatricial contraction or by the bulk of the newly formed inflammatory infiltrate or of pus collections. Typhoid fever (q. v.) is also associated with necrotic processes in some instances.

Tuberculosis. In the rare cases in which laryngeal tuberculosis of such severe type as to demand tracheotomy is cured, decannulation usually presents little difficulty after the infiltrations are reduced. Should cicatricial stenosis from ulceration persist, it is, of course, to be treated in the same way as cicatrices in other cases, by laryngostomy. The author has seen but a single case of this kind. In the non-cicatricial forms, which are relatively common, laryngostomy is not necessary, and direct application of the cautery will give such a degree of reduction of infiltration as to give an ample lumen.

Lues. Swain reports a case of luetic immobility of both cords in which the intermittent wearing of an intubation tube gained sufficient lumen in the larynx for respiration until general medication cured the patient. Under the careful watchfulness of Dr. Swain, such a procedure was safe, but as a rule patients are far safer with a tracheotomy. Luetic cicatrices are proverbially prone to return, and are particularly vicious in contraction. Prolonged stretching with oversized intubation tubes following either incision with the galvano-cautery or excision with cutting forceps is sometimes successful, but usually laryngostomy is required. In those old cases of chronic luetic fibrosis, which are, in a sense, paraluetic conditions little, if at all, amenable to the older methods of medication, salvarsan has accomplished wonders. It has even been claimed that cicatrices of luetic origin have been benefited. It would seem, however, that in such cases there must have been an underlying fibrosis of the nature of a luetic lesion, and not purely and simply a cicatricial condition following such a lesion. Scar tissue is scar tissue, regardless of what produced it, and we must rely upon laryngostomy for the cure of most of these scarred conditions.

Scleroma. Dr. Emil Mayer recommends the use of radiotherapy in the treatment of scleroma. If the stenosis is severe, doubtless it would be well to open the larynx externally and keep it open as in laryngostomy, so that the applications of the ray could be direct to the scleromatous tissue. Previously the results of treatment of scleroma were unsatisfactory, and those unamenable to ray treatment probably constitute the only cases of chronic laryngeal stenosis in which decannulation is impossible.

Diphtheria. Diphtheritic cases may be of the panic, spasmodic or, rarely, the paralytic types; but more often the stenosis is of either the hypertrophic or cicatricial forms. After intubation, especially if prolonged, there may be a hypertrophic condition, which is manifest in two ways: 1. An edematous condition of the upper orifice of the larynx, usually worse anteriorly around the base of the epiglottis, but also in some instances extending backward over the glossoepiglottic fold and the ventricular band, either or both. (Fig. 11, Plate I.) To this form, the author has given the name supraglottic hypertrophy. It resembles somewhat the ordinary acute laryngeal edema, except that it is firmer, seems to be chiefly anteriorly, is more sharply limited than the latter lesion usually is, and it has somewhat of a tendency to overhang and occlude inspiration more than expiration. The supraglottic hypertrophy the author has found, in some instances, to be due to the wearing of an intubation tube which has a sharp angle at its upper anterior edge. In one instance, the tube was smooth and rounded in this position, but was entirely too thick in the neck for the age of the child. Where these or any other defects in the tube are suspected of being responsible for the trouble, it is wise to change the tube for one of correct model and size and await results before attempting any more radical treatment, though local applications of the galvano-cautery can be made while testing out the effect of a correct tube. Excessive polypoid supraglottic hypertrophy should be excised. (Fig. 11, Plate I.) The infraglottic type is usually bilateral. (Fig. 87.) The masses encroach upon the lumen from each side like hypertrophic turbinals. Patients with either the supraglottic or infraglottic forms, if intubated, should be tracheotomized and the intubation tube thus dispensed with. They are very much safer with a tracheotomic cannula in place than intubated. In the infraglottic type of hypertrophy, the most wonderful results have followed the author's method of direct applications of the galvano-cautery (q. v.) With care there is no need of injuring any of the muscles or either of the crico-arytenoid joints. The author and Dr. Ellen J. Patterson have never yet failed to cure a subglottic hypertrophic post-diphtheritic stenosis by the galvanocauterant treatment.

In the cicatricial type of post-diphtheritic stenosis the fibrous tissue may take many forms. In some cases there is a band running across the larynx from one side to the other, it may be between the two ventricular bands, between the two cords, or from one band to the opposite cord, or to the same cord of the same side. Occasionally the cicatrix is in the form of a funnel with a minute opening at the bottom of the funnel. (Fig. 1, Plate I.) In some instances there is a web anteriorly (Fig. 4, Plate I), which very much diminishes the air space and may interfere with phonation or may not, depending on the degree of approximation possible. In two instances the author has seen a cicatricial mass between the arytenoids posteriorly with ankylosis of both joints, leaving only a very small opening close to the anterior commissure. This is unusual. More frequently the opening is somewhere in the posterior two-thirds. The management of the panic and spasmodic types of post-diphtheritic stenosis has been previously herein considered. The cicatricial forms require dilatatory intubation or laryngostomy or both. (q. v.)

Typhoid fever. About ten years ago, when typhoid fever was very prevalent in Pittsburgh, the author made an investigation of the laryngeal complications (Am. Journal Med. Sciences, Nov. 1905) with the aid of Dr. Ralph Duffy and Dr. Joseph H. Barach. It was found that the ulcerative lesions in the larynx were practically always the result of a mixed infection, and in some instances they were due to thrombosis of a small vessel with subsequent necrosis. When the ulcerative processes reached the perichondrium cicatricial stenosis was almost certain to follow, and practically all of the cases with perichondritis resulted in necrosis and required tracheotomy for acute edematous stenosis. The decannulation of these cases was chiefly by prolonged intubation, with special intubation tubes, the author's T-shaped cannula, and in some instances, laryngostomy. The detailed results have been previously reported. (Bib. 248 and 252). Ankylotic and paralytic post typhoid stenoses were treated with excellent results by Dr. Ellen J. Patterson and the author, by endoscopic evisceration of the larynx. (q. v.) (See also Figs. 86 and 452.)

Scarlatina may be followed by acute laryngeal stenosis, due to infection with either strepococcic or other pyogenic organisms. There may be cellulitus of the neck, chondritus and necrosis, but these are rare. In any event, the stenosis following is cicatricial and is handled like any other cicatricial stenoses.

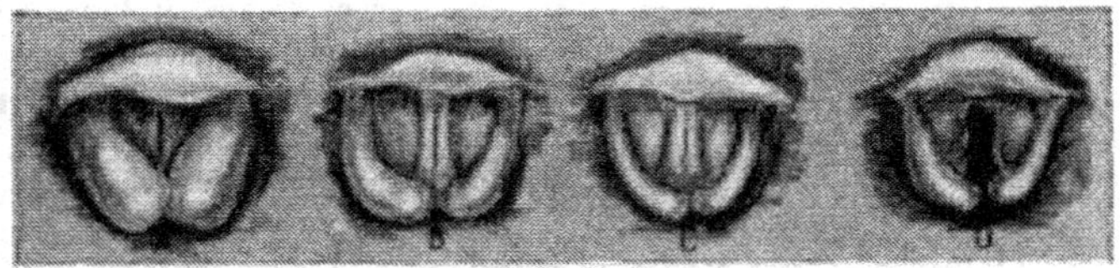

FIG. 452.—Post-typhoid ankylotic stenosis. A, infiltration of aryepiglottic folds and arytenoid region with fixation of cricoarytenoid articulations. B, three months later; infiltration disappeared, arytenoids immobile. C, twelve months later; tissues shrunken but no abduction possible. D, result of endoscopic evisceration, six months after decannulation. No mobility and no tendency to formation of an adventitious cord in the absence of a motile arytenoid.

Trauma. Occasionally foreign bodies, by a prolonged sojourn may ulcerate through from the esophagus into the trachea, causing cicatricial stenosis as elsewhere herein mentioned. Trauma, during the procedure of intubation, is very often charged with producing stenosis, which prevents the abandonment of the intubation tube. In the author's experience, this is exceedingly rare, the stenosis being due to other causes incidental to the disease for which the intubation is done. Diphtheria is essentially a necrotic process, that with or without intubation is apt to leave cicatricial stenosis, and, in the author's experience, stenosis has followed tracheotomy about as frequently as intubation. Decubitus is frequently referred to as though it were the presence of the tube that caused ulceration. It is doubtful if a properly fitting intubation tube will cause any ulceration, no matter how long it remains if it be free from roughness or sharp edges, and is removed sufficiently frequently to be cleaned. A tube left in too long may be crusted with concretions that will produce ulceration. Lynah reports fatal trauma from intubation tubes forced into the tissues of the neck by unskilled attempts at intubation. Tracheotomy is so commonly postponed until the very last moment that it is most frequently an emergency operation. Consequently the incision in the trachea is often very much misplaced, running off at an angle, or even slicing the side off the trachea like a slab from a log. Often also damage is done with dilating forceps tearing through the interannular tissue, and at times even denuding the cartilage of the rings. Then again, for one reason or another, various newly devised incisions with trap doors and even with excisions of cartilage are tried experimentally, nearly always resulting in more or less stenosis after cicatricial contractions set in. (Fig. 12 and 16, Plate I, and Fig. 443.) Undoubtedly in the insertion of a tracheotomic cannula, especially if it be done without a pilot, it is very easy to denude the posterior wall of the trachea, and in time an ulceration may follow, which may be attributed to decubitus, when really it is simply oft-repeated trauma. A properly fitted tracheotomic cannula should not produce decubitus, or even erosion of the epithelium. Neglect of cleanliness produces diseased granulations that result in building up a great mass of inflammatory infiltrate, which later becomes fibrous, and a thick dense scar results. Operations for malignancy and other conditions in the neighborhood of the trachea and larynx may cause stenosis, and in one instance the author has seen a compression stenosis in the trachea due to cicatricial contraction following a burn with a band of hot iron externally on the neck.

Attempted suicide occasionally results in serious damage to the cartilage, and if very careful work is not done, stenosis may follow. Usually an intubation tube should be worn in the larynx and trachea until the wound inflicted in attempted suicide has healed.

Abscesses have been the cause of the stenosis in two cases sent to the author for decannulation. Necrosis of the cricoid cartilage during pneumonia, in one case, was the fundamental process. In the other direct study discovered an old abscess in the "party wall." Treatment of these conditions by the direct method is easy, once the lesion is located but the location is not always easily determined unless careful search is made. If the original cords are destroyed by the abscess, good adventitious bands can be formed in some cases from the resultant scar tissue as elsewhere herein explained.

Treatment of cicatricial stenosis. In deciding the method of treatment to be used in a given case, it is very essential that a very careful bronchoscopic and direct laryngoscopic examination be made in addition to ordinary indirect laryngoscopy. With the direct laryngoscope and the esophageal speculum the party wall can be accurately studied. In many instances granulation tissue about the tracheal cannula should be removed in order to determine to what extent this is a factor in the stenosis. Occasionally a case is encountered where the nature of the stenosis which has required a tracheotomy has not been determined, and where it is exceedingly difficult to determine it. In some instances there is nothing to be seen but a large, smooth, rounded swelling on all sides of the larynx, suggesting tuberculosis, lues, or an inflammatory condition. In such instances, before planning a procedure, it was at one time necessary to do an exploratory thyrotomy, but since the development of the direct method where ample specimens can be accurately taken, it is possible to make an accurate diagnosis of conditions, if not of their etiology, in every instance. A sliding punch forceps should be used for this purpose, the distal end being inserted between the cords and a large mass of the tissue removed, always avoiding injury to the cricoarytenoid joints.

The treatment of all the different forms of stenosis is much the same if cicatrices have formed. In cases which have not yet cicatrized, cicatrization must be brought about by excision of exuberant granulations and argyrol applications, as the very first step. The fungating granulations from necrotic cartilage are particularly troublesome. In these cases the quickest and best method is to lay open the larynx and trachea to facilitate drainage and resorcin applications. Such cases require laryngostomy anyway, but dilatation must not be commenced until the cartilaginous necrosis has ceased and healing is complete. In intubated cases which show a tendency to close within a few hours or a few days after the removal of the intubation tube, it is safer to do a tracheotomy and remove the intubation tube. In a few instances, however, it may be well to try intubational dilatation. Webs and bands of cicatricial tissue should be excised. Should intubational dilatation fail, laryngostomy will cure almost every case. The treatment is prolonged but not painful and, by the author's method, the patient has the use of the whispered voice during the entire treatment.

CHAPTER XXXIX.

Intubational Dilatation of Chronic Laryngeal Stenoses.

Intubational dilatation of chronic stenoses is advisable as the first means of treatment of all post inflammatory chronic laryngeal stenoses. It is also indicated when there is a slight recurrence of stenosis after apparent cure by laryngostomy. It is best adapted to comparatively recent cases in which there is not a thick deposit of cicatricial tissue. Theoretically, it should yield better results than it does clinically, because the longer cicatricial tissue is held on the stretch the less tendency it has to recur and conversely the shorter the duration of the stretching the more prompt the recurrence. Its percentage of cures, however, is sufficiently high to warrant giving it first trial. Delavan has had a large experience with, and excellent results from, intubation in chronic stenosis. (Bib. 108, 109, 110, 111, 455.) Emil Mayer (Bib. 372) and W. Kelly Simpson (Bib. 498) have had excellent results. All of these reports show that great patience and prolonged treatment, usually a number of years, are necessary for results.

Intubational dilatation should not be used in post-intubational post-diphtheritic subglottic edema, because this form of stenosis yields more readily to the author's method of galvano-cauterization (q. v.) Intubational treatment is not satisfactory when tracheal stenosis coexists with the laryngeal stenosis. Laryngostomy is preferable for such cases.

Intubation tubes and instruments. To be of any benefit in cicatricial cases dilatation must be prolonged, and for this purpose nothing equals the large size intubation tube modeled after the tube of O'Dwyer. In cases in which the coughing out of the tube involves risk of closure of the larynx with serious dyspnea, the subglottic retaining swell must be large, and in most cases the author's personal preference is for a device suggested to the author by a patient with a luetic cicatricial stenosis. It was a great comfort to this patient to know that the tube could not be coughed out, and the author and Dr. Patterson have subsequently used the same plan in a number of other cases with similar good results. It is made of silver-plated brass, which is preferable to the hard rubber. The post-tube also has the advantage of maintaining a large tracheal fistula which is a great safeguard because the patient can learn to spread the wound orifice himself if need be. The first ones were made of aluminum because of the lightness. But as aluminum is corroded by boiling and

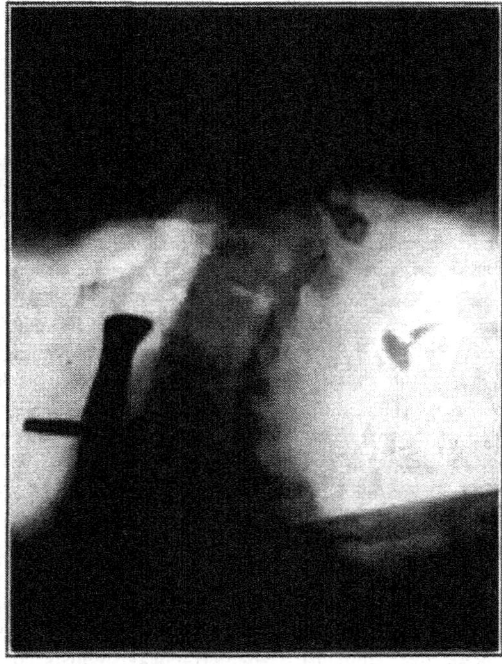

Fig. 453.—Radiograph of the living patient, showing the author's self retaining dilating intubation tube in position in a man of eighteen years, afflicted with post-typhoid laryngeal stenosis.

even by secretions, we have now abandoned it in favor of silvered brass. The author has tried the wearing of soft rubber tubes because of the effect of soft rubber in softening cicatricial tissue, but as the procedure is not safe without tracheotomy, it is better to do a laryngostomy when the effect of soft rubber is desired. Our screw-post tube was illustrated (Fig. 453) in the Laryngoscope, September, 1909, without knowing that

Schmiegolow had used the principle in the tube, Fig. 454, in 1894 (Bib. 480, 481). John Rogers also developed a very ingenious self retaining tube and his methods and results are excellent (Bib. 455, 456, 457). Priority in the self retaining principle, therefore, rests with Schmiegolow, and the Rogers tube antedated that of the author.

For palpatory insertion of his tubes (Fig. 455) the author has found the instrument shown in Fig. 456 to be preferable to the form of instrument used by O'Dwyer. Parenthetically, it should here be stated that the author in referring to tubes and intubation instruments refers only to such as are used in the dilatatory treatment of chronic stenosis of the larynx. For diphtheria and like conditions the author has never seen any improvement on the original O'Dwyer apparatus. For intubation and extubation by the direct method the author uses the instrument shown in Fig. 457.

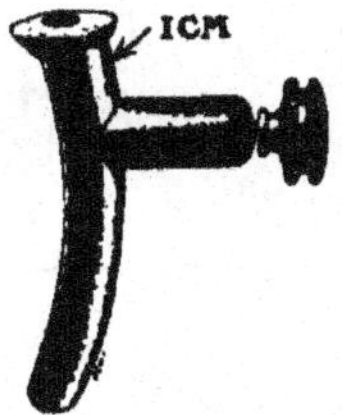

FIG. 454.—Self retaining intubation tube of Schmiegelow (Bib. 480, 481.)

Intubation and extubation. The method of palpatory introduction is precisely the same as taught by O'Dwyer and fully described and illustrated in the text books. In children palpatory introduction is quite easy but in adults it is, in some cases, quite difficult until after much practice. The larynx is usually so far down, especially when the patient is retching, that the arytenoids cannot be reached by the finger, and in many cases these landmarks have been destroyed by previous necrosis. The right aryepiglottic fold is generally present in some form and will serve as a palpatory landmark. The direct method of intubation is usually quite satisfactory though the supraglottic swell of the large adult tubes will not go through any but an open laryngoscope. No special instrument is necessary for extubation. The post is unscrewed and removed, and then the tube is pushed up into the pharynx with a hemostat, being careful not to scratch the tube. The patient can usually eject the tube from the pharynx, but, if not, the neck of the tube can be seized in the pharynx with the operator's first and second fingers.

Care of patients under intubational treatment for laryngeal stenosis. The tendency of an intubation tube in the intubational treatment is to sink lower and lower and also to bury itself below the epiglottis anteriorly. This must be combatted at first by the support afforded by the block (C, Fig. 455) and later by keeping the tube up into its place with gauze packing below the post in the cervical fistula. The post must be screwed tightly with a hemostat to prevent its accidental unscrewing. The block (C, Fig. 455) is usually dispensed with after the establishment of a long well epidermatized trough.

It is quite essential that the tubes shall be of large size and that they shall be worn constantly. The size should be increased up to the

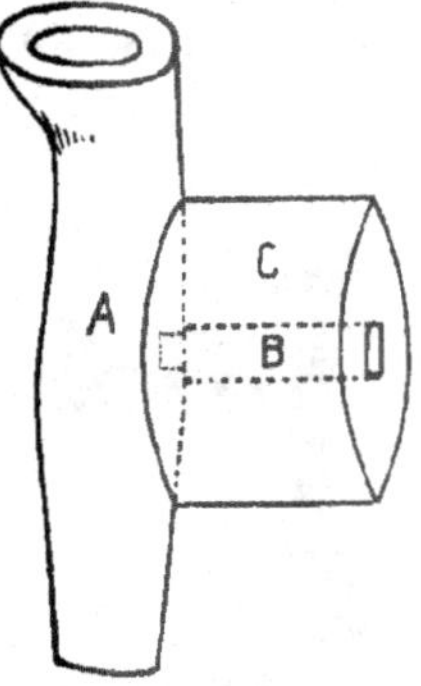

FIG. 455.—The author's self retaining intubation tube for the treatment of chronic laryngeal stenosis. The tube (A) is introduced through the mouth, then the post (B) is screwed in through the tracheal wound. Then the block (C) is slid into the wound, the square hole in the block guarding the post against all possibility of unscrewing. If the threads of the post are properly fitted and tightly screwed up with a hemostat, however, there is no chance of unscrewing and gauze packing is used instead of the block to maintain a large fistula. The shape of the intubation tube has been arrived at after long clinical study and trials, and cannot be altered without risk of falling into errors that have been made and eliminated in the development of this shape.

point where it requires a slight degree of force for insertion. Great care must be taken, however, not to increase size too rapidly nor to carry it too far. lest chondrial necrosis set in and make matters worse than before. Usually once a month is often enough to substitute the next larger size. The tube must be removed for cleansing every alternate day at first. After a few weeks the duration may be increased until it can remain in a week or even two weeks. Should swelling and tenderness develop around the wound the tube should be removed and cleansed. Should the inflammatory signs persist it may be necessary to substitute a tracheotomic cannula for a few days. The position of the supraglottic swell of the tube should be watched daily preferably by the laryngeal mirror. Overhanging granulations, if any, should be removed with tissue forceps, Fig. 35, by the direct method. Once every week, when the tube is removed, a bronchoscope should be passed to note progress and to remove deeper granulations, treat ulceration by applications, or

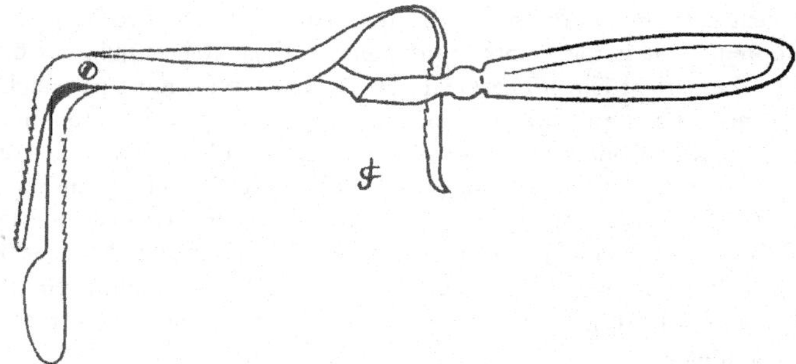

FIG. 456.—Introducer for the author's self-retaining intubation tubes, when it is desired to use the palpatory method of introduction. This instrument is for adults. For children the O'Dwyer principle is preferable, if an indirect instrument is desired.

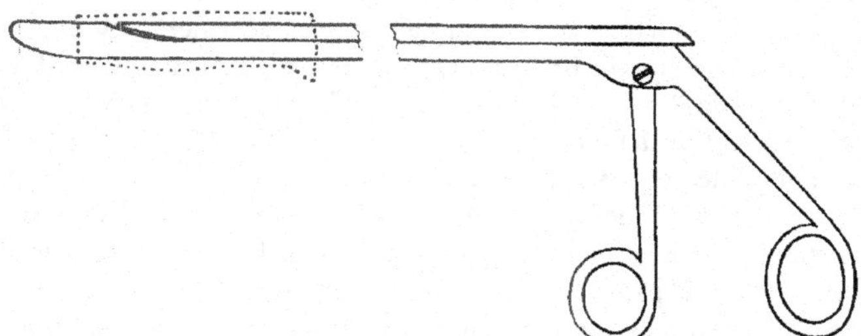

FIG. 457.—Introducer for placing the author's intubation tubes by the direct method. For children the introducer of Mosher is better.

by change of tubal shape, or by temporary tubal discontinuance as may be indicated. For this inspection the bronchoscope should always be passed through the larynx; thus the approach is in what should be the normal laryngeal and tracheal axes. In no case should the tracheal fistula be allowed to close while the patient is under intubational dilatation of a chronic laryngeal stenosis. Should an intubation tube become obstructed suddenly a good tracheal nurse can extubate the patient by the method described, and if needed for breathing, insert an ordinary tracheotomic cannula temporarily.

From time to time, after the first few months, the tube may be left out for a few hours to note with the mirror and by the breathing what gain is being made in the area of cross section of the laryngeal lumen. The duration of the extubation test period may be increased if the improvement warrant, until finally the tube can be abandoned altogether. The supreme test is the breathing at night. When this is quiet without the tube the patient is a probationary cure. His larynx must be watched and, if need be, intubation resumed before his larynx gets too much contracted. Six months without the tube may be called a cure. Fortunately the fistula will usually stay patent during this time because it is epithelialized with dermal epithelium. If it show any tendency to close completely it must be kept open by the wearing of an obturator, which consists in a silver plug long enough barely to reach the trachea, the plug being metallically attached to a tape holder after the manner of a tracheotomic cannula.

The treatment may require from three months to four years. During this time the patient has a good whispered voice but cannot phonate. He can attend to any work, even hard labor, provided his work does not require a voice; and provided he could, in case of emergency, extubate himself and put in a tracheotomic cannula. In only a few cases is the secretion of such a nature as to bring about such an emergency after the first three or four months of treatment. A few patients are afflicted with a tubal accumulation of a thick, gummy, adherent secretion which they cannot cough out of the tube.

The ultimate vocal results in the successful cases is excellent in proportion as arytenoid motility remains. In ankylotic and necrotic arytenoid conditions the patient will get a loud though rough and inflexible phonation. Many patients acquire a peculiar sidewise dipping of the head, with working of the platysma myoides and other cervical muscles just as they commence to speak. The ultimate voice in adults is usually lower in pitch than before treatment. In children time will work wonders in the development of flexible, almost unimpaired voice.

CHAPTER XL.

Laryngostomy.

Definition. Laryngostomy is the name given to the surgical procedure of laying open the larynx anteriorly and keeping it open for a long period of treatment. More or less of the trachea is usually included in the opening and the procedure is then laryngotracheostomy.

History. It was done for stenosis first by Heryng in 1894 (Bib. 215) and by Ruggi for recurrent papilloma in 1898 (Bib. 461). It has since been elaborated and developed by Sargnon (Bib. 472, 473, 474), Canapel, Melzi, Cagnola, Barlatier, Baratoux, Vignard and others. Sargnon's methods and results are especially worthy of study.

The author first performed it in 1900, reporting five successful cases, with exhibition of two of the patients at the meeting of the American Laryngological, Rhinological and Otological Society, February, 1904. (Bib. 268). In these cases the author used the T-shaped silver cannula shown at A and B, in Fig. 458, and a laryngostomy cannula (Fig. 459). In two of the cases the stenosis subsequently recurred. In 1906 Killian demonstrated a vastly better method by post-operative dilatation, that made of laryngostomy an operation that has now a permanent place in the surgery of the larynx. He also made use of a T-shaped cannula (C, Fig. 458), but it was made of soft rubber and was used in successively increasing sizes for dilatation. He had discovered that the contact and elastic pressure of the soft rubber caused a softening and absorption of the obstructive endolaryngeal tissue. Taking advantage of the effect of the contact of rubber tubing, the author fitted the rubber tubing in increasing sizes and of proper length for the particular case (Figs. 461 and 475) over the upright branch of his old laryngostomy cannula. (Fig. 459). The results of this have been ideal. Sargnon suggested tying the rubber drain to an ordinary cannula as shown in Fig. 462. Under his skilful care this produced excellent results, but in the hands of others great care has been necessary to combat its tendency to the development instead of the obliteration of the spur (E, Fig. 460), which all old cannula wearers have. Fournier suggested using an ordinary tracheotomic cannula, the tubing having a side-opening through which the cannula was placed. This also produced good results, but it does not obliterate the spur (E, Fig. 460) like the author's apparatus, Fig. 461. Mr. Walter G. Howarth has had excellent results from dispensing altogether with a cannula. (Fig. 464). The rubber tubing is cut long enough to

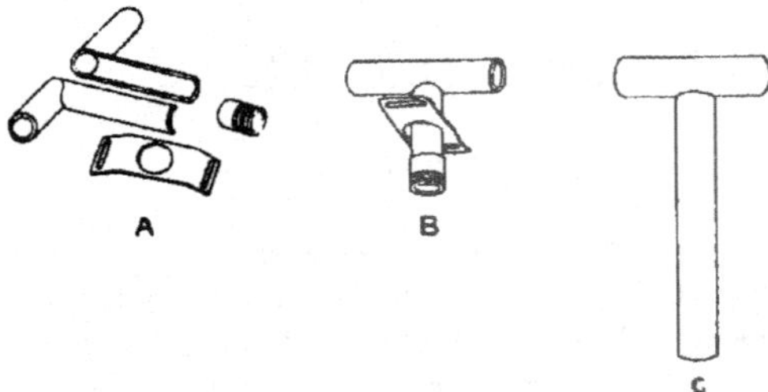

Fig. 458.—A. B., T-shaped separable tracheal cannula of the author. Each section is inserted separately, then the two are held together by the ring. (Bib. 268). The tape holder retains the tube and dressings. C, T-shaped soft rubber tube of Killian.

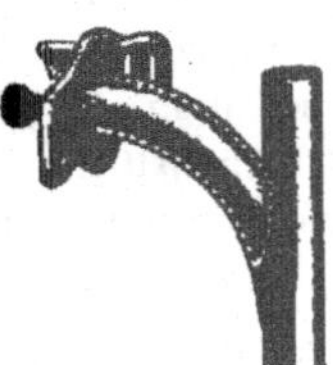

Fig. 459.—Author's laryngostomy cannula originally used without rubber tubing. After Killian's discovery of the effect of rubber dilatation, rubber tubing in increasing sizes and of proper length has been placed over the upright branch tube, as shown in the radiograph, Fig. 475, and the schema, Fig. 461.

extend down the trachea past the fistula and is held in place by ligatures which are fastened to the middle of the tubing, opposite the fistula, by passing the sutures through the wall of the tubing with a needle, before the tubing is put in place. This method seems excellent, and is readily placed without discomfort to the patient. Thost does not use the soft rubber softening and absorbing method. He inserts a smooth, hard-rubber plug, or wedge, above the ordinary tracheal cannula as shown in Fig. 466. His results are excellent. Much careful work, however, is

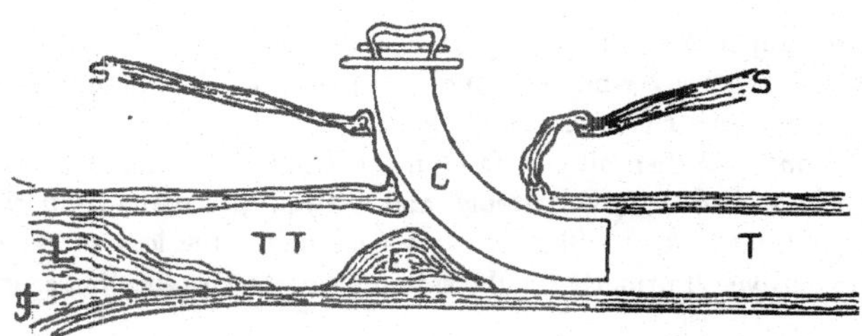

FIG. 460.—Schematic representation of the problem involved in laryngeal stenosis when the patient has been wearing a cannula for a long time. In addition to the original stenosis (L) in the larynx, the wearing of the cannula (C) has built up the stenotic mass (E) in the trachea. S represents the skin and T, TT, represent the trachea.

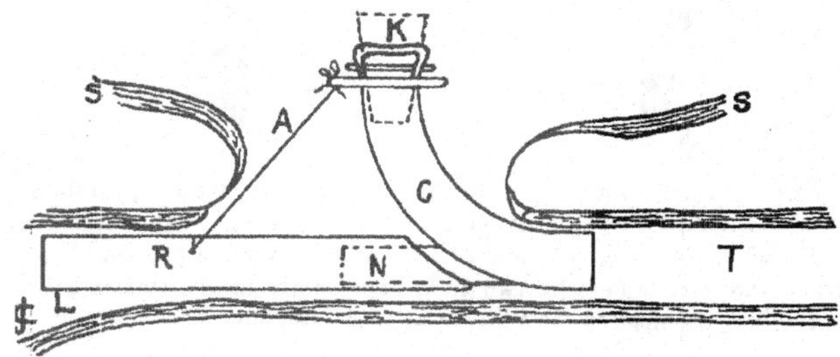

FIG. 461.—Schema showing the author's method of laryngostomy. The hollow upward metallic branch (N) of the cannula (C) holds the rubber tube (R) back firmly against the spur (E) on the back wall of the trachea. Moreover, the air passing up through the rubber tube (R), permits the patient to talk in a loud whisper, the external orifice of the cannula being occluded most of the time with the cork (K).

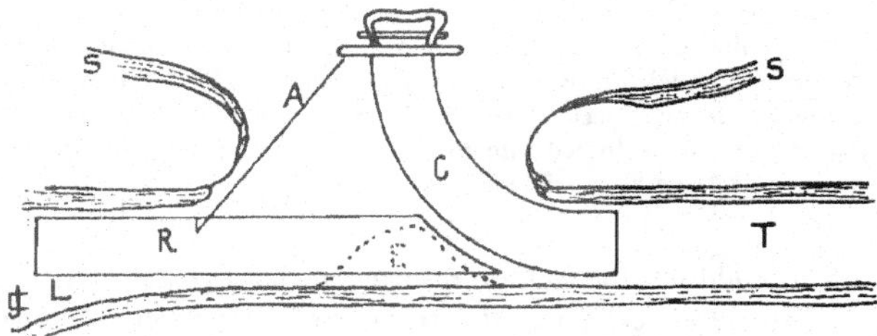

FIG. 462.—Schema showing the method of Sargnon for after-treatment of laryngostomy Excellent results have followed this method. The tendency of the cicatricial spur (E) to push forward the lower end of the rubber tube (R) should be combated The tubing, R, is plugged with gauze at each dressing.

needed to combat the spur, shown at E, Fig. 460. The patient has not even a whispered voice while the plug is in place, but doubtless this could be remedied by an air canal in the plug.

Indications. When all else fails in a case of cicatricial stenosis, recourse must be had to laryngostomy, and with proper patience in carrying out the treatment, it will cure every case unless the loss of cartilage is very extensive. Formerly, in the stenosis due to chronically recurring

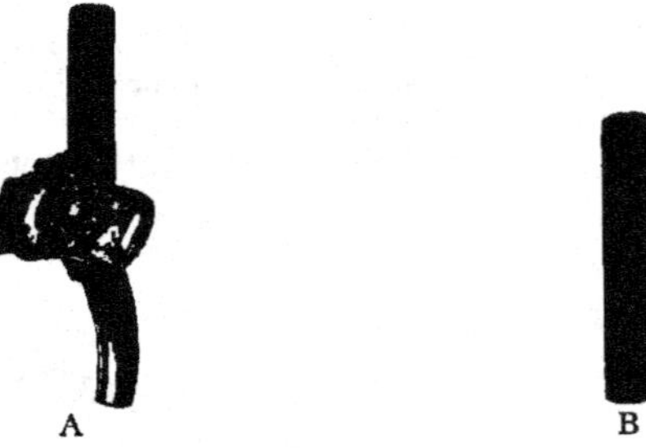

Fig. 463.—Fournier's method of holding the rubber dilatatory drain in position. B, rubber drain with side opening cut in lower end. A, tracheal cannula attached to drain by passing the tube of the cannula through the side hole of the rubber drain, where it is held by two ends of a suture to the staples of the tape plate. The tubing is plugged with gauze at each dressing.

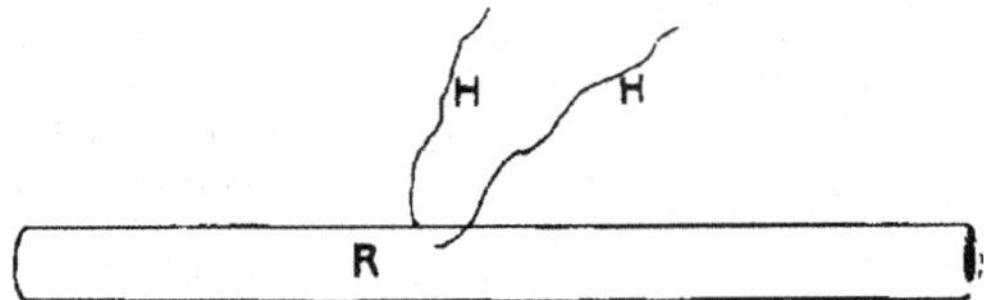

Fig. 464.—Method of Mr. Walter G. Howarth in laryngostomy. The cords (H, H) transfixed through the wall of the rubber tubing (R). After the tube is in place in the larynx and trachea the free ends of the cords are tied over the large plug of gauze that is forced into the laryngostomy opening in the effort to keep this opening as large as possible.

papillomata in children, the author resorted to laryngostomy in intractable cases, but since perfecting the technic of direct removal, he has found that by persistence with the extirpation and alcohol applications, it is possible ultimately to cure every case. There are a number of stenotic conditions such as scleroma that doubtless would be benefited by laryngostomy, but the author has had no personal experience with them.

Contraindications. Pyrexia is an absolute contraindication. Active lues and active tuberculosis, local or elsewhere, do also. Bronchial and pulmonary disorders greatly increase the risks and if irremediable, they are contraindications. Serious organic disease anywhere is prohibitive. Excessive loss of laryngeal and tracheal cartilage will preclude a successful result. A purulent focus, as in the nasal accessory sinuses, increases the risk but is not an absolute contraindication.

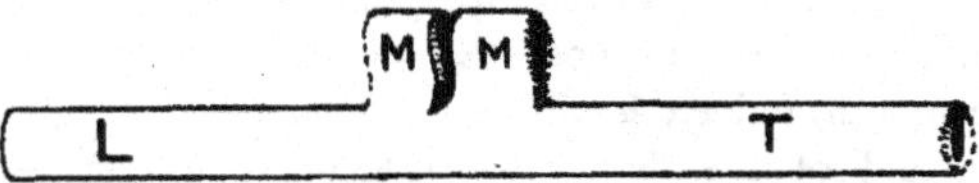

Fig. 465.—Special rubber tube of Moure for laryngostomy. The tubular parts (L and T) are in the larynx and trachea, respectively, while the loops (M, M) project through the external wound to keep it patulent.

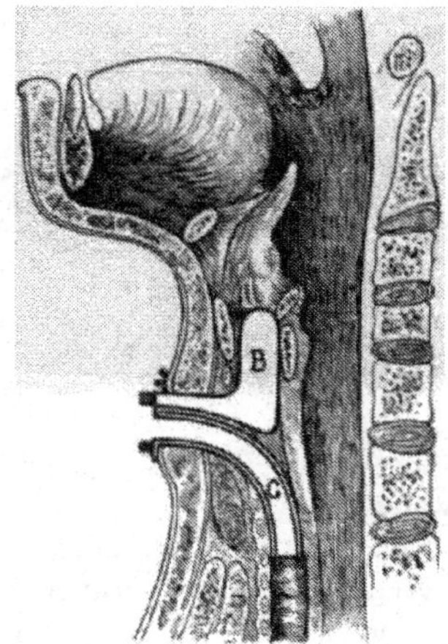

Fig. 466.—Thost's apparatus for the dilatation of cicatricial laryngeal stenosis. The hard rubber plug, B, is inserted from below upward before the ordinary tracheal cannula, C, is inserted.

Instruments. Besides general operating instruments, the requisites are a blunt pointed bistoury, Moure's thyrotomy shears or the turbinotome (Fig. 467), small retractors, silk for suturing the mucosa to the skin. As in all external laryngeal surgery a small electric light, worn between the operator's eyes (not on top of the head) is essential. The illuminating and the visual axes must almost coincide. For the postoperative dilatatory dressings, soft rubber tubing evenly graduated in sizes from 15 to 45 French scale sizes is needed. These are unobtainable in drainage tubing, but veterinary catheters answer admirably. These tubes must be cut in length to suit the case, the cut edges being rounded with sand paper or by singeing in the flame of an alcohol lamp, being careful not to burn the rubber, only to melt off the sharp angle of the cut edge.

Preliminaries. The patient's health, if improvable, must be improved. Luetic cases should have at least one month's treatment, whether active lesions are present or not. As in all operations about the air passages, the mouth and teeth should be put in the best possible condition with the aid of the dentist if necessary. Alcohol 25 per cent strength is the best non-toxic antiseptic mouth wash. All proprietary preparations are a delusion, unless they contain alcohol; though they

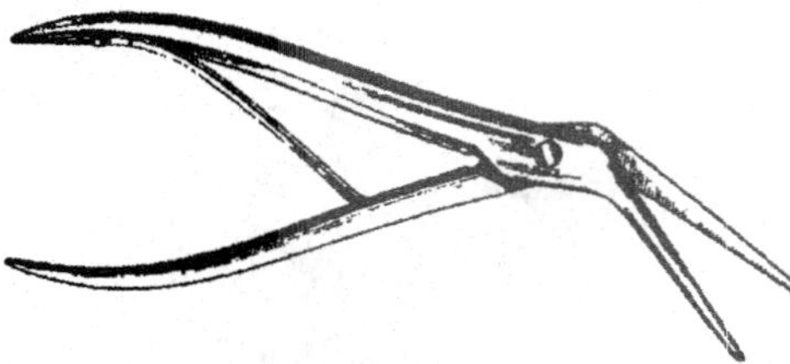

FIG. 467.—Turbinotome of the author, originally devised for turbinotomy but found excellent for thyrotomy and laryngotomy.

may be used to flavor the wash. Diseased tonsils should be removed radically and healing awaited.

Position of the patient. The patient is placed in the combined Trendelenberg-Rose position to prevent aspiration of blood and secretions. If the wound be not allowed to close during the operation, the retractors being always kept in place, the blood cannot be aspirated up hill. If the edges of the wound be allowed to approximate there is no longer an open trough, but a tube, continuous with the trachea, up which fluids can be aspirated.

Anesthesia. Local infiltration anesthesia is far the best and safest anesthetic. The solution we use is the same as for tracheotomy (q. v.). The intradermatic, not hypodermatic, injection of this solution along the line of incision, will produce absolute analgesia of the skin and partial anesthesia of scar tissue. The interior of the larynx can be anesthetized in adults by the local swabbing with a 20 per cent. cocaine solution. This must be applied through the tracheal fistula before commencing to operate. It will have no effect afterward. The only really painful part is the thyrotomic clip (Fig. 468) and this is over in an instant.

Operation. For clearness the operation may be described in four steps:

1. Opening of the larynx.
2. Incision of the posterior wall.
3. Suture of the mucosa to the skin.
4. Placing of the dilating tube and the dressing.

1. *Laryngotomy.* This step is described as dividing the tissues layer by layer, skin, cellular tissue, fascia, thyroid gland, etc. Such procedure is a great waste of time. The simplest method, requiring but a second or two, is to insert the lower blade of the inverted turbinotome

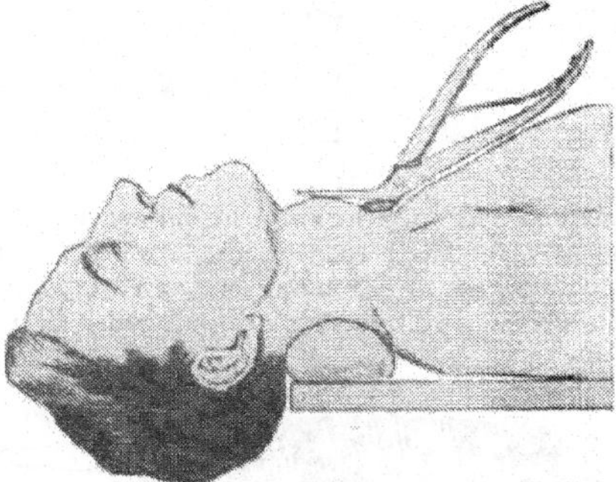

Fig. 468.—Turbinotome in position to make the thyrotomic clip. The table is not shown steeply inclined toward the head as it should be before the turbinotome is inserted.

(Fig. 467) in the tracheal fistula, as shown in Fig. 468, and to divide all the tissues, including the skin, at one clip. The incision must always extend to the tracheotomic fistula, no matter how low, in order that all the conditions within to be dealt with may be exposed to view and treatment. This applies with especial force to the granulatory or hyperplastic spur (E, Fig. 460), which is so often a factor in preventing decannulation. In making this clip in cases in which the thyroid cartilage has been divided before, as is often the case in the cases that come to the author, great care should be taken to follow the line of fibrous union. The thyroid cartilage rarely, if ever, unites with cartilaginous tissue, and the island of cartilage (E, Fig. 469) produced by a cut in a new location, is very likely to die. This is a disaster because it diminishes the already deficient size of the laryngeal framework.

2. *Incision of the posterior wall* is best done with a sharp scalpel, vertically, exactly in the median line, clear through the scar tissue, but with great care not to incise the anterior esophageal wall. In intubated cases the scars are usually on the posterior wall in the cricoid region, and they should be divided through to the cartilage; remembering, of course, that above the cricoid cartilage the posterior laryngeal wall is soft, otherwise the esophagus might be penetrated. Now we come to the essential technical improvement of Killian. Instead of excising the cicatricial tissue, and eviscerating the larynx, he took advantage of the

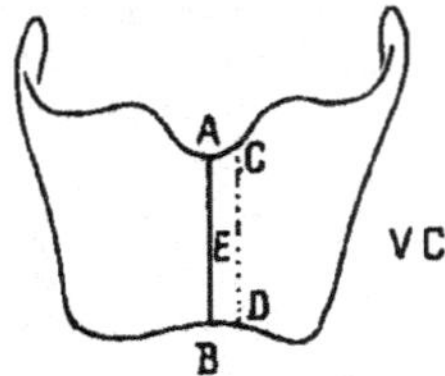

Fig. 469.—Schema showing error to avoid in opening the larynx in any case in which the thyroid cartilage has been previously divided. If the new incision (as at C, D) does not follow the line of fibrous union, A, B, the island of cartilage, E, will likely become necrotic, still further narrowing the larynx and rendering cure extremely difficult.

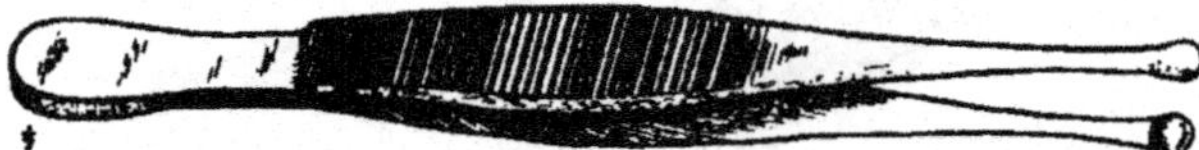

Fig. 470.—Author's grasping forceps for external laryngeal operations. They hold firmly large or small, protruding or flat tissues, and do not tear out like all forms of toothed forceps do.

tendency of the tissues to absorb and melt away under the contact and elastic pressure of soft rubber tubing. The linear median incision is to form a trench in which to lay the tube. Lateral cicatrices are not incised, but left to disappear in the post-operative treatment. Sargnon and Barlatier advise excision in cases of limited membranous cicatrices, plugging the wound for a few days with vaselined gauze. In some cases the author has found it advantageous to excise with curved scissors web-like cicatrices, and also to excise very thick cicatricial infiltrations, thus shortening the after treatment. For grasping tissues within the larynx the forceps, Fig. 170, are the best.

4. *Placing of the dilating tube, the cannula and the dressing.* The patient is now asked to cough, if, indeed, he has not been coughing freely.

If the reader uses general anesthesia, he is urged never to have the patient so deeply under that the *tracheal* cough reflex is completely abolished. The laryngeal cough reflex may be more or less controlled as desired by the preliminary use of cocaine. The tracheal cough reflex

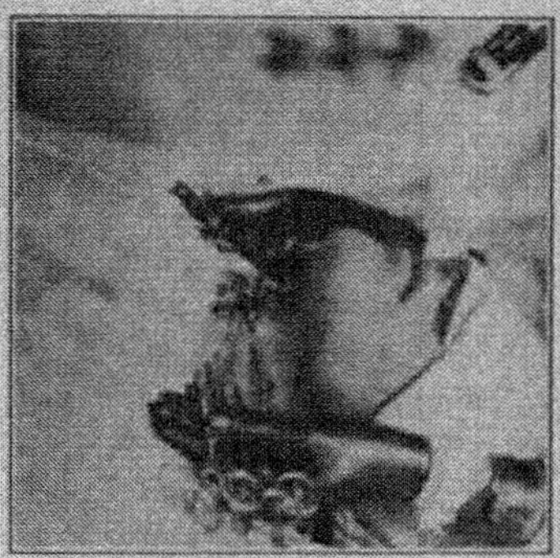

FIG. 471.—Photograph of wound immediately after laryngostomy, before the placing of the cannula, rubber dilating tube, dilatatory drain, and dressings. The silk-worm gut sutures uniting the skin to the lining of larynx have hemostats attached to them. The suture ends were cut off afterward.

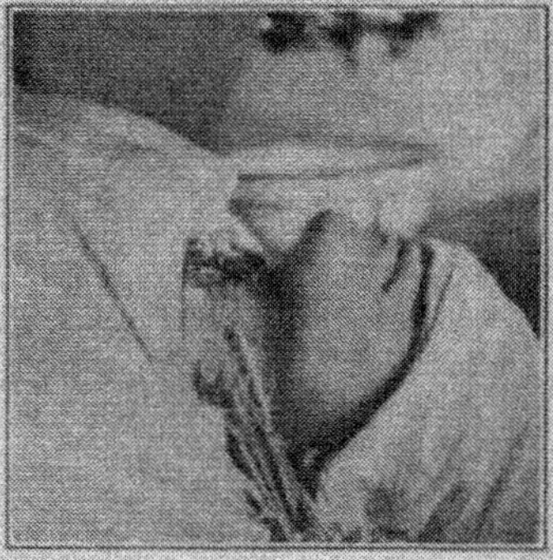

FIG. 472.—Rubber tube and cannula in place ready for the application of the dressings.

is the watch-dog of the lungs, as the author has so often urged, and should never be abolished in the surgery of the air passages. The rubber dilating drain is now cut to length. It should extend upward as high as possible without interfering with epiglottic closure and downward over all of the vertical branch of the cannula. Its upper end is plugged with gauze securely stitched to the rubber, lest it escape into the trachea. The two ends of a braided silk cord, previously transfixed through the wall of the lower end of the rubber tubing and tied, are now carried outward and made fast, one end to the right and the other to the left end of the tape holder of the tracheal cannula. They are drawn taut in such a way that the soft rubber tubing cannot slide upward off the vertical branch of the cannula.

3. *Suture of the mucosa to the skin.* The mucosa, or the cicatricial tissue of each lateral wall of the larynx, is sutured to the skin by three or more deeply placed silk-worm gut sutures which pass through

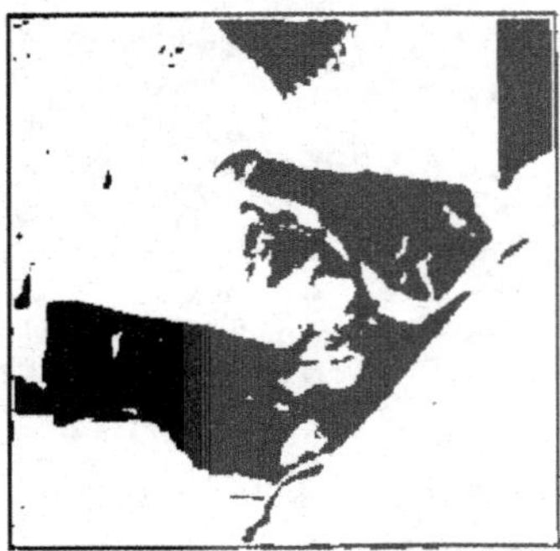

FIG. 473.—A case of laryngostomy one month after operation. The epidermatization of the laryngeal cavity is progressing.

the laryngeal lining and intervening tissues to and through the skin. Superficial stitches slough out in a few days. Care must be taken not to lacerate the edges of the tracheal or laryngeal cartilages. Preservation of the cartilage is of primary importance in all stages. If there is no cicatricial tissue at the divided edges to support sutures they had better be dispensed with, because normal tracheal or laryngeal edges will be lacerated.

In placing the apparatus it must be borne in mind that if the tube were to slide upward even slightly it would ride above the spur (E, Fig. 460). The great efficiency of the author's method is due to its keeping the soft rubber in perfect pressure contact with this spur, and giving the straight up and down line to the posterior tracheal wall as shown in the radiographs, Figs. 474 and 475. In placing the apparatus the rubber tubing with braided silk cords attached by suture to its lower

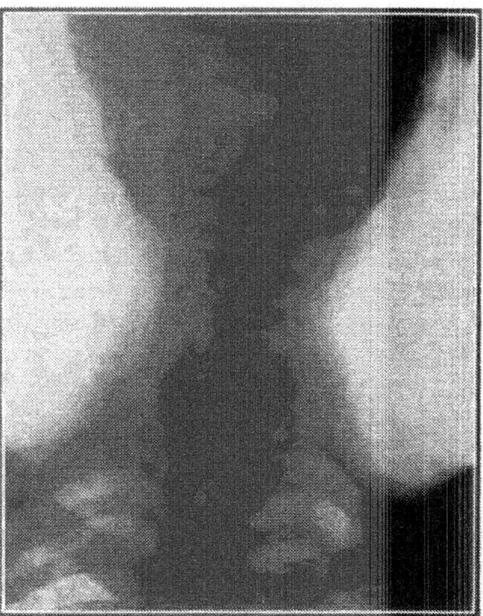

Fig. 474.—Anteroposterior radiographic view of the author's laryngostomy apparatus in situ, in a woman 27 years of age, affected with post-typhoidal cicatricial laryngeal stenosis.

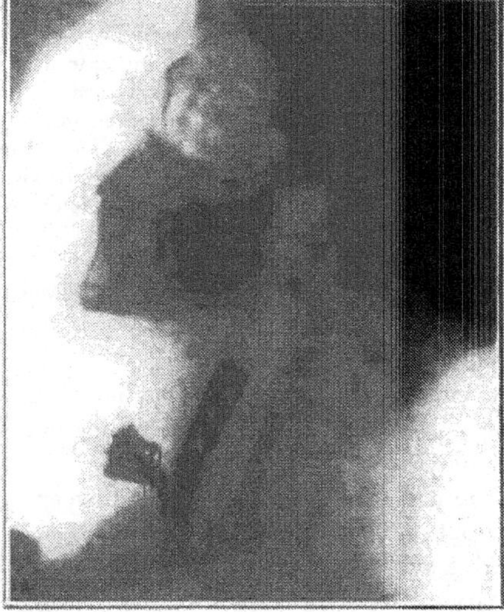

Fig. 475.—Lateral radiographic view of the same patient as shown in Fig. 474.

end, is inserted through the laryngostomy wound and pushed upward into the larynx, the outer ends of the silk being prevented from escaping by clamping a hemostat on them. The special laryngostomy cannula is then inserted into the tracheal trough. The rubber tubing is then pulled down and made fast.

With this, or any other form of apparatus, if increased pressure at one point is desired, the diameter of the dilating rubber tube may be increased at the corresponding point, as suggested by Sargnon and Barlatier, by slipping over the tube another bit of tubing of the proper diameter to be telescoped over, and of a length to correspond with the

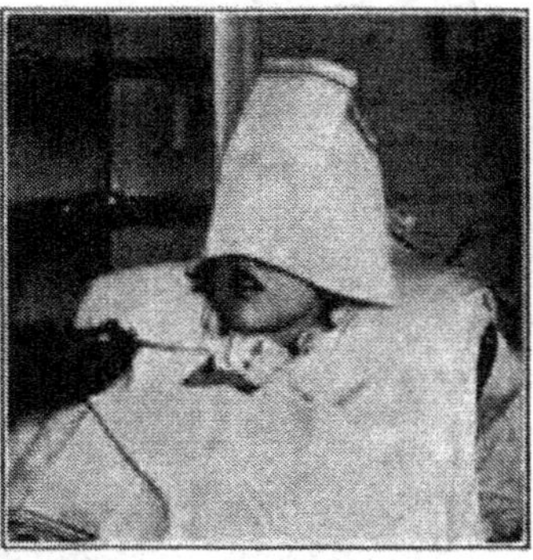

Fig. 476.—Author's method of packing tracheal and external laryngeal wounds to keep them open. A double thickness of gauze is spread over the whole front of the neck. The portion over the wound is then tucked into the wound. Then a little hard roll of gauze is forced into the wound, carrying the double layer with it. This form of dressing prevents any ends from getting down into the trachea. Useful in dressing laryngostomies, thyrotomies and tracheotomies.

vertical extent of the portion of the laryngeal or tracheal lumen that requires the additional pressure.

After the tube is placed the gauze dressing, in the form of a tight roll of proper size, is smeared with sterile vaseline, and forced into the wound in such a way as to keep it open. Our preference is for the form that we use in thyrotomy dressings. (Fig. 476.)

After-care. The dressing should be changed every three hours, the gauze being wrung out of bichloride of mercury 1:10,000 solution. This is contrary to routine surgery, but routine surgery has a high mortality if applied to the larynx. Nurses trained in this laryngeal and tracheal work attend to the dressing under the supervision of Dr. Ellen J. Patterson, who dresses the wound once daily herself. In laryngostomies she puts in place the increasing sizes of dilating tubes. If sloughing or too great pain should supervene, it is well to omit increasing the size and let the patient wear the same size or the next smaller size for a week or more, as seems best. It is absolutely necessary to observe the utmost vigilance to prevent any loss of what dilatation has been gained. A few days without any dilating tube may seriously retard the cure.

After the first few days, the gauze plug stitched inside the upper end of the rubber dilating tube is omitted and the patient can then speak in a whisper, and can breathe through the mouth, the external orifice of the cannula being corked. This is one of the great advantages of the author's method.

The success of the operation, like all laryngeal surgery, is dependent almost entirely upon the care, patience and skill with which this after-

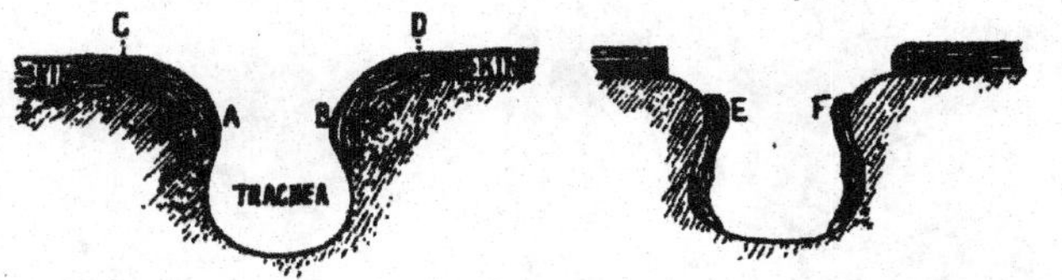

Fig. 477.—Schema illustrating the author's method of hastening epidermatization of a laryngostomy wound. An incision through the skin is made on each side as shown by the dotted lines, C, and D. The skin is dissected loose from the subcutaneous tissue (except at the edges of the laryngostomy opening) so as to allow it to slide. If packing is put under to prevent it healing back into its old position, it will be found in a few days that the skin has been drawn down into the wound as shown at E, F, thereby satisfying the tendency to contract.

treatment is carried out. The dilatation should be slow, making progress no faster than the tissues will tolerate. Sloughing or excessive fetor is a warning to ease up on the pressure. The sloughs and exudates are usually infections of buccal origin. They are usually thin and may be cleared away by mopping with hydrogen peroxid solution. They may surround the stitches, which may have to be removed if the sphacelic process is too severe.

The purpose is to get rid of the cicatricial tissue and to cover the newly formed lumen of the larynx first with small firm granulations, then with epidermal epithelium. This must be kept in mind in the after care as it is the keynote to success. This epidermatization may take two months or longer. It is claimed by some that some regeneration of cartilage takes place. In many cases the wound seems to be shallower though larger. That is, it is nearer the surface of the skin. A few remain deep. In these deep cases we have found it advantageous to slide a section of skin on each side down into the wound as shown in Fig. 477. Where the skin and subcutaneous tissue are not too cicatricial from repeated operation and the healing of open granulating wounds, this method has also been very efficacious in preventing cicatricial contraction in shallow cases. The method will be readily understood from Fig. 477. At A and at B are seen the normal skin edges dipping down into the

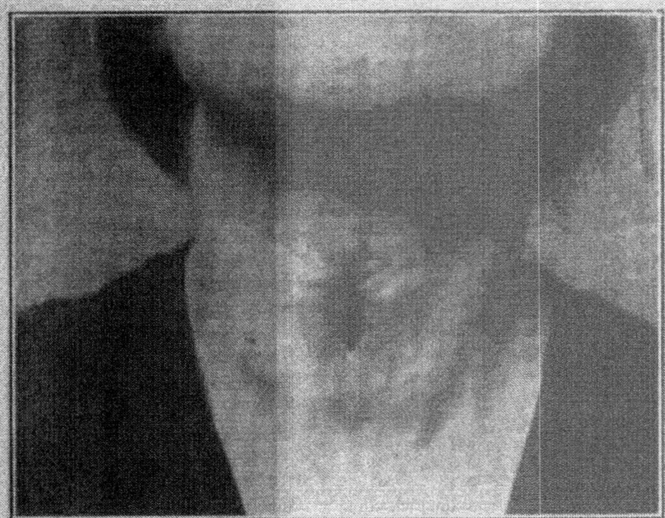

FIG. 478.—From a photograph illustrating the ideal result in laryngostomy. When the after-treatment has been properly carried out, the skin will be pulled down into the wound in a funnel-like shape as here shown. It is an elongated funnel, not a circular one. The actual skin surface should be drawn in, not simply an epithelialized cicatricial tissue.

tracheal wound. To obtain this dipping down of normal skin (not cicatricial tissue covered with epidermal epithelium) it is necessary to have normal skin to begin with, and the possibility of obtaining this will depend somewhat upon the position of the original tracheotomy. If the laryngostomy has gone through perfectly normal skin and the after-packing has been carefully attended to, the skin surface should dip down into the wound as shown at A, B, Fig. 477, and in the photograph, Fig. 478. If, however, granulations have been allowed to rise higher than the edges of the skin the object will be defeated. But having obtained the condition shown in Fig. 478, the author's method of preventing contraction has yielded excellent results. Not only does it satisfy the tendency of the cicatricial tissue to contract but it also furnishes a good dermal lining for the trachea, or, rather, for the new adventitious lumen that is to supply the place of the old stenosed trachea.

Epidermatization is favored by the use of a ten per cent ointment of scarlet red.

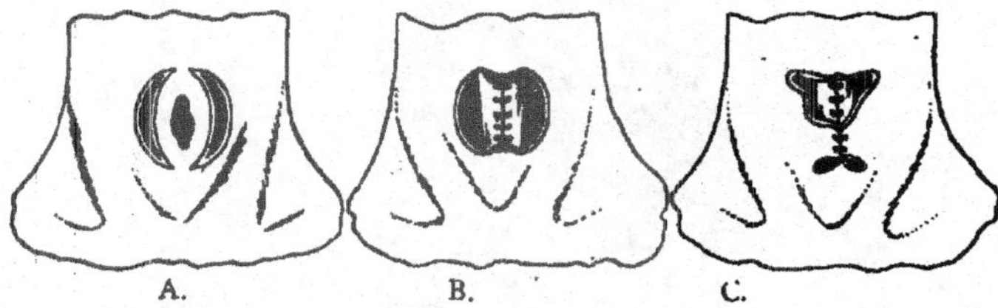

Fig. 479.—Schema of the autoplastic operation of Berger for closing a tracheodermal fistula. A, elliptic incisions around the fistula. B, flaps turned epidermis inward and sutured. C, manner of drawing together and suturing the skin to cover the flaps. (After Molinie).

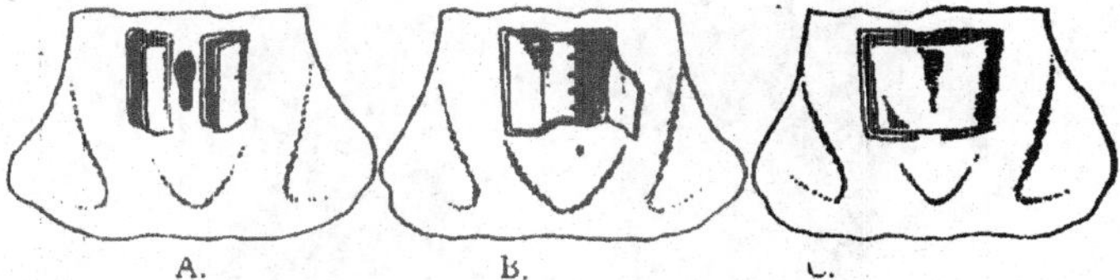

Fig. 480.—Schema of the autoplastic operation of Gluck for the closure of a tracheo-dermal fistula. A, form of incisions and flaps, one on each side of the fistula. B, one flap turned back and sutured, epidermal surface inward. C, the other flap dragged over to close the wound. (After Molinie.)

Duration of the treatment varies from three to six months, occasionally longer. At the end of this time, it is in most cases possible to close the laryngostomy by a plastic operation, but it is better not to do so. No matter how promising the result appears, the small opening should be allowed to remain patulous for a few months longer to facilitate the watch for recurrence. In rare cases a number of years have been required for complete cure. No case should be called cured until six months have elapsed.

Autoplasty. The laryngostomy opening will rarely unite without autoplasty because of its epidermatization. When autoplasty is required, the Berger or Gluck operations, clearly shown in Figs. 479 and 480, will usually close the opening perfectly, though a number of minor secondary operations are at times necessary to close little fistulae which occur, usually at the corners of the flaps. Like all plastic operations, success depends upon large well nourished flaps, placed without too much tension. It is necessary, in males, to modify the shape of the flaps to avoid if possible the turning in of skin bearing coarse hair. The outer surface of the skin flap is always turned in toward the trachea. In one

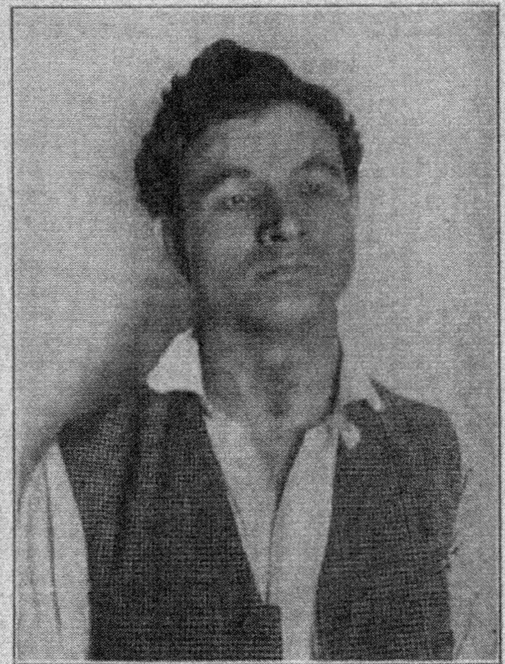

FIG. 481.—From a photograph of a patient taken two years after complete cure of obstinate cicatricial post-typhoid laryngotracheal stenosis, by laryngostomy. (Four years have elapsed since complete cure and plastic closure. Voice and breathing are excellent. Patient was originally tracheotomized, *in extremis*, by Dr. Joseph H. Barach).

of our cases, three plastic operations failed to close a fistula. The entire front of the neck was a mass of scar-tissue. After each operation, a small fistula would persist. We discovered that it was the pressure during cough that forced a small opening and forced the secretion out, thus causing a leak. By doing a tracheotomy very low in the neck, the pressure on the plastic above at the site of the laryngostomy during coughing was completely prevented. After healing of the laryngostomy opening was complete, the cannula below was removed and the lower wound packed in the usual way until it closed from the bottom up. This new tracheal wound, not being epidermatized, healed in about ten days. This patient, now four years after complete closure and six years after the lumen was enlarged to the desired point, remains absolutely free of stenosis and has now a good, though rough, voice. Figure 481 was made from a photograph taken two years ago. In some instances we took the tension off the plastic stitches by the use of the lacing, Fig. 482.

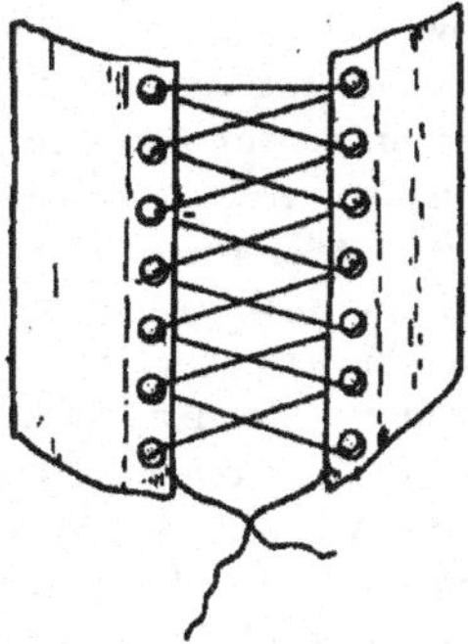

Fig. 482.—Lacing adhesive strips for lessening the tension on the sutures of autoplastic flaps.

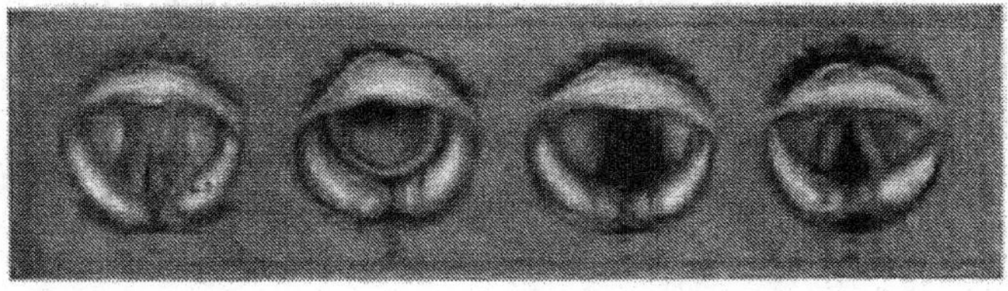

Fig. 483.—Illustrating the result of laryngostomy in a boy of sixteen years. A, post-typhoid laryngeal stenosis. The entire subglottic region is filled with inflammatory tissue, fixing the cords. B, laryngostomy tube in situ. C, after four months' treatment with the author's apparatus. D, two years after the tracheal fistula was closed by autoplasty. (Laryngeal mirror views sketched from life by the author.)

Results. Of the author's eighteen cases, two are still under treatment. Two were cured by laryngostomy without dilatation, two recurred and were afterward cured by the author's method, as described. The other fourteen cases are well. The vocal results in all were very satisfactory, and especially so in the cases with some degree of arytenoid mobility at the start. Pitch was more or less altered, being in most instances deeper.

CHAPTER XLI.

Decannulation After Cure of Laryngeal Stenosis.

Abandonment of the cannula. When a tracheotomized case reaches the stage, by whatever mode of treatment, when the patient is to be trained to breathe again through the mouth, it is necessary to occlude the cannula. The best method, in our experience, is to insert a rubber cork in the inner cannula. It is quite unnecessary, with a properly fitting cannula, to have a fenestrum in the tube. The fenestrum causes no end of irritation and favors the formation of granulation tissue, because it is impossible to have the fenestrum in the lumen clear of contact with the walls of the trachea. It is, anyway, unnecessary, because plenty of air will pass the cannula if it be of the proper size, and breathing can be unimpeded without a fenestrum. If an attempt is made to leave the cannula out, no matter how well the patient may be able to breathe, there is apt to be panic, because the removal of the tube is associated with dyspnea in the earlier history of the case; and associated ideas, terror and nerve habit cause the panic. On the other hand, when a cork is used for two or three weeks, the patient becomes accustomed to breathing through the mouth and realizes that he can do so. When this confidence is acquired there will be no panic. In cases that cannot get sufficient air through the mouth, a slot may be made in the cork for air leakage as shown in Fig. 484. All decannulation cases must be closely watched at night. A patient will be quite dyspneic with a cork that can be comfortably worn in day time. In most instances where laryngostomy has not been done the fistula into the trachea will close very rapidly. This should be retarded all that is possible, and the wound should be packed firmly open until the tracheal cartilage has united completely. Otherwise, there will be a mass of granulation tissue projecting into the trachea at the site of the unhealed wound. In an acute case where a tracheotomy has been done for temporary stenosis, if the wound is allowed to heal promptly the cartilage will heal very, very slowly and all the time will be throwing granulations into the trachea, as the author had abundant opportunity to observe with the bronchoscope some years ago. (Bib. 269). These may become so large as to demand a second tracheotomy. Of course, the granulations can be removed bronchoscopically and resorcin or other applications thus made, but as a rule it is better in such a case to open the tracheal wound again and deal with

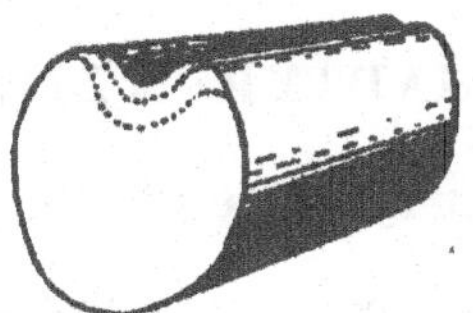

FIG. 484.—Enlarged illustration of cork used to occlude the cannula in training patients to breathe through the mouth again, before decannulation. The groove allows air leakage, the amount of which is regulated by the use of different corks having various sizes of grooves as indicated by the dotted lines. A smaller and still smaller air leak is permitted until finally an ungrooved cork is tolerated.

it properly by getting healing of the cartilage first. In cases in which the cannula has been worn a great length of time the cartilage is, usually, covered with fibrous tissue and possibly some extension of the tracheal epithelium, but not enough to prevent a prompt union. It usually takes but a short period of packing until the tracheal wound is united, and the wound will begin to fill up from the bottom, when the packing will be gradually, of necessity, less and less deep, until none can be inserted.

CHAPTER XLII.

Malignant Disease of the Larynx.

A therapeutic cure for cancer remains to-day, as it always has been, a hope long deferred. As applied to the larynx, there has, as yet, been no result from the roentgen ray, radium, mesothorium, or other radio-active substances, vaccines, diathermy, foetal autolytic products, or ionic surgery, that renders their use advisable instead of operation in an operable case; but as post-operative measures to lessen recurrence and for palliation, some of these measures seem to have value. Well planned, careful, external operation followed by painstaking after-care, is the only cure so far known and it is a cure only in a properly selected case. Endolaryngeal operation (q. v.) is contraindicated except in minute growths limited to the tip of the epiglottis, which are not strictly endolaryngeal.

Prophylactic treatment. Whether we regard the influence of irritation as a factor or not, and whether or not we regard the continuance of chronic inflammatory processes as resulting in segregation of ephethelium with subsequent proliferation as a factor in the etiology of cancer, there can be no question in the mind of any one who will review all the evidence, that there is, in many parts of the body, a certain precancerous condition at the site of cancer. The author's case records afford abundant evidence that it is exceedingly rare for cancer to develop in a previously normal larynx. The history of almost every cancer case indicates more or less annoyance referable to the larynx for so long a period of time that we cannot ignore the influence of chronic laryngitis as at least a predisposing cause of cancer of the larynx. Specific ulcerations and benign growths can prepare a soil more favorable than normal tissues for the invasion of cancer, and a rapid cure of any form of curable laryngeal disease is a prophylactic measure.

Palliative treatment. The four conditions that we must combat with palliative treatment, are: (1) Odor. (2) Pain. (3) Dysphagia.

(4) Dyspnea. Odor is due largely to the saprophytes. To hold these in check, the local use of antiseptics and, above all, the removal of secretions before there is time for decomposition, are necessary. Hydrogen peroxid to remove secretions, and dilute alcohol as an antiseptic, are among the very best for these purposes. Pain may be, to some extent. controlled by insufflation of orthoform and menthol. In dysphagia, intubation of the esophagus will postpone gastrostomy until near the end. When gastrostomy is indicated, however, it should be done at once and not delayed until the patient has become moribund from starvation. For odynphagia when due to ulceration of the epiglottis, the author's experience coincides with that of Sir St. Clair Thomson, in the relief afforded by the amputation of the projecting portion of this structure. Amputation is a relatively minor procedure. For dyspnea, tracheotomy should be done early before the patient's general condition suffers. It should always be done low in the neck, else it will soon be invaded by the cancerous process.

CHAPTER XLIII.

Malignant Disease of the Larynx.— Continued.

CURATIVE OPERATIONS.

Contraindications to attempted cure by operation. The contraindications to any operation other than palliative are: metastatic foci, organic disease, feebleness, alcoholism, pyorrhea alveolaris, suppurative disease of the accessory sinuses. A very high grade of malignancy is an absolute contraindication to any operation other than palliative. This seems to be the contraindication least often recognized. When the relatively rapid increase of the growth in size, or the laboratory findings, indicate a high degree of malignancy, or a very vulnerable soil (which is probably the same thing) no operation whatever other than palliative is permissible, because recurrence is certain. Impossibility of entire removal here, as elsewhere, is an absolute contraindication. Impossibility of removal *en masse* of the cancerous tissue, involving the necessity of incision through cancerous tissue or infected lymph channels, is an absolute contraindication often ignored. It is useless to remove infected nodes and leave behind the channels by which the infection was carried from the original focus to the nodes. Not only will infection spread from the unremoved channels, but the cutting through them will scatter the infection which will be taken up by the open mouths of both lymph and blood vessels. Careful esophagoscopy will often reveal infiltration of the periesophageal glands, and when this condition is present, operation is absolutely contraindicated, even if the glands are cervical. Within the past year, the author has seen eighteen cases of malignant disease of the larynx, in only one of which did he think operation advisable. Of the seventeen cases in which he advised against any operation other than palliative, five cases were laryngectomized by other surgeons and all five are now dead. The contraindications to operation in every one of these cases was extension of the disease to the lower deep cervical and mediastinal glands, and in four of the cases it was the bronchoscope and the esophagoscope that served to point out the probability of deep mediastinal glandular involvements and disease of the party wall below the larynx. One of the cases showed a very high degree of malignancy, the growth quite evidently having extended from the larynx downward and involving the trachea and party wall in a period of about four or five months. In such a case recurrence is certain, no matter how radical the removal, and any operation is inadvisable; but this patient found a surgeon who would operate. The wound never completely healed, malignancy being found in the granulations and rapid extensions soon terminated the case. Any operation other than palliative is absolutely contraindicated when there is involvement of the party wall below the second ring of the trachea. This is not because the second ring of the trachea cannot be removed, but simply because the bronchoscope and esophagoscope in our clinic have shown that when any malignant growth has gone below the second ring of the trachea, there is involvement of the mediastinal lymphatics. There is only one way in which to select the cases suitable for operation, and that seems exceedingly difficult to do, for most men. If every one were to approach every problem of operability with these two things in mind; namely, (a) mortality, (b) recurrence, the general average of the published statistics would be vastly better. The tendency is to go on the principle of "We will give him a chance, anyway."

Choice of operation. In an early intrinsic malignancy of very limited extent, not involving the posterior portion of the larynx, the results of thyrotomy have been positively brilliant. Nowhere in the whole realm of the surgery of malignant diseases have such results been obtained as in thyrotomy in such cases. But unfortunately, thyrotomy is being done on cases in which it is doubtful if even laryngectomy could save the patient's life. Cases have come under our observation where we advised against thyrotomy, but the patients afterward were thyrotomized by other surgeons, and in every single instance the disease recurred. In two of the cases, laryngectomy was afterwards done, followed by a second recurrence and fatal termination, one case within twelve months, and the other fourteen months from the time of the original thyrotomy. The author hopes that he will not be considered egotistical in making these statements. He claims no originality whatever in the matter; simply having followed the initiative of Sir Felix Semon and Sir Henry Butlin, who, seconded by Sir St. Clair Thomson, Mr. Tilley, Dundas Grant, Richard Lake, Prof. Moure and others, have very clearly defined the limits of operability and have conclusively proven that it is only in intrinsic malignancy of very limited extent that good results can be expected of thyrotomy. Notwithstanding this, thyrotomies are to-day being done upon patients in whom there is very extensive disease, which has gone beyond the limits not only of the intrinsic area, but of the entire larynx. If operators wish to operate upon such cases, they at least should not report them as thyrotomies and befog the issue and mar statistics by operations upon unsuitable cases. The author hopes that he will be pardoned for speaking thus plainly about these matters, but he feels very strongly upon the subject, for the reason that his own work has convinced him of the beautiful results obtainable by thyrotomy in a properly selected case.

It is frequently stated that the larynx is poorly supplied with lymphatics, and this is given as the reason for the good results obtainable by thyrotomy in properly selected cases. This is an error. The larynx is very abundantly supplied with lymphatics and they anastomose with each other very freely, but instead of leading out by many channels they empty into two small glands on each side without any anastomosis with neighboring lymphatic systems (Cuneo). To this peculiar lymphatic arrangement is due the success of thyrotomy in the hands of the few operators who have limited its use strictly to a properly selected case and who have had the most brilliant results in the surgical treatment of malignancy in any part of the body. The statement sometimes made that cancer will not invade hyaline cartilage and that this is the reason for favorable results in early and radical laryngeal operations, is an error. Malignant epithelial proliferation will not primarily invade cartilage; but when cancerous processes proceed to ulceration with consequent secondary mixed pyogenic infections, the cancerous processes will follow the suppurative processes through the damaged cartilage. Thus we not infrequently see cancer, in its later stages, perforate the thyroid cartilage. The real reason for the success of early operation in laryngeal malignancy is that, because of the peculiar lymphatic arrangement mentioned above, the anteriorly located, intrinsic cancerous process does not, for a long time after its incipiency, reach the cartilage. Another phase of the subject, lost sight of by those who state that hyaline cartilage is not invaded by cancer, is that sarcoma is a form of malignancy that occurs in the larynx and it may invade the cartilage early. In one case seen by the author the origin was in the perichondrium and the cartilage was probably involved almost from the incipiency. In another case a laryngeal endothelioma had its origin apparently from the perichondrium, with early cartilaginous involvement.

Indications for thyrotomy. Thyrotomy is indicated in any instance in which the involvement is intrinsic and is so slight that there is a practical certainty that all of the growth may be removed by cutting through normal tissue and not through neoplastic tissue. In other words, the cancer must not only be intrinsic, but it must be of very limited extent. If it be quite extensive, even though still intrinsic, it is reasonably certain that at thyrotomy all of the tissue cannot be removed. Fixation of the cricoarytenoid joint renders party wall invasion probable and if long continued a recurrence will probably follow operation.

Indications for laryngectomy. Laryngectomy is indicated in any operable case of *intrinsic* cancer of too great an extent to be dealt with by thyrotomy without cutting into neoplastic tissue. Laryngectomy is indicated in laryngeal cancer *extrinsic* by origin or extension, if there is little or no adenopathy, provided there are no contraindications (q. v.).

Hemilaryngectomy. As stated some years ago, the author rarely advises the operation of hemilaryngectomy, because of the much greater infective risk as compared with total laryngectomy. In such cases as are deemed operable, and in which the disease cannot be completely removed by thyrotomy, it has seemed better to do a total operation, which is safer because the trachea is entirely cut off and brought forward through the skin, so that infection cannot set up septic bronchitis.

Hemicricoarytenoidectomy has, in our hands, been followed by recurrence requiring the total operation.

Subhyoid pharyngotomy was formerly a very useful method of gaining access to the upper orifice of the larynx. It has been entirely supplanted for all benign conditions by direct endoscopic methods. For malignancy it seems rarely justifiable because of prompt recurrence after removal in this region.

MORTALITY AND RESULTS OF OPERATION.

Three things have, in the past, rendered records worthless and have very much befogged the statistics of the mortality and of the end-results of radical operation for cancer of the larynx.

1. The operation of thyrotomy has been confused with the operation of laryngectomy.

2. Nearly all of the cases operated upon for thyrotomy were not suitable cases for this operation. In fact very few were operable at all by any method.

3. The difficulty not only in discovering the disease early, but of getting the opportunity to operate early. Both of these difficulties are less than in the author's early days. Then patients did not so frequently consult the laryngologist for seemingly minor ailments; then, also, when malignancy was discovered early, the patient started on a search for

some one who would tell him he had no cancer. Such were almost always found in those days and the patient's only opportunity for cure was lost by delay.

One thing stands out clearly in the results of to-day as compared to those of many years ago; namely, the relatively slight operative mortality of total laryngectomy. When the author took up the surgical treatment of laryngeal malignancy, laryngectomy was still under the blight of the pre-aseptic days. Even after the general establishment of surgical asepsis in practically all other fields of general surgery, aseptic technic, especially in the dressings, was neglected because of the impossibility of absolute sterilization of the field and prevention of its subsequent contamination. To-day the average operative mortality in the large clinics is about ten per cent and this can be greatly reduced by refusal to operate except upon the most favorable cases. Though largely freed of its operative risk, laryngectomy cannot be said to be frequently curative of cancer, and is rarely advisable. As pointed out by Delavan (Bib. 116 and 118) the exact curative value of total laryngectomy has not yet been determined statistically because the literature is entirely made up of glittering generalities, incomplete statistics and cases reported too soon after operation.

Causes of death in laryngectomy. The operation of laryngectomy is necessarily associated with a certain degree of shock. Therefore, organic disease or lowered vitality of the patient, necessarily assumes first position as a factor in mortality. Injury to parathyroids has undoubtedly been a factor in some instances, and injury to both vagi doubtless has occurred. Infection of one vagus leading to an acute infective vagitis, may produce marked symptoms of depression, and may even prove fatal. Sloughing of the esophagus and other infective conditions, together with all forms of sepsis, and especially septic mediastinitis have been reported by a number of operators as causes of death in laryngectomy.

Excessive traction upon the esophagus, as demonstrated by sphygmomanometric tracings (Fig. 485) made upon some of the author's cases by Dr. Boyce (Bib. 254) introduces a serious factor through cardiac inhibition as will be understood from the following notes of Dr. Boyce:

"In regard to your last thyrotomy (for epithelioma of the larynx) in which I took sphygmomanometric readings, they never fell below what I take to be the patient's ordinary tension. He was at no time deeply anesthetized, and frequently struggled. The high readings I attribute rather to muscular effort than to operative irritation. In regard to the two laryngectomies of yours in which I took sphygmomanometric readings, I may say that the most interesting feature of the blood-pressure chart in the case of Mr. P. was the fall that occurred when the larynx was turned upward. A subsequent fall occurred when the upper end of the esophagus was drawn on just previous to incising it. In the subsequent case of laryngectomy, that of Mr. M., the blood pressure was seen to fall steadily as long as the esophagus was being manipulated. In this latter case the fall went almost to the danger point I had fixed on in my mind as the one at which the operation should be stopped. This fall of pressure is so remarkable, and so out of proportion to the apparent severity of the operation, that it suggests the theory that the de-

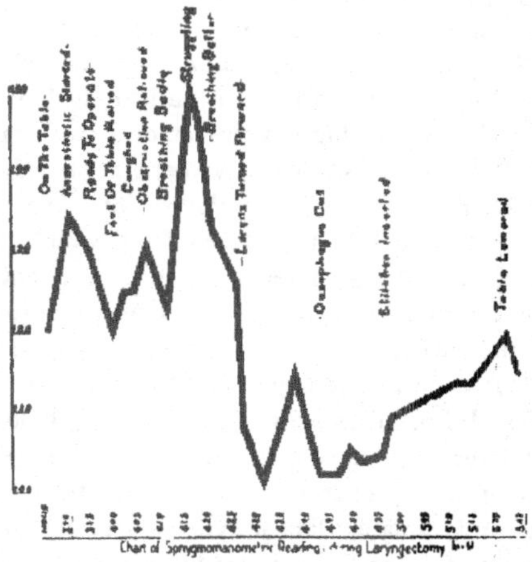

FIG. 485.—Chart of sphymomanometric readings recorded by Dr. John W. Boyce during laryngectomy by the author.

pressor nerve mechanism of the human heart runs in the substance of the esophagus. If so, it might account not only for death on the table, said to occur in these operations, but also, by the profound prostration induced, for some of the inhalation pneumonias that are reported as following. Whether other observation shall confirm this theory or not, the practical effect indicates most extreme caution in making traction on the esophagus, and that incisions into it should be made with the part as nearly as possible in its natural position."

The author has had only two deaths from any cause whatever within a month after the operation of laryngectomy. One of these was due to sloughing of the esophagus, and the other to exhaustion produced by a severe therapeutic test, in which enormous doses of potassium iodid and mercury had figured. Since this instance, it has been the author's practice invariably to insist upon full recuperation after all therapeutic tests, before undertaking operation.

Recurrence. The deficiency of the lymphatic drainage from the larynx renders extension exceedingly slow, so that laryngeal cancer is, in its early stages, a purely local process, and as such is curable by sufficiently wide removal. Recurrence within a year after operation may mean that the operative removal was inadequate, but it seems quite certain that in some instances, at least, it may be due to infection at the time of operation owing to cutting through malignant tissue, as evidenced by a point of recurrence in the midst of cicatricial tissue. Recurrences either at the original site, or in remote locations after a period of a year, may be looked upon as reinfections on a vulnerable soil. In one previously reported case of the author, a patient died of cancer of the stomach seven years after laryngectomic removal of a cancer from the larynx. This well known case is everywhere regarded as reinfection upon a vulnerable soil rather than repullation of the primary process. Had it recurred in the neck in the region from which the larynx had been removed, it would have been regarded as a recurrence. (See comment of Sir Felix Semon, Bib. 494.) It seems that, for the practical determination of the adequacy of an operation, we may say that freedom from recurrence for a period of one year after operation indicates adequate removal though not necessarily a cure. Everything in the clinical history of cancer indicates that it requires a vulnerable soil. We cannot cure vulnerability of soil by operation nor by any other known means.

For statistics and valuable data proving the remarkable curative efficiency of thyrotomy the reader is referred to the Bibliography for references to various articles by Sir Felix Semon, to whom the world is indebted for the discovery of a cure for that dreadful affliction, malignant disease of the larynx. Convincing data will also be found in the writings of Sir Henry Butlin (Bib. 63), Sir St. Clair Thomson (Bib. 538), Mr. Tilley, Dundas Grant, Richard Lake, Mr. Barwell, Adam Brown Kelly, Logan Turner, E. J. Moure, Watson Williams, Dan McKenzie, Sir W. Milligan, William Hill, Stuart-Low, Jobson Horne, Hunter Tod, Douglas Harmer and others.

Statistics. In publishing, herewith, statistics of every case he has ever radically operated upon, the author acknowledges that he has always refused to operate on any but the most hopeful cases, and the results are not claimed to be due to any superiority of organization or of technic, but just simply to the firm resolution to say "No" in any but the most hopeful cases. This has been done with the object of determining what may be accomplished by the operation of thyrotomy when strictly limited to properly selected cases. Of the 211 cases of malignancy in the larynx, four were sarcomata, one was an endothelioma, and the balance were all carcinomata. In eight instances, the malignancy was concurrent with lues, in three with tuberculosis; and in two instances tuberculosis, lues and carcinoma all were present in the form of a mixed lesion (Bib. 253). Since thyrotomy is such an ideal operation for intrinsic malignancy, it may be wondered why out of 118 apparently intrinsic cases only 27 were thyrotomized. The cases not thyrotomized were in five classes. 1. Cases seen in consultation with other operators who themselves did the operation. 2. Cases in which the patient refused operation. 3. Cases in which, though the growth still remained intrinsic, it was of too great an extent. 4. Cases in which organic disease elsewhere contraindicated operation. 5. Cases in which at thyrotomy the disease was found to have gone down the party wall, or elsewhere invaded the tissues of the neck to such an extent that a more radical operation than thyrotomy was indicated. In our later cases, such discoveries at thyrotomy have not been made because bronchoscopy, esophagoscopy and direct laryngoscopy have enabled us to exclude involvements lower down, such as subglottic infiltrations, and particularly involvement of the party wall not visible by ordinary indirect examination. In May, 1909, in a paper read, by invitation before the New York Academy of Medicine (Bib. 250), the author reported the statistics of all the malignant laryngeal cases in his clinic to that date. The cases seen since are incorporated with that report in the following complete record of all cases seen by the author:

Of 14 laryngectomies, two died within thirty days, giving a 14 per cent operative mortality. Four died within a year of local recurrence, three lived one year and were thereafter lost to observation, two lived two years, dying of recurrence, one two and one-half years, dying of recurrence, one three years, dying of cerebral hemorrhage, one seven years, dying of cancer of the stomach. Recapitulating this, of fifteen complete laryngectomies, eight of the patients were free from recurrence at the end of one year, yet all are dead now, and the average duration of life is but little over one year. These statistics were based on a complete report of all the author's cases five years ago, and he has not since done a total laryngectomy. By this it is not meant that such operations are deemed altogether unjustifiable, but cases where he felt that he could honestly advise laryngectomy have not since come under the author's care for operations, though he has seen two operable cases in consultation that were very successfully done by another operator, both being alive now at the end of one year and of fourteen months, respectively. Tabular reports of all cases in the author's clinic follow.

TABLE I.

CANCER OF THE LARYNX.

Cases of malignant disease of the larynx seen in 27 years, 1886 to 1913	211
Of these the disease was apparently intrinsic in	118
The disease was extrinsic by origin or extension in	93
Of the extrinsic cases the growth had extended beyond the limits of the larynx in	36
Number of patients operated upon (94 operations)	88
These operations were:	
Palliative tracheotomies, esophageal intubations, etc	36
Thyrotomies	27
Complete laryngectomies	14
Subhyoid pharyngotomies	9
Hemicricoarytenoidectomies	2
Partial laryngectomies included under laryngectomies (done later)	3
Partial laryngectomies included under thyrotomies	3
Of the laryngectomies and pharyngotomies there were extirpations of the cervical esophagus in	6
Of the laryngectomies and pharyngotomies there were extirpations of other portions of neck, including the external, internal and common carotid arteries, pneumogastric nerve, jugular vein, submaxillary gland, lymph nodes, tongue, hypo-pharynx, etc.	8

TABLE II.

THYROTOMY.

Number of operations	27
Alive and well after thirteen years	1
Alive and well after ten years	1
Alive and well after eight years	1
Alive and well after seven years	3
Alive and well after six years	3
Alive and well after five years	4
Alive and well after four years	2
Alive and well after three years	2
Alive and well after one year	1
Died of general diseases after one year	2
Lost trace of after one year	4
Died of recurrence (in spite of subsequent laryngectomy)	3
Died within thirty days	0

Recapitulation: Of twenty-seven thyrotomies, twenty-four of the patients were free from recurrence at the end of one year. No operative mortality.

It will be noted in the table that the extensive operations upon the neck and esophagus and tissues adjacent to the larynx are just the same in number in the statistics published in 1909. They are included here simply for completeness. The reason that none of these operations has been done in our clinic in the past five years is that in none of the cases that we have seen did conditions seem to justify such extensive operation, for the reason that in practically all of them that might have been so operated, we have discovered, endoscopically, deep cervical or mediastinal lymphatic extension which rendered operation unjustifiable.

Vocal results after operation for malignant disease of the larynx. In all of our cases of thyrotomy, the patients have been able to phonate. The voice has been really a good voice for all practical purposes. In twenty of the cases, the voice had a considerable degree of flexibility.

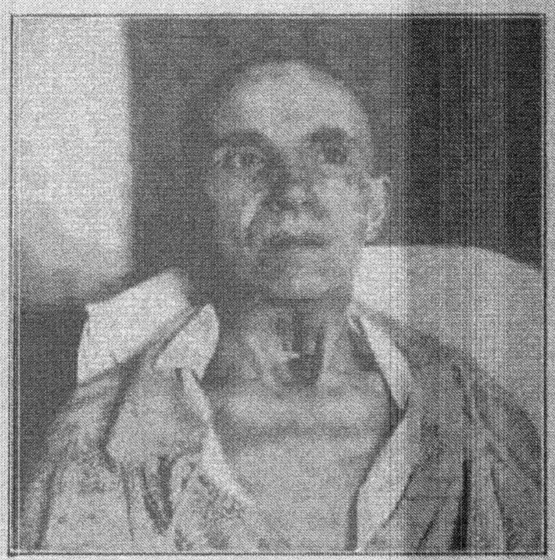

FIG. 486.—From a photograph of a man of fifty-four years, taken six months after laryngectomy for cancer of the larynx. About 5 cm. (vertically) of the involved anterior esophageal wall was removed, the edges being stitched to the skin. The upper aperture seen opens into the esophagus; by drawing it together with the fingers swallowing was easily accomplished. The lower opening is the orifice of the amputated trachea which was stitched to the skin. By placing a rubber colostomy pad over both openings the tracheal expiratory blast went through the mouth, giving the patient a loud whispered voice.

In two, the voice was very rough and lacking in flexibility, though quite loud. In four other cases, it was necessary to damage the arytenoid joint in order to make sure of getting enough peri-neoplastic normal tissue. The voice, though useful, was not loud in any of these but was more of the nature of what is commonly known as a "stage whisper." In two of these cases, removal of one arytenoid was required to get the necessary width of normal. In both cases there was no attempt to form an adventitious vocal cord, corroborating the author's previously published original observation that the traction by the arytenoid is the chief factor in the formation of adventitious vocal bands. In two cases the ventricular bands phonated excellently, there being no tendency to the generation of adventitious bands after removal of both arytenoids. In another instance both ventricular bands and the normal and the adventitious bands, all four vibrated on phonation. In the laryngectomic cases, one failed to develop a buccal voice, because he would

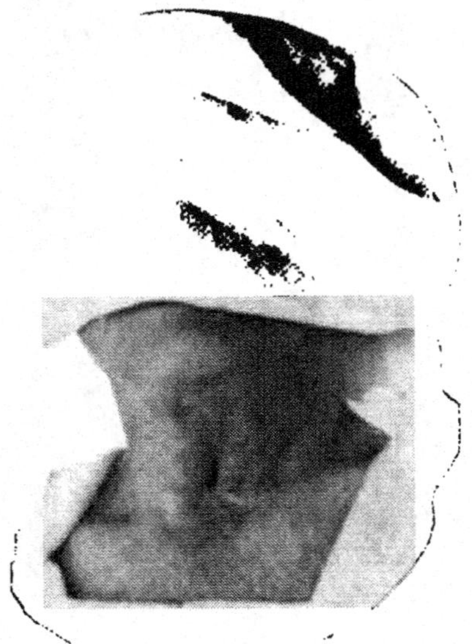

Fig. 487.—From a photograph of a man of 68 years, taken nine months after laryngectomy for endothelioma of the larynx. The trachea was stitched to the skin and the pharynx closed. (Author's case. For interior view of pharynx see Fig. 9, Plate II.)

not try, with sufficient patience and persistence. In one, a very good useful voice resulted from the use of a colostomy pad, which connected the two openings, the pharyngeal and the tracheal, externally on the skin surface (Fig. 486) as previously reported (Bib. 254).

Undoubtedly the stitching of the trachea to the skin, as first done by Solis Cohen, decreases the mortality of laryngectomy; but on the other hand, as pointed out by Sir St. Clair Thomson, the patient's condition, should he survive, is very much better and more enjoyable if the upper and lower air passages can be connected. In Sir St. Clair Thomson's case, the patient used an artificial larynx for breathing and speaking, and needed to remove the cork only when unusual exertion called for extraordinary respiration. In one of our cases a secondary operation to open the pharynx above the tracheo-dermal opening was very successful as to breathing and voice with a prothetic apparatus, but buccal and pharyngeal secretions caused considerable annoyance.

Summing up, the vocal results after external operation for malignant disease of the larynx, it is well to keep in mind, as mentioned in connection with endolaryngeal evisceration, the vocal results depend upon the degree of arytenoid mobility present after operation, because, as previously demonstrated by the author, it is the tugging of the arytenoid that is the chief factor in the development of an adventitious cord. While the ventricular bands may, and often do, assume the function of the lost cords, yet their phonatory result is nothing like as good as an adventitious cord with good arytenoid mobility. Moreover, the ventricular band of one side may require extirpation in the wide removal necessary for the cure of malignancy, for under no circumstances should any of the foregoing considerations of vocal results lead the operator into the error of insufficiently wide removal. It is well also to remember that at best the buccal voice and the artificial larynx are incomparable to even a whispered laryngeal voice, therefore, laryngectomy is warranted only when nothing less will offer good hope of cure. But, finally, no consideration of conservation of voice should weigh against life-saving thoroughness of extirpation.

CHAPTER XLIV.

Technic of Thyrotomy for Malignant Disease of the Larynx.

Preparation of the patient. Oral sepsis is the greatest element of risk in any laryngeal operation, therefore the most important part of the preparation of the patient is to have carious teeth filled or removed and to have the entire mouth put in as clean and as healthy a condition as possible by the dentist, and there must be no hesitation in removing questionable teeth. Frequent brushings of the teeth with a good paste or powder of which chalk is the base, together with frequent rinsings with alcohol 25 per cent, which is the best non-toxic antiseptic, should be kept up before as well as after operation. The usual general surgical preparations should be carried out in every detail as to bath, laxative, fast, etc. The beard and moustache should be removed, if the patient have these, and the face should be freshly shaven the morning of the day of operation.

Anesthesia. When the author had developed a local anesthetic technic to the point where thyrotomy in any man of normal courage could be done under local anesthesia, he felt that a very distinct advance had been made in his work, but since operating upon the last few cases under intratracheal insufflation anesthesia with ether, using the Elsberg apparatus, there seem to be five great advantages in favor of ether, when used by insufflation. In the first place, the return flow of air and ether vapor remove from the trachea, and keep out of the lower air passages, all blood and secretions. (2) The cough reflex can be abolished for a few moments at a time, whenever desired, and as promptly brought back by switching from ether to pure air. (3) When the insufflation tube is inserted, there is no more concern about the anesthetic, save to ask the anesthetist to increase or lessen the depth of anesthesia, as desired. (4) The great saving of operative duration over tracheotomy.

which formerly was used by some operators for the dual purpose of administering the anesthetic and of tamponning the trachea with a tampon cannula. (5) The anesthetist is removed far from the operator's way. Should it later be found necessary to abandon the thyrotomy and do a laryngectomy, all that is necessary is to incise the trachea below the involvement and insert a fresh sterile insufflation catheter through the incision, the insufflation nozzle being transferred to the new catheter. In doing the Gluck operation of laryngectomy from above downward, the catheter can be inserted into the upper orifice of the larynx through the upper part of the skin incision, and the peroral tube removed. In either case the result is the same. The anesthetizing tube is entirely out of the operator's way, and combined with the Trendellenberg position, the flow of blood is entirely upward. It cannot reach the lower air passages because of the return flow of air. It is surprising how little space the insufflation catheter occupies in the larynx. One would have anticipated that it would be considerably in the way in the operation of thyrotomy, but on the contrary it remains closely in the posterior portion of the larynx (Fig. 488) and could easily be moved a little to one side, if it were necessary to excise any part of the posterior wall. As a matter of fact, if it is necessary to excise any part of this wall, the operation of thyrotomy is contraindicated anyway, for reasons already mentioned. Another great advantage of insufflation anesthesia in thyrotomy is that the operative incision need be only long enough to expose the thyroid and cricoid cartilages, consequently, the isthmus of the thyroid gland need not be divided, thus saving much time in arresting oozing, etc., as compared to the long incision required for the insertion of a tracheotomy tube for anesthesia below the thyrotomic wound. In the use of local anesthesia for thyrotomy, the interior of the larynx should be thoroughly cocainized through the direct laryngoscope. This is done with two pairs of operating gloves, one pair being removed after the cocainization so as to lose no time starting the external operation. The skin is now infiltrated as advised for tracheotomy (q. v.). If the stages of the operation are now done with a proper degree of facility, the entire operation can be completed within about ten minutes, and no further anesthesia will be necessary. If a longer time is occupied, it will be necessary to infiltrate the endolarygeal structures with the previously mentioned infiltration solution. The reason for making the endolaryngeal application is that a much more profound effect can be obtained before an incision is made than afterward. It is necessary in the endolaryngeal application, to use a 20 per cent solution of cocaine, and adrenalin may be added if desired in order to intensify the effect of the cocaine, and also to cause a sharp limitation of the growth, as advised by Sir St. Clair Thomson. It is necessary to hold the solution in contact for twenty or thirty seconds; simply brushing is not sufficient. Of course the patient must be warned that he cannot breathe during this time, and it is necessary to get his confidence in order that he will not struggle or become alarmed. If it is desired to administer chloroform, two methods are available. (1) The old method with a tampon cannula inserted through a tracheotomic wound, as the first step in the operation, or using an ordinary cannula and tamponning the trachea after the larynx is open, with a gauze sponge, to which a silk cord is attached. This is pushed down through the laryngeal opening, completely occluding the trachea above the cannula. The chloroform inhalation tube, or, better, the hand ball insufflation apparatus, may be attached to the tracheal cannula for the administration of chloroform. (2) The other method is to have the anesthetist hold a sponge saturated with chloroform over the wound intermittently. Neither of these methods is in any way comparable to the intratracheal insufilation of ether. A general anesthetic by the ordinary open method is dangerous in any case with even the slightest dyspnea, but thyrotomy is rarely, if ever, justifiable in any malignant case that is so far advanced as to produce the slightest evidence of dyspnea.

To forestall excessive coughing the trachea may be punctured and 2 cc. of a 2 per cent cocaine solution may be injected into the tracheal interior with a hypodermic syringe before incision.

Operative technic of thyrotomy. The technic of thyrotomy for cancer, is quite simple. The insufflation catheter being in place, and the patient anesthetized, the operator's headlamp in place, the skin surface being sterilized by the usual iodine method, an incision is made in the skin from the level of the hyoid bone to about the level of the second ring of the trachea. The long incision previously made when a tracheotomy tube was to be inserted, is unnecessary, but, of course, an ample length of incision is always wise in any operation about the neck. The thyroid and cricoid cartilages are quickly laid bare without elevating or otherwise damaging the outer perichondrium. It being necessary to remove the inner perichondrium, the removal of any of the outer perichondrium would result in chondrial necrosis with consequent laryngeal stenosis. The thyroid cartilage is split up the median line with the turbinotome (Fig. 468). In making this clip with the turbinotome, it is essential in cases of growths that are close to the anterior commissure, to make the cut sufficiently to one side to avoid cutting through the growth, in compliance with the well known surgical principle that it is necessary to avoid cutting through malignant tissue. For this purpose it is always necessary to have previously made an accurate localization by laryngoscopy, direct or indirect. In some instances, it may be found necessary to split the cricoid cartilage, though, as a rule, this should be avoided. In reoperations the old incision must be followed (See Fig. 469). The lateral wings of the thyroid cartilage are easily spread with retractors, giving a good view of the interior of the larynx. The cricoid cartilage, because it is a

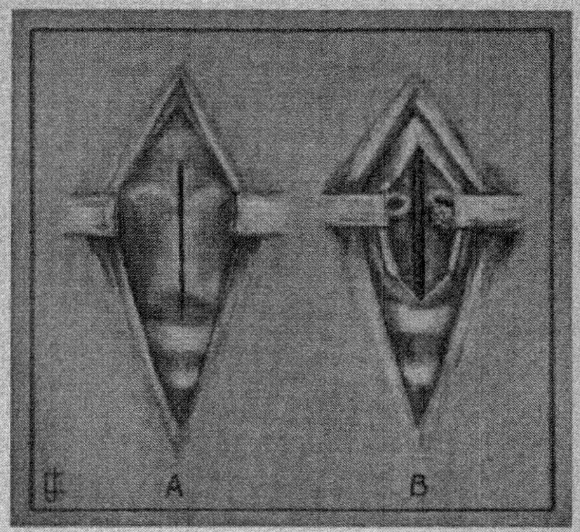

Fig. 488.—Illustration of thyrotomy or laryngofissure. A, shows the line of incision through the thyroid cartilage. The tubinotome is inserted at the cricothyroid membrane, the points passing upward (Fig. 468). B, shows retractors placed inside the larynx to hold back the wings of the divided thyroid cartilage. In the median line is seen the insufflation anesthesia catheter. The growth is on the left vocal cord. Perichondrial dissection begins at the divided edge of the thyroid cartilage, the retractor being shifted to the bared cartilage as soon as sufficient perichondrium has been separated. It will be noted that the cords do not look like the thin bands seen perorally. They are identified by their position below the ventricle.

complete ring, spreads less easily if partially ossified, as it often is. Care must be taken not unnecessarily to injure the divided ends of any of the cartilages, in using retractors or otherwise.

The most astonishing thing to the operator who opens the larynx for the first time is the totally different appearance of the larynx as compared to the laryngoscopic image. He expects to see two white ribbon-like vocal bands, and instead has great difficulty in identifying anything resembling a vocal cord. The landmark for which the operator must look is the ventricle. The ridge bounding the ventricle above is the ventricular band, and the ridge bounding it below is the vocal cord. This ridge, of broad base and triangular cross section, has a thick rounded crest and this crest is the vocal cord. (Fig. 488).

Observation of the size and position of the growth in the open larynx will determine the plan of excision. The first step will be to plug the pharyngeal orifice with a tethered tampon. In every instance, it is necessary to remove the inner perichondrium, and the incisions of the overlying soft parts must be in the normal widely out from the diseased area. The perichondrium is best raised with a periosteum elevator, such as Freer uses for septal work, after a start is made with the knife. Toothed forceps lacerate and do not hold as well as the author's grasping forceps. (Fig. 470). After the removal of the growth, close inspection of it will determine whether or not a sufficiently wide area of the normal has been removed. If it has not, it is unfortunate, but the best thing to do is to excise an additional portion of the normal, and if it is found that the initial clipping has been done too close to the growth, it is necessary to attack the opposite side of the larynx and do a perichondrial dissection of a sufficient area. The reason for perichondrial dissection is that cartilage and bone as before stated are not readily involved, while perichondrium is in some cases attacked by malignant disease, and it should be removed though apparently normal, lest it be invaded. If it is found that the cartilage itself has been invaded by the mixed pyogenic infections, the case is not one for thyrotomy, and the entire larynx and trachea should be removed, unless it is found, on exploration, that the deep lymphatics of the neck are involved all the way down to the level of the clavicle, in which case it is far better to abandon the operation and insert a tracheotomic cannula after removing whatever tissue has been detached in the larynx. The patient will live longer with the tracheotomic cannula by way of palliation, than he would if the entire larynx were removed in such a case, for involvement of the deep cervical lymphatics, as mentioned, means almost invariably that the mediastinal lymphatics are also involved, rendering complete extirpation impossible. In practically all instances that are adapted to the operation of thyrotomy, the dissection will need to be begun at the divided edge of the thyroid cartilage. The ideal operation is the one in which a relatively large mass of normal tissue is removed with the malignant growth, standing up as an island in the center, with an area of at least 6 mm. (preferably more) of apparently normal tissue in every direction. Should the growth by any mischance be cut through, all instruments that have been used in the cutting should not be used again unless resterilized and the growth should be removed with the greatest possible rapidity; for regardless of our theories as to the infectiousness of cancer, the fact remains that there is a sound basis for the opinion that recurrences in the scar are due to wound infection at the time of operation, quite as often as to incomplete removal. Great care should be taken to avoid unnecessary injury to the cricoarytenoid joint because the formation of an adventitious cord, as demonstrated by the author, depends largely upon the traction of the corresponding arytenoid to pull out a new cord from the scar tissue. Obviously, this must not be considered if complete removal of a sufficiently wide area of normal requires removal even of the entire arytenoid. Bleeding is carefully arrested at each step of the operation so as to keep the wound as dry as possible. After the excision of the growth with its normal surrounding tissue, there may be considerable oozing, and in a few instances, it may be necessary to twist or even tie vessels. Ordinarily, however, the bleeding soon ceases under pressure with gauze sponges and the exposure to the air. When satisfied as to completeness of removal, and all hemorrhage having been stopped, a stitch may be put at the upper ends of the skin incision, if the incision has been rather long. Dr. Patterson and the author are convinced that to make any attempt to stitch together the divided wings of the thyroid cartilage, or the perichondrium covering the outside of the thyroid cartilage, is a great mistake. Every swallowing movement, which is, of course, unavoidable, will separate the cut edges of the thyroid cartilage so strongly that it will tear out any suture that can be placed, resulting in needless damage to the important laryngeal framework. It is far better for safety and from every other point of view to pack the wound widely open until the cartilages have united by fibrous union, which they will do in exactly the right position without any stitches whatever, if the patient lie on his back with his head straight almost constantly during the after-treatment. The method of dressing developed by Dr. Patterson, is ideal. (Bib. 208). A large triple layer of gauze is spread over the wound and the entire front of the neck. A firm roll of gauze is then forced down into the wound pushing ahead of it the triple layer of gauze. (Fig. 476). By this method the wound is kept widely open, and yet there is no risk of any ends of packing getting down into the trachea thus causing irritating cough, or even asphyxia. This gauze should be wrung out of bichloride solution 1:10,000, and the dressing should be changed every three hours. Any tendency of the skin to dip down into the wound, must be combated by elevation of the skin edges at each dressing. When the cartilages have united by good firm fibrous union, the wound may be allowed to close from the bottom. If the larynx is closed, and the skin closed over it, as advised by some operators, not only is there danger from endolaryngeal swelling after primary union of the skin; but, undrained externally, the cartilage will fungate as it always does in healing, and fungations will occlude the interior of the larynx and trachea, not only misleading the operator into suspecting recurrence, but the fungations may be so exuberant as to occlude the larynx and require tracheotomy, to say nothing of the risks of septic bronchitis from the discharges thrown off by the granulating surface into the interior of the air passages. Cartilage is slow to heal and it is much slower in the absence of external drainage.

After-care of thyrotomic cases. It is wise to put elevating blocks under the foot of the bed for 48 hours, and during this time, the patient should lie upon his back with sand pillows on each side of his head in order to keep the head straight in the median line so that there will be no twist on the laryngeal cartilages from traction by the tissues of the neck. After 48 hours, there will be little risk of permanent displacement of the divided thyroid cartilage. Patients sit up in bed on the third day, and get out and move about on the fourth. It is absolutely necessary to have an abundance of fresh air at all times. The windows should be widely open, or better still, the patient should be in a fresh-air room It is absolutely necessary to have nurses skilled in tracheal work in order that the wound shall be dressed every third hour, and also to meet any emergencies that may arise. Ordinarily, however, emergencies and complications are rare. If the arytenoids and sphincter are injured and there is no undue reaction and no excision of any part of the upper orifice of the larynx, the patient will have no difficulty in swallowing without leakage. The first test should be made with sterile water, and all foods should be sterile liquids for a week, by which time granulations will protect.* Vocal rest is necessary. It is, however, not wise to keep the patient silent too long, for some vocal effort will prevent stiffening of the arytenoid joints, and an occasional attempt to speak will do no harm, provided there are long intervals of rest between. About three or four times a day, the patient should ask for any requirements, in order to give a few moments use to the laryngeal motor mechanism. After healing of the wound the larynx should be examined once a week with the mirror. It is usually best not to remove any little suspicious fungation that may appear after a few weeks. It will be found usually that what appeared to be a recurrence is only a fungating granuloma that will disappear spontaneously. Healing is usually complete in three or four weeks.

*Sir Felix Semon advises feeding the patient in the horizontal position on the operated side, the head hanging slightly over the edge of the bed.

Modifications of the foregoing technic. The foregoing, is, in brief, the method of operation and of after care followed by Dr. Patterson and myself. We do not use a curette because if it remove any infected tissue, it will simply stir the infection about and implant it in the soil to cause a recurrence, later. If it remove no infected tissue, it is unnecessary to use it, and as compared to a clean cut, it leaves a surface which is slower healing. No other plan than clean cutting is, in our opinion, satisfactory. The use of the galvano-cautery knife for the excision of malignancy elsewhere has proven advantageous; and may, eventually prove satisfactory for laryngeal malignancy. Operators, who prefer general anesthesia and are without an intratracheal insufflation ether apparatus, do a preliminary tracheotomy as low as possible and insert an ordinary tracheal cannula through which the anesthetic is given. The Hahn and Trendelenberg cannulae are no longer used.. Instead, after the larynx is opened gauze packing is firmly placed down in the trachea above the cannula to prevent trickling down of blood and secretions.

Complications. Necrosis of cartilage with subsequent stenosis may result from damaging the cartilage of both perichondria, or from insertion of stitches, both of which are avoidable. In case of reoperations an island of cartilage may die if the line of fibrous union of the previous incision be not followed as mentioned under "Laryngostomy" (Fig. 469). Lung complications after thyrotomy by the methods herein given are exceedingly rare.

CHAPTER XLV.

Technic of Laryngectomy.

Preparation of the patient is the same as for thyrotomy.

Position of the patient. As advised for thyrotomy the best position of the patient is a combined Trendelenberg-Rose position. The inclination of the table need not be extreme if the intratracheal insufflation anesthesia be used.

Anesthesia. It is quite feasible to remove the larynx with local anesthesia, by infiltrating first the skin and then the deeper tissues as they are approached. But much operative time will be saved and shock diminished by intratracheal insufflation anesthesia. If this be not used, the only safe way of using general anesthesia without prolonging the operation is to administer the anesthetic through a preliminarily inserted tracheal cannula. A gauze sponge is kept saturated continuously by very small drops of ether as advocated by Ferguson. Under no circumstances should etherization be attempted by the ordinary method through the mouth if there is the slightest degree of dyspnea, for reasons given in Chapter XXXVII. If the operation is done by the Keen or Gluck methods, from above downward without tracheotomy, the insufflation is started with the catheter inserted through the mouth in the usual way. When the stage is reached where it is desired to draw the larynx forward, a fresh sterile insufflation catheter can be inserted into the upper orifice of the larynx and the anesthetic thus continued until the trachea is amputated, when the catheter is removed and a fresh one inserted into the lower trachea after the removal of the amputated larynx.

Operative technic of laryngectomy. Two classes of procedure have been followed. In one the extirpation of the larynx, without tracheotomy, begins above, at the thyrohyoid membrane, the larynx being drawn forward as it is separated from the party wall, and the amputation from the trachea being done when sufficient of the larynx and trachea have been thus dissected loose and drawn out. During the operation the

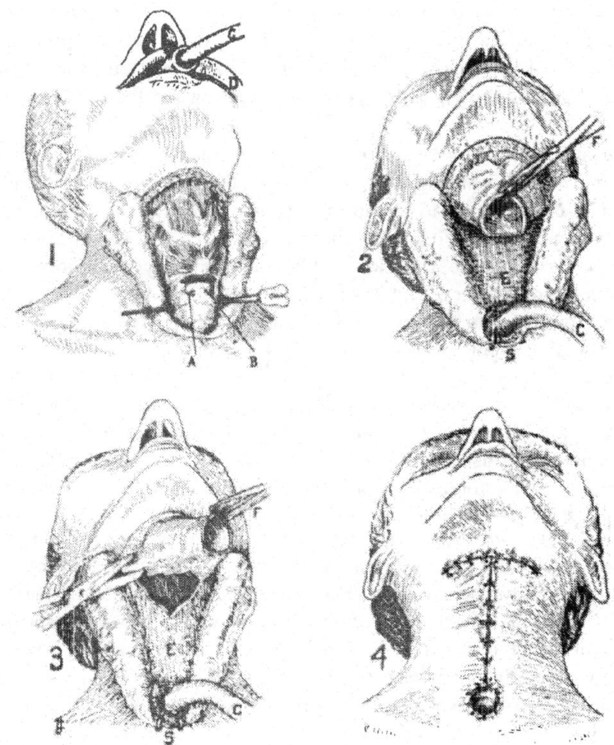

FIG. 480.—Schematic illustration of laryngectomy with the aid of intratracheal insufflation anesthesia. At 1 is shown the trachea and larynx exposed during anesthesia administered with the Elsberg apparatus through the silk-woven catheter, C, held in place with the Janeway bite block D. The incision has been made of T-shape, as will be understood by the sutured wound in 4. The trachea is elevated forward by means of the grooved director inserted carefully between the trachea and the esophagus. Two anchor sutures are inserted around the first ring of the trachea as shown at A, B, after preliminary incision of the interannular membrane.

2. The trachea has been severed between the cricoid and the first ring, drawn forward, and firmly fastened with the anchor sutures (A, B) at S. A fresh insufflation catheter (C) has been inserted for the continuation of the anesthetic. The larynx has been dissected free from the esophageal wall (E) and is held forward with the forceps, F.

3. The scissors are shown dividing the cornu of the thyroid cartilage. The pharyngeal wall has been divided so as to free the larynx posteriorly and this clipping will be continued around over the front so as to free the entire larynx, by severing the thyrohyoid membrane.

4. The wound is stitched together throughout its entire extent after suturing the pharynx, putting in supporting sutures, and securely anchoring the trachea to the skin (Modified from Molinié).

anesthetic, which has been started through the mouth, is given through the outdrawn larynx. The other method is used after preliminary tracheotomy. The trachea is divided below the cricoid and the larynx is dissected away from the party wall by working upward from below. (Fig. 489).

The author prefers to do a preliminary tracheotomy about a week beforehand so as to permit firm adhesions between the trachea and the soft tissues of the neck to anchor the trachea firmly, thus avoiding the tendency to retraction within the thorax, when the trachea is afterwards cut off and stitched to the skin. The inflammatory adhesions in the neighborhood of the trachea close various avenues by which infection could find its way into the mediastinum, and this barrier can be increased as desired by a blunt dissection around the sides of the trachea. One week later, the trachea is amputated (as low as previous bronchoscopy has indicated) through a T-shaped incision, the transverse portion of which is at about the level of the thyroid notch, the vertical portion extending downward as far as may be needed, but preferably not into the preliminary tracheotomy wound. The tracheal end of the larynx is raised very carefully without undue traction upon the esophagus, and is carefully freed from the esophagus from below upward, until the arytenoids are reached. The vagi and the parathyroids should be carefully avoided, especially the latter. The author has a number of times removed without ill effect part of one vagus when it was suspiciously close to the involved area. The pharyngeal wall is carefully cut away with the scissors, being careful to save all of the mucosa and submucosal tissues possible, in order to make the strongest possible wall when the pharynx is sutured after removal of the larynx. Usually the tips of the horns of the thyroid cartilage are cut off and left. The thyrohyoid membrane is incised and the aryepiglottic folds are clipped free with the scissors. All hemorrhage is carefully arrested at each stage of the operation: a clean, dry wound being essential to accurate work. The pharynx is now sutured with silk, being careful not to perforate the mucosa, the edges of which are inverted. Then each layer of the soft tissue is carefully stitched into place so as to afford the greatest possible support to withstand the strain of deglutition. Before stitching the skin, the Elsberg insufflation catheter, or the anesthesia cannula, either of which, up to this time, has been in place in the preliminary low tracheotomy wound, is removed and the cut end of the trachea above the old tracheotomic wound is brought forward and inserted through a button-hole in the skin below the laryngectomic incision. If this incision has been so long as to extend into the tracheotomic skin incision, this part of the incision must be very carefully and firmly stitched with tension sutures deep as well as superficial. The trachea is then stitched all around to the skin surface. The preliminary tracheotomic incision is drained by a wick of gauze inserted into the old wound below the new tracheal orifice. The skin is then accurately stitched and a large gauze dressing wrung out of mercuric bichloride 1:10,000 is applied.

As with malignancy, everywhere, it is useless to do a laryngectomy and leave involved glands in the neck. The most favorable time for the removal of the glands is at the preliminary tracheotomy, because a rather extensive neck dissection at that time has the advantage of forming a barrier against infection of the mediastinum at the laryngectomy later, and if the glandular involvement is such that there is reason to be-

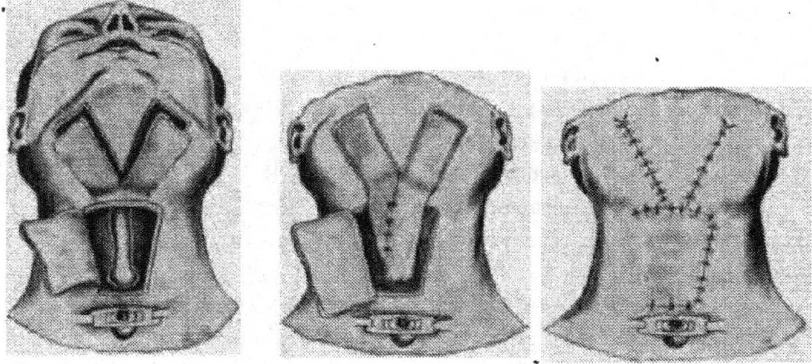

Fig. 490.—Plastic operation for repair of the esophagus after very extensive esophageal resection at laryngectomy. The two upper flaps are turned epidermal surface inward. Ordinarily the pharyngeal walls can be drawn together without these autoplastic dermal flaps. (After Molinie.)

lieve that the mediastinal glands are also infected, it is better to abandon all hope of cure and leave the tracheotomy tube in or not, according to conditions. If dyspnea is present at all, it is better to leave the tube in, for it will shortly be required, and it is better done early than late. The histologic examination of suspicious lymph nodes is always advisable. If a lymph node taken from near the upper thoracic aperture shows malignant involvement, laryngectomy is rarely, if ever, justifiable. The author has in a number of cases been able to discover malignant nodes along the side of the party wall, and in the mediastinum by esophagoscopy (q. v.).

After-care. Antibechics and all opium derivatives must be forbidden. Feeding should be by a soft rubber catheter or very small stomach tube passed through the mouth. Plenty of fluid must be given. The external dressings are renewed every three or four hours, because it is impossible to prevent their being soiled by the contiguous tracheal opening. The tracheal dressings are of separate pieces of gauze, renewed as advised under tracheotomy. The tracheal cannula is kept in place in the end of the amputated trachea, but as the latter is stitched to the skin there is no wound to pack open. The wick of gauze in the lower end of the laryngectomic incision is removed and renewed with the dressings every three hours, and discontinued when drainage is no longer needed. If the pharyngeal wound break down, the lower stitches of the skin wound must be opened and free drainage of pharyngeal secretions by fresh dressings inserted every hour. The patient should be propped up in bed on the second day and gotten out of bed on the fourth or fifth day. Ordinarily the feeding tube may be abandoned and the patient permitted to swallow strained sterile liquid food in small sips at the end of a week or ten days.

Esophageal resection. If removal of much of the anterior esophageal wall is required autoplastic repair with dermal flaps (Fig. 490) may be required. The esophagus is, surgically, one of the most intolerant organs in the body; and, moreover, recurrence of malignancy is almost certain. Therefore esophageal resection is rarely advisable.

The dermal flap operation (Fig. 490) is best adapted to female patients. In males, hair from the epidermal flaps may require frequent endoscopic removals.

Complications. Operative complications are now relatively rare. Streptoccemia and pulmonary complications which by older methods were so frequent are now seldom seen. Profound shock, weak and rapid pulse, slight temperature elevation, profound depression, white or ashy gray complexion, out of all proportion to the usual post-operative reaction are symptoms denoting acute esophagitis, vagitis or septic mediastinitis. Beyond stimulants and local drainage of necrotic areas, treatment is of little avail.

Artificial larynx. Most patients abandon the use of a prothetic apparatus and devote themselves to the development of a buccal voice. The most satisfactory apparatus is that of Sir Robert Woods of Dublin. Next to this in efficiency is that of Gluck.

CHAPTER XLVI.

Bibliography.

1. ABRAHAM, JOSEPH H. Direct Laryngoscopy, Tracheobronchoscopy and Esophagoscopy with Demonstrations. Ala. Med. Jour., July, 1908.

2. ABRAND, DR. Diagnosis of Foreign Bodies in the Respiratory Tract. Archiv. Gen. de Med., Vol. XCI, No. 9, Sept. 1912, p. 782.

3. ADAM, JAMES. Asthma. Published by Henry Kimpton. London, 1913.

4. ALBRECHT, W. Surgical Treatment of Tuberculosis of the Larynx. Ztschr. f. Ohrenh., u. f. Krankh. der Luftw., Bd. 61, Heft 2, 1910.

5. ALBRECHT, T. Die Direkte Laryngo-Tracheo-Bronchoskopie und ihre Bedeutung für Diagnose und Therapie. Med. Klinik, Dec. 12, 1909.

6. ALBRECHT. A Modification of Suspension Laryngoscopy. Berl. Klin. Woch., July 8, 1912, Vol. XLIV, No. 28, p. 1331.

7. ARROWSMITH, H. Case of Apparently Primary Intra-Laryngeal Actinomycosis. The Laryngoscope, Oct., 1910.

8. ARROWSMITH, H. Angioneurotic Edema of the Esophagus. Transactions Amer. Laryngol., Rhinol. and Otol. Soc., 1915. Also, Proceedings Amer. Med. Assn., Laryngologic Section, 1914.

9. ARROWSMITH, H. (Brooklyn.) Certain Aspects of Rhinolaryngology and their Relation to General Medicine.* N. Y. Med. Journ., Dec. 17, 1910. Read at the Nov. 1910 meeting of the Med. So. of County of Kings.

10. ARSLAN. Removal of Foreign Body from Bronchus by Direct Bronchoscopy. (Broncoscopia Diretta con Estrazione di Corpo Estraniero del Broncho). Rev. Crit. di Clin. Med., Sept. 24, 1910.

11. ANDERS AND BOSTON. Text book. Med. Diag. Article on Gastroscopy, p. 417.

12. AUER AND MELTZER. Insufflation Anesthesia. Med. Record, Vol. LXXVII, p. 477. Also Bulletins Rockefeller Institute.

13. ARROWSMITH, H. Intralaryngeal Actinomycosis. The Laryngoscope, Oct., 1910.

14. ALBRECHT, W. Suspension Laryngoscopy in Children. Journal of Laryngology, February, 1914.

19. BOYCE, JOHN W. Foreign Bodies in the Lungs Simulating Pleural Effusion. Med. Record, Oct. 14, 1911.

20. BAR, LOUIS. Traitement Galvanoplastique de la Tuberculose du Larynx. Proc. Belgian Laryngological Society. 1913.

21. BALLENGER, W. L. Diseases of the Nose and Throat. Pub. by Lea and Febiger.

22. BANNES, F. The Diagnosis of Foreign Bodies in the Bronchi, with Report of a Case of Wandering of a Foreign Body from the Right into the Left Bronchus. Med. Klinik, No. 7, Feb. 18, 1912, p. 276.

23. BARACH, JOSEPH H. Anaphylaxis. Archives of Diagnosis. New York, Oct., 1911.

24. BARACH, JOSEPH H. Observations on Sound Production and Sound Conduction along the Respiratory Tract. Amer. Journ. of the Med. Sciences. Oct., 1911.

25. BARLATIER. Les Pansements dans la Laryngostomie. La Pratique Med., No. 1, 1909.

26. BARNHILL, J. F. Report of Case of Foreign Body in the Respiratory Tract. Indianapolis Med. Jour., March, 1909.

27. BASSLER, ANTHONY. Dis. of Stomach. F. A. Davis.

28. BAYSSIERE, M. E. Aneurysm of the Arch of the Aorta. Dangers of Esophagoscopy. Le Larynx, Nov., Dec., 1911, p. 175.

29. BECK, J. C. Cyst of Epiglottis. The Laryngoscope, Sept., 1909.

30. BIRKETT, HERBERT S. Report of a Case of Primary Lupus Vulgaris of the Oropharynx and Nasopharynx Treated by X-Rays. N. Y. Med. Record. 1904, p. 1013.

31. BIRKETT, HERBERT S. Further Report of a Case of Primary Lupus Vulgaris of the Oropharynx and Nasopharynx Treated by X-Rays. N. Y. Med. Rec., 1905, p. 739.

32. BENHAM, E. W. Foreign Body Removed from Bifurcation of Trachea by Lower Bronchoscopy. Journ. Lancet, Vol. XXXII, No. 15, Aug. 1, 1912, p. 414.

33. BERENS, T. P. A Case of Primary Carcinoma of the Trachea. Ann. of Otol., Rhinol. and Laryngol., Dec., 1909.

34. BISCOE, F. L. Diphtheria. Virginia Med. Semi-Monthly, Oct. 11, 1907.

35. Blegvad, N. Rh. (Copenhagen.) Foreign Body in the Esophagus; its Removal with the Esophagoscope. Ugeskrift for Laeger, No. 48, Nov. 30, 1911, p. 1775.

36. Blondiau. Woman Tracheotomized Fifteen Years Ago for Suffocating Papilloma of Larynx Still Under Treatment. Presse Oto-Laryngologique Belge, July, 1910.

37. Boggs, Russel H. The Treatment of Multiple Glandular Tumors. Medical Record, Dec. 23, 1911.

38. Boland, F. K. and Ridley, R. B. Removal of Whistle from Esophagus after Five Weeks. Charlotte Med. Journ., March, 1910.

39. Botella, E. Neuva technica simplificada para las exploraciones esophagoscopias, Bol. de Laringol., Otol. y Rhinol., Nov.-Dec., 1909.

40. Botella, E. Foreign Bodies in the Left Bronchus Removed by Bronchoscopy. Rev. Espanola de Laringol., No. 1, 1910, and Arch. Internat. de Laryngol., d'Otol et de Rhinol., March-April, 1910.

41. Boston and Anders. Text Book. Med. Diagnosis. Article on Gastroscopy, p. 417.

42. Botey. Casuistica Esofagoscopica. Arch. de Rinol., No. 156, 1909.

43. Botey. Some Cases of Esophagoscopy. Arch. de Rinol., Laringol., etc. March-April, 1910.

44. Botey. Treatment of Tracheotomized Patients by Elastic Dilatation and Laryngostomy. Arch. de Rinol., May, June, July, Aug., 1910.

45. Bourack, C. M. Case of Foreign Body in the Esophagus with Fatal Termination. Arch. Internat. de Laryngol., d'Otol. et de Rhinol., May-June, 1910.

46. Bowen, Chas. F. (Columbus, Ohio.) Removal of Foreign Bodies from the Esophagus and Bronchus. (Read before the Ohio State Med. Ass'n., May 9, 1911.

47. Boyce, J. W. Diaphragm in Tone-Production. A Fluoroscopic Study. The Laryngoscope, April, 1910.

48. Brewer, G. E. Operative Procedures from the Standpoint of the General Surgeon. The Laryngoscope, Aug. 1909, and Ann. of Surg., Nov., 1909.

49. Brewer, George E. Surgery Larynx and Trachea. Keens Surgery. Vol. VI, p. 364.

50. Bruel, Leon. Concomitant Stenoses of the Esophagus and Pylorus through the Injection of Caustic Fluids. These de Paris, 1910.

51. Bruenings. Use of Tracheobronchoscopy and Esophagoscopy in the Oto-laryngological Clinic of the University of Jena. Ztschr. f. Ohrenh. u. f. Krankh. der Luftw., Bd. 62, Heft 3-4, 1910.

52. Bruenings. Simple Method for Diagnosing Esophageal Cancer. Muench. med. Wchnschr., Nov. 22, 1910.

53. Bruenings, W. Uber Fortschritte in der Esophagoskopischen Behandlung Verschluckter Fremdkörper. Deutsche med. Wchnschr., April 29, 1909.

54. Brun and Molinie. Corps Etranger de la Bronche Droite (tube de verre). Bronchoscopie; Extration; Guerison. Le Larynx, No. 5, 1909.

55. Brunetti, F. Recherche Anatomische ed Anatomopatologiche sulle Terminazioni Nervose nei Muscoli Intrinseci dela Laringe Umana. Arch. Ital. di Laringol., April, 1909.

56. Bryan, J. H. Perichondritis of the Larynx in Typhoid Fever. Proc. Am. Laryngol. Soc., 1913.

57. Bulson, Albert E., Jr. Bronchoscopy and Esophagoscopy Jour. Ind. State Med. Assn., Vol. VI, No. 4. April 15, 1913, p. 150.

58. Burckhardt, A. S. Tuberculosis of the Esophagus. Arch. f. Verdanungs-Krankh., Aug., 1910.

59. Butlin, Henry T. Operations for Cancer of the Larynx. Journal of Laryngology, Rhinol. and Otol., 1908.

60. Burger, H. Ein Tödlich Verlaufener Bronchoskopischer Fremdkörperfall. Ztschr. f. Laryngol., Rhinol. u. ihre Grenzgebiete, Bd. 1, p. 785, 1909.

61. Bronner, Adolph. Fissure of the Mouth of the Esophagus. Brit. Med. Journ., Oct. 19, 1912.

62. Bruenings, W. Die Direkte Laryngoskopie, Bronchoskopie und Oesophagoskopie. Text book. Pub. by J. F. Bergman Wiesbaden.

63. Butlin, Sir Henry. Indications for Early Radical Treatment of Malignant Disease of the Larynx. Brit. Med. Journ., Oct. 26, 1895.

69. Carpenter, E. W. Broncho-Esophagoscopy. The Laryngoscope, May, 1914.

70. Carpenter, E. W. Death of Infant Caused by Fragment of Peanut in the Lung. The Laryngoscope, March, 1914.

71. Cauzard, P. Oesophagoscopie. Arch Internat de Laryngol. etc., XXV, p. 1066, 1908.

72. Cauzard, P. Oesophagoscopie et Tracheobronchoscopie. Rev. hebd. de Laryngol., p. 417, 1908.

73. Carpenter, E. W. Bronchoscopy. Journ. S. Car. Med. Assn., Vol. VIII, No. 8, Aug., 1912, p. 222.

74. Carrel, A. Experimental Intrathoracic Surgery by the Meltzer and Auer Method of Intratracheal Insufflation. Med. Record, March 19, 1910, and Berl. Klin. Wchnschr., March 28, 1910.

75. CASSELBERRY, W. E. The Cutting in Two of a Large Steel Pin, while Transfixed in the Left Bronchus and Its Removal by Lower Bronchoscopy. Transactions Amer. Laryngol. Soc., 1910.

76. CASTEX. Total Laryngectomy in the Practice of Prof. Jeannel. (La Laryngectomie Totale dans le Service de M. le Professeur Jeannel). These de Toulouse, 1910.

77. CHAPPEL, W. F. Early Diagnosis of Malignant Disease of the Larynx. N. Y. Med. Record, Oct. 16, 1909.

78. CHAPMAN, G. H. Some Different Terminations of Foreign Bodies in the Wind-Pipe. L'ville Monthly Journ. of Med. and Surg., June, 1910.

79. CHAUVEAU, C. Cannula Used and Broken in the Trachea. (Canule usee et beisee dans la trachee). Arch. internat de Laryngol. d'Otol. et de Rhinol., Jan.-Feb., 1910.

80. CHENERY, W. E. Case of Paralysis of the Left Vocal Cord Caused by Peritracheal Tumor. The Laryngoscope, Jan., 1909.

81. CHIARI, O. Death in Case of Superior Bronchoscopy. (Ein Todesfall bei der Bronchoscopia Superior). Monatschr. f. Ohrenh. u. Laryngo-Rhinol., Bd. 44, Heft. 8, 1910.

82. CHIARI, O. Two Cases of Foreign Bodies Removed by Bronchoscopy Several Years after their Entrance. (Ueber zwei Fälle von Fremdkörpern welche mehrere Jahre nach ihrem Eindringen Bronchskopisch entfernt wurden). Monatschr. f. Ohrenh. u. Laryngo-Rhinol., Heft 1, 1910.

83. CISNEROS, JUAN. Results of Operative Treatment of Laryngeal Cancer. (Resultados del tratamiento operatori del cancer laringo.) Bol. de Laringol., Otol. y Rinol., May-August, 1910.

84. CLAOUE, R. Study of Foreign Bodies in the Esophagus and Bronchus. Gaz. hebd. des Sci. med. de Bordeaux, March 20, 1910.

85. CLARKE, THOMAS WOOD AND MARINE, DAVID. Pulmonary Gangrene following Foreign Bodies in the Bronchi. Med. and Pathological Services of the Lakeside Hospital.

86. CLARK, J. PAYSON AND RICHARDSON, OSCAR. Case of Foreign Body in the Trachea. Status Lymphaticus. Death. Autopsy. Boston Med. and Surg. Journ., Jan. 26, 1911.

87. COCKS, GERHARD HUTCHISON. Status Thymo-lymphaticus and its Relation to Sudden Death. The Laryngoscope, St. Louis, July, 1910.

88. COMPAIRED. Nos Interventions dans le Cancer du Larynx. Arch. Internat. de Laryngol., d'Otol. et de Rhinol., March, 1909.

89. COOLIDGE, A., JR. Annals of Otology, Rhinology and Laryngology, Dec., 1906. (Also Proceedings Am. Laryngol. Soc., 1906.)

90. COLE. Demonstration of X-Ray Plates of Esophagus, Stomach and Colon. Post-Graduate, April, 1910.

91. CRILE, GEO. W. The Identity of Cause of Aseptic Wound Fever and So-Called Post-Operative Hyperthyroidism and their Prevention. Read before the So. Surg. and Gyn. Ass'n., Dec. 17, 1912.

92. CULP, J. F. Foreign Body in the Bronchus. Proc. Amer. Laryngol. Rhin. and Otol. Soc. 1913, p. 318.

93. COLE, L. G. Localization of Foreign Bodies. Med. News, March 15, 1902.

94. COAKLEY, CORNELIUS G. Foreign Bodies in the Esophagus. Trans. Am. Laryngol. Ass'n., 1913.

95. COAKLEY, CORNELIUS G. Fatal Case of Asphyxia. Trans. Am. Laryngol. Ass'n., 1910. (Very interesting as bearing on "status lymphaticus.")

96. COATES, GEORGE M. Jackstones in the Esophagus. Arch. Pediatrics, Aug., 1914.

100. DAVIS, EDWARD D. Relief of Pain of Laryngeal Tuberculosis. Lancet, Oct. 18, 1913.

101. DA COSTA, JOHN C. Modern Surgery. (Text book pub. by Saunders & Co.)

102. DAVIS, EDWARD D. Observations on Suspension Laryngoscopy, with the Notes of a Few Cases. British Med. Jour. No. 2716, Jan. 18, 1913, p. 115.

103. DAVIS, H. J. Case of Laryngeal Vertigo. Jour. of Laryngol., Rhinol. and Otol., March, 1910.

104. DAVIS, J. L. Laryngeal Neoplasms. The Laryngoscope, May, 1908.

105. DAVIS, J. L. Laryngeal Neoplasms—A Later Review. The Laryngoscope, April, 1910.

106. DELALANDE, H. De la Gastroscopie. Pub. by Imprimerie Commerciale 56 Rue du Hautoir, Bordeaux. In collaboration with E. J. Moure, 1908.

107. DELAVAN, D. BRYSON. Foreign Bodies in the Air Passages. Reference Handbook of the Medical Sciences, Vol. I, p. 168.

108. DELAVAN, D. BRYSON, AND JOHN ROGERS. Treatment of Chronic Laryngeal Stenosis. Transactions Am. Laryngol. Soc., 1905.

109. DELAVAN, D. BRYSON. Intubation in Chronic Stenosis of the Larynx. Med. News, March 19, 1898.

110. DELAVAN, D. BRYSON. Treatment of Cicatricial Stenosis of the Larynx. Journ. Laryngology 1909, Nov., p. 585.

111. DELAVAN, D. BRYSON. Treatment of Cicatricial Stenosis of the Larynx. Laryngoscope, Nov., 1909.

112. DENKER, ALFRED. Tracheobronchial and Pulmonary Syphilis Diagnosed by Means of the Bronchoscope. Deutsche Med. Woch., No. 1, Jan. 4, 1912, p. 11.

113. DENNIS, F. L. Laryngeal Fissure for Intrinsic Laryngeal Carcinoma. Colo. Med., June, 1909.

114. DUPUY, HOMER. (1) Foreign Body in the Esophagus Removed by Esophagoscopy; (2) Foreign Body in Bronchial Tract. New Orleans Med. and Surg. Journ., May, 1913—LXV—815.

115. DOWNIE, WALKER. Syphilis as a Cause of Esophageal Stenosis. Brit. Med. Journ. Oct. 19, 1912.

116. DELAVAN, D. BRYSON. Withholding of Reports of Operations for the Relief of Cancer of the Throat. New York Med. Journ., Oct. 14, 1893.

117. DELAVAN, D. BRYSON. Primary Epithelioma of the Epiglottis.

118. DELAVAN, D. BRYSON. Statistics for Relief of Malignant Disease of the Larynx.

125. ELSBERG, CHAS. A. Anesthesia by the Intratracheal Insufflation of Air and Ether. Annals of Surgery, Feb., 1911.

126. ELSBERG, C. A. Value of Continuous Intratracheal Insufflation of Air (Meltzer) in Thoracic Surgery; With Description of an Apparatus. Med. Record, March 19, 1910, and Ann. of Surg., July, 1910.

127. ELSBERG, C. A. AND LILIENTHAL, H. General Anesthesia by Means of Meltzer's Continuous Intratracheal Insufflation. Berl. Klin. Wchr., May 23, 1910.

128. ELSNER, H. Gastroscopie, 1911. Pub. by George Thieme, Leipzig.

129. EPHRAIM, A. The Importance of Bronchoscopy in Internal Medicine. Berl. Klin. Wchnschr., Oct. 25, 1909.

130. EPHRAIM, A. C. (Breslau.) Anesthesia in Bronchoscopy. Arch. Intern. de Laryngol. d'Otol. et de Rhin., May-June, 1912. Vol. XXXIII, No. 3, 690.

131. EPHRAIM, A. Endobronchial Therapy. Berl. Klin. Wchnschr., July 4, 1910.

132. EPHRAIM. Significance of Bronchoscopy for Internal Medicine. Deut. med. Wchnschr., No. 5, 1910.

133. EPHRIAM, A. Local Treatment of Chronic Bronchial Diseases. Arch. f. Laryngol. u. Rhinol., Bd. 24, Heft 1, 1910, and Arch. Internat. de Laryngol. d'Otol. et de Rhinol, Nov.-Dec., 1910.

134. EMERSON, LINN. Perforation of Esophagus and Aorta by a Chicken Bone. Discussion. Proc. Amer. Laryngol., Rhinol. and Otol. Soc., 1913, p. 321.

135. EDINGTON. Abstract by Guthrie. Congenital Occlusion of the Esophagus. Laryngoscope, Jan., 1914.

144. FAULDER, T. JEFFERSON. Direct Esophagoscopy. Brit. Med. Journ., Aug. 27, 1910.

145. FERRERI, G. Technic of Tracheobronchoscopy. The Laryngoscope, April, 1910.

146. FORBES, HENRY H. Direct Laryngoscopy. Post-Graduate, Vol. XXVIII, No. 1, Jan., 1913, p. 28.

147. FOSTER, H. Report of Two Unusual and Interesting Cases of Acute Edema of the Larynx. The Laryngoscope, St. Louis, Feb. 1910.

148. FOURNIER, G. Contribution l'Etude de la Dilatation Caoutchoutee dans la Laryngostomie. Rev. hebd. de Laryngol., d'Otol. et de Rhinol., Oct. 9, 1909.

149. FRASER, J. S. Direct Laryngoscopy, Tracheobronchoscopy and Esophagoscopy. Edinburg Med. Jour., Vol. X, No. 1, Jan., 1913, p. 6.

150. FRESC. Traction Diverticula of the Gullet Diagnosed by Esophagoscopy. Monatschr. f. Ohrenheilk., Nov., 1911, p. 1323.

151. FREUDENTHAL, WOLFF. Personal Observations with Suspension Laryngoscopy. Medical Record, February 22, 1913.

152. FREUDENTHAL, W. Endobronchial Treatment of Asthma. N. Y. Med. Journ., June 24, 1911.

153. FREUDENTHAL, WOLFF. The Removal of Foreign Bodies from the Esophagus and the Bronchi with the Aid of the Fluoroscopic Screen. Intern. Journ, of Surg., Sept., 1910.

154. FREUDENTHAL, WOLFF. A Plea for Systematic Use of Bronchoscopy in Our Routine Work, with Description of a Modified Bronchoscope. N. Y. Med. Journ., May 23, 1908.

155. FRIEDBERG, S. A. Bronchoscopy and Esophagoscopy. Illinois Med. Journal, March, 1911.

166. GAREL, J. Cancer du Larynx Siegeant sur le Repli Aryteno-epiglottique Gauche; Operation Endolaryngeal: Guerison. Rev. hebd. de Laryngol., d'Otol. et de Rhinol., Sept. 18, 1909.

167. GAUB, O. C. AND JACKSON, C. Bronchoscopic Aid in Thoracotomy. The Laryngoscope, Feb., 1910.

168. GLEITSMANN, J. Cordectomy for Bilateral Abductor Paralysis with Demonstration of Specimen. The Laryngoscope, April, 1910. Arch. f. Laryngol. u. Rhinol., Vol. 23, Heft 1, 1910, and Arch. Internat. de Laryngol. d'Otol et de Rhinol., March-April, 1910.

169. GLUCKSMANN, GEORGE. The Newer Methods of Extraction of Foreign Bodies from the Upper Air and Food Passages. Berl. Klin. Woch., XLIX, No. 23, June 3, 1912, p. 1081.

170. GOLDBACH, L. J. Direct Laryngo-Tracheo-Bronchoscopy and Esophagoscopy. Report of Cases. The Laryngoscope, Sept., 1910.

171. GOLDSTEIN, M. A. Lipoma of the Larynx. The Laryngoscope, 1909. (Excellent resumé of the subject.)

172. GRAY, A. L. Remarks on X-Ray Technic in the Treatment of Laryngeal Papillomata in Children. Ann. of Otol., Rhinol. and Laryngol., June 25, 1910.

173. GREENE, D. C. Laryngotomy and Laryngectomy for Cancer. Boston Med. and Surg. Jour., Jan. 28, 1909.

174. GREEN, A. S. AND LACK, H. L. Subglottic Laryngeal Tumor. Proc. Soc. Med., Vol. 1, No. 8, 1909.

175. GRIFFITH, J. P. C. AND LAVENSON, R. S. Case of Congenital Malformation of the Esophagus with Report of a Case. Arch. of Pediatr., March, 1909.

176. GRISWOLD, W. C. Five Cases of Foreign Bodies, for which Bronchoscopy or Esophagoscopy was performed. Post-Graduate, Vol. XXVII, No. 5, May, 1912, p. 397.

177. GROVE, W. E. Tracheobronchoscopy in Diagnosis and Treatment. Wisconsin Med. Jour., Vol. XI, No. 11, April, 1913, p. 346.

178. GUISEZ, J. Maladies de l' Esophage. Paris, 1911.

179. GUISEZ. New Cases of Diagnosis by Means of Direct Laryngoscopy not Possible with Mirror. (Neue Fälle von Diagnosen mittels Direkter Laryngoskopie die mit dem Spiegel nicht Gestellt werden Konnten.) Ztschr. f. Laryngol. Rhinol. u. ihre Grenzgeb., Bd. 2, Heft 6, 1910.

180. GUISEZ AND ABRAND. Physiology of the Esophagus. Ann. des Mal. de l'Oreille, du Larynx, du Nez et du Pharynx, Sept., 1910.

181. GUISEZ. Two Unusual Cases of Tuberculosis of the Esophagus Diagnosed and Treated by Esophagoscopy. Gaz. des Hopit., March 8, 1910.

182. GUISEZ. Removal by Bronchoscopy of Foreign Bodies in Bronchi of Two Infants. Bull. de La Soc. de Ped., June, 1910.

183. GUISEZ. Broncho-Esophagoscopy in Diagnosis of Aneurism of the Aorta. Arch. des Mal. du Coeur, etc., April, 1909.

184. GUTHRIE, THOMAS. Twelve Cases of Foreign Body in the Larynx and Esophagus, in Most of Which Removal Was Effected by Direct Endoscopy. Liverpool Med. Chir. Journ., July, 1912, No. 62, p. 459.

185. GOLDSTEIN, M. A. Discussion on Foreign Bodies in the Trachea. Proceedings Am. Lar., Rhin. and Otol. Soc., 1913, p. 388.

186. GREEN, NATHAN W. An Esophagoscope with Direct Outside Illumination. Annals of Surgery, Feb., 1914.

194. HARRIS, THOMAS J. Radium for Papilloma of the Larynx in Children. Proceedings International Medical Congress, London, 1913.

195. HALSTED, T. H. Practicality of Bronchoscopy and Esophagoscopy. The Laryngoscope, July, 1909.

196. HARET AND JAUGEAS. Tumor of the Trachea Cured by Radiotherapy. Soc. of Radiol., May 11, 1909.

197. HAUSTED. Asphyxia Caused by the Lumbricoid Ascarides in Trachea. Hospitalstidende, May 18, 1910.

198. HAYS, HAROLD. The Pharyngoscope. The Laryngoscope, July, 1909.

199. HICKEY, P. M. Foreign Bodies in the Esophagus and Lower Air Passages. Jour. Mich. State Med. Soc., Jan., 1910.

200. HILL, WILLIAM. On Gastroscopy, 1912. Pub. by John Bales and Sons and Danielson, Oxford St., London.

201. HILL, WILLIAM. On Gastroscopy: A Plea for its Routine Employment by Gastric Experts. Brit. Med. Journ., Oct., 1911, p. 1074.

202. HOLINGER, J. Papilloma of the Larynx Combined with Open Foramen Ovale in Heart. Trans. Chicago L. and O. Soc., May 17, 1910.

203. HOPKINS, F. E. A Case of Multiple Foreign Bodies in the Smaller Bronchi. Ann. of Otol., Rhinol. and Laryngology, Vol. XX, No. 4, Dec., 1911, p. 825.

204. HORAND. Total Laryngectomy for Syphilitic Stenosis of Larynx. Lyon Med., July 24, 1910.

205. HORNE, W. J. Specimens showing the Pathogenesis of Pachydermia Laryngis Verrucosa et Diffusa. Proc. R. Soc. Med., Vol. 1, No. 9, 1909.

206. HORN, HENRY. The Bronchoscopic Treatment of Bronchial Asthma. Read in the Section on Laryngology and Otol. of the A. M. A. at 61st Annual Session held at St. Louis, June, 1910.

207. HORSLEY, J. S. Suture of Recurrent Laryngeal Nerve with Report of a Case. Trans. of South. Surg. and Gynecol. Ass'n., Dec., 1909.

208. HOWARTH, W. G. Direct Laryngoscopy, Bronchoscopy and Esophagoscopy. (Translation of Brünings' text book.)

209. HUBBARD, THOMAS. Esophagoscopy and Bronchoscopy; Reports of Cases of Foreign Bodies in the Esophagus and Bronchi Operated by the Killian Method. Transactions of the Amer. Laryngol. Assn., 1911.

210. HUBER, FRANCIS. Removal of Foreign Bodies from the Bronchi. Surg. Gyn. and Obstetrics, May, 1910, pages 524-529.

211. HUNT, JOHN G. (Fort William.) Report of a Case of Aspiration of a Silver Tracheotomy Cannula Removed by Lower Bronchoscopy. Canadian Med. Ass'n. Journ., Vol. XI, No. 5, May, 1912, p. 414. Also Annals Otol., Rhinol. and Laryngol., June, 1912, p. 355.

212. HOWARTH, W. G. Foreign Bodies in the Air Passages. Lancet, Oct. 4, 1913.

213. HILL, WM. Idiopathic Spasm of the Esophagus as a Common Diagnostic Error. Journ. Laryngol., Rhinol. and Otol. (Very interesting discussion.)

214. HERYNG, THEODORE. Laryngeal Arthritis. (Gosiec Krtani) Medycyna, No. 26, 1910.

215. HERYNG, THEODORE. Soft Rubber Dilatation of the Stenosed Larynx. Discussion Proc. Eleventh Internat. Med. Congress, Rome, 1894.

216. HOWARD, C. P. Etiology and Pathogenesis of Bronchiectasis. Amer. Journ. Med. Sciences, March, 1914.

219. INGERSOLL, J. M. Primary Malignant Growth of the Trachea. Transactions Amer. Laryngol. Soc., 1914. Also Annals Otol., Rhinol. Laryngol., June, 1914.

220. IWANOFF, A. Technic of Laryngostomy. Ztschr. f. Laryngol. Rhinol. u. ihre Grinzgeb., Bd. 3, Heft 2, 1910.

221. IGLAUER, SAMUEL. Electro-Magnets in the Extraction of Foreign Bodies from the Trachea and Bronchi. Proc. Am. Acad. Opthal. and Oto-Laryngol., 1913.

222. IGLAUER, SAMUEL. Three Cases of Foreign Body in the Bronchi. Lancet-Clinic, Vol. CII, No. 22, June 1, 1912.

223. IGLAUER, SAMUEL. Tracheobronchoscopy—With Report of Cases. Ohio State Med. Journ., April, 1911.

224. IGLAUER, SAMUEL. Foreign Body in Larynx and Trachea Removed by the Aid of the Suspension Laryngoscope. The Laryngoscope, June, 1913.

225. INGALS, E. F. Tacks and Nails in the Air Passages: Bronchoscopy. Journ. of A. M. A., Feb. 17, 1912, pp. 467-469.

226. INGALS, E. F. Treatment of Foreign Bodies in the Esophagus. The Laryngoscope, Jan., 1912, Vol. XXII, No. 1, p. 47. Also Am. Journ. Surgery, Jan., 1912.

227. INGALS, E. F. Bronchoscopy and Esophagoscopy: The Technic, Utility and Dangers. The Laryngoscope, July, 1909, and Ann. of Otol., Rhinol. and Laryngol., March, 1909.

228. INGALS, E. F. Bronchoscopy for Removal of Foreign Bodies from the Lungs. N. Y. Med. Journ. and Phila. Med. Journ., July 8 and 15, 1905.

229. JACKSON, CHEVALIER. Anesthetic Attachment for the Bronchoscope. The Laryngoscope, February, 1910.

230. JACKSON, CHEVALIER. A New Bronchoscope. Laryngoscope, March, 1908.

231. JACKSON, CHEVALIER. A Foreign Body Extractor (mechanical spoon). The Laryngoscope, July, 1908.

232. JACKSON, CHEVALIER. Drowning of the Patient in His Own Secretion. Editorial. The Laryngoscope, Dec., 1911.

233. JACKSON, CHEVALIER. Foreign Bodies. The Aid of Esophagoscopy, Bronchoscopy and Magnetism in Their Extraction. The Laryngoscope, April, 1905.

234. JACKSON, CHEVALIER. Endothelioma of the Larynx. Report of a Case. Pennsylvania Med. Journ., June, 1907.

235. JACKSON, CHEVALIER. Insufflation Anesthesia. Editorial. The Laryngoscope, Sept., 1913.

236. JACKSON, CHEVALIER. Bronchoscopy and Esophagoscopy. Journ. A. M. A., Sept. 25, 1909, Vol. LIII, pp. 1009-1013.

237. JACKSON, CHEVALIER. Statistics of Seventy Cases of Gastroscopy. American Journ. of the Med. Sciences, July, 1908.

238. JACKSON, CHEVALIER. The Dilatation of Bronchial Strictures. Journ. of the A. M. A., Sept. 21, 1912, Vol. LIX, pp. 1123-1126.

239. JACKSON, CHEVALIER. Gastroscopy. Archives Internationales de Laryngologie.

240. JACKSON, CHEVALIER. Voluntary Aspiration of a Foreign Body into the Bronchi. Removal by Bronchoscopy. The Laryngoscope. St. Louis, Dec., 1909.

241. JACKSON, CHEVALIER. Esophageal Stenosis Following the Swallowing of Caustic Alkalies. Journ. of A. M. A., Nov. 26, 1910, Vol. LV, pp. 1857-1858.

242. JACKSON, CHEVALIER. Laryngeal, Bronchial and Esophageal Endoscopy. Editorial. Laryngoscope, Vol. XXI, No. 12, Dec., 1911, p. 1183.

243. JACKSON, CHEVALIER. The Bronchoscope as an Aid in General Diagnosis. Archives of Diagnosis, April, 1908.

244. JACKSON, CHEVALIER. Tracheotomy. The Laryngoscope, April, 1909.

245. JACKSON, CHEVALIER. Position for Endoscopy. (Editorial) The Laryngoscope, May, 1912.

246. JACKSON, CHEVALIER. Influenzal Tracheitis. (Editorial) The Laryngoscope, February, 1912.

247. JACKSON, CHEVALIER. Direct Methods of Examination of the Larynx, Trachea, Bronchi, Esophagus and Stomach. International Clinics, Vol. 11, Twenty-second Series.

248. JACKSON, CHEVALIER. Laryngostomy. The Laryngoscope, Sept., 1909.

249. JACKSON, CHEVALIER. Tracheobronchoscopy. Annals of Surg. for March, 1908.

250. JACKSON, CHEVALIER. Clinical Diagnosis and Operative Procedure in Intralaryngeal Carcinoma, from the Standpoint of the Laryngologist. The Laryngoscope, Aug., 1909.

251. JACKSON, CHEVALIER. Direct Laryngoscopes. The Laryngoscope, June, 1913.

252. JACKSON, CHEVALIER. The Larynx in Typhoid Fever. Am. Journ. Med. Sci., Nov., 1905.

253. JACKSON, CHEVALIER. Primary Malignant Disease of the Larynx. The Laryngoscope, August, 1904.

254. JACKSON, CHEVALIER. Thyrotomy and Laryngectomy for Malignant Disease of the Larynx. Brit. Med. Journ., Nov. 24, 1906.

255. JACKSON, CHEVALIER. Thymic Tracheostenosis, Tracheoscopy, Thymectomy, Cure. Journ. of the Amer. Med. Ass'n., May 25, 1907, Vol. XLVIII, pp. 1753-1756.

256. JACKSON, CHEVALIER. Esophagoscopic Removal of Open Safety-Pins by New Method. The Laryngoscope, April, 1910.

257. JACKSON, CHEVALIER. The Surgery of the Esophagus, Laryngologically considered. The Laryngoscope, Oct., 1909.

258. JACKSON, CHEVALIER. Anesthesia for Peroral Endoscopy. Proc. Amer. Laryngol. Ass'n., 1912, p. 88. (Interesting discussion).

259. JACKSON, CHEVALIER. Some Problems of Direct Laryngoscopy and Bronchoscopy. Am. Acad. Opthal. and Oto-Laryngol., 1912.

260. JACKSON, CHEVALIER. Laryngeal, Bronchial and Esophageal Endoscopy. The Laryngoscope, Vol. XXII, No. 2, Feb., 1912, p. 130.

261. JACKSON, CHEVALIER. Bronchoscopic Aid in Thoracotomy, 1910.

262. JACKSON, CHEVALIER. Esophagoscopy and Gastroscopy. The Laryngoscope, St. Louis, Sept., 1911.

263. JACKSON, CHEVALIER. Decannulation and Extubation after Tracheotomy and Intubation, Respectively. Proc. Am. Laryngol. Soc., 1913. (Interesting discussion).

264. JACKSON, CHEVALIER. Tracheobronchoscopy. Journal of Laryngology, Rhinology and Otology. London, Dec., 1907.

265. JACKSON, CHEVALIER. Esophagoscopy and Gastroscopy. Ref. Handbook Med. Sci., Vol. III. Wm. Wood and Co.

266. JACKSON, CHEVALIER. Technic of Insertion of Intratracheal Insufflation Tubes. Surgery, Gynecology and Obstetrics. Oct., 1913.

267. JACKSON, CHEVALIER. Bronchoscopy. Ref. Handbook Med. Sci., Vol. II. Wm. Wood and Co.

268. JACKSON, CHEVALIER. Laryngeal Stenosis from Post-typhoid Perichondritis. Annals of Otology, Rhinology and Laryngology, March, 1904.

269. JACKSON, CHEVALIER. Tracheobronchoscopy, Esophagoscopy and Gastroscopy. Text book. Pub. by The Laryngoscope, St. Louis, 1907.

270. JACKSON, CHEVALIER. Recent Advances in Endoscopy of the Larynx, Trachea, Bronchi, Esophagus and Stomach. (Report to the International Medical Congress, London, 1913, Section XV). Also published in The Laryngoscope, July, 1913.

271. JACKSON, CHEVALIER. Obstructions in the Trachea and Bronchi. Musser-Kelly Hand book of Treatment. Saunders and Co., Philadelphia.

272. JANEWAY, H. H. Gastroscopy. Journal Am. Med. Ass'n., Oct. 11, 1913.

273. JANEWAY, H. H. AND GREEN, N. W. Esophagoscopy and Gastroscopy. Surg., Gyn. and Obst., Sept., 1911, p. 245.

274. JERVEY, J. W. Nail Occluding Third Bronchial Ramus; Upper Bronchoscopy Recovery. Southern Med. Journ., Vol. VI, No. 3, March, 1913, p. 191-193.

275. JOHNSTON, R. H. Esophagoscopy in the Removal of Foreign Bodies. N. Y. Med. Jour., Sept. 4, 1909.

276. JOHNSTON, R. H. Extension and Flexion in Direct Laryngostomy. A Comparative Study. Ann. of Otol., Rhinol. and Laryngol., March, 1910.

277. JOHNSTON, R. H. Straight Method of Direct Laryngoscopy. The Laryngoscope, Dec., 1910.

278. JOHNSTON, R. H. Direct Laryngoscopy in the Removal of Laryngeal Tumors. The Laryngoscope, Vol. XXII, No. 10, Oct., 1912, p. 1214.

279. JOHNSTON, R. H. Esophagoscopy. Laryngoscope, Vol. XXI, No. 12, Dec., 1911, p. 1156.

280. JOHNSTON, R. H. Some Esophageal Cases. Md. Med. Jour., Feb., 1909.

281. JOHNSTON, R. H. Some Original Endoscopic Methods. Laryngoscope, May, 1913, XXIII, 607.

282. JOHNSTON, R. H. Straight Direct Laryngoscopy and Esophagoscopy. Am. Acad. Ophthal. and Oto-Laryngol., 1912.

283. JOHNSTON, R. H. The Removal of Foreign Bodies from the Upper End of the Esophagus. Am. Acad. Ophthal. and Oto-Laryngol., 1912.

284. JOHNSTON, R. H. Direct Laryngoscopy in Diagnosis and Treatment of Papillomata of the Larynx. The Laryngoscope, Nov., 1909.

285. JOHNSTON, R. H. Removal of Laryngeal Tumors in the Left Lateral Position. The Laryngoscope, May, 1909.

286. JOHNSTON, R. H. Direct Laryngoscopy. Cincinnati Lancet-Clinic, Sept. 18, 1909. (An interesting series of cases reported in this article).

287. JANEWAY, HENRY. Intratracheal Anesthesia from the Standpoint of the Nose, Throat and Oral Surgeon. The Laryngoscope, Nov., 1913.

288. JANEWAY, H. H. AND GREEN, N. W. Cancer of the Esophagus and Cardia. Ann. of Surg., July, 1910.

296. KAHLER, OTTO. Scabbard Trachea and Pulmonary Emphysema. Proc. Stuttgart Laryngological Society, May, 1913.

297. KAHLER, OTTO. Chirurgische Behandlung der Kehlkoptuberculose. Monats. f. Ohrenheilkunde 47 Jahrgang, x heft.

298. KAHLER, OTTO. Esophagoscopy and Bronchoscopy. Pub. by Montz Perles. Vienna, 1909.

299. KAHLER, OTTO. Bronchoscopy and Esophagoscopy. Laryngoscope, Sept., 1911.

300. KAHLER, OTTO. Diverticulum of the Tracheo-Bronchial Tree. Monatschr. f. Ohrenheilk. und Laryngo-Rhinol., Heft 1, 1911.

301. KAHLER, OTTO. Zur Bronchoskopie bei Fremkörpern. Monatschr. f. Ohrenh. u. Laryngo-Rhinol., Heft 2, 1909.

302. KAHLER, OTTO. Bronchoscopy and Esophagoscopy; Their Indications and Contraindication. Arch. f. Laryn., Vol. XXV, No. 2, 1911, p. 371.

303. KELLY, A. BROWN. Some Experiences in the Direct Examination of the Larynx, Trachea and Esophagus. Brit. Med. Journ., Sept. 26, 1908, p. 896.

304. KELLY, A. BROWN. Perforation of Esophagus due to Ulceration Produced by Foreign Bodies. Proc. Royal Soc. Med., Vol. V, No. 7, May, 1912.

305. KELLY, A. BROWN. Stenoses at the Lower End of the Esophagus, with Special Reference to those of Spastic Origin. Brit. Med. Jour., Oct. 19, 1912.

306. KILLIAN, GUSTAV. Laryngoscopy. Berl. Klin. Woch., No. 13, March 25, 1912, p. 581.

307. KILLIAN, GUSTAV. Short Hints for Examining the Esophagus, Trachea and Bronchi by Direct Methods. Printed as MS.

308. KILLIAN, GUSTAV. Suspension Laryngoscopy. Archiv. f. Laryngol. und Rhin., Bd. XXVI, No. 2, p. 278.

309. KILLIAN, F. The History of Bronchoscopy and Esophagoscopy. Deutsche Med. Woch., 1911, No. 35, Aug. 31, p. 1585.

310. KILLIAN, G. Tracheobronchoscopy in its Diagnostic and Therapeutical Aspects. The Laryngoscope, St. Louis, Dec., 1906.

311. KILLIAN, GUSTAV. Die Directen Methoden in den Jahren, 1911 und 1912. Proc. Internat. Med. Congress, 1913.

312. KILLIAN, GUSTAV. Improved Technic for Laryngoscopy. Berliner Klinische Wochenschrift, March 25, XLIX, No. 13, pp. 581-628.

313. KOSCHIER, H. Operative Treatment of Carcinoma of the Larynx. Wien. Klin. Woch.. Vol. XXII, No. 27.

314. KUBO, INO. (Japan). Stenosis of the Trachea and Esophagus due to Pressure from an Abscess of a Thoracic Vertebra, Diagnosed by Means of Tracheoscopy and Esophagoscopy; Operation; Improvement. Arch. f. Laryng., Vol. XXV, No. 3, 1911, p. 506.

315. KUBO, INO. The Present Status of the Direct Method in Japan. Semon's Internat. Centralblatt f. Laryngol., Rhin., etc., No. 10, 1913.

316. KUHN, F. AND MELTZER, S. J. Intra-tracheal Insufflation and Peroral Intubation. Berl. Klin., Wchnschr., Sept. 19, 1910.

317. KYLE, D. BRADEN. Diseases of the Nose and Throat. W. B. Saunders.

318. KYLE, JOHN J. Direct Laryngoscopy and Tracheobronchoscopy. Journ. of the Indiana State Med. Ass'n., Feb. 15, 1908.

319. KYLE, D. BRADEN. Removal of a Toothplate that had Remained in the Esophagus Seventeen Years. Transactions Am. Laryngol. Soc., 1913. Also Proc. Internat. Med. Congress, Section XV, London, 1913.

320. KYLE, D. BRADEN. Surgical Treatment of Tubercular Lesions of the Upper Respiratory Tract. Proc. Sixth International Congress on Tuberculosis.

321. KYLE, D. BRADEN. Nose and Throat (Text book). Saunders Co., Philadelphia.

322. KNEEDLER, G. C. Tracheotomy. Pgh. Med. Journ., Jan., 1914.

323. KIRSTEIN, A. Autoscopy. Berlin Klin. Woch., No. 22, 1895.

324. KIRSTEIN, A. Autoscopy. (Monograph). Coblentz, 1906.

325. KOB AND WADSACK. Echinococcus of the Left Lung. Berlin. Klin. Woch., p. 1097, No. 33, 1906.

328. LEVY, ROBERT. Tuberculosis of the Mouth. (Excellent colored illustrations.) The Laryngoscope, Dec., 1907.

329. LIEBAULT, G. A. M. Chronic Inflammatory Stenoses of the Esophagus. Thesis 191. Faculty of Medicine. University of Paris. 1913.

330. LABOURE. Esophagoscopy for Foreign Bodies. Arch. Intern. de Laryng., Jan.-Feb., 1912, p. 83.

331. Lack, H. L; Delsaux, V., and Delavan, D. B. Treatment of Cicatricial Stenosis of the Larynx. Brit. Med. Jour., Oct. 16, 1909.

332. Landon, L. H. Practicability of the Meltzer-Auer Method of Continuous Intra-tracheal Insufflation. University of Pa. Med. Bull., July-August, 1910.

333. Lange, S. The Roentgen Examination of the Esophagus. N. Y. Med. Jour., Jan. 23, 1909.

334. Lange, S. Early Recognition of Esophageal Stricture. Med. Record, Jan. 16, 1909.

335. Large, S. H. Pathological Lesions and Trachea. Lantern Slides. Am. Acad. Ophthal. and Oto-Laryngol., 1912.

336. Large, S. Some of My Mishaps in Seventy-five cases of Tracheobronchoscopy and Esophagoscopy. The Laryngoscope, Nov., 1910.

337. Large, S. H. Foreign Body in Right Bronchus. Cleveland Med. Jour., Nov., 1909.

338. Laurent, F. V. Respiration for Tone-Production. The Laryngoscope, Dec., 1910.

339. Lazarraga. Complete Removal of Larynx Under Local Anesthesia. Its advantages. Arch. Internat. de Laryngol., d'Otol. et de Rhinol., Nov.-Dec., 1910.

340. Leavy, Chas. A. Chronic Stenosis of Larynx and Trachea. Report of Case. The Laryngoscope, 1913.

341. Lederman, M. D. Edema of the Larynx Following an Infection of the Lower Pharynx. The Laryngoscope, May, 1909.

342. Lerche, Wm. A Contribution to the Surgery of the Esophagus. Surg. Gynecology and Obstetrics. Oct., 1910, pages 345-361.

343. Lewisohn, Richard. A New Principle in Esophagoscopy and Gastroscopy. Annals of Surgery, Vol. LVII, No. 1, Jan., 1913, p. 28.

344. Lewisohn, Richard. A New Esophagoscope. Journ. Amer. Med. Ass'n., Nov., 1911, p. 1681.

345. Lilienthal, H. First Case of Thoracotomy in a Human Being under Anesthesia by Intra-tracheal Insufflation. Ann of Surg., July, 1910

346. Lockard, L. B. Amputation of Epiglottis in Laryngeal Tuberculosis. Denver Med. Times and Utah Med. Jour., Oct., 1910.

347. London, Julius. A New Gastro-Esophagoscope. Medical Record, Vol. LXXXII, No. 25, Dec. 21, 1912, p. 1125.

348. Loeb, Hanau W. Fibropapilloma of the Larynx. Ann. Otol., Rhinol. and Laryngol., Nov., 1902.

349. Lynah, Henry L. Diphtheritic Stenosis of the Larynx. The Laryngoscope, Dec., 1913.

350. LYNCH, R. C. · Magnetic Extraction of a Foreign Body from the Bronchus. Proc. Amer. Acad. Ophthalmol. and Oto-Laryngol., 1913.

351. LEVINGER. Multiple Osteomata of the Trachea Clinically Diagnosticated by Means of Direct Tracheoscopy. Muench. med. Wchnschr., Nov. 15, 1910.

352. LITCHFIELD, LAWRENCE. Abuse of Normal Salt Solution. Journ. A. M. A., July 25, 1914.

356. MELTZER. Intratracheal Insufflation Anesthesia. Bulletins Rockefeller Institute, New York City, 1910, 1911, 1912.

357. MACNIE, JOHN S. Removal of a Stick-Pin from the Second Bifurcation by Direct Bronchoscopy under Local Anesthesia. Journal Lancet. August 15, 1913.

358. MACDONALD, W. A. Congenital Membrane Between Vocal Cords. Can. Jour. of Med. and Surg., Dec., 1909.

359. MAKUEN, G. HUDSON. Respiratory and Vocal Symptoms in Papillomata of the Larynx. Ann. of Otol., Rhinol and Laryngol., Sept., 1910.

360. MAKUEN, G. HUDSON. Removal of an Open Safety-Pin from the Trachea by Upper Bronchoscopy. Journ. of the Amer. Med. Ass'n., July 22, 1911, Vol. LVII, p. 286.

361. MANN, M. Atlas of Killian's Tracheobronchoscopy. (Excellent colored plates of pathological specimens of trachea, mediastinal tumors, etc.). Pub. by Curt Kabitzsch, Würzburg. (Lehrbuch der Bronchoskopie, by same author and publisher just published as we go to press, is an excellent practical manual).

362. MANN, R. H. T. Removal of a Grain of Corn from the Entrance of the Left Bronchus of a Child Four Years Old. Jour. Arkans. Med. Soc., April, 1910.

363. MANN, R. H. T. Foreign bodies in the Air Passages and the Esophagus. Jour. Kansas Med. Soc., Vol. XIII. No. 4, April, 1913, p. 155.

364. MARSCHIK, H. AND VOGEL, R. Fremkörper in den oberen Luft und Speisenwegen mit besonderer Berücksichtigung der Esophagotomie. Wien Klin. Wchnschr., Oct. 14, 1909.

365. MARSCHIK, H. Larynxcarcinom bei Jugendlichen Personen. Monatschr. f. Ohrenh. u. Laryngo-Rhinol., Heft 9, 1909.

366. MASON, N. R. AND INGLIS, H. J. Acute Edema of the Larynx Following Etherization for Forceps Delivery. Report of a Case. Boston Med. and Surg. Jour., June 2, 1910.

367. MASSEI. Complete Review of the Clinical Laryngological Work for 1909. Monograph Naples. 1910.

368. MASSEI, F. Direct and Indirect Laryngoscopy. Monat. f. Ohrenheilk. Laryng. Rhin., Vol. XLVI, No. 5, p. 595.

369. MATTHEWS. The Relation of Nasal Conditions to Asthma Journ. Amer. Med. Ass'n., Oct. 12, 1912.

370. MAYER, EMIL. Treatment of Cicatricial Stenosis of the Larynx. The Laryngoscope, Jan., 1912.

371. MAYER, E., AND YANKAUER, J. Further Bronchoscopic Observations. Zeitschr. f. Laryng., Vol. IV, No. 3, 1911, p. 395.

372. MAYER, E. Stenosis of the Larynx Cured by Intubation. Med. Record, Dec. 25, 1909.

373. MAYER, E. Esophageal Diverticula. Proceedings Am. Laryngological Association, 1910.

374. MAYER, E. Further Report of a Case of Tracheal Scleroma. Am. Jour. of Med. Sci., Feb., 1909.

375. MAYO, C. H. Diagnosis and Surgical Treatment of Esophageal Diverticula. Ann. of Surg., June, 1910.

376. McKENZIE, DAN. The Laryngectomy. Journ. Laryngol. Rhinol., Oct., 1913.

377. McKINNEY, R. Esophagoscopy in the Removal of Foreign Bodies from the Esophagus. Laryngoscope, Oct., 1912.

378. McREYNOLDS, J. O. Mastoiditis Complicated by Ulceration and Rupture of the Esophagus. Texas State Jour. of Med., Oct., 1906.

379. MELTZER, S. I. Method of Respiration by Intratracheal Insufflation; its Scientific Principle and its Practical Availability in Medicine and Surgery. Med. Record, March 19, 1910, and Berl. Klin. Wchnschr., March 21, 1910. (Excellent resume by same author in Berl. Klin. Woch., No. 15 and 16, 1914).

380. MILLER, CLIFTON M. Chronic Nasal Diphtheria. Virginia Med. Semi-Monthly, April 12, 1912.

381. MILLER, MORRIS B. Perforation of the Ileum by Foreign Bodies. Annals of Surgery, Nov., 1913, p. 707.

382. MILLSPAUGH, W. P. Interesting Esophageal Cases. The Laryngoscope, Sept., 1913.

383. MILLSPAUGH, W. P. Esophagoscopy for Removal of Foreign Bodies. Southern Cal. Practitioner, Vol. XXVII, No. 6, June, 1912, p. 265. Also April, 1912.

384. MERMOD, (Lausanne). Hemorrhagies dans les Interventions Endo-laryngees. Archives Internationales, 1913.

385. MERMOD (Lausanne). Propulsion of the Tongue in Direct Laryngoscopy. Archives Internat. de Laryngol., d'Otol. et de Rhinol., 1912

386. Monson, S. H. Foreign Body in the Larynx. Cleveland Med. Jour., June, 1910.

387. Moorhead, Robert L. Foreign Body in the Trachea Removed by Means of the Bronchoscope. Long Island Med. Journ., Vol. VI, No 7, July, 1912, p. 251.

388. Mosher, H. P. Three Esophageal Cases. The Laryngoscope, Oct., 1909.

389. Mosher, H. P. Direct Intubation of the Larynx. The Laryngoscope, Oct., 1909.

390. Mosher, H. P. The Direct Examination of the Larynx and of the Upper End of the Esophagus by the Lateral Route. Boston Med. and Surg. Journ., Vol. CLVIII, No. 6, pp. 189-191, Feb. 6, 1908.

391. Mosher, H. P. A Tube for Closing and Removing an Open Safety-Pin. The Laryngoscope, Oct., 1911.

392. Moure, E. J. De l'examen Gastroscopique. La Presse Medicale, February 3, 1912.

393. Munch, F. Technic of Direct Visual Inspection of Upper Air Passages, Esophagus and Stomach. Presse Med., March 31, 1909.

394. Munch, F. Bronchoscopie et Esophagoscopie. Rev. hebd. de Laryngol., d'Otol. et de Rhinol., Sept. 11, 1909.

395. Murphy, J. Direct Examination of the Larynx, Trachea, Bronchi and Esophagus. Australian Med. Jour., Oct., 1910.

396. Murphy, J. W. Bronchoscopy, with the Report of Two Cases. Lancet-Clinic, Sept. 30, 1911, p. 338.

397. Murphy, J. W. Tracheobronchoscopy, Esophagoscopy and Gastroscopy. Cincinnati Lancet Clinic, July 11, 1908.

398. Murphy, J. W. Removal of Foreign Bodies from the Trachea and Esophagus. Ky. Med. Jour., Oct. 1, 1909.

399. Myer, Jesse S. Cardiospasm with Dilatation of the Esophagus. Journ. of the Amer. Med. Ass'n., Oct. 29, 1910, Vol. LV, pp. 1544-1550.

400. Myer, J. S. Cardiospasm with Dilatation of the Esophagus. Jour. A. M. A., Oct. 29, 1910.

401. Musson, Emma E. Endoscopic Treatment of Bronchiectasis Penn'a. Med. Journ., Jan., 1914.

402. McKinney, R. Comparison of the Technic of Broncho-Esophagoscopy with Jackson's and Brunings' Methods. (Favors Brunings).

403. Mosher, H. P. Some Observations on Esophageal Cases The Laryngoscope, June, 1909.

404. Mehnert. Anatomy of the Esophagus. Archiv. fur Klin. Chir., Bd. 27, p. 76.

405. MOSHER, H. P. Esophagoscope in Esophageal Surgery. Boston Med. and Surg. Journ., Sept. 14, 1911.

406. MOURET, J. Laryngo-Tracheo-Bronchoscopy and Esophagoscopy in the Sitting Position. Bulletin Soc. Francaise d'Oto-rhino-laryngologie, 1913.

407. MERMOD, (Lausanne). Traitement de la Tuberculose par le Galvano-cautere. Archives Internationales (Chauveau) Oct. to Dec., 1904.

408. MAYER, EMIL. Report of a Case of Tracheal Tumor. Proceedings Am. Med. Assn., Sect. Laryngol. and Otol., 1912, p. 183.

409. MACKLESTON. Osteomata of the Trachea. The Laryngoscope, Dec., 1909.

410. MCKENZIE, DAN. Removal of a Foreign Body From the Larynx. Lancet, July 14, 1914.

411. NEUMANN, FRIEDR. Endolaryngeal and Endobronchial Operations. Monatschr. f. Ohrenheilk., Oct., 1911, p. 1113.

412. NORRIS, R. T. Pin Removed from Ascending Division of Left Bronchus with Aid of Fluoroscopic Screen. Surg., Gynecol. and Obstetrics, May, 1910.

413. NOWOTNY. Uber die Bronschoskopie als Heilmethode bei Bronchialstenose. Przeglad Lekarski, No. 24 and 25, 1909.

419. O'DWYER. Chronic Stenosis of the Larynx Treated by a New Method. N. Y. Med. Rec. June 5, 1886.

420. O'DWYER. Intubation for Chronic Stenosis of the Larynx. N. Y. Med. Journ., March 10, 1888.

421. O'REILLY, CHARLES A. Demonstration of the Kahler Bronchoscope. The Laryngoscope. Aug., Sept., 1913. (Interesting discussion on Instruments.)

427. PACKARD, F. R. History of a Case of Recurrent Papilloma of the Larynx, Extending over Thirty Years, During which two Thyrotomies were Performed. Ann. of Otol., Rhinol. and Laryngol., Sept., 1910.

428. PARKER, CHARLES. Surgery of the Thymus Gland. Thymectomy. Report of Fifty Operated Cases. Amer. Jour. of Diseases of Children. Feb., 1913, Vol. 5, pp. 89-122.

429. PATTERSON, ELLEN J. Hyoid Bone Elevation in General Anesthesia. Annals of Surgery, Nov., 1913.

430. PETIT DE LA VILLEON. Foreign Body in Esophagus. Fatal Hemorrhage Through Perforation of Aorta. Gaz. hebd. des Sci. med., Oct 23, 1910.

431. PFAHLER, G. Diagnosis of Carcinoma of the Esophagus by the Roentgen Rays. Arch. of Diag., Jan., 1909.

432. PHILLIPS, WENDELL C. Diseases of the Ear, Nose and Throat. F. A. Davis, Philadelphia.

433. PLUMMER, H. Silk Thread as a Guide in Esophageal Technic. Surg. Gynecol. and Obstetrics, May, 1910.

434. PRATT, JOHN A. Direct Laryngeal Examination. New York Med. Journ., May 24. 1913—XCVII—1076.

435. PUTNAM, C. R. L. Foreign Bodies in Esophagus or Stomach Causing Obstruction. Post-Graduate, Feb., 1910.

436. PRATT, J. P. Apparatus for Intratracheal Insufflation. Journ. Am. Med. Ass'n., Jan. 3, 1914.

437. PATTERSON, D. R. Direct Examination of the Esophagus and Upper Air Passages. Brit. Med. Journ., Aug. 18, 1906.

438. PATTERSON, D. R. Papillomata in Children. Lancet, July 21, 1906.

439. PATTERSON, D. R. Removal of Foreign Bodies from the Air and Food Passages. Brit. Med. Journ., Feb. 8, 1908.

440. PATTON, JAMES M. Localization and Extraction of Foreign Bodies from the Lower Air Passages. Western Med. Review, Sept., 1913, p. 463.

446. REEDE, E. H. Syphilitic Tracheal Stenosis. Washington Medical Annals, Vol. II, No. 5.

447. RENON, E., GERAUDEL AND MARRE, L. Modern Diagnostic Methods Applied to a Cancer of the Bronchus and Lungs. Presse Med., May 28, 1910.

448. RICHARDSON, C. W. Unusual Foreign Body in Right Bronchus Removed by Lower Bronchoscopy. The Laryngoscope, Oct., 1910.

449. RICHARDSON, OSCAR. Foreign Body in Trachea. Status Lymphaticus. Death. Boston Med. and Surg. Journ., Jan. 26, 1911.

450. RICHARDS, GEO. L. Report of a Case of Phlegmon Starting as a Peri-tonsillar Abscess and Extending Downward as far as the Second Ring of the Trachea. The Laryngoscope, August, 1913.

451. RIO, A. DEL. Nineteen Foreign Bodies Removed from the Air Passages by Tracheobronchoscopy. Ztschr. f. Ohrenh. u. f. Krankh. der Luftw., Bd. 62, Heft 1, 1910.

452. ROBINSON, SAMUEL. Intratracheal Ether Anesthesia, 1400 Cases from 15 Surgical Clinics. Surg., Gynecol. and Obstetrics, March 1913.

453. ROCHE, G. AND MOLINIE, J. A Foreign Body in the Left Bronchus. Extraction with the Bronchoscope. Recovery. The Larynx, Jan.-Feb., 1912, p. 20.

454. ROGERS, JOHN R. Report of a Case of Tracheobronchoscopy for Removal of Foreign Body. Jour. of Mich. State Med. Soc., Vol. XII, No. 4, April, 1913, p. 216.

455. ROGERS, JOHN. Treatment of Chronic Stenosis of the Larynx by Intubation. Am. Jour. Med. Sci., April, 1908.

456. ROGERS, JOHN. Treatment of Chronic Stenosis of the Larynx. Am. Journ. Med. Sci., Nov., 1905.

457. RIDPATH, ROBERT F. Routine Use of the Bronchoscope. The Laryngoscope, Nov., 1914.

458. ROSS, GEORGE G. Perforation of the Ileum by a Foreign Body. Annals of Surgery, Nov., 1913, p. 707.

459. ROSS, G. W. Traumatic Esophageal Stricture in a Two-Year-Old Child. Albany Med. Annals, Jan., 1910.

460. RUDGERS, D. W. Case of Foreign Body in the Trachea. N. W. Lancet, May 1, 1909.

461. RUGGI, G. Treatment of Stenosis of the Larynx by Laryngostomy with Dilatation. Semaine Med., Feb. 17, 1909.

462. RENDU, ROBERT. Speculum for Gastroscopy. Rev. Hebdom. de Laryngol., d'Otol., Nov. 16, 1912.

463. REICH, A. Amyloid Tumors in the Trachea. Beitr. zur Klin. Chir., Jan., 1910.

464. RICHARDS, GEORGE L. Two Cases of Abductor Paralysis. Journ. Laryngol., Rhinol. and Otol., Oct., 1906.

469. SEELIG, M. G. Carcinoma of the Esophagus. Annals of Surgery. Dec., 1907.

470. SMITH, HARMON. Fulguration in the Treatment of Papilloma of the Larynx in Children. The Laryngoscope, October, 1913.

471. SEMON, SIR FELIX. Malignant Disease of the Thyroid Gland Perforating the Trachea. Proc. Royal Soc. Med., Vol. V, No. 8, June, 1912.

472. SARGNON, L. Contribution to the Study of Laryngotracheal Stenoses. (Interesting resume with statistics of 135 cases). Bull. d'Oto-Rhino-Laryngeal. Jan. 1, 1912.

473. SARGNON AND BARLATIER. Surgical Treatment of Laryngo-Tracheal Stenosis. Arch. Internat de Laryngol. d'Otol et de Rhinol., Jan.-Oct., 1910.

474. SARGNON, L. Contributions to Laryngostomy. (Contributions a la Laryngostomie). Bull. de Laryngol., Otol. et Rhinol., July, 1910.

475. SARGNON, L. AND ALAMARTINE, H. Cicatricial Stenoses of the Esophagus. Revue de Chir., Aug. 10, 1912.

476. SARGNON AND VIGNARD. Pin Stuck in Right Bifurcation of Right Bronchus. Removed by Lower Bronchoscopy; Cure. Lyon Med., April 13, 1913—XLV—782.

477. SARGNON AND BARLATIER. Etat Actuel de la Laryngostomie. Rev. hebd. de Laryngol., d'Otol. et de Rhinol., Sept. 11, 1909.

478. SARGNON AND BARLATIER. Traitement Chirurgical des Stenoses Laryngo-Tracheales. Arch. Internat. de Laryngol., d'Otol., et de Rhinol., Sept., Nov.-Dec., 1909.

479. SCHLEIFSTEIN, J. D. Laryngostomy in Scleroma. Monatschr. f. Ohrenh. u. Laryngo-Rhinol., Heft 12, 1910.

480. SCHMIEGELOW, E. Laryngeal Tubage in Adults with a Special Self-Retaining Intubation Tube. Revue de Laryngologie, d'Otol. et de Rhinol., 1894.

481. SCHMIEGELOW, E. Intubation of the Larynx in Adults. Proceedings Eleventh Internat. Congress at Rome, 1894. (Interesting discussion).

482. SCHNELL AND MOLINIE. Corps Etrangers de la Trachee (Haricot). Bronchoscopie; Extraction; Guerison. Le Larynx, No. 5, 1909.

483. SCHMIEGELOW, E. A Case of Corpus Alienum Pulmonis Removed by Bronchoscopy. Med. Selskabs, March 9, 1909.

484. SCHMIEGELOW, E. Cicatricial Stenosis of the Larynx After Attempted Suicide. Trans. Dan. Oto-Laryngol. Ass'n., 1910.

485. SCHMIEGELOW, E. Clinical Contributions to the Pathology of Cancer of the Larynx. (Klinische Beiträge zur Pathologie des Kehlkopfkrebses) Arch. f. Laryngol. u. Rhinol., Bd. 23, Heft 3, 1910, and Ugeskr. f. Laeger, July 14 and 21, 1910.

486. SCHOONMAKER, PERRY. The Bronchoscope, Esophagoscope and Gastroscope in Diagnosis and Treatment. American Med, Vol. VI, No. 6, Pages 323-326, June, 1911.

487. SCHOUSBOE. Case of Obliteration of Esophagus. Trans. Dan. Oto-Laryngol. Ass'n., 1909-1910.

488. SCHROTTER, H. V. Bronchoscopy for Foreign Bodies. Wien. Klin. Woch., XXV, No. 12, March 21, 1912, p. 417.

489. SCHWARTZ, ANSELME. Foreign Bodies in the Respiratory Tract. Archiv. Gen. de Medicine, Vol. CCI, June, 1912, p. 422.

490. SCHWINN, J. Thymic Asthma. Thymectomy. Journ. Am. Med. Ass'n., June 20, 1908.

491. SARGNON, A. Contribution a l'Endoscopic Direct. Commun. Congress Societe Francaise d'Oto-Rhino-Laryngol., 1913.

492. SEMON, SIR FELIX. Congenital Malformation of the Larynx, with a Diverticulum of the Esophagus. Trans. Clin., Soc., London, Vol. XXV.

493. SEMON, SIR FELIX. Operative Treatment of Malignant Disease of the Larynx. Brit. Med. Journ., Oct. 31, 1903.

494. SEMON, SIR FELIX. Diagnosis and Treatment of Laryngeal Cancer. Brit. Med. Journ., Feb. 2, 1907.

495. SHURLY, BURT R. Manifestations of Thyroid Disease in the Upper Respiratory Tract. The Laryngoscope, St. Louis, March, 1911.

496. SHURLY, BURT R. An Investigation of Postoperative Conditions Five to Ten Years after Intubation. Annals of Otology, Rhinology and Laryngology, Dec., 1910.

497. SIEUR AND PERIER, C. Progressive Dilatation of Stenosis of the Larynx after Laryngostomy. Bull. de l'Acad. de Med., April 13, 1909.

498. SIMPSON, W. K. Laryngeal Stenosis in the Adult, Successfully Treated by Intubation; Continuous Wearing of Tube for Four Years. Am. Jour. of Surg., April, 1909.

499. SMITH, HARMON. Case of Laryngeal Carcinoma Under Observation for Thirteen Years—Ultimate Laryngectomy. The Laryngoscope, Feb., 1910.

500. SIMPSON, W. LIKELY. Some indications for Direct Methods for Examination of Larynx. Memphis Med. Mo., No. 12, Vol. XXXII, Dec., p. 563.

501. SMITH, HARMON. Multiple Papilloma of the Larynx in Children. The Laryngoscope, St. Louis, Feb., 1909.

502. STEIN, OTTO J. The Laryngo-Tracheal Manifestations of Thyroid Disease. The Laryngoscope, March, 1913.

503. SPEESE. Perforation of the Ileum by a Foreign Body. Annals of Surgery, Nov., 1913, p. 706.

504. STILLMAN, F. L. Direct Inspection of the Esophagus and Bronchial Tubes. Ohio State Med. Journ., March, 1906.

505. STOLTE, H. Demonstration of a Foreign Body in the Esophagus Removed by Escophagoscopy. Jour. Ophth. and Oto-Laryngol., March, 1909.

506. STUCKY, J. A. AND WILLIAM. Report of an Unusual Case of Multiple Papilloma of the Larynx, Necessitating Tracheotomy and Thyrotomy; and Two Cases of Foreign Body in Lower Trachea. Lancet-Clinic, May 3, 1913, CIX, 481.

507. SWAIN, H. L. Cysts, Abscess and Edema of the Epiglottis. Proceed. Am. Laryngol. Ass'n., 1908.

508. SWAIN, HENRY L. The Use of the Bronchoscope and Esophagoscope for the Location and Removal of Foreign Bodies in the Air and Food Passages. Trans. of the Conn. State Med. Soc., 1908, pp. 158-170.

509. SMITH, HARMON. Safety Pin Removed from the Larynx by Direct Laryngoscopy. The Laryngoscope, Nov., 1913, p. 1097.

510. STUCKY, J. A. Two Cases of Foreign Body in the Trachea. Proc. Amer. Lar. Rhin. and Otol. Soc., 1913, p. 383.

511. SEMON, SIR FELIX. Recurrence of Papillomata after Seventeen Thyrotomies. Proc. Laryngol. Soc., London, Jan. 1, 1894, p. 62.

512. STUCKY, J. A. Papilloma of the Larynx. Proc. Amer. Lar. Rhinol. and Otol. Soc., 1913, p. 383.

513. VON SCHRÖTTER, H. Bronkoskopie bei Fremdkörper. Wiener Klin. Woch., March, 1912, p. 447.

514. SEBILEAU, P. AND LEMAITRE, F. Present Status of Broncho-Esophagoscopy. (Etat Actuel de la Broncho-Esophagoscopie). Presse Med., Jan. 15, 1910.

515. SAUER, W. E. Fibroma of the Trachea. The Laryngoscope, April, 1908.

516. SEMON, SIR FELIX. Results of Radical Operation for Malignant Disease of the Larynx. Lancet, Dec. 15, 22, 29, 1894.

517. SEMON, SIR FELIX. Alleged Liability of Benign Laryngeal Growths to Undergo Malignant Degeneration. New York Med. Journ., Sept. 1, 1894.

518. SEMON, SIR FELIX. Allbutt and Rolleston's System of Medicine. Vol. IV, 1908, p. 251.

524. TANTURRI, D. Diagnosis and Cure of Two Cases of Esophageal Spasms by Esophagoscopy. Arch. Ital. di Laringol., Bd. 29, Heft 1, 1910.

525. TAPIA. Case of Syphilitic Tracheal Stenosis Diagnosed by Indirect Tracheoscopy. Rev. Clin. de Madrid, Feb., 1910.

526. TAPIA. Dental Plate Remaining in Esophagus about Ten Years. Rev. Espanola de Laringol., No. 1, 1910.

527. TAPIA. Two Cases of Foreign Bodies in the Bronchi. Rev. Hebd. de Laryn., d'Otol. et de Rhin., Nov. 23, 1912. Vol. XXXIII, No. 47, p. 612.

528. TEXIER, V. Foreign Bodies in the Esophagus for Seventy-two days; Esophageal Abscess; Extraction by Esophagoscopy; Cure, Rev. Hebd. de Laryn., et d'Otol., Aug. 24, 1912, Vol. XXXIII, No. 34, p. 209.

529. THIGPEN, C. A. Foreign Bodies in Bronchus; Bronchoscopy. Southern Med. Journ., Vol. V, No. 1, Feb., 1912, p. 28.

530. THOMAS, H. W. Pathologic Report of Esophagostomiases in Man. Ann. of Trop. Med. and Parasitol., June, 1910.

531. THOMAS, BENJAMIN A. Esophagoscopy and Gastroscopy in Diagnosis. Surg. Gynecol. and Obstetrics, Oct., 1909, pp. 427-431.

532. THOMAS, B. A. Esophagoscopy and Gastroscopy in Diagnosis. Surg., Gynecol. and Obstetrics., Oct., 1909.

533. THOMAS, B. A. Tracheobronchoscopy and Its Merit in a Case of Foreign Body in the Bronchus. New York Med. Journ., Oct. 9, 1909.

534. THOMSON, SIR ST. CLAIR. Extensive Tuberculosis of the Larynx in Woman, aged 40, Completely Cicatrized After Treatment with Galvano-Cautery and Tracheotomy. Proc. R. Soc. Med., Vol. 1, No. 5, 1909.

535. THOMSON, SIR ST. CLAIR. Four Cases of Epithelioma of the Larynx Following Operation. Proc. Roy. Soc. Med., Vol. 3, No. 5, 1910.

536. THOMSON, SIR ST. CLAIR, AND HALL, F. DE H. Removal Through the Mouth of a Shawl-Pin Impacted in a Secondary Bronchus. Lancet, May 7, 1910.

537. THOMSON, SIR ST. CLAIR. Removal Through the Mouth of a Tooth-Plate. Impacted in the Esophagus for Two and One-half years. Lancet, Vol. CLXXXIV, No. 4662, p. 16.

538. THOMSON, SIR ST. CLAIR. Intrinsic Cancer of the Larynx. Brit. Med. Journ., Feb. 17, 1912.

539. THOMSON, SIR ST. CLAIR. Diseases of the Nose and Throat London, Appleton and Co.

540. TILLEY, H. Direct Esophagoscopy; A Unique Experience. Lancet, March 27, 1909.

541. TODD, FRANK C. Removal of Foreign Body from the Right Bronchus. Journ. A. M. A., March 9, 1912, p. 692.

542. TURNER, A LOGAN. The Submucous Areolar Tissue of the Larynx, and its Significance in the Spread of Edema. Edinburg Med. Journal, May, 1902.

543. TURNER, A. LOGAN. Direct Laryngoscopy and Tracheo-bronchoscopy and Esophagoscopy. Edinburg Med. Journ., Jan. and Feb., 1913, Vol. X, No. 2, p. 126.

544. TURNER, O. W. Simple Method by Which an Open Safety-Pin was Removed from the Bronchus Without Closing the Pin. The Laryngoscope, Dec., 1910.

545. TILLEY, HERBERT. Direct Bronchoscopy. Lancet, April 22, 1911.

546. TILLEY, HERBERT. Removal of a Green Pea from the Right Bronchus by an Improvised Method. Proceedings (Section XV) International Congress of Medicine, London, 1913.

547. THOMSON, JOHN A. Large Fibroma of the Larynx. Lancet Clinic, March 7, 1914.

548. THEISEN, CLEMENT F. Tumors of the Trachea. Annals Otol. Rhinol. and Laryngology, Dec., 1906.

561. VIANNAY, C. Eight Cases of Laryngostomy with Dilatation. Lyon Chir., Nos. 1 and 2, 1910.

562. VIGNARD, SARGNON AND ARNAUD. Stenoses Cicatricielles, Esophagoscopie. Esophagotomie et Dilatation Retrograde. Lyon Med., March 28, 1909.

563. VON EICKEN, CARL. Radiography and Bronchoscopy for Foreign Bodies. Zeit. f. Ohren. und die Erkrankungen dur Luftwege, Aug., 1912, Vol. LXV, Nos. 2 and 3, p. 103.

564. VON EICKEN, CARL. Die Klinische Verwertung der direkten Untersuchungsmethoden der Luftwege und der Oberen Speisewege. Archiv. für Laryngologie. 15 Bd. 3 Heft.

567. WAGGETTE, ERNEST B. Direct Laryngoscopy, Bronchoscopy and Esophagoscopy. Brit. Med. Journ., Sept. 26, 1908, p. 897.

568. WAGGETTE, ERNEST B. Malignant Disease and Pouches in the Esophagus. Brit. Med. Journ., Oct. 19, 1912.

569. WAGGETTE, ERNEST B. Direct Laryngoscopy, Bronchoscopy and Esophagoscopy. Allbutts System of Medicine.

570. WALLER, P. G. Fatal Esophageal Hemorrhage Eight Days After Swallowing Foreign Body. Albany Med. Ann., Jan., 1910.

571. WARTHIN. Status Lymphaticus. Archives of Pediatrics. Aug., 1909.

572. WELLS, W. A. On the Various Affections of the Voice and their Local Causation. The Laryngoscope, March, 1909.

573. WHITE, JOSEPH A. Laryngo-Esophageal Fistula. Proc. Am. Laryngol., Rhinol. and Otol. Soc., 1911.

574. WILSON, NORTON L. Early Operation in Bilateral Abductor Paralysis. The Laryngoscope, 1900.

575. WINSLOW, J. R. Report of a Case of Bronchoscopy for Multiple Foreign Bodies (Almond Shell and Pulp) in a Child, Two Years of Age, with Some Observations Upon Bronchoscopy in Infants and Young Children. Transactions Am. Laryngol. Soc., 1912.

576. WINSLOW, JOHN R. Membraneous Synechia of Vocal Cords. Journ. Eye, Ear and Throat Diseases. Nov., 1905.

577. WISHART, D. J. G. Esophagoscopy and Tracheobronchoscopy. Dom. Med. Monthly, Sept., 1909.

578. WOIATCHEK, V. Experiences d'Introduction de Corps Etranger dans les Bronches chez les Animaux. Archiv. Internat. de Laryngol., etc. (Chauveau) July-August, 1911.

579. WOOD, GEO. B. The Actual Cautery in the Treatment of Localized Tuberculous Lesions. Annals of Otology, Rhinology and Laryngology, Sept., 1911.

580. WOODS, SIR ROBERT. Two Cases of Subglottic Tumor. Journ. Laryngology, Rhinol. Otol., Oct., 1913.

581. WOOLSEY, WM. Intratracheal Insufflation Anesthesia. Read before the N. Y. Society of Anesthetists, March 6, 1912.

582. WRIGHT, J. Microscopical Diagnosis of the Intralaryngeal Growths from a Practical Standpoint. The Laryngoscope, Aug., 1909, and N. Y. Med. Jour., July 17, 1909.

583. WISHART, D. J. G. Bronchoscopy and Esophagoscopy. Canada Lancet, Feb., 1909.

584. WHERRY, W. P. Removal of Foreign Bodies from the Respiratory Tract by Laryngoscopy and Esophagoscopy. Western Med. Rev., Sept., 1913.

585. WOOD, GEORGE B. Pathology of Foreign Bodies in the Lungs. Philadelphia Monthly Med. Journ., June, 1899.

586. WELLS, WALTER A. Thyroid Gland Tumors of the Larynx. Journ. of Laryngology, Oct., 1902.

587. WADSACK AND KOB. Echinococcus of the Left Lung. Berlin Klin. Woch. p. 1097, No. 33, 1906.

593. YANKAUER, S. Foreign Body Removed from the Bronchus. The Laryngoscope, Nov., 1910.

594. YANKAUER, SIDNEY. A New Safe Procedure in Bronchoscopy. Arch. f. Laryn. u. R., Bd. XXVI, Heft 3, p. 708.

595. YANKAUER, SIDNEY. Three Cases of Foreign Body in the Bronchus. The Laryngoscope, Oct., 1912, Vol. XXII, No. 10, p. 1218.

596. YANKAUER, S. Foreign Body Cases. Discussion. Proc. Am. Laryngol. Rhinol. and Otol. Soc., 1913, p. 321.

600. ZIMMERMAN, ALFRED (Heidelberg). Inspired Foreign Bodies. Zeit. f. Laryn., u. f. Krank., etc., Bd. LXVII, No. 1-2, p. 49.

BIBLIOGRAPHY OF SUSPENSION LARYNGOSCOPY.

ALBRECHT: Suspension-laryngoscopy in Children.
Association of Charite Physicians. Meeting May 2, 1912. *Berliner Klin. Wochenschr.*, No. 27, 49, Vol. 1, July, 1912, p. 1295-96.

ALBRECHT: A Modification of Suspension-laryngoscopy.
From the University Polyclinic for Nose and Throat Patients in Berlin. *Berlin. Klin. Wochenschr.*, No. 28, 49, Vol. 8, July, 1912, p. 1331-32.

ALBRECHT: A New Spatula for Suspension-laryngoscopy.
Berliner Klin. Wochenschr., No. 44, 1912. *Semon's Internat. Centralbl. f. Laryngol., Rhinol. u. verw. Wissensch.*, Vol. XXIX, January, 1913, No. 1, p. 5.

ALBRECHT: The Importance of Suspension-laryngoscopy for Children.
Archiv. f. Laryngologie u. Rhinologie, Vol. 28, p. 1.

BLUMENFELD: Control of Haemorrhage in the Larynx by means of Clamp-stitch.
Zeitschr. für Laryng. u. Rhinol., Vol. IV, 1912, p. 389.

BRIEGER: Demonstrates Suspension-laryngoscopy in Association with Miodowski and Seiffert.
Discussion. *Medizin. Sektion d. Schles. Gesell. für vaterland Kultur zu Breslau. Klin. Abend im Allerheiligenhospital v.* Nov. 8, 1912. *Berlin. Klin. Wochenschr.*, Vol. 50. Jan. 20, 1913, No. 3, p. 133.

BRIEGER: Suspension-laryngoscopy.
Med. Klinik., Vol. 50, 1912. *Semon's Internat. Centralbl. f. Laryngol., Rhinol u. Verw. Wissensch.*, Vol. XXIX, Mar., 1913, No. 3, p. 114.

BRIEGER: Transact. of Society of German Laryngol., 1913, p. 142.

DAVIS, L. D.: Observations on Suspension-laryngoscopy, with Notes of a Few Cases. *British Med. Journ.*, January 18, 1893. *Semon's Internat. Centralbl. f. Laryngol., Rhinol. u. verw. Wissensch.*, April, 1913, No. 4, Vol. XXIX, p. 188.

DENKER-BRUENINGS: Textbook of the Diseases of the Ear and Respiratory Passages, p. 489.

FREUDENTHAL: Suspension-laryngoscopy with Demonstration of Method Page 131 Transactions of the Americ. Lar., Rhin. and Otol. Society, 1913.

FREUDENTHAL: Personal Observations with Suspension-laryngoscopy.
Medical Record, February 22, 1913.

FREUDENTHAL: Concerning Suspension-laryngoscopy.
Arch. f. Laryngologie, Vol. 27, p. 459.

FRONING: Suspension-laryngoscopy.
General Medical Society of Cologne. *Muench. med. Wochenschr.*, 1913, p. 1742.

GERBER UND FRITZ HENK (II): The Modern Methods of Examination of the Respiratory Passages, Incl. Suspension-laryngoscopy.
Society of Scientific Therapeutics, *Koenigsberg i. Pr. Official Minutes*, 13, I. 1913. *Deutsche Medizin. Wochenschr.*. Mar. 27, 1913, Vol. 39, No. 13, p. 626.

HENRICH: Contribution to the Clinic of Direct Methods of Examination.
Muenchn. Medizin. Wochenschr., No. 48, 1913.

HEYMANN: Transactions of the Society of Charite-physicians, Vol. 18, 1912.

HOELSCHER: Experiences with Suspension-laryngoscopy.
Society of Charite Physicians. Meeting of May 2, 1912. *Berliner Klin. Wochenschr.*, No. 27, Vol. 49, July 1, 1912, p. 1294-95.

HOELSCHER: About Clinical Experiences with Killian's Suspension-laryngoscopy.

Med. Corresp. Bl. d. Wuertemberg. aerztl. Landesvereins. No. 24, 1912. *Semon's Internat. Centralbl. f. Laryngol., Rhinol. u. verw. Wissensch,* Vol. XXVIII, Sept., 1912, No. 9, p. 483.

HOELSCHER:

Transactions of the Society of German Laryngologists, 1913, p. 144.

HOPMANN:

Muenchn. Med. Wochenschr., 1913, p. 1742.

HOWARTH, W.: A Hook-spatula for Suspension-laryngoscopy.

Lancet, July 19, 1913. *Semon's Internal. Centralbl. f. Laryngol., Rhinol. u. verw. Wissensch,* Vol. XXIX, Nov. 1913, No. 11, p. 550.

IGLAUER, SAMUEL: Foreign Bodies in Larynx and Trachea Removed by the Aid of Suspension-laryngoscope.

The Laryngoscope, June, 1913. *Semon's Internal. Centralbl. f. Laryngol., Rhinol. u. verw. Wissensch,* Dec., 1913. Vol XXIX, No. 12, p. 601.

KAEMPFER. LOUIS G.: Suspension-laryngoscopy.

New York Medical Journal, Jan. 4, 1913. *Semon's Internat. Centrbl. f. Laryngol., Rhinol. u. verw. Wissensch,* Vol. XXIX, June 1913, No. 6, p. 285.

KAHLER, OTTO: The Chirurgical Intra and Extra Laryngeal Treatment of Laryngeal Tuberculosis.

Ref. Delivered at the 85th Meeting of Naturalists in Vienna (p. 1275). *Monatsschr. f. Ohrenheilkunde u. Laryngo-Rhinologie,* Vol. XLVII, 1913, pp. 1269-1283.

KATZENSTEIN:

Transactions of the Society of German Laryngologists, 1913, p. 143.

KILLIAN: Suspension-laryngoscopy. A Modification of the Direct Method.

Transactions of the III International Laryngo-Rhinological Congress. Berlin, August 30-September 2, 1911, p. 112, Part II: Transactions.

KILLIAN: On Suspension-laryngoscopy.

Berlin. Klin. Wochenschr., No. 13, 1912. *Semon's Internat. Centrbl. f. Laryngol., Rhinol. u. verw. Wissensch,* Vol. XXIX, January, 1913, No. 1, p. 5.

KILLIAN: On Suspension-laryngoscopy.

Society of Charite Physicians, Meeting of May 2, 1912. *Berliner Klin. Wochenschr.,* No. 27, Vol. 49, July 1, 1912, p. 1293-94.

KILLIAN, GUSTAV: Suspension-laryngoscopy.
Reprint from the *Arch. of Laryngol. and Rhinol.*, Vol. 26, No. 2, Berlin, 1912.

KILLIAN: On Suspension-laryngoscopy.
Berlin. Klin. Wochenschr., No. 27, p. 1293, 1912. *Semon's Internat. Centrbl. f. Laryngol., Rhinol. u. verw. Wissensch.*, Vol. XXIX, January, 1913, No. 1, p. 5.

KILLIAN: The Suspension-hook in its Newest Form.
Transactions of the Society of German Laryngol., 1913, p. 25.

KILLIAN: Demonstrations of Suspension-laryngoscopy.
Transactions of the Internat. Med. Congress, London, 1913.

KILLIAN:
Naturalists' Meeting, Vienna, 1913, Laryngol. Section.

KILLIAN: On Suspension-laryngoscopy.
1913, *Berliner Klin. Wochenschr.*

KLESTADT:
Berlin. Klin. Wochenschr., 1913, No. 3, p. 133.

LAUTENSCHLAEGER:
Berlin. Klin. Wochenschr., 1913, p. 448.

MANN:
Transactions of the Society of German Laryngologists, 1913, p. 144.

MAYER, E.: Removal of a Carcinoma of the Epiglottis by Suspension-laryngoscopy.
Arch. f. Laryngol., p. 592, Vol. 27, No. 3.

POLLATSCHEK: Direct Operations upon the Larynx.
Orvosi hetilap., No. 49, 1912.

SEIFFERT: The Killian Suspension-laryngoscopy.
Zeitschr. f. Laryngologie u. Rhinologie, VI, H. 4, 1913.

SIEGEL: Twilight Sleep in Obstetrics with Solutions of Skopolamine.
Muenchn. Mediz. Wochenschr., 1913.

SIMOLEKI: Laryngeal Scleroma Treated by Suspension-laryngoscopy.
Monatschr. f. Ohrenheilk. u. Laryngo-Rhinologie, Vol. XLVII, No. 7, p. 989.

STEINER: On Suspension-laryngoscopy.
Prager Medizin. Wochenschr., 1913, No. 28.

STORATH:
Muenchn. Mediz. Wochenschr., 1913, p. 325.

STRAUB: On Decomposition and Conservation of Skopolamine Solutions.
Muenchn. Med. Wochenschr., 1913, No. 41.

WOLFF, J. H.: Demonstration of an Apparatus for Suspension-laryngoscopy.
Laryngological Society of Berlin, Meeting of April 19, 1912. *Berlin. Klin Wochenschr.*, June 10, 1912, No. 24, Vol. 49, p. 1151.

Description of Colored Plates.

PLATE I.

LARYNGEAL AND TRACHEAL STENOSES.

1. Direct view. Sitting position. Male, aged 14 years. Post-diphtheritic cicatricial stenosis cured by endoscopic evisceration. (See Fig. 5.) Known to be well two years after decannulation.

2. Direct view. Sitting position. Male, aged 18 years. Post-typhoid cicatricial stenosis. Mucosa was very cyanotic because cannula was removed for laryngoscopy and bronchoscopy. Cured by laryngostomy (See Fig. 6). Still well four years after decannulation and plastic closure.

3. Direct view. Sitting position. Male, aged 27 years. Post-typhoid infiltrative stenosis. Left arytenoid destroyed by necrosis. Cured by laryngostomy. Failure to form adventitious band (Fig. 7) because of lack of arytenoid activity.

4. Direct view. Recumbent position. Male, aged 40 years. Post-typhoid cicatricial stenosis. Cured of stenosis by endoscopic evisceration with sliding-punch forceps. Anterior commissure twice afterward cleared of cicatricial tissue as in other case shown in Fig. 15. Ultimate result shown in Fig. 8.

5. Same patient as Fig. 1. Sketch made two years after decannulation and plastic.

6. Same patient as Fig 2. Sketch made four years after decannulation and plastic.

7. Same patient as Fig. 3. Sketch made three years after decannulation and plastic.

8. Same patient as Fig. 4. Sketch made one year after decannulation, fourteen months after clearing of the anterior commissure to form adventitious cords.

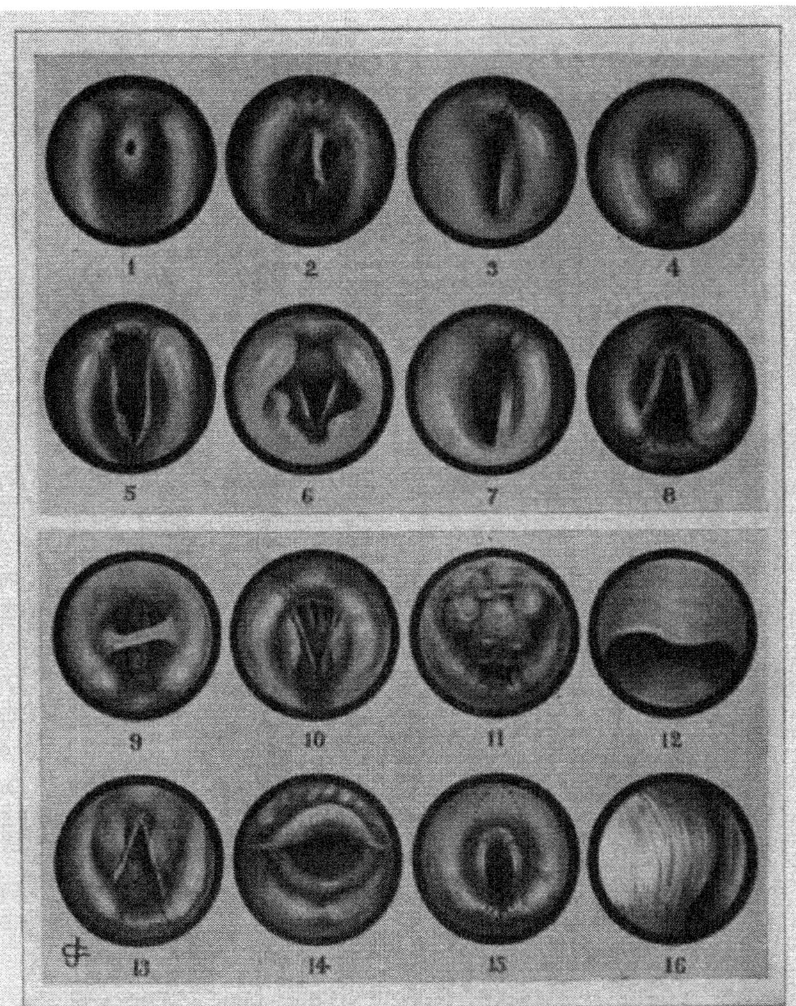

PLATE I.

Direct laryngoscopic views. Photographic reproduction of oil color-drawings from life by the author. For description, see previous pages.

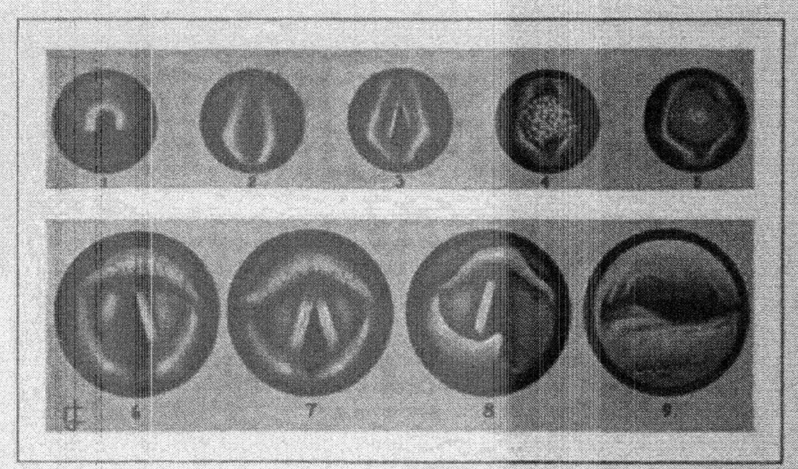

PLATE II.

Direct and indirect laryngeal views. Photographic reproduction of oil color-drawings from life by the author. For description, see previous pages.

9. Direct view. Recumbent. Female, aged 16 years. Web post-diphtheritic (?) or congenital (?). "Rough voice" since birth but larynx never examined until stenosed after diphtheria. Web removed and larynx eviscerated with punch forceps. Recurrence of stenosis (not of web). Cure by laryngostomy. This view also illustrates the true depth of the larynx which is often overlooked because of the misleading flatness of laryngeal illustrations.

10. Direct laryngoscopic view. Child, aged 22 months. Post-diphtheritic hypertrophic subglottic stenosis. Cured by galvano-cauterization.

11. Direct laryngoscopic view. Child, aged three years. Post-diphtheritic hypertrophic supraglottic stenosis. Forceps excision. Extubation one month later. Still well four years later.

12. Bronchoscopic view of post-tracheotomic stenosis following a "plastic flap" tracheotomy done for acute edema. Male, aged 47 years. (Not treated because of advanced nephritis).

13. Direct laryngoscopic view. Anterolateral thymic compression stenosis in a child of 18 months. Cured by thymopexy. Seen six months later. Still well.

14. Indirect laryngoscopic (mirror) view. Laryngostomy rubber tube in position in treatment of post-typhoid stenosis. Woman, aged 30 years.

15. Direct view. Post-typhoid stenosis after cure by laryngostomy. Male, aged 30 years. Dotted line shows place of excision for clearing out the anterior commissure to restore the voice.

16. Endoscopic view of post-tracheotomic tracheal stenosis from badly placed incision and chondrial necrosis, in a child of three years. Tracheotomy originally done for influenzal tracheitis. Cured by tracheostomy.

PLATE II.

DIRECT AND INDIRECT LARYNGEAL VIEWS.

Fig. 1. Epiglottis of child as seen by direct laryngoscopy in the recumbent position. 2. Normal larynx spasmodically closed as is usual on first exposure without anesthesia. 3. Same on inspiration. 4. Supraglottic papillomata as seen on direct laryngoscopy in a child of two years. 5. Cyst of the larynx in a child of four years, seen on direct laryngoscopy without anesthesia. 6. Indirect view of larynx eight weeks after thyrotomy for cancer of the right cord in a man of fifty years. 7. Same after two years. An adventitious band indistinguishable from the original one has replaced the lost cord. 8. Represents the condition of the larynx three years after hemilaryngectomy in a patient fifty-one years of age. Thyrotomy revealed such extensive involvment, with an open ulceration which had reached the perichondrium that the entire left wing of the thyroid cartilage was removed with the left arytenoid. A sufficiently wide removal was accomplished without removing any part of the esophageal wall below the level of the crico-arytenoid joint. There is no attempt on the part of nature to form an adventitious cord on the left side. The normal arytenoid drew the normal cord over, approximately to the edge of the cicatricial tissue of the operated side. The voice, at first a very hoarse whisper, eventually was fairly loud, though slightly husky and inflexible. 9. Mouth of the esophagus one year after laryngectomy for endothelioma in a man aged sixty-eight years. The purple papillae anteriorly are at the base of the tongue and from this the mucosa slopes downward and backward smoothly into the esophagus. There are some slight folds toward the patient's right (to the left in the illustration) and some of these are quite cicatricial. The epiglottis was removed at operation. The trachea was sutured to the skin and did not communicate with the pharynx. Indirect view.

PLATE III.

ESOPHAGOSCOPIC VIEWS.

1. Direct view of the larynx and laryngopharynx in the dorsally recumbent patient, the epiglottis and hyoid bone being lifted with the direct laryngoscope, or the esophageal speculum. The spasmodically adducted vocal cords are partially hidden by the overhang of the spasmodically adducted ventricular bands. Posterior to this the aryepiglottic folds ending posteriorly in the arytenoid eminences are seen in apposition. The esophagoscope should be passed to the right of the median line into the right pyriform sinus, represented here by the right arm of the dark crescent.

2. The right pyriform sinus in the dorsally recumbent patient. The eminence at the upper left border corresponds to the edge of the cricoid cartilage.

3. The cricopharyngeal constriction of the esophagus in the dorsally recumbent patient, the cricoid cartilage being lifted forward with the esophageal speculum. The lower (posterior) half of the lumen is closed by the fold corresponding to the orbicular fibers of the cricopharyngeus, which advances spasmodically from the posterior wall. (Compare Fig. 10). This view is not so clearly obtained with an esophagoscope.

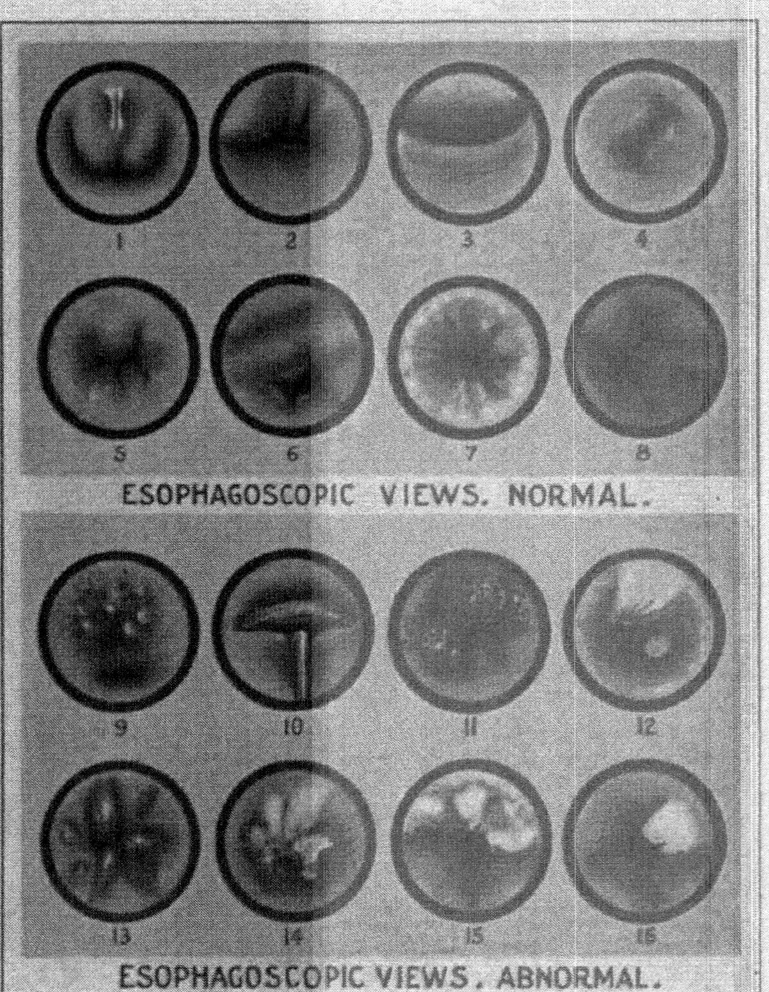

PLATE III.

Photographic reproductions of the author's oil color-drawings from life. **For description, see previous pages.**

4. Passing through the right pyriform sinus with the esophagoscope; dorsally recumbent patient. The walls seem in tight apposition, and, at the edges of the slit-like lumen, bulge toward the observer. The direction of the axis of the slit varies, and in some instances it is like a rosette, depending on the degree of spasm.

5. Cervical esophagus. The lumen is not so patulent during inspiration as lower down; and it closes completely during expiration.

6. Thoracic esophagus. Dorsally recumbent patient. The ridge crossing above the lumen corresponds to the left bronchus. It is seldom so prominent as in this patient, but can always be found if searched for.

7. The esophagus at the hiatus. This is often mistaken for the cardia by esophagoscopists. It is more truly a sphincter than the cardia itself, and in the author's opinion it is questionable if there is any truly sphincteric action at the cardia. It is the spasmodic closure of this hiatal sphincter that produces the syndrome called "cardiospasm."

8. View in the stomach with the open-tube gastroscope. The forms of the folds vary continually.

9. Sarcoma of the posterior wall of the upper third of the esophagus in a woman of thirty-one years. Seen through the esophageal speculum, patient sitting. The lumen of the mouth of the esophagus, much encroached upon by the sarcomatous infiltration, is seen at the lower part of the circle.

10. Coin (half-dollar) wedged at the upper thoracic aperture of a boy aged fourteen years. Seen through the esophageal speculum, recumbent patient. Forceps are retracting the superjacent cricopharyngeal fold preparatory to removal of foreign body.

11. Fungating, squamous-celled epithelioma in a man of seventy-four years. Fungations are not always present, and are often pale and edematous. The appearance of malignancy may be masked by inflammation due to mixed infections.

12. Cicatricial stenosis of the esophagus following the swallowing of lye in a boy of four years. Below the upper stricture is seen a second stricture. A third one, not shown, was located eccentrically farther down. An ulcer surrounded by an inflammatory areola and the granulation tissue together illustrate the etiology of cicatricial tissue. The fan-shaped scar is really almost linear but it is viewed in perspective. Patient was cured by esophagoscopic dilatation.

13. Angioma of the esophagus in a man of forty years. The patient had hemorrhoids and varicose veins of the legs.

14. Luetic ulcer of the esophagus, 26 cm. from the upper teeth, in a woman of thirty-eight years referred for dysphagia. Two scars from

healed ulcerations are seen in perspective on the anterior wall. Branching vessels are seen in the livid areola of the ulcers.

15. Tuberculosis of the esophagus in a man of thirty-four years. No vessels are visible near the grayish-white patches. A specimen of tissue removed esophagoscopically was reported by Dr. Ernest W. Willetts to be tuberculous.

16. Leucoplakia of the esophagus near the hiatus in a man aged fifty-six years.

PLATE IV.

Fig. 122 and Fig. 123. Views obtained by suspension laryngoscopy. For descriptions see Chapter VIII.

PLATE V.

Upper illustration. A, gastroscopic view of a gastrojejunostomy opening drawn patulous by the tube mouth. (Gastrojejunostomy done by Dr. George L. Hays.) B, carcinoma of the lesser curvature. (Patient afterward surgically explored and diagnosis verified by Dr. John J. Buchanan.) C, healed perforated ulcer (patient referred by Dr. John W. Boyce).

Lower illustration. Drawn from a case of post-diphtheritic subglottic stenosis cured by the author's method of direct galvano-cauterization of the hypertrophies. A, immediately after removal of the intubation tube, hypertrophies like turbinals are seen projecting into the subglottic lumen. B, five minutes later. The masses have now closed the lumen almost completely. The patient became so cyanotic that a bronchoscope was at once introduced to prevent asphyxia. C, the left mass has been cauterized by a vertical application of the incandescent knife. D, completely and permanently cured after repeated cauterization.

PLATE VI.

Endoscopic views through the Janeway gastroscope. A. Looking in the direction of the pylorus. B. View toward the fundus. From illustrations furnished by Henry Janeway.

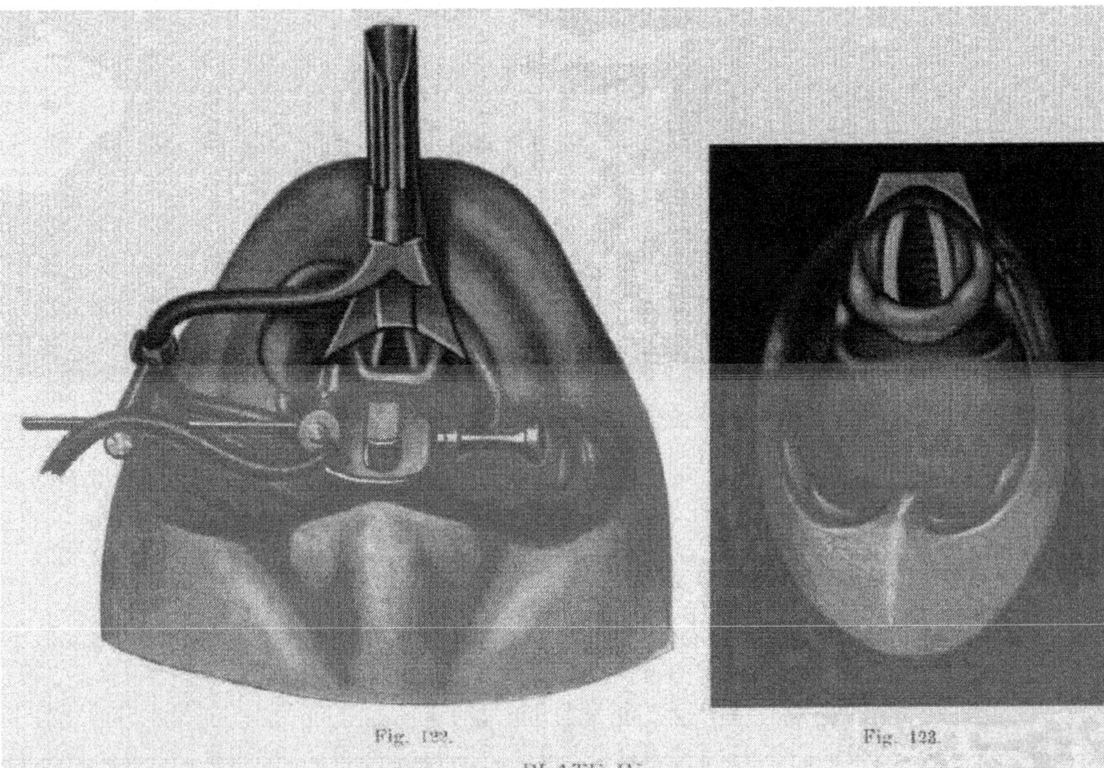

Fig. 122. Fig. 123.

PLATE IV.

Reproduction of colored plates furnished by Prof. Killian. For description, see Chapter VIII.

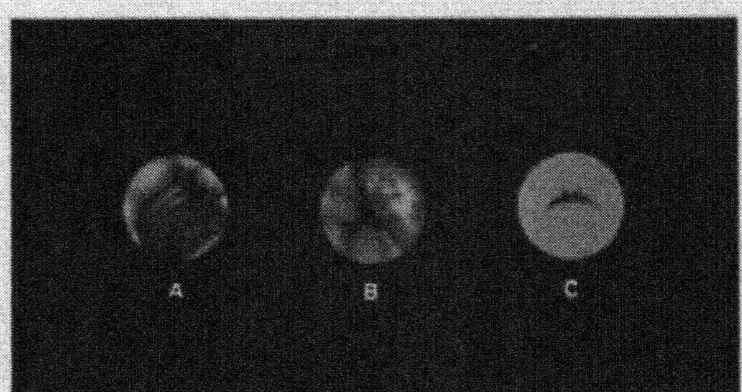

Gastroscopic Views.

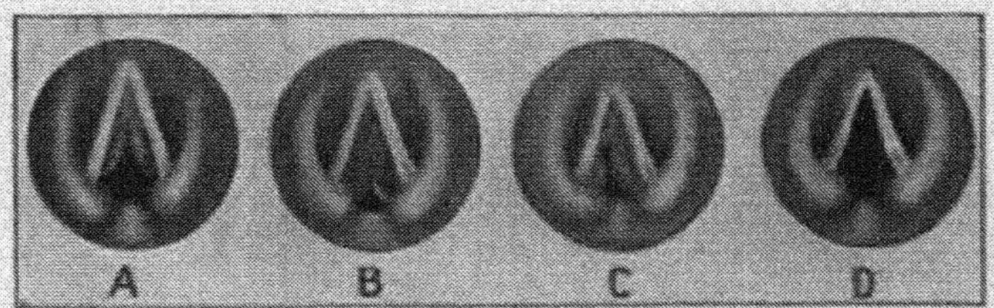

Direct Laryngoscopic Views.

PLATE V.

Reproductions of oil color-drawings from life by the author.

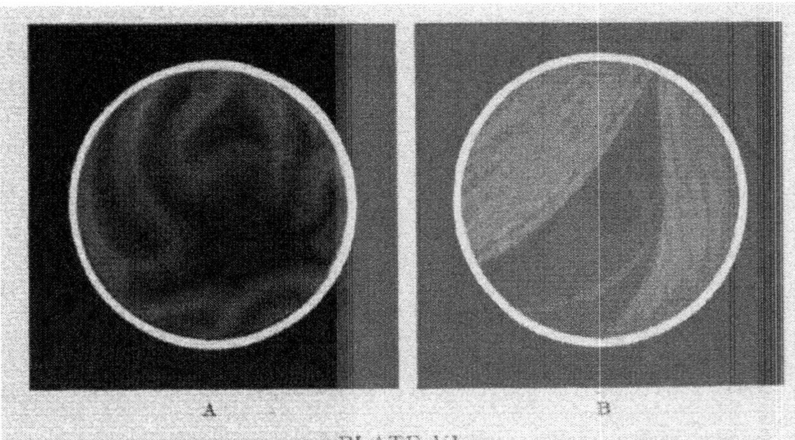

A B

PLATE VI.

Views through the lens-system gastroscope. For description, see previous pages.

INDEX

CPSIA information can be obtained at www.ICGtesting.com
Printed in the USA
LVOW03s1341030815

448646LV00015B/271/P